SECOND EDITION

toward a moral horizon

NURSING ETHICS FOR LEADERSHIP AND PRACTICE

EDITED BY

JANET L. STORCH
UNIVERSITY OF VICTORIA

PATRICIA RODNEY
UNIVERSITY OF BRITISH COLUMBIA

ROSALIE STARZOMSKI
UNIVERSITY OF VICTORIA

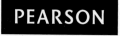

PEARSON

Toronto

Vice-President, Editorial Director: Gary Bennett
Senior Acquisitions Editor: Lisa Rhan
Marketing Manager: Julia Jevmenova
Supervising Developmental Editor: Madhu Ranadive
Project Manager: Patricia Ciardullo
Manufacturing Coordinator: Susan Johnson
Production Editor: Mohinder Singh/Aptara®, Inc.
Copy Editor: Melissa Churchill
Proofreader: Aptara®, Inc.
Compositor: Aptara®, Inc.
Art Director: Miguel Acevedo
Cover Designer: Miguel Acevedo
Interior Designer: Miguel Acevedo
Cover Image: Getty Images

10 9 8 7 6 5 4 3 2 1 [CRW]

Library and Archives Canada Cataloguing in Publication

Toward a moral horizon: nursing ethics for leadership and practice / edited by Janet L. Storch,
Patricia Rodney, Rosalie Starzomski.—2nd Ed.

Includes index.
ISBN 978-0-13-507494-7

1. Nursing ethics.   I. Storch, Janet L., 1940-   II. Rodney, Patricia Anne, 1955-
III. Starzomski, Rosalie Catherine, 1956-

RT85.T68 2013   174.2'9073   C2011-906673-4

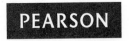

ISBN 978-0-13-507494-7

Contents

Foreword   xi

Preface   xv

About the Editors   xix

Contributors   xxi

Reviewers   xxv

Part 1   BACKGROUND ON THE MORAL TERRAIN   1

Chapter 1   Nursing Ethics: The Moral Terrain   1

Being Ethically Fit   2

The Approach   2

Changes in Nursing Roles and Responsibilities Impacting Ethics   4

Our Research, Practice, and Leadership in Ethics   5

Widening the Language/Vocabulary of Ethics   6

The Context of Health Care and Nursing in 2012   7

Toward an Ethical or Moral Climate   11

Moral Communities and Inter-Professional Practice   14

    Summary 14 • *For Reflection 15* • *Endnotes 15*
    • *References 15*

Chapter 2   A Historical Perspective on Nursing
and Nursing Ethics   20

A Glimpse at Ancient Nursing History   20

Religion, Spirituality, Ethics, and the Development of Nursing   21

Values in Early Nursing Practice   22

Altruism and Nursing Ethics   23

Responses to Constraints on Ethical Practice   24

Ethics in Nursing Education   25

From Character to an Ethics of Nursing   27

Professional Obligations   28

Human Rights and Nursing Ethics   28

Biotechnology and Bioethics   29

Nursing Philosophy, Feminist Ethics, and Nursing Ethics   30

Organization of the Profession and Codes of Ethics   31

*Summary 32 • For Reflection 33 • Endnotes 34
• References 34*

Chapter 3   Philosophical Contributions to Nursing Ethics   41

What is Nursing Philosophy?   42

Philosophical Influences on Nursing Ethics   44

The Contested Boundaries of Nursing Ethics and
Nursing Science   45

Challenges of Unity in Nursing Ontology and
Nursing Ethics   46

Unresolved Ethical Nursing Issues   49

The Nature of Good Nursing Practice   50

*Summary 54 • For Reflection 54 • Endnote   55
• References 55*

Chapter 4   Our Theoretical Landscape: A Brief History of Health
Care Ethics   59

A Brief History of Health Care Ethics   60

A Conflicted Landscape? Challenges in Theory and Application
in Health Care Ethics   71

*Summary 75 • For Reflection 75 • Endnotes 75
• References 77*

Chapter 5   Our Theoretical Landscape: Complementary
Approaches to Health Care Ethics   84

Contextual Ethical Inquiry   84

*Summary 95 • A Wider Terrain: Toward Relational
Ethics 96 • For Reflection 97 • Endnotes 97
• References 99*

Chapter 6   Narrative Ethics in Health Promotion and Care   107

The Value of Narrative   107

Types of Narrative in Health Ethics   109

Uses of Narrative in Health Ethics   111

Narratives in Health Ethics Research   117

*Summary 120 • For Reflection 121 • Endnotes 121
• References 121*

Chapter 7   Relational Ethics for Health Care   127

Relational Ethics   127

Relational Themes   129

Environment   129

Embodiment   131

Mutual Respect   133

Engagement   134

Relational Ethics Through Dialogue   138

Relational Ethics: Knowing Ourselves as We Engage
with Others   139

For Reflection 141 • Endnote 141 • References 141

Chapter 8   Relational Practice and Nursing Obligations   143

Connecting Relationships, Ethics, and Nursing Effectiveness   144

Relationships, Ethics, and Nursing Obligations   147

Obligations as External Entities   148

Reframing Obligation   149

Bringing a Relational Inquiry Lens to Relationships   150

Relational Inquiry and Nursing Obligations   151

Summary 156 • Endnotes 157 • References 157

Chapter 9   Moral Agency: Relational Connections
and Support   160

Conceptualizing Moral Agency   161

Nurses' Voices   163

Nurses' Knowledge and Nurses' Work   164

Nurses' Enactment of Their Moral Agency   165

Supporting Nurses as Moral Agents   173

*Summary 180 • For Reflection 180 • Endnotes 180
• References 181*

Chapter 10   The Moral Climate of Nursing Practice:
Inquiry and Action   188

Moral Climate Change   188

Taking Action to Improve the Moral Climate of
Nursing Practice   198

*Summary 204 • For Reflection 205 • Endnotes 205
• References 207*

Chapter 11   Building Moral Community: Fostering Place Ethics in Twenty-First Century Health Care Systems for a Healthier World   215

Introduction   215

Generating Place Ethics in Twenty-First Century Health Systems   217

Creating Healing Places: A Restorative Task   221

Expanding Moral Horizons: Fostering Ecologically Literate Moral Imaginations to Strengthen Systems of Care   225

Locating Place Ethics in the Health Care Ethics Landscape   226

Advancing Place Ethics: Charting a Path to Reinhabitation   228

Summary 229 • For Reflection 230 • Endnotes 230 • References 230

Part 2   CURRENT APPLICATIONS OF HEALTH CARE ETHICS/NURSING ETHICS   236

Chapter 12   Ethics and Canadian Health Care   236

Canada's Health Insurance System: The Background   237

Limitations of the Canadian System   239

Public Needs/Problems: Private Solutions?   240

Values in Tension in Health Care Provision   242

What is Fair?   243

Toward Informed Ethical Choices   244

Take Home Message for Nurse Leaders   245

Summary 247 • For Reflection 248 • Endnotes 248 • References 248

Chapter 13   Working Within the Landscape: Ethics in Practice   254

Addressing Diversity   255

Reflections on Interests   256

Ethical Action for Individuals   259

Organizational Ethics Resources   271

Summary 273 • For Reflection 274 • Endnotes 274 • References 276

Chapter 14   Research Ethics and Nursing   282

Background: Evolution of Research Ethics in Canada   283

Responsibility of Research Ethics Boards   286

Roles for Nurses in Research Ethics   288

Responsibility of Nurses as Leaders in Research Ethics 296
Summary 297 • For Reflection 298 • Endnotes 298 • References 299

Chapter 15 Educative Spaces for Teaching and Learning Ethical Practice in Nursing 302

Introduction 302

Our Intent 303

Nursing Ethics Pedagogy in Context 303

Principles and Practices: Creating Educative Spaces for Nursing Ethics Pedagogy 308
Summary 312 • For Reflection 312 • References 313

Chapter 16 Listening Authentically to Youthful Voices: A Conception of the Moral Agency of Children 315

Narratives of Moral Experience 315

Examining the Conventional Framework 317

From Moral Subject to Moral Object 319

What about the Voice of the Child? 320

What about Moral Responsibility? 323

Agency Within a Moral World 324

Revisiting the Ethics in Practice Narratives 327
Summary 328 • For Reflection 328 • Endnotes 328 • References 330

Chapter 17 Ethics and End-of-Life Decisions 333

A Moral Imperative for Nurses 334

Good Care at the End of Life 339

Relief of Pain and Discomfort 342

Information and Truthfulness 343

Fostering Family and Friend Support 345

Listening, Reflecting, and Developing Trust 346

Nurses and Palliative Care 347

Assisted Suicide and Euthanasia in Canada 348

Nurses Leading and Influencing Change in End-of-Life Care 349
Summary 351 • For Reflection 351 • Endnotes 352 • References 353

Chapter 18   A Further Landscape: Ethics in Health Care Organizations and Health/Health Care Policy   358

The Context: The Malaise of Modernity   359

Ethics in Health Care Organizations   362

Ethics in Health/Health Care Policy   366

Democratic Policy Processes   369

Further Reflections: Ecological and Political   371
> *Summary 372 • For Reflection 373 • Endnotes 373 • References 375*

Part 3   BROADENING THE VIEW OF HEALTH CARE ETHICS/NURSING ETHICS   384

Chapter 19   Home Health Care: Ethics, Politics, and Policy   384

The Political Context: Neo-Liberalism   385

Ethical Implications: The Everyday Lives of Clients, Families, and Home Care Nurses   388

Recommendations   392
> *Summary 394 • For Reflection 395 • Endnote   395 • References 395*

Chapter 20   Ethics of Public Health   398

What is Public Health?   398

Who is the "Public" in Public Health?   400

What is Public Health Ethics?   400

What are the Philosophical and Theoretical Underpinnings of Public Health Ethics?   405

What about Ethics and Public Health Nursing?   414

Pandemic Ethics   416
> *Summary 419 • For Reflection 421 • Public Health Ethics Case Study Resources 421 • References 421*

Chapter 21   Challenging Health Inequities: Enacting Social Justice in Nursing Practice   430

Health Inequities   431

Intersectionality: Social Positioning and Systems of Oppression   432

Systemic Processes: Neo-Liberalism and Biomedicine   433

Perspectives on Social Justice   435

Nursing Practice and Promotion of Social Justice   437

Summary 440 • For Reflection 440 • References 440

Chapter 22   Opening Pandora's Box: The Ethical Challenges of Xenotransplantation: A Biotechnology Exemplar   448

Biotechnology—Promises and Pitfalls   449

Xenotransplantation: An Illustration of the Benefits and Challenges of Biotechnology   450

Public Participation in Decisions About Xenotransplantation   460

Opening Moral Space for Discussion About Biotechnology: Implications for Nurses   463

Summary 465 • For Reflection 466 • References 466

Chapter 23   Ethical Issues in Pregnancy and Reproduction   473

Induced Abortion   474

Assisted Human Reproduction   477

Prenatal Testing and Screening   481

Summary 485 • For Reflection 485 • Endnotes 486 • References 486

Chapter 24   Genetics and Identity: Diagnosis, Management, and Prevention of Health Conditions   491

Social, Familial, and Ethical Implications of New Genetic Advances   492

Genetics and Complex Disorders: Psychiatric Illness as an Illustrative Example   496

Practical Challenges and Opportunities for Nursing   498

Genetic Counselling and Nurses   500

Summary 502 • Website Resources 503 • Book Resource 503 • For Reflection 504 • Endnotes 504 • References 505

Chapter 25   Neuroethics: An Emerging Field of Scholarship and Practice   509

Introduction   509

Part One: Definitions of and Perspectives on Neuroethics   509

Part Two: From Bench Neurotechnology to Bedside
Neuroscience-Based Care   512

Part Three: Neuroscience of Ethics   517

*Summary 520 • For Reflection 521 • Endnotes 521
• References 522*

Chapter 26   To Boldly Go Forward: Epilogue and
Future Horizons   527

What We Have Offered   528

On the Horizon   529

References 534

Appendix A   537

Appendix B   539

Appendix C   542

Index   543

Foreword

Readers of the second edition of *Toward a Moral Horizon: Nursing Ethics for Leadership and Practice* are in for a treat. Once again the editors and authors were most ethical in designing and executing this text. Its length, a hefty 592 pages, should surprise no one as each theme is carefully contemplated, related to the whole, elaborated, and ultimately presented to the reader as but one tempting course of a delicious and memorable feast. The editors faithfully fulfill their promise to provide substantive background in ethics and to critique and advance the state of health care and nursing ethics. While those new to nursing ethics will find a comprehensive introduction to the ethical dimensions of nursing practice and the state of nursing ethics, those familiar with nursing ethics will find themselves thinking as they read, *"I never thought about that," or "I never read that author," or simply, "What a great insight."* In short, this text is designed to stretch our moral reasoning about the practice of nursing and health care and to challenge each nurse's everyday moral activities, what we value, how we make decisions and behave, and who we are becoming by virtue of our moral choices. The editors challenge their readers to make ethical fitness in service of benefiting others their goal and offer incomparable resources to achieve this goal.

The structure of the book is well conceived. I particularly enjoyed the 11 chapters in Part 1, which aimed to provide substantive background in ethics, to critically examine ethical principles and theories, and to focus on key concepts of ethical practice—specifically relational practice, moral agency, and moral climate. While many writings in nursing ethics offer critiques of the adequacy of the Beauchamp and Childress principles of common morality (autonomy, beneficence, nonmaleficence, and justice), few are as nuanced—and as challenging—as what this book offers as alternatives: narrative ethics, relational ethics, and ecological ethics—all as part of a "A Peace Proposal" intending to integrate new approaches to theorizing in health care ethics.

- Jeffrey Nisker's chapter on narrative ethics is a particular delight to read. His personal sharing and practical examples of how to use narrative ethics makes this chapter much more than the usual introduction to the use of narratives in health care."For almost 20 years the wise fox's words in *The Little Prince*, 'It is only with the heart that one can see rightly' (de Saint-Exupéry 1943) has informed not only the way I engage in health ethics education, research, and policy development, but the way I live my life. I hope you will consider using story to delve deeper into the ethical issues in which we are immersed than a theories-and-principles-based approach allows. I hope you will use narratives to approximate empathy for the persons at the centre of the ethical issue, their families, and their health professionals. I hope you will use narratives to bring the beauty of persons, too often confined within a clinical diagnosis, to classrooms, conference auditoria, and policy tables. For narratives can 'help compassion happen'."

- In Chapter 7, "Relational Ethics for Health Care," Vangie Bergum uses a six-part clinical example to illustrate four themes of relational ethics: environment, embodiment, mutual respect, and engagement, as well as the importance of dialogue and the caregiver's self-knowledge. The critical message of this chapter, "If relationships are the focus of understanding and examining moral life, it is important to attend to the *quality* of relationships in all practice, whether with patients and their families, with other health care professionals, or with administrators and politicians," is yet another example of what distinguished this text.

- Chapters 8–10 richly describe the relational obligations of nurses and analyze how the moral climate in our practice settings and society's values facilitate or compromise the nurse's moral agency. Not to be missed are the five critical changes that need to occur if nurses are to be effective moral agents, which include the challenges for leadership and educators.

- Finally, Patricia Marck's chapter on ecological ethics re-echoes the above themes while promoting moral communities using place ethics. "As with many schools of ethical thinking, place ethics may be easy to admire, less easy to fully imagine, and much more difficult to practise and critique in our daily work and lives. Enacting a full commitment to place ethics is, like restoration itself, 'a work in progress—never finished, never "corrected".' While many with a stake in health care may be initially drawn to a place ethic by its promise of improving the eco-efficiency and sustainability of tomorrow's health systems, there is a much deeper and even more vital reason to continue exploring the potential for place ethics in the years ahead. That reason is to rediscover more ethical relations with each other as we reestablish more ethically justifiable relations with the places we share."

Part 2 describes applications of health and health care ethics and nursing ethics related to practice, research, education, and policy, and highlights the particular nursing challenges of giving voice to children and working in partnership with people at the ends of their lives. Chapter 18 concludes, "We are, indeed, diverse people experiencing diverse realities, but sharing existential vulnerabilities. Throughout this book we have made the case that health care ethics therefore needs to draw on diverse sources of wisdom—sources that we hope will continue to evolve and flourish." This book is a valuable guide to these diverse sources of wisdom. Part 3 examines more recent areas of ethical focus, such as home health care, public health, challenging health inequities, and the various biotechnologies of xenotransplantation, reproductive health, genetics, and neuroethics.

Strengths of the book include the following:

Scholarship. This revision makes a significant contribution to the ethics literature by continuing to highlight the work of Canadian ethicists. Those familiar with health care ethics and nursing ethics, however, will discover ample discussion of all the leading scholars addressing the text's themes. The references at the end of each chapter alone are a reason to read the text, as they will position readers wanting to delve deeper with the perfect beginning sources.

Uniform Excellence. A common flaw of edited volumes is a lack of cohesiveness and uneven quality. The editors here have worked diligently to ensure that each chapter is a piece of a whole and that each delivers the highest quality treatment of its theme. Related themes in previous or subsequent chapters are referenced.

Clarity and Assimilation. Great care is taken in each chapter to alert readers to what the authors are intending to achieve in both the opening paragraphs and chapter summaries. Recurrent features include Ethics in Practice boxes and For Reflection. The Ethics in Practice boxes apply the content being described to actual practice situations and illustrate ways in which ethics is an integral part of practice in all health care practice settings as well as in policy development, education, administration, and research. The reflection questions concluding each chapter prompt each reader to assess her assimilation of essential content and ability to relate this to current practice.

Authenticity and Modeling. There is no doubt that the authors know nursing practice and ethics. Perhaps more important is the fact that they continue to care passionately about nursing's ability to make health care "work" for those who need it. Every page of this book examines what needs to change at the level of the individual, institutions/professions, and society to support nurses' ability to do just this. Amply modeled is the type of research, scholarship, practice, education, leadership, policy development, and personal and professional transformation needed to effect these changes.

Groundbreaking. Chapter 1 begins with the claim that the direction of nursing ethics can never be complacent. The book's last four chapters devoted to biotechnological development, pregnancy and reproduction, genetics, and neuroethics, by design, address a "wide array of ethical concerns and challenges that have major implications for scholarship and practice—and that [the authors] consider to be highly relevant to emerging frontiers in nursing ethics." The authors challenge readers to identify areas where nurses need to develop greater knowledge and ethical awareness to care for people in the twenty-first century. They have most certainly demonstrated why this matters and how to do it well.

Conclusion. It is not often that an ethics book leaves one wanting to read more. The second edition of *Toward a Moral Horizon: Nursing Ethics for Leadership and Practice* does just that. I hope its editors are already working on the next edition.

To the editors and authors, "I salute you. Thank you." To readers, "Enjoy!"

Carol Taylor, Ph.D., RN
Professor of Nursing
Georgetown University

Preface

Welcome to the second edition of *Toward a Moral Horizon: Nursing Ethics for Leadership and Practice*. We believe that this enhanced edition will meet the needs of many, since this entire text is constructed to help nurses and all health care providers to take up the challenge of embedding ethics in health care practice, education, research, and policy at all levels—from local to global.

In 2004, we developed the first edition of this book to serve as a text for a graduate course in nursing ethics and to provide practicing nurses with content to enhance their roles as leaders within diverse health care settings. We had the opportunity to use the book in teaching both graduate and undergraduate students in nursing as well as practicing nurses and other health care providers. We learned a great deal in the development and use of the first edition. We thank our contributors, reviewers, and students past and present, for adding to our understanding of what is needed in a text of this nature.

We are deeply indebted to our current contributors whose manuscripts have added breadth and depth to the study of nursing ethics. Both contributors and reviewers include Canadians from almost every province in Canada as well as individuals from the United Kingdom, the United States, and Australia. We are grateful that nurse ethicists, educators, administrators, practitioners, and researchers gave so generously of their time; and we are also delighted that physicians, philosophers, clinical ethicists, medical educators, chaplains, health care ethics consultants, political scientists, sociologists, and research ethicists responded so readily to our requests for writing or for review of chapters for this second edition.

As was the case with our first edition, we have divided the book into three main sections titled: Background on the Moral Terrain; Current Applications of Health Care Ethics/Nursing Ethics; and Broadening the View of Health Care Ethics/Nursing Ethics.

The first section includes 11 chapters, some new to this section, and others significantly revised and updated. The content of the early chapters in this section is related to situating nursing within the current health care environment by recording a history of past influences on health care, nursing, and ethics. The authors in Chapters 4 and 5 focus on the theoretical development in ethics pointing to further theory in chapters that follow (Chapters 6 to 8). Chapters 9, 10, and 11 on moral agency and moral climate provide a rich approach to theory in practice, and conclude this first section.

Section II begins with a chapter on Canadian health care to remind readers of the structures, policies, and underlying values that have shaped and are shaping health care policy and practice in Canada. The remaining six chapters focus on ethics in nursing practice, research ethics and nursing, ethics education in nursing, ethics involving youth, ethics and end-of-life decision making, and a final chapter on ethics in health care organizations and in health/health care policy. This final chapter is part of the set of theoretical chapters that begins with Chapters 4 and 5, includes Chapter 13, and ends with Chapter 18. Each chapter carries the title of "Landscape" to indicate their relatedness to each other. The intent of providing this depth of conceptual thinking and theorizing about ethics is to indicate the variety of ethical theorizing, how this applies to practice (including education and research), and how it assists us to apply ethics to enhancing the environment of organizations.

In Part 3, which includes eight chapters, newer areas involving health care ethics and nursing ethics are investigated in some depth. The revised chapter on home health care provides important scholarship on this emerging, yet largely unattended field of endeavour. A review of the ethics of public health, with the attached table of public health ethics frameworks, is courageously new, as is the chapter on challenging health inequities where the author focuses on poverty and addictions. Following are several seminal chapters dealing with new technologies and their application in transplantation, human reproduction, and genetics. The authors of the new chapter on neuroethics chart a course for the ethical reflection needed as this emerging field evolves. All the chapters in Part 3 provide nurses and other health care professionals with background they will require to provide leadership in important and evolving fields of application.

In the appendices, we include three ethical decision-making models as examples of the types of models available for clinical or policy decision making.

In completing this book, we want to thank family and friends who have patiently given us time and support to focus on this work. Jan particularly wants to thank her husband Don who has put up with piles of books, articles, manuscripts, as well as her anxiety and impatience to bring this book to completion. Jan also wants to say what a thrill it was to connect with so many people who are committed to health care ethics and nursing ethics, and to hear their readiness to be involved with this edition. In addition to her amazing family and friends, Rosalie wants to pass on a heartfelt thanks to her graduate students and the health care practitioners at the Vancouver Coastal Health Authority whose clinical conundrums and ideas for resolution provided direction for this book.

Paddy is deeply indebted to colleagues in nursing and other disciplines who have been so generous with their time and expertise. These colleagues have included long-term mentors, academic experts, practice leaders, co-researchers, and graduate students. Further, she is most thankful for her family, particularly John.

In closing, we want to recognize the Canadian Bioethics Society and the Canadian Nurses Association (as well as the International Center for Nursing Ethics) as organizations that have been fundamental to our continuing networking opportunities.

Janet L. Storch, Rosalie Starzomski,
and Patricia (Paddy) Rodney

SUPPLEMENTS

Text Enrichment Site (www.pearsoncanada.ca/storch)

A Text Enrichment Site has been created for this edition at www.pearsoncanada.ca/storch. This site is available to readers and instructors. It includes a copy of the Code of Ethics for Registered Nurses from the Canadian Nursing Association and additional case studies that will help students to apply the material they have learned for further study.

CourseSmart for Instructors (ISBN 0135074959)

CourseSmart goes beyond traditional expectations—providing instant, online access to the textbooks and course materials you need at a lower cost for students. And even as students save money, you can save time and hassle with a digital eTextbook that allows you to search for the most relevant content at the very moment you need it. Whether it's evaluating textbooks or creating lecture notes to help students with difficult concepts, CourseSmart can make life a little easier. See how when you visit www.coursesmart.com/instructors.

CourseSmart for Students (ISBN 0135074959)

CourseSmart goes beyond traditional expectations—providing instant, online access to the textbooks and course materials you need at an average savings of 50 percent. With instant access from any computer and the ability to search your text, you'll find the content you need quickly, no matter where you are. And with online tools like highlighting and note-taking, you can save time and study efficiently. See all the benefits at www.coursesmart.com/students.

Technology Specialists

Pearson's Technology Specialists work with faculty and campus course designers to ensure that Pearson technology products, assessment tools, and online course materials are tailored to meet your specific needs. This highly qualified team is dedicated to helping schools take full advantage of a wide range of educational resources, by assisting in the integration of a variety of instructional materials and media formats. Your local Pearson Education sales representative can provide you with more details on this service program.

About the Editors

Dr. Janet L. Storch

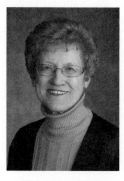

Janet (Jan) Storch, RN, BScN, MHSA, Ph.D., is a professor emeritus at the University of Victoria School of Nursing. She has been a scholar in ethics since the mid-1970s. She served as president of the Canadian Bioethics Society (1992–1993), and of the National Council on Ethics in Human Research (1999–2001). Currently, she chairs the Research Ethics Board of Health Canada and the Public Health Agency of Canada, and serves on clinical ethics committees with the B.C. Ministry of Health and within several Victoria health agencies. She continues an active program of publication in health care ethics and nursing ethics and in research on patient safety in home care.

During her career Dr. Storch has received research funding (for and with teams) from most of the national health funding bodies (NHRDP, SSHRC, CHSRF/CIHR, HC, and CPSI), as well as from provincial funding agencies in Alberta and B.C., and from Associated Medical Services. In 2001–2002 she was ethics scholar in residence at the Canadian Nurses Association and she has led the past three revisions of the CNA Code of Ethics. She is also a member of the editorial board of *Nursing Ethics*. In Alberta, Dr. Storch was a founding member of the John Dossetor Bioethics Center and of the Provincial Health Ethics Network. Dr. Storch has been honoured by several provincial and national nursing associations (the Alberta Association of Registered Nurses Abe Miller Award Nurse of the Year, the Registered Nurses Association of British Columbia Award of Distinction, the Canadian Nurses Association 1 of 100 Centennial Awards, the Canadian Association of Schools of Nursing Ethel Johns Award), and by three universities (an Alumni Honor Award from the University of Alberta, a DSc from Ryerson University, and a LLD from the University of Western Ontario).

Dr. Rosalie Starzomski

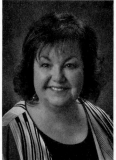

Rosalie Starzomski, RN, BN, MN, Ph.D., is a professor and associate director for research and scholarship at the University of Victoria School of Nursing. She is a clinical ethicist at the Vancouver Coastal Health Authority and a faculty associate at the W. Maurice Young Centre for Applied Ethics at the University of British Columbia. Her research, practice, teaching, and publications are focused on health care and nursing ethics, organ donation, transplantation, nephrology, influencing change in the health care system, and health care decision making.

Dr. Starzomski's clinical background includes over 30 years as a nephrology/transplant advanced practice nurse. She teaches undergraduate and graduate nursing and health care professional students and consults on ethics and health policy for a number of health care agencies. Dr. Starzomski has been actively involved in the community as the chairperson of several health care ethics committees and has taken on volunteer leadership roles for many organizations including the Kidney Foundation of Canada, Canuck Place, the Canadian Nurses Association, Health Canada, the World Council for Renal Care, and the Canadian Council for Donation and Transplantation (CCDT). She chaired the Diverse Communities Initiative and the National Organ Donation Collaborative for CCDT. She is a member of the Board of Directors of the Canadian Organ Replacement Registry and a member of the Canadian Institutes of Health Research (CIHR) Standing Committee on Ethics. She has been the recipient of numerous awards including an Award of Excellence for Nursing and an Award of Excellence for Nursing Practice from the College of Registered Nurses of British Columbia, the Queen Elizabeth II Golden Jubilee Medal for outstanding and exemplary achievement and service to the community and to Canada, and the University of Victoria School of Nursing Award of Excellence for Nursing Education.

Dr. Patricia (Paddy) Rodney

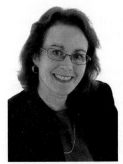

Patricia (Paddy) Rodney, RN, MSN, Ph.D., is an associate professor at the University of British Columbia (UBC) School of Nursing where she teaches undergraduate, masters, and doctoral students. Dr. Rodney has been extensively involved in education, leadership, and practice in health care ethics over the past 20 years. She is a faculty associate with the W. Maurice Young Centre for Applied Ethics at UBC and a research associate with Providence Health Care Ethics Services. She is also an ethics consultant on the B.C. Provincial Advisory Panel on Cardiac Health and she is a member of the Provincial Forum for Clinical Ethics Support and Coordination in British Columbia. Dr. Rodney's former positions have included membership on the B.C. Women's Hospital and Health Centre Ethics Committee and president of the Canadian Bioethics Society (2007–2009).

Dr. Rodney's research and publications focus on the moral climate of health care delivery and end-of-life decision making. She has a particular interest in moral agency and the difficulties that nurses and other health care professionals experience in the current moral climate of health care delivery. Dr. Rodney has therefore been engaged in a program of research as a co-principal applicant with academic and practice-based colleagues (using participatory action and qualitative methodologies) aimed at improving the moral climate of health care delivery. This research has been funded by the Canadian Health Services Research Foundation, the Canadian Nurses Foundation, and the B.C. Cancer Agency. Further, she has been a co-applicant with diverse interdisciplinary colleagues on a number of CIHR funded studies exploring inequities in health care delivery, particularly for Aboriginal peoples. This research has been co-led by Aboriginal researchers. Dr. Rodney's past awards include the Sigma Theta Tau Region I Dissertation Award and the Registered Nurses Association of British Columbia Award of Distinction. Commencing in May 2010, Dr. Rodney became a founding interim board member of the newly formed Association of Registered Nurses of B.C.

Contributors

Gayle Allison, RN, MN, CCHN (C)
Clinical Specialist, Fraser Health Authority
Surrey, British Columbia

Joan Anderson, RN, MSN, Ph.D.
Professor Emeriti
University of British Columbia, School of Nursing
Vancouver, British Columbia

Jehannine C. Austin, Ph.D., CGC/CCGC
Assistant Professor, MSFHR Scholar and CIHR New Investigator
Psychiatry and Medical Genetics, University of British Columbia
Vancouver, British Columbia

Francoise Baylis, Ph.D., FRSC, FCAHS
Professor and Canada Research Chair in Bioethics and Philosophy
Dalhousie University, Novel Tech Ethics
Halifax, Nova Scotia

Vangie Bergum, RN, MEd, Ph.D.
Professor Emerita
Faculty of Nursing, University of Alberta
Edmonton, Alberta

Helen Brown, RN, MSN, Ph.D.
Assistant Professor
School of Nursing, University of British Columbia
Vancouver, British Columbia

Barbara Buckley, RN, MSN
Doctoral Student and CIHR Doctoral Trainee
School of Nursing, University of British Columbia
Vancouver, British Columbia

Michael M. Burgess, Ph.D.
Principal, College for Interdisciplinary Studies and Professor, W. Maurice Young Centre
for Applied Ethics and Department of Medical Genetics
University of British Columbia
Vancouver, British Columbia

Franco A. Carnevale, RN, Ph.D.
Associate Professor and Assistant Director Master's Program
School of Nursing, McGill University
Montreal, Quebec

Susan Cox, Ph.D.
Associate Professor and MSFHR Scholar
W. Maurice Young Centre for Applied Ethics
University of British Columbia
Vancouver, British Columbia

Lori d'Agincourt-Canning, MSc, MA, Ph.D.
Clinical Ethicist, Clinical Ethics Service
Children's and Women's Health Centre of British Columbia
Vancouver, British Columbia

Gweneth Doane, RN, BSN, MA, Ph.D.
Professor, School of Nursing and Associate Dean, Graduate Studies
University of Victoria
Victoria, British Columbia

Cynthia Forlini
Ph.D. Student, Neuroethics Research, IRCM
Integrated Program in Neurosciences, McGill University
Montreal, Quebec

MaryLou Harrigan, Ph.D.
Health Care Consultant and Editor
Vancouver, British Columbia

Bashir Jiwani, Ph.D.
Ethicist and Director, Fraser Health Ethics Services
Surrey, British Columbia

Joy Johnson, RN, Ph.D., FCAHS
Professor School of Nursing, University of British Columbia
Vancouver, British Columbia

Susan Kadyschuk, RN, MSN, CNN(c)
Neuroscience Nurse, Fraser Health Authority
Vancouver, British Columbia

Christopher (Chris) Kaposy, Ph.D.
Assistant Professor, Health Ethics
Division of Community Health and Humanities
Faculty of Medicine, Memorial University of Newfoundland
St. John's, Newfoundland

Marianne Lamb, RN, MN, Ph.D.
Professor and Graduate Coordinator
School of Nursing, Queen's University
Kingston, Ontario

Joan Liaschenko, RN, Ph.D., FAAN
Professor, Center for Bioethics and School of Nursing, University of Minnesota
Minneapolis, Minnesota

Marjorie MacDonald, RN, MSN, Ph.D.
Professor, School of Nursing, University of Victoria
Victoria, British Columbia

Patricia Marck, RN, MN, Ph.D.
Professor and Director, School of Nursing
Associate Dean, Faculty of Health & Social Development
University of British Columbia-Okanagan Campus
Kelowna, B.C., Canada

Lee Ann Martin, MD
Medical Oncologist
Fraser Valley Cancer Centre
Surrey, British Columbia

Michael McDonald, Ph.D.
Professor Emeritus
W. Maurice Young Centre for Applied Ethics
University of British Columbia
Vancouver, British Columbia

Gladys McPherson, RN, MSN, Ph.D.
Assistant Professor
School of Nursing, University of British Columbia
Vancouver, British Columbia

Lynn Corinne Musto, RN/RPN, MN
Doctoral Student
School of Nursing, University of British Columbia
Surrey, British Columbia

Jeffrey Nisker, MD, Ph.D., FRCSC, FCAHA
Professor, Obstetrics-Gynecology and Oncology and
Coordinator Health Ethics and Humanities
Schulich School of Medicine and Dentistry
University of Western Ontario
London, Ontario

Kathleen (Kathy) Oberle, RN, MEd, Ph.D.
Professor Emeritus
Faculty of Nursing, University of Calgary
Calgary, Alberta

Bernadette (Bernie) Pauly, RN, MN, Ph.D.
Associate Professor, School of Nursing and Scientist,
Centre for Addictions of British Columbia, University of Victoria
Victoria, British Columbia

Barbara Pesut, RN, MN, Ph.D.
Assistant Professor
School of Nursing, University of British Columbia, Okanagan
Kelowna, British Columbia

Elizabeth Peter, RN, Ph.D.
Associate Professor and Associate Dean, Academic Programs
Lawrence S. Bloomberg Faculty of Nursing
University of Toronto
Toronto, Ontario

J. Craig Phillips, RN, PMHCNS-BC, Ph.D., LLM, ARNP
Assistant Professor
School of Nursing, University of British Columbia
Vancouver, British Columbia

Eric Racine, Ph.D.
Assistant Research Professor IRCM and Director, Neuroethics Research Unit
Department of Medicine and Department of Social and Preventive Medicine
Université de Montréal Department of Neurology and Neurosurgery and
Biomedical Ethics Unit, McGill University
Montreal, Quebec

Elena Serrano, RN, MA
Professional Practice Leader, Nursing
British Columbia Cancer Agency
Vancouver, British Columbia

Nickie Snyder, RN, BSN, CCRN
Doctoral Student, Nursing
University of Washington
Ferndale, Washington

Annette Street, Ph.D.
Professor
Health Clinical School of Nursing, La Trobe University
Heidelberg West, Australia

Colleen Varcoe, RN, MEd, MN, Ph.D.
Professor and Acting Director, School of Nursing
University of British Columbia
Vancouver, British Columbia

Reviewers

We are very grateful to the following reviewers for the excellent feedback on chapters they provided during the development of this edition.

Joan Anderson, RN, Ph.D.
Professor Emeriti, School of Nursing
University of British Columbia
Vancouver, British Columbia

Jeanne Besner, RN, Ph.D.
Former Director, Health Systems and Workforce Research Unit
Alberta Health Services
Calgary, Alberta

Victoria Bungay, RN, Ph.D.
Assistant Professor, School of Nursing
University of British Columbia
Vancouver, British Columbia

Jane Chambers-Evans, RN, MSc.A., MSc. (Bioethics)
MUHC Clinical Ethicist and Professor
School of Nursing, McGill University
Montreal, Quebec

Paula Chidwick, Ph.D.
Ethicist
William Osler Health Centre
Brampton, Ontario

Philip Crowell, Ph.D., MA, MDiv.
Director Department of Spiritual Care
Children's and Women's Health Centre of British Columbia
Vancouver, British Columbia

Lori d'Agincourt-Canning, MSc., MA, Ph.D.
Clinical Ethicist
Children's and Women's Health Centre of British Columbia
Vancouver, British Columbia

Anne Davis, RN, Ph.D., DSc. (Hon.), FAAN
Professor Emerita, University of California in San Francisco and
Part Time Professor, Nagano College of Nursing, Japan
University of California
San Francisco, California

Raisa Deber, Ph.D.
Professor, Department of Health Policy, Management and Evaluation
Faculty of Medicine, University of Toronto
Toronto, Ontario

Shafik Dharamsi, Ph.D.
Assistant Professor, Department of Family Practice
Faculty of Medicine, University of British Columbia
Vancouver, British Columbia

John B. Dossetor, OC, BM, Bch, Ph.D., FRCPC
Professor Emeritus, Medicine/Bioethics
University of Alberta
Ottawa, Ontario

Jonathan Down, MB, BS, MHSc., FRCPC
Developmental Pediatrician
Queen Alexandra Centre for Children's Health
Victoria, British Columbia

Marie Edwards, RN, Ph.D.
Assistant Professor, Faculty of Nursing
University of Manitoba
Winnipeg, Manitoba

Andrea Frolic, Ph.D.
Clinical and Organizational Ethicist, Hamilton Health Sciences
Assistant Professor, Faculty of Health Sciences McMaster University Medical Center
Hamilton, Ontario

Ann Heesters, MA
Director of Ethics and Spiritual Care
Toronto Rehabilitation Institute, University Centre
Toronto, Ontario

July Illes, Ph.D.
Professor, National Core for Neuroethics
University of British Columbia
Vancouver, British Columbia

Pamela Khan, BN, MSc. (A)
Senior Lecturer, Lawrence S. Bloomberg Faculty of Nursing
University of Toronto
Toronto, Ontario

Rosella Jefferson, RN, MN
Clinical Nurse Specialist, Critical Care Program
Children's and Women's Health Centre of British Columbia
Vancouver, British Columbia

Patrick Loftus, RN, R.Psych.N, BScN
Medical Services Coordinator
Canadian Blood Services, British Columbia/Yukon Centre
Vancouver, British Columbia

Karen MacKinnon, RN, Ph.D.
Assistant Professor
School of Nursing, University of Victoria
Victoria, British Columbia

Susan MacRae, RN, BN, BA
Fellowship Clinical Medical Ethics
University of Chicago and Picker Institute

Barbara Mildon, RN, Ph.D., CHE, CCHC(C)
Vice President, Professional Practice and Research, and
Chief Nurse Executive, Ontario Shores Centre for Mental Health Services
President-Elect, Canadian Nurses Association
Courtice, Ontario

Maureen Mooney, RN, CCRP
Clinical Research Coordinator, Clinical Trials, British Columbia Transplant
Provincial Health Services Authority
Vancouver, British Columbia

Anne Moorhouse, RN, Ph.D.
Professor
Seneca-York Collaborative Nursing BScN Program
Toronto, Ontario

Col. John Murray, RN, Ph.D., CPNP, CS, FAAN
Director, Nursing Research Surgical Programs and Emergency Department
Children's Hospital
Boston, Massachusetts

We wish to acknowledge and thank the following reviewers who provided feedback during the early planning stages of this edition:

Charlotte Pooler
Grant MacEwan

Kathleen Stephany
Douglas College

Wanda Pierson
Langara College

Aroha Page
Nipissing University

Cindy Milner
Langara College

Sylvia Burrow
Cape Breton University

Charlotte Thompson
Camosun College

Barney Hickey
Langara College

Donna Romyn
Athabasca University

Nancy Walton
Ryerson University

Jane Chambers-Evans
McGill University

Kathleen Oberle
University of Calgary

Sherrill Conroy
University of Alberta

Billie Hilborn
University of Toronto

Susan Young
University of British Columbia

Mitzi Mitchell
York University

Rita Schreiber
University of Victoria

PART 1

Background on the Moral Terrain

CHAPTER 1

Nursing Ethics: The Moral Terrain

Janet L. Storch

. . . . the direction of nursing ethics . . . is never complacent, it takes cultural contexts seriously, it is always concerned with the betterment of health care practice, and necessarily seeks philosophical and empirical insights that go beyond the current state of the art. (Gallagher 2010, 156)

Our purpose in revising this book is to celebrate and update the important progression of nursing ethics. Our book is written for senior undergraduate students, graduate students, educators, administrators, and for all nurse leaders as well as other health professionals in practice, policy, and research everywhere. Our key goal is to enable nurses, and other health professionals, to become ethically fit (Kidder 2009), to maintain ethical fitness, and to continue to push the boundaries of health care ethics and nursing ethics outward.

The progression of nursing ethics is well stated in the above quote by Ann Gallagher, editor of the journal *Nursing Ethics*. In 1932, Goodrich published a book titled *The Social and Ethical Significance of Nursing* in which she described professional nursing as "an essential factor of the social order" (7). Later, Jameton (1984), in his landmark text, applauded nurses as being the "inspiration and hope for progress in health care" (xvi) and as those health professionals who have the greatest commitment to the people they serve—their clientele (xvi).

Ethical issues have continued to change over the decades and also since 2004 when our first book, *Toward a Moral Horizon: Nursing Ethics for Leadership and Practice*, was published. Eight years ago we titled this first chapter, "A Developing Moral Terrain." This revised chapter is called simply "The Moral Terrain." This is not to suggest that nursing ethics has arrived, as much as to state that we perceive many of the pressing ethical issues in nursing in previous decades and in the mid-1980s as foundational to many of the issues today, even while many new ethical concerns are developing. Also, nurses have taken great steps toward enhancing their ethics in practice to uphold their commitment to the people in their care and the public they serve.

We know that our fellow health professionals, including physicians, social workers, and many other colleagues, are concerned about ethical leadership and practice as well. But as the quote that introduces this chapter suggests, nurses have often led the way in enlarging the focus on improving health and health care practice, and going beyond what has been considered the purview of traditional health ethics and nursing ethics. They have done so because they have generally "...tended to work with a broader understanding of health than have most other health professions" (Yeo 2010a, 16). They have also responded to a changing context of nursing practice. Some of these changes will be highlighted later in this chapter. Meanwhile, we turn to the overall goal of this chapter and book.

BEING ETHICALLY FIT

Rushworth Kidder, president and founder of the Institute for Global Ethics in the USA, coined the concept of "ethical fitness," which he described as similar to physical fitness. He explains that we are not born with physical fitness, rather, it is reached by giving a little effort each day, and it needs to be maintained. So too, ethical fitness needs to be developed and maintained. It requires being mentally engaged—thinking, reasoning, grappling with difficult situations or their potential, on a regular basis, as well as a commitment to finding better ways to reach good outcomes (Kidder 2009).

> Ethics is not a blind impartiality, doling out right and wrong according to some stone-cold canon of ancient and immutable law. It's a warm and supremely human activity that cares enough for others to want right to prevail. And it's not mere analysis. . . ." (50–51)

Being ethically fit is about how one prepares to make good choices and take actions that benefit others. Similarly, Yeo has suggested that big problems start off with small problems in health and health care; therefore, nurses are urged to "become vigilant about proactively raising questions of value" in their everyday nursing practice (2010a, 27), thus anticipating ethical situations that might lie ahead, in advance (2010b, 41–42).

Ethical fitness means that we take time for reflection on our practice, and that we take time to learn more about ethics. It involves having conversations with colleagues about ethics in our practice, as well as learning and engaging in joint learning and problem solving to tackle barriers that detract from ethical practice (Storch et al. 2009a). It also includes paying attention to, and working to enhance the ethical climate of our workplaces (Corley et al. 2005; Gershon et al. 2004; Hart 2005; Olson 1998; Pauly et al. 2009; Rodney et al. 2006; Ulrich et al. 2007).

THE APPROACH

The approach in this book is designed to provide substantive background in ethics (in Part I), including a historical sketch of nursing in order to locate our current philosophical and ethical thinking; to critically examine ethical principles and theories (including foundational theories as well as narrative ethics, relational ethics, and ecologically informed ethics); and to focus on concepts of ethical practice, specifically moral agency and moral climate. Following this background, in Part II we turn to applications of health and health care ethics and nursing ethics related to practice, research, education, organizational leadership, and policy. We also address particular areas of practice that are challenging to the enactment of nursing values such as hearing the voice of children and working in partnership with people at the end of their life. In the final section of the book (Part III) we examine specific and more recent areas of ethical focus, such as home health care, public health, health inequities, and the various biotechnologies of xenotransplantation, reproductive health, genetics, and neuroethics. We conclude the text with imagining the yet-to-be-explored areas of ethical practice. Within these various areas of practice, changes in inter-professional and inter-provider relationships impact ethical care as well. For example, no longer are physicians considered in traditional ways as captain or head of the team: other professionals are more fully involved in what has been called the "circle of care" (Yeo and Moorhouse 2010, 252).

Within the chapters, "Ethics in Practice" situations are provided to illustrate ways in which ethics is an integral part of practice in all health care practice settings, as well as in policy development, education, administration, and research. Questions for reflection are also provided along with key references for the continued exploration of ethics in leadership and practice.

Our design for this text is based upon our own research and engagement in ethics work in health care and nursing. Throughout the book we highlight leadership in health ethics and nursing ethics. We believe that leadership for ethical policy and practice arises from

> ". . . nurses in senior leadership positions, from nurses in practice and from academics, all working in collaboration, each contributing within the limitations of their own contexts, but bringing unique knowledge, skills and energy essential to the provision of ethical nursing practice." (Storch et al. 2009b, 78)

In this introductory chapter, we begin with a sketch of changes in nursing roles to illustrate why ethics has become more clearly situated in everyday practice as well as in health and society more broadly. We then provide a brief overview of our own program of research in nursing ethics over a decade. During this time, the importance of developing an ethics vocabulary to allow nurses and other health professionals to be more specific about the nature of their ethical concerns was receiving increased attention (Webster and Baylis 2000; Canadian Nurses Association 2008) and began to impact conversations amongst nurses and between nurses and other health professionals, allowing them to "name" ethics issues. Knowing other terms besides *an ethical dilemma* to describe an ethical situation is critical to enhancing and deepening the dialogue about ethical matters.

As we continue in this introductory chapter, we then briefly summarize debates about whether there is a distinct nursing ethics. We analyze the context of health care and nursing in 2012, using patient safety as one example of an ethical challenge. Clarification of ethical terms and concepts through use of practice examples are then provided, followed by reflections on the value of codes of ethics. We conclude this chapter with an emphasis on the need for ethical leadership and dialogue with health professional colleagues to promote greater teamwork in health care. It is our intent that this chapter set the stage for the chapters that follow.

CHANGES IN NURSING ROLES AND RESPONSIBILITIES IMPACTING ETHICS

In 1966, Davis edited a book titled, *The Nursing Profession: Five Sociological Essays.* None of these essays were written by nurses, but all reflected the situation of being a nurse as hospitals became places for diagnosis and treatment, and as other health professionals began to emerge on the health care scene. Up until that time, RNs were "trained" to do the work of physiotherapy, respiratory therapy, social work (to some degree), occupational therapy, and essentially to function as treating the "whole person" required. As these specific roles in health care, and their accompanying educational programs developed, nurses and nursing as a profession faced new challenges. Mauksch (1966), one of the five authors of Davis' book, compared the predicament of nursing to "a sheet of rolled-out cookie dough from which the housewife has cut many cookies . . . which are baking in the oven" (124). Left on the table is "a network of dough which still suggests the entire scope and area of the previously solid surface" (124). Mauksch used this analogy to point out that other health care professions have become independent, but nursing's role remains the "unity and scope of total patient care." Concluding this analogy, he maintained that this is so because after hours the other "cookies" go home and nursing picks up these various duties.

This was an accurate description of nursing training and nursing practice in the 1960s and 1970s. Following that period, the growing emphasis on inter-professional work and, increasingly, on collaborative team work amongst all health professions has gradually molded many working teams of health professionals and other health care providers. That includes some other health care professionals now being available after hours, often on a 24/7 assignment pattern, particularly in emergency departments and critical care units.

Thirty years later, another sociologist described the situation of nursing in hospitals (Chambliss 1996). Based on a 15-year study to explore the "moral geography of hospital nursing" (10), Chambliss concluded that because many nurses continue to be employees in hospitals, they do not deal mainly with tragic choices as much ". . . as with practical, often political, issues of cajoling, tricking, or badgering a recalcitrant system into doing what ought to be done. Nurses continue to admire Florence Nightingale because she did what should be done, and did so without being fired" (7). He emphasized that ethical issues are embedded in complexes of routine care and emergency care, and nurses may forget their ethical commitments in the face of conflict (see also Varcoe and Rodney 2009). Among the many insights arising from his study, Chambliss (1996) stated,

> The great ethical danger, I think, is not that when faced with an important decision one makes the wrong choice, but rather that one never realizes that one is facing [an ethical] decision at all. (59)

That reality, and the fact of differing perspectives about ethics embodied in different professions, can create serious challenges for nurses and others who struggle to be moral agents in twenty-first century health care environments (see Chapter 9). We have found significant evidence of these challenges in our research.

OUR RESEARCH, PRACTICE, AND LEADERSHIP IN ETHICS

Over the past 14 years, we have been involved in a program of research about ethics in nursing leadership and practice. During that period we have undertaken three major funded studies that we named "Ethics in Practice" (a one-year study), "Ethics in Action" (a three-year study), and "Leadership for Ethical Policy and Practice" (a second three-year study).[1] Through that research we have come to better understand the concerns nurses face on a daily basis, the ethical issues that beset them, and the strength they can find in working together to address the challenges of their work environments.

More specifically, we have come to understand the meaning of moral agency, moral distress, and ethical or moral climates more deeply. In this book, we will draw from that research as substance for Ethics in Practice situations, and for critical analyses of health care. Our first collaborative funded study ("Ethics in Practice") was a study that involved focus groups of nurses in 19 settings across the health care spectrum. We simply asked nurses two key questions: What does ethics mean to you in your nursing practice? And, what do you do when you face an ethical situation? (Doane et al. 2004; Rodney et al. 2002; Storch et al. 2002; Varcoe et al. 2004).

The degree of perceived isolation and ethical or moral distress that nurses reported in this first study, and their testimonies of needing to rely on each other to deal with ethical situations, led us to a second funded study ("Ethics in Action"). This study involved working intensively with nurses on two different clinical units—an emergency department and a medical oncology unit. We worked with nurses through buddy shifts, over quick coffee discussions in ER, in small and large group meetings, retreats, joint presentations, and so on. "Ethics in Action" was designed to determine how nurses might work together (collectively) to assist each other towards the goal of good ethical practice (Hartrick Doane, Storch, and Pauly 2009; Rodney et al. 2006; Varcoe and Rodney 2009).

On the strength of that second study, we engaged in our third funded study ("Leadership for Ethical Policy and Practice" [LEPP]) to bring together formal nursing leaders and front line nurses from various regions and practice settings in British Columbia (B.C.) in the pursuit of ethical or moral climates in their work environments and in the development of moral communities (Storch et al. 2009a; 2009b). Work continues from the LEPP study—for example, the "Participatory Action Research on Ambulatory Oncology Care in the British Columbia Cancer Agency" (Rodney et al. 2010)—with the intent of examining and positively affecting the moral climate of interdisciplinary workplaces to optimize practice. Meanwhile, our interest in understanding moral distress in nursing and health workplaces has led to a further quantitative and qualitative study of moral distress (Pauly et al. 2009; Varcoe et al. in review). Corley (2001; Corley et al. 2005), a pioneer in researching moral distress, served as our consultant and joined us for a research conference where she noted that while many researchers were studying moral distress, few were trying to determine how to deal with it in practice such as we were in our LEPP study (M. Corley, personal communication, October 27, 2006). We will say more about the insights we have gained through our research in this book, particularly in Chapters 9 and 10.

In addition to this research, all three author/editors of this book have served and continue to serve on clinical ethics committees, research ethics committees, as ethics consultants, in professional association ethics development, and in continuing education programs on health care ethics, nursing ethics, and research ethics. The first edition of this text was designed for use in a graduate course in nursing at the University of Victoria. Apart from our graduate teaching in ethics in several universities, we have each been involved in undergraduate and graduate teaching of nursing students, medical students, health administration students, and a range of inter-professional ethics education teaching and research activities. As importantly, we have been advocates for enhanced ethical health policies and the goal of ethical climates in health agencies. In doing so, we've been involved with others in shaping a more inclusive ethics vocabulary.

WIDENING THE LANGUAGE/VOCABULARY OF ETHICS

For most nurses, a wider vocabulary of ethics has allowed them to see more clearly how ethics is part of their everyday practice. For example, in the past two revisions of the Canadian Nurses Association *Code of Ethics for Registered Nurses* (2002; 2008) types of ethical experiences and situations have been defined and an ever-widening use of ethical terms employed in outlining nursing obligations and endeavors. These include ethical problems, ethical or moral uncertainty, ethical dilemmas or questions, ethical or moral distress, ethical or moral residue, ethical or moral disengagement, ethical violations, and ethical or moral courage. Given the use of both ethical and moral as part of the definition of the situations to be described in this book, a distinction between *moral* or *morality* and *ethics* is in order. Generally, *moral* or *morality* is concerned with what "ought to be" while *ethics* is focused on reflective analysis about how the "oughts" can be put into action (Yeo 2010b, 40). Other scholars combine concepts of morality and ethics to suggest that ethics itself is about thinking and doing, and that it is culturally constructed (Caldwell, Lu, and Harding 2010, 191). In this text, the editors, who are also authors and co-authors of several chapters, use *ethics* and *morals* interchangeably. The reason to incorporate both is because health care ethics literature includes the use of both terms; also in searches of studies in nursing and other disciplines using both terms can be helpful in canvassing a wider array of literature.

Ethical dilemmas are an important part of health care ethics and will continue to be a priority for ethics consultation. Yet, even the term *dilemma* may incorrectly pre-suppose win-lose situations. Further, because dilemmas represent only a fraction of situations encountered in the field of practice, the focus on ethical dilemmas alone has allowed many health professionals to miss or ignore the importance of ethics in their every-day practice.

A range and variety of moral and ethical theories exist. Many of these will be presented in Chapters 4 to 8 and 11 in the first part of this text and they are also discussed in other chapters of this book as well as in other nursing ethics and health care ethics texts (e.g., Baylis et al. 2004; Oberle and Raffin Bouchal 2009; Yeo et al. 2010). However, as Hanssen and Alpers (2010) note,

Although ethicists compare different theories and point out where they conflict, nurses work in practical settings in which they tend to combine different philosophies to solve ethical problems and dilemmas at hand. (206)

(See Chapters 5 and 13 for more about the importance of combining approaches to ethical problems.)

Is There a Distinct Nursing Ethics?

There has been a long-standing debate about whether nursing ethics is a distinct area of ethics. In attempting to respond to this question, Fry (1989) contrasted the views of those who suggested there was very little that was morally unique about nursing and those who claimed that nursing ethics is distinct (i.e., it is not just another species of applied ethics) (11). In considering models of nursing ethics, Fry pointed to the unique role of nurses in health care and the "social significance of nursing" (12).

During the late 1980s and 1990s attention was focused on finding answers to the above question about ethics for practice by comparing and contrasting models of relationships between health professional and patient. For example, in 1984, Childress and Siegler (1999) wrote about metaphors and models of doctor-patient relationships. Their metaphors and models included those of paternalism, partnership, rational contractor, friendship, and technician analogies. Similarly, moral relationships between nurse and client were categorized as metaphors that *limited nurses* (such as nurse as parent, nurse as servant, and nurse as friend); *misguided metaphors* (such as nurse an engineer or technician); and *helpful metaphors* (such as nurse as in a covenantal relationship, as healer, and as advocate) (Storch 1999).

As with previous explorations about the uniqueness of nursing ethics (Fry 1989; Twomey 1989; Wainwright 2009), the relationships amongst bioethics, medical ethics, and nursing ethics continue to be a matter of debate (see Chapter 3, 4 and 5). At the same time, over the past two decades, nurses have continued to explore and act upon an approach to nursing ethics that focuses on the everyday nature of nursing ethics while holding the larger vision of social justice in focus (Canadian Nurses Association [CNA] Code of Ethics 2008, Part 2, Ethical Endeavours). Throughout this book, our various authors trace diverse elements of this history and address implications for the future.

THE CONTEXT OF HEALTH CARE AND NURSING IN 2012

The world of health care and nursing has changed rapidly and envisioning the challenges of the current decade has been both imaginative in the visioning, and already a step behind practice. In 2007, when the Canadian Nurses Association (CNA) extended an invitation to nurses across Canada to identify anticipated influences on nursing and nursing ethics in the decade ahead, the response was massive in amount and diverse in content.

This 2007 input about the context of nursing practice formed the basis of attention to value and responsibility statements in the 2008 revision of the CNA Code of Ethics for Registered Nurses (CNA Code 2008, Appendix B). These contextual influences were then grouped into three areas: challenges and opportunities *affecting the public*, those *affecting nurses and other health professionals*, and challenges within *the socio-political context* of the health care system. The public's greater access to health information of all types, their increasing expectations of the health care system, and their sense of increasing inequities in the system, were considered key challenges. Rising rates of infection, including new infectious agents and old agents re-emerging (e.g., tuberculosis), and human-made and natural disasters were also high on this list. Challenges for health professionals and nurses included issues arising from the increased diversity of people receiving health care, the shortage of human and financial resources, and a paucity of well-prepared managers. Also included were positive challenges such as broadened scopes of practice for nurses, and a growing cadre of nurse researchers able to research the salience of change from a nursing perspective. The list of socio-political challenges included the sustainability of the Canadian health care system, as well as rapid changes in technology and its appropriate introduction, as key concerns. Other concerns were the changing modes of practice (such as early discharge of patients from hospital care leading to hardship for them and their families); the complexity of care in all settings, the accelerating trend toward public-private sector delivery, and concerns for attention to patient safety (see Chapter 12).

Patient Safety

Perhaps nowhere is the impact of the social, economic, and political contexts of health care illustrated as clearly as in the emergence of the patient safety movement, which began in Canada in the late 1990s. This movement was preceded by extensive and deep cutbacks in health care funding that began in the late 1980s. The cuts were in keeping with an emerging free market economy (neo-liberalism) and a rights-based ideology in Canadian society that persists today (see Chapter 18). Using this one challenge of health care (patient safety), as an example, may help us to better appreciate the impact of the multitude of these health care delivery changes on nursing.

For many years, statistics had been kept about nosocomial infections (hospital acquired illnesses) and some iatrogenic illnesses (illnesses caused by medical treatment), but these were largely for internal use. The realization of the extent of these adverse events in health care (Baker and Norton 2004; Baker et al. 2004) caught policy makers, health care providers, and the public off guard. How care was being delivered, the lack of appropriate implementation and monitoring of some newer technologies in practice, how old and new infectious agents were spreading through health care facilities and the community, and many taken-for-granted notions about the essential "goodness" of health care were examined and found wanting.

Despite these revelations, governments at all levels were reluctant to concede that the drastic health care cuts of the late 1980s and early 1990s might be related to patient safety. Yet, it seemed clear that those cutbacks, along with current financial constraints and a shifted balance of power in health policy from evidence to ideology, have been instrumental in shaping the current dilemmas of the system, including patient safety (Storch 2005; Varcoe and Rodney 2009). For example, there have been numerous reports of patients experiencing harmful effects of improperly sterilized equipment with suggestions that substituting staff not properly trained in sterilization techniques for formerly well-prepared technicians led to this harm. Such mishaps also occurred within health professional groups, including improperly experienced pathologists who made mistakes in diagnosing cancerous tumours, leading to either earlier than expected deaths or improper and harmful treatment for patients with low risk tumours (see, for example, Gregory and Parfrey 2010).

To compound the problem, the move toward less local governance of health services with a shift in responsibility from local boards and councils to large regional boards, along with a simultaneous shift down from provincial ministries of health to these same health regional boards, has made it difficult to hold anyone responsible for unsafe practices that lead to increased morbidity and mortality (see Chapter 12 and 18). Nevertheless, nurses have been seriously impacted by these ongoing cutbacks in health care and by the significant task-shifting involving nurse displacement still in progress (Gottlieb 2009). The current shortage of nurses can be seen as the collateral damage of the cutbacks (e.g., a drop in interest in nursing as a profession in the 1990s, lack of full-time employment for RNs, devaluation of nursing knowledge and skills). Given the nursing shortage, administrators have used other, less educated (or uneducated) individuals to do "nursing tasks" as if those tasks were all that constituted the nursing care needed. Based upon a review of studies involving 16 countries, Horton, Tschudin, and Forget (2007) found that nurses have been devalued to a significant degree worldwide (see also Allan, Tschudin, and Horton 2008). When nurses' knowledge is not valued, and when other less- or un-trained workers are substituted for RNs, near misses can become errors and the increased likelihood of rising errors in medical and health care persist. These kinds of challenges are addressed in Chapters 9, 10, and 11 of this book.

As will be discussed by authors in Part II of this book, inadequate attention paid to the social determinants of health, home health care, and to creating a strong public health service has also lead to preventable hospitalizations making more people vulnerable. Early discharges, without adequate community support through home care and other services, often adds to the lack of patient safety (McDonald et al. 2009). In continued attempts aimed at cost reduction, health executives have been involved in persistent re-structuring of their agencies with an impact on the workflow of nursing, reporting patterns, and other important communication processes. In commenting on similar work pressures for efficiency on other executives, Goodpaster (2007) noted,

> Under stress they ignored certain higher values (like honesty and concern) in favor of lesser values (like security and efficiency). (21)

As "Ethics in Practice 1-1" illustrates, attention to developing leaders who are moral agents has never been more critical.

ETHICS IN PRACTICE 1-1

Being a Moral Agent

In meetings designed to include discussion about the quality of care, three nurse managers in a large health care agency repeatedly raised concerns about the shortage of professional nursing staff due, they believed, to the agency's current hiring practices. They often cited instances where potential (near misses) and actual errors occurred with less prepared staff engaging in nursing tasks. At first, their concerns were greeted with a polite silence, and then by occasional suggestions that those managers were neither receptive to change nor to "the better" use of less costly personnel. Eventually they were not told the time and location of meetings that had been a routine part of their work expectation. They concluded that they might have to limit their advocacy for the patients under their supervision. so that they might receive critical details .about other proposed changes in delivery of care. (From "Ethics in Practice" study.)

These nurse managers were each attempting to fulfill their responsibilities as moral agents. A **moral agent** is someone who has the capacity to direct his or her actions to some ethical end—in this case, good outcomes for patients (see Chapter 9).

Health care professionals are moral agents since their commitment to being a professional requires them to use their knowledge and skills for the good of those in their care. Nurses have taken this concept seriously (Rodney 1997) and are beginning to recognize that almost every decision they make about, for example, which call bell they will respond to first, how much time they will devote to listening to a troubled patient while two other patients require their attention, and so on, are everyday ethical decisions.

As we see in Ethics in Practice 1-1, nurse managers are not immune to making difficult ethical decisions, nor are other health care managers or administrators (Gaudine and Beaton 2002; Mitton et al. 2010). In exercising their moral agency, they also encounter moral distress. Although some practitioners and managers suggest that moral distress should be expected when an individual chooses to be a nurse, another health professional, or a manager, the difference between moral stress (anticipated) and moral distress (a compromised action or decision) needs to be understood (Pauly, Storch, and Varcoe 2010).

Being a moral agent requires moral reflection, which, according to Goodpaster (2007), is synonymous with conscience (4). He notes that individual and organizational consciences are critical to harm prevention, and that these "internal moral compasses can be more reliable than external sanctions—legal or economic" (5). Vision and strength in a corporate culture are not mere sentiments as is often portrayed (12). "True leaders add ethical value to value-added" (258).

Experiencing Moral Distress

ETHICS IN PRACTICE 1-2

Dealing with Moral Distress

When a co-ed hospital room policy was put in place in some provinces and regions in Canada, it was implemented in some areas with little regard for the type of hospital unit on which male and female patients might share a room without loss of privacy or dignity. Nurses on one unit in an older part of an urban hospital were alarmed and increasingly distressed when they found a young man placed in a room with four elderly women awaiting placement in long-term care. They believed that all patients in that room were subject to loss of dignity and that their care of each patient was compromised by this placement. They spoke to the bed utilization manager about their moral distress. When their advocacy was not heeded, they decided as a team that they would preserve patient dignity by moving beds to accommodate male and female patients in separate rooms. While this added to their workload, they felt strongly about what they perceived as a violation of ethical responsibility and took action to decrease their own moral distress, while continuing their advocacy for their patients ("Ethics in Action" study).

Moral distress is not just feeling some stress or some distressing situation, but includes a sense of feeling compromised in fulfilling a duty of care. In Ethics in Practice 1-2 the nurses met together to discuss this ethical problem, engaged their nurse manager, and raised their concerns with the bed utilization manager. Meanwhile, to lessen the patients' loss of privacy and dignity, they took action to create a more dignified environment for all concerned. Their action led to changes in policy to recognize that some hospital units are not suitable for co-ed occupancy.

Developing a Moral Community

ETHICS IN PRACTICE 1-3

"We Have No Ethical Issues in our Practice"

A group of registered nurses and licensed practical nurses in a small community hospital began meeting, at the invitation of researchers, to discuss the ethical concerns they were facing in their practice. When first approached to see if they wished to be part of the study, some were not certain that they had any ethical issues. They confessed to having communication issues, issues with their assignments, and issues in emergency care, but could not see ethical concerns as part of their problems. However, they agreed to meet to "see how it goes," particularly when their senior administrators provided financial and moral support for their patient assignments to be covered by relief staff while they met. As they commenced discussion about issues impacting the everyday care they provided they began to see those issues through an "ethics lens." For example, as they discussed issues of task shifting amongst staff members, they began to hear what others were saying, particularly about the fear of those less well prepared for the tasks they were required to take on, and they understood how this was a matter of relational ethics (see Chapters 7 and 8). Since all professed to be there for the benefit of the patients, they could see how even minor resentments amongst them about staffing became major ethical problems for safe, competent, and ethical care ("Leadership for Ethical Policy and Practice [LEPP]" study).

TOWARD AN ETHICAL OR MORAL CLIMATE

The moral distress nurses and other health professionals experience in health care today can be addressed by working toward a moral community, as illustrated in Ethics in Practice 1-3. A moral community is ". . . a workplace where values are made clear and are shared, where these values direct ethical action and where individuals feel safe to be heard" (CNA Code 2008, 27) (see Chapter 10). Such a moral community can enhance the ethical climate or culture of the workplace (Rodney et al. 2006; Storch et al. 2009a). Extensive studies have been undertaken in Canada in the past decade with a focus on healthy workplaces for health workers (Laschinger and Finegan 2005; Lowe 2006; Lowe and Chan 2010; Shamian and El-Jardali 2007). Notably absent from this focus are studies that include discussion about *ethics in the workplace*. If, for example, nurses and other health professionals are repeatedly forced to compromise their professional and personal values, their mental and spiritual health is likely to be in serious jeopardy (Ford, Fraser, and Marck 2010).

Goldman and Tabak (2010) adopted Ulrich's definition of an ethical climate for their research on moral climate:

> An ethical climate represents the shared perceptions of organizational practices related to ethical decision-making and reflection, including issues of power, trust and human interactions within an organization (233).

Thus, an ethical climate profoundly influences both decision making and subsequent behavioural responses to ethical problems (see Chapter 10). The way in which difficult patient care problems are defined, discussed, and decided is in large part a function of the ethical climate of the organization (Schluter et al. 2008). Gradually, codes of ethics have been developed for guidance for organizations, including regional health authorities, provincial health services, and national health organizations to complement professional codes of ethics. Examples of these codes are provided in the following section.

Can Codes of Ethics Help?

The purpose and impact of codes of ethics on ethical actions has long been debated. Codes can serve a number of functions and their utility depends on how they have been developed and their uptake by those within the organization or professional body for which they are intended.

Recent organizational codes of ethics in health care are normally intended for all who work in the organization including contract workers, physicians from private practice, and volunteers. For example, one regional ethics committee developed a code of ethics based on six values: respect, honesty, integrity, collaboration, justice, and accountability. These values were presented in three iterations: a one-page statement of the values, a five-page bulleted statement with each value described along with examples, and a detailed discussion about each value with references for further study. The declared purpose was to "help the organization and individuals recognize and think clearly about the ethical issues in what they do."[2]

The Alberta Health Services Draft Code of Ethical Conduct (October 2009) is one example of a code of ethics designed to apply to health services throughout an entire province. The code makes reference to being principle-based with four values (respect, accountability, transparency, engagement) and five principles. Details about the five principles, with examples, were provided in the code, along with rights and responsibility statements for implementing the code.

The *Health Ethics Guide* developed by the Catholic Health Association of Canada (2002) is an example of a national organizational code. This code sets out the context of ethical reflection as focused on the "healing relationship" after which Christian moral values are identified. Fundamental values are the dignity of the human person and the interconnectedness of every human being. Based upon those two values, stewardship and creativity, respect of human life, the common good, charity, and solidarity are added values (Catholic Health Association of Canada 2002). This guide also includes a section on creating an ethical environment (22–23).

Professional codes of ethics for numerous health professionals are also important. Since health care in Canada is largely a provincial responsibility, some of these codes are provincially oriented. Others are national in development and in nature. The Canadian Nurses Association code is one example of a national code developed by nurses, for nurses, as ethical guidelines for practice. It has been revised every five to seven years. During its last revision (2008), the development of this code became controversial due to changing governmental influences on professional self-regulation in many provinces. Those provincial colleges and associations most impacted by provincial governments believed they needed a "regulatory code" they could use for their purposes, while the remaining provinces and the national association favoured a relational ethics approach to this code with a strong emphasis on social justice. For example, Peter (2011) urged that, codes of ethics and standards of practice need to address social justice to promote its acceptance as a collective responsibility. A regulatory code would include only enforceable, measureable standards, whereas a relational ethics code includes aspirational statements and visionary ethical endeavours that (although difficult to measure) serve to guide nurses toward higher ethical standards (Storch 2008).

The only way that the 2008 value-based Canadian Nurses Association code could be approved by the 10 provinces and two territories was to create a part A (which regulator-oriented representatives could support) and a part B (which social justice and relational ethics oriented representatives could support). The underlying threat leading to the creation of this unique code was that each province might choose to create its own code of ethics for registered nurses. For some time, both Ontario and Quebec have had their own codes of ethical conduct but nurses across Canada seemed reluctant to allow this "splintering" of ethical codes to proceed further.

It is no surprise that widespread skepticism about codes of ethics exists. Wainwright and Pattison (2004) have summarized the opposition to codes of ethics well. Essentially, they point out that ". . . people expect both too much and too little from codes, often assuming meaning, clarity, and unity that is not there" (111). They summarize the purposes of codes of ethics as follows: to offer guidance, substance for regulation, for discipline, for information sharing (about what the profession stands for), and for stating how the profession will protect the public. Yet, they maintain that codes usually contain impossible ideals and conflicting values, without showing how such conflicts might be dealt with. For individuals and for organizations, conflicts often arise due to areas beyond their control (e.g., limitations of the built environment and confidentiality, imbalances of power and authority between members of the health care team).

We believe that codes of ethics have a place and a purpose. At a minimum they serve to make nurses aware of the meaning of safe, compassionate, competent, and ethical care, while also serving as a means to alert colleagues in practice to maintain an "ethics lens" in their everyday practice.[3] As Brown and Allison point out in Chapter 15, ethics education for practice should extend beyond knowledge and reliance on codes. Yet, codes can provide benchmarks against which practitioners can assess their "ethical fitness." The conflicting obligations that are part of most codes can also provide a basis for discussion amongst nurses and other health professionals as they try to sort out difficult issues to balance toward "the good" in their practice. In 2010 the Canadian Nurses Association (CNA) released a set of eight e-learning modules on using the code of ethics, available to all through the CNA website. These ethics modules provide an excellent resource for individual or group study and discussion. They are available on the public CNA website and their usefulness can well extend to discussions with other health professionals in practice.

MORAL COMMUNITIES AND INTER-PROFESSIONAL PRACTICE

Since other health professionals have codes of ethics and other ethical guidelines they might use, there is room for conflicting priorities amongst a health care team. Such conflicting ideals underscore the importance of health care team members working together to build moral communities. Such communities help create the environmental climate for ethical reflection and for dialogue to learn and to resolve difficult situations that stand in the way of good ethical practice. Further, they serve as a forum for advocacy for better ethical policies and procedures for patient care. Interdisciplinary education is also needed so that health professionals and other health care providers, both at the basic level of their college or university education and as continuing collaborative ethics education, can learn to engage in ethical discussion within work units (Storch and Kenny 2007).

Along with ethical guidelines, ethical decision-making models can also be helpful. Appendices A to C of this book provide such models, one developed by Storch and the others by McDonald. In Chapter 13, the use of the McDonald model for ethical decision-making is provided. All chapters in this book point to diverse strategies that can help nurses and other health care professionals strengthen the moral communities in which they work.

Summary

Within this chapter, the purpose and design of *Toward a Moral Horizon: Nursing Ethics for Leadership and Practice* has been described, along with reference to the organization of nursing roles past and present. The importance of "ethical fitness" has been emphasized, and the place of an ethics vocabulary in developing that fitness is outlined. The context of health and health care has been discussed briefly, focusing on current challenges nurses face. The editors' research in nursing ethics and practice, with the intention of finding ways to *embed ethics* in organizations and provide better ways for nurses to practice ethically, has also been reviewed. Being a moral agent, dealing with moral distress, and working toward an enhanced ethical climate continue to be advocated.

Codes of ethics have been promoted as one tool to assist health care providers, including nurses in direct care and in formal leadership positions. Emphasized throughout the chapter is the importance of ethics discussions with nursing colleagues, physicians, and all health care professionals and health care providers. Ethics discussions build trust, a vital element in the provision of safe, compassionate, competent, ethical care.

We trust that the chapters in this book will provide rich grounding to promote discussion amongst health care professionals, and to equip nurses and other health professionals for practice that involves using an "ethics lens."

For Reflection

1. In your nursing practice, have you considered yourself to be a moral agent?

2. Have you encountered situations that you might call morally distressing? At the time, did you consider those situations as having anything to do with ethics?

3. What moral concepts might be particularly helpful to nurse leaders?

4. How might you initiate discussion of ethics among health team members?

5. Do you consider yourself to be ethically fit?

Endnotes

1. We acknowledge with gratitude initial funding for our first study; then complementary funding from Associated Medical Services, Inc.; and the Social Sciences and Humanities Research Council of Canada for our second study. Our third study was funded by the Canadian Health Services Research Foundation, the First Nations and Inuit Branch (B.C.), and the Office of Nursing Policy of Health Canada. A full list of authors of the article describing the LEPP study is as follows: J. Storch, P. Rodney, C. Varcoe, B. Pauly, R. Starzomski, L. Stevenson, L. Best, H. Mass, T. R. Fulton, B. Mildon, F. Bees, A. Chisholm, S. MacDonald-Rencz, A. Sanchez-McCutcheon, J. Shamian, C. Thompson, K. Schick-Makaroff, and L. Newton (2009) plus nurses involved in direct care on six sites as well as nursing supervisors, a physician, and several other health care providers.

2. The Vancouver Island Health Authority Draft Code of Ethics. 2007. Victoria, B.C.: Author.

3. See also the American Nurses Association (ANA) booklet that provides an interpretation and application of the ANA Code of Ethics for Nurses (Fowler 2008).

References

Alberta Health Services. 2009. *Alberta Health Services Draft Code of Ethical Conduct*. Edmonton: Author.

Allan, H., Tschudin, V., and Horton, K. 2008. The devaluation of nursing: A position statement. *Nursing Ethics, 15* (4), 549–556.

Baker, G.R. and Norton, P.G. 2004. *Patient safety and healthcare error in the Canadian healthcare system: A report to Health Canada*. Ottawa: Health Canada.

Baker, G.R., Norton, P.G., Flintoft, V., Blais, R., Brown, A., Cox, J., Etchells, E., Gahli, W.A., Hebert, P., Majumdar, S.R., O'Beirne, M., Palacois-Derlingher, I., Reid, R.J., Sheps, S., and Tamblyn, R. 2004. The Canadian adverse events study: The incidence of adverse events among hospital patients in Canada. *Canadian Medical Association Journal, 170* (11), 1678–1687.

Baylis, F., Downie, J., Hoffmaster, B., and Sherwin, S. (Eds.). 2004. *Health care ethics in Canada.* Toronto: Thomson Canada Ltd.

Caldwell, E.S., Lu, H., and Harding, T. 2010. Encompassing multiple moral paradigms: A challenge for nursing educators. *Nursing Ethics, 17* (2), 189–199.

Canadian Nurses Association. 2002. *Code of ethics for registered nurses.* Ottawa: Author.

Canadian Nurses Association. 2008. *Code of ethics for registered nurses.* Ottawa: Author.

Catholic Health Association of Canada. 2002. *Health ethics guide.* Ottawa: Author.

Chambliss, D.F. 1996. *Beyond caring: Hospitals, nurses and the social organization of ethics.* Chicago: University of Chicago Press.

Childress, J.F. and Siegler, M. 1999. Metaphors and models of doctor-patient relationships: Their implications for autonomy. In E-H Kluge (Ed.), *Readings in biomedical ethics: A Canadian focus* (2nd ed.; pp. 133–144). Scarborough, ON: Prentice Hall Allyn and Bacon Canada.

Corley, M. 2006. Personal communication, October 27.

Corley, M., Elswick, R., Gorman, M., and Clor, T. 2001. Development and evaluation of a moral distress scale. *Journal of Advanced Nursing, 33* (2), 250–256.

Corley, M., Minick, P., Elswick, R., and Jacobs, M. 2005. Nurse moral distress and ethical work environment. *Nursing Ethics, 12* (4), 381–390.

Davis, F. (Ed.). 1966. *The nursing profession: Five sociological essays.* New York: John Wiley and Sons.

Doane, G., Pauly, B., Brown, H., and McPherson, G. 2004. Exploring the heart of ethical nursing practice: Implications for ethics education. *Nursing Ethics, 11* (3), 240–253.

Ford, N.J., Fraser, K.D., and Marck, P.B. 2010. Conscientious objection: A call for nursing leadership. *Nursing Leadership, 23* (3), 48–55.

Fry, S.T. 1989. Towards a theory of nursing ethics. *Advances in Nursing Science, 11* (4), 9–22.

Fowler, M.D.M. (Ed.). 2008. *Guide to the Code of Ethics for Nurses: Interpretation and application.* Silver Spring, MD: American Nurses Association.

Gallagher, A. 2010. Editorial. The trouble with "transcultural nursing ethics." *Nursing Ethics, 17* (2), 155–156.

Gaudine, A. and Beaton, M. 2002. Employed to go against one's own values: Nurse managers' accounts of ethical conflict within their organization. *Canadian Journal of Nursing Research, 34* (2), 17–34.

Gershon, R., Stone, P.W., Bakken, S., and Larson, E. 2004. Measurement of organizational culture and climate in healthcare. *Journal of Nursing Administration, 34* (1), 33–40.

Goldman, A. and Tabak, N. 2010. Perception of ethical climate and its relationship to nurse demographic characteristics and job satisfaction. *Nursing Ethics, 17* (2), 233–246.

Goodrich, A.W. 1932. *The social and ethical significance of nursing.* New York: The Macmillan Company.

Goodpaster, K.E. 2007. *Conscience and corporate culture.* Oxford, UK: Blackwell Publishing.

Gottlieb, L.N. 2009. Putting health care during the past decade in context: An interview with Dr. Judith Shamian. *Canadian Journal of Nursing Research, 41* (1), 21–30.

Gregory, D.M. and Parfrey, P.S. 2010. The breast cancer hormone receptor testing controversy in Newfoundland and Labrador, Canada: Lessons for the health system. *Healthcare Management Forum, 23* (3), 114–118.

Hanssen, I. and Alpers, L-M. 2010. Utilitarian and common-sense morality discussions in intercultural nursing practice. *Nursing Ethics, 17* (2), 201–211.

Hart, S.E. 2005. Hospital ethical climates and registered nurses' turnover intentions. *Journal of Nursing Scholarship, 37* (2), 173–177.

Hartrick Doane, G., Storch, J., and Pauly, B. 2009. Ethical nursing practice: Inquiry-in-action. *Nursing Inquiry, 16* (3), 1–9.

Horton, K., Tschudin, V., and Forget, A. 2007. The value of nursing: A literature review. *Nursing Ethics, 14* (6), 716–740.

Jameton, A. 1984. *Nursing practice: The ethical issues.* Englewood Cliffs, NJ: Prentice Hall.

Kidder, R.M. 2009. *How good people make tough choices: Resolving the dilemmas of ethical living.* New York: Harper.

Laschinger, H.K.S. and Finegan, J. 2005. Empowering nurses for work engagement and health in hospital settings. *Journal of Nursing Administration, 35* (10), 439–449.

Lowe, G.S. 2006. *Making a measurable difference: Evaluating quality of work life interventions.* Ottawa: Canadian Nurses Association.

Lowe, G. and Chan, B. 2010. Using common work environment metrics to improve performance in healthcare organization performance. *HealthcarePapers, 10* (3), 8–23.

Mauksch, H.O. 1966. The organizational context of nursing practice. In F. Davis (Ed.) *The nursing profession: Five sociological essays* (pp. 109–137). New York: John Wiley and Sons, Inc.

Mitton, C., Peacock, S., Storch, J., Smith, N., and Cornelissen, E. 2010. Moral distress among healthcare managers: Conditions, consequences and potential responses. *Healthcare Policy, 6* (2), 99–112.

Oberle, K. and Raffin Bouchal, S. 2009. *Ethics in Canadian nursing practice: Navigating the journey.* Toronto: Pearson Canada.

Olson, L.L. 1998. Hospital nurses' perceptions of the ethical climate of their work setting. *Image: Journal of Nursing Scholarship, 30* (4), 345–349.

Pauly, B.M., Storch, J.L., and Varcoe, C. 2010. *Moral distress in health care symposium, Sept 18-19, 2010.* Final Report. Ottawa: Canadian Institutes of Health Research.

Pauly, B., Varcoe, C., Storch, J., and Newton, L. 2009. Registered nurses' perceptions of moral distress and ethical climate. *Nursing Ethics, 16* (5), 561–573.

Peter, E. 2011. Fostering social justice: The possibilities of a socially connected model of moral agency. *Canadian Journal of Nursing Research, 43* (2), 11–17.

Rodney, P. 1997. *Towards connectedness and trust: Nurses' enactment of their moral agency within an organizational context.* Unpublished doctoral dissertation, University of British Columbia, Vancouver.

Rodney, P., Doane, G., Storch, J., and Varcoe, C. 2006. Toward a safer moral climate. *Canadian Nurse, 102* (8), 24–27.

Rodney, P., Martin, L.A., Serrano, E., Housden, L., Moody, E., Vandenberg, H., Asher, M., Lamasan, M., and Young, M. 2010. *Collaborative practice in ambulatory oncology care: Working with insights from a participatory action research project.* Abstract for presentation at the 21st Canadian Bioethics Society Annual Conference, *Voices of communities,* Kelowna, B.C. June 9–12, p. 37.

Rodney, P., Varcoe, C., Storch, J.L., McPherson, G., Mahoney, K., Brown, H., Pauly, B., Hartrick Doane, G., and Starzomski, R. 2002. Navigating toward a moral horizon: A multi-site qualitative study of nurses' enactment of ethical practice. *Canadian Journal of Nursing Research, 34* (3), 75–102.

Schluter, J. Winch, S., Holzhauser, K., and Henderson, A. 2008. Nurses' moral sensitivity and hospital ethical climate: A literature review. *Nursing Ethics, 15* (3), 305–321.

Shamian, J. and El-Jardali, F. 2007. Healthy workplaces for health care workers in Canada: Knowledge transfer and uptake in policy and practice. *HealthcarePapers, 7* (Sp), 6–25.

Storch, J.L. 1999. Moral relationships between nurse and client: The influence of metaphors. In E-H. Kluge (Ed.), *Readings in Biomedical Ethics: A Canadian Focus* (2nd ed.; pp. 145–154). Scarborough, ON: Prentice-Hall Allyn and Bacon Canada. Also included in Baylis et al. 2004, (pp. 178–186) see above.

Storch, J. 2005. Patient safety: Is it just another bandwagon? *Canadian Journal of Nursing Leadership, 18* (2), 39–55.

Storch, J. 2008. Codes of ethics: Aspirational or regulatory? *Canadian Journal of Nursing Leadership, 21* (2), 31–33.

Storch, J.L. and Kenny, N. 2007. Shared moral work of nurses and physicians. *Nursing Ethics, 14* (4), 478–491.

Storch, J., Rodney, P., Pauly, B., Brown, H., and Starzomski, R. 2002. Listening to nurses' moral voices: Building a quality health care environment. *Canadian Journal of Nursing Leadership, 15* (4), 7–16.

Storch, J.L., Rodney, P., and Starzomski, R. (Eds.) 2004. *Toward a moral horizon: Nursing ethics for leadership and practice.* Toronto: Pearson Prentice Hall.

Storch, J., Rodney, P., Pauly, B., Stevenson, L., Fulton, T., Newton, L., and Schick Makaroff, K. 2009a. Enhancing ethical climates for nursing work environments. *Canadian Nurse, 105* (3), 20–25.

Storch, J., Rodney, P., Varcoe, C., Pauly, B., Starzomski, R., Stevenson, L., Best, L., Mass, H., Fulton, T., Mildon, B., Bees, F., Chisholm, A., MacDonald-Rencz, S., McCutcheon, A., Shamian, J., Thompson, C., Schick Makaroff, K., and Newton, L. 2009b. Leadership for ethical policy and practice: Participatory action project. *Canadian Journal for Nursing Leadership, 22* (3), 68–80.

Twomey, J.G. 1989. Analysis of the claim to distinct nursing ethics: Normative and non-normative approaches. *Advances in Nursing Science, 11* (3), 25–32.

Wainwright, P. 2009. *Is transcultural nursing ethics viable?* Paper presented at the ICNE Pre-ICN Workshop. Durban, South Africa, June 30, 2009.

Wainwright, P. and Pattison, S. 2004. What can we expect of professional codes of conduct, practice and ethics? In S. Pattison and R. Pill (Eds.), *Values in professional practice: Lessons for health, social care and other professionals* (pp. 109–122). Oxford: Radcliffe Medical Press.

Webster, G. and Baylis, F. 2000. Moral residue. In S.B. Rubin and L. Zoloth (Eds.), *Margin of error: The ethics of mistakes in the practice of medicine* (pp. 217–232). Hagerstown, MD: University Publishing Group.

Ulrich, C., O'Donnell, P., Taylor, C., Farrar, A., Danis, M., and Grady, C. 2007. Ethical climate, ethics stress, and the job satisfaction of nurses and social workers in the United States. *Social Science and Medicine, 65,* 1708–1719.

Varcoe, C., Doane, G., Pauly, B., Rodney, P., Storch, J. L., Mahoney, K., McPherson, G., Brown, H., and Starzomski, R. 2004. Ethical practice in nursing: Working the in-betweens. *Journal of Advanced Nursing, 45* (3), 316–325.

Varcoe, C., Pauly, B., Storch, J., Schick-Makaroff, K., and Newton, L. in review. Nurses' perceptions of and responses to situations of moral distress: Qualitative findings.

Varcoe, C. and Rodney, P. 2009. Constrained agency: The social structure of nurses' work. In B.S. Bolaria and H.D. Dickinson (Eds.), *Health, illness, and health care in Canada* (4th ed.; pp. 122–151). Toronto: Nelson.

Vancouver Island Health Authority. 2007. *Clinical ethics: Health ethics handbook.* Victoria, BC: Author.

Yeo, M. 2010a. Introduction. In M.Yeo, A. Moorhouse, P. Khan, and P. Rodney (Eds.) *Concepts and cases in nursing ethics* (3rd ed.; pp. 11–36). Peterborough, ON: Broadview Press.

Yeo, M. 2010b. A primer in ethical theory. In M. Yeo, A. Moorhouse, P. Khan, and P. Rodney (Eds.), *Concepts and cases in nursing ethics* (3rd ed.; pp. 37–72). Peterborough, ON: Broadview Press.

Yeo, M. and Moorhouse, A. 2010. Confidentiality. In M. Yeo, A. Moorhouse, P. Khan, and P. Rodney (Eds.) *Concepts and cases in nursing ethics* (3rd ed.; pp. 245–272). Peterborough, ON: Broadview Press.

Yeo, M., Moorhouse, A., Khan, P., and Rodney, P. 2010. *Concepts and cases in nursing ethics* (3rd ed.). Peterborough, ON: Broadview Press.

CHAPTER 2

A Historical Perspective on Nursing and Nursing Ethics

Marianne Lamb and Janet L. Storch

It is clear that since the beginning of "modern" nursing in the 1800s, nurses have believed that their role in society brought with it specific moral obligations.

In this chapter we take a backward glance at nursing and nursing ethics as it has developed over time. Reflecting upon these historical roots can assist us in understanding changes in the ethical beliefs and values of nursing. Connecting to our past helps us to appreciate the social, spiritual, economic, political, and religious changes that have shaped health care and nursing as well as health care ethics and nursing ethics. We can more clearly see issues of gender (the role of women), social class, and the role of religion as significant in nursing's history. Thus, we can learn from the past and connect our past to our future.

We begin this reflection by considering glimpses of the development of nursing worldwide, including depictions of the role of women, by considering the spiritual influences upon nursing, as well as the influence of the organization of health care and the practice of nursing. Following this synopsis, we look briefly at education and nursing ethics, nursing ethics and the influence of medical and biomedical ethics, and the development of professional associations and codes of ethics. The nursing literature is a major source of information about the evolution of ethics over time, and although we have drawn on international literature, a majority of the early sources are North American, with a focus on Canadian nursing.

A GLIMPSE AT ANCIENT NURSING HISTORY

In writing about nursing and "primitive peoples," Goodnow (1942) notes that in early history, religion and healing (medicine) were closely united (14–17). When healing was not possible, provision was made for care, particularly for travellers, servants, and soldiers. In Egypt numerous hygienic laws had been developed dating back to 2900 B.C., with some type of housing for the sick in temples. Historical documents from India make reference to nurses who were required to exhibit three main qualities of character—"high standards, skill and trustworthiness" (Donahue 1985). Further requirements of these nurses were specified as the following:

> After this should be secured a body of attendants of good behaviour, distinguished for purity or cleanliness of habits, attached to the person for whose service they are engaged, possessed of cleverness and skill endued with kindness, skilled in every kind of service that a patient may require, endued with general cleverness, competent to cook food and curries, clever in

bathing or washing a patient, well conversant in rubbing or pressing the limbs, or raising the patient or assisting him in walking or moving about, well skilled in making or cleaning beds, competent to pound drugs or ready, patient, and skilful in waiting upon one that is ailing, and never unwilling to do any act that they may be commanded (by the physician or patient) to do. (Donahue 1985, 62, citing Charaka-Samhita, vol. 1, 168–169)

In roughly this same time period (1500 B.C.E.), the Hebrew people, who "learned much of their hygiene from the Egyptians," migrated to Canaan and during their journey developed some of the "highest attainments in hygiene." They also emphasized providing care for all, rich and poor alike (Nutting and Dock 1974, 1–62).

In other parts of the world, such as China, little mention is made of hospitals or nursing as families were responsible for care of the sick according to Confucian teaching. In Korea, where recorded medical history dates back to 1406, nursing was ascribed to females in the family, notably the wife and mother who was responsible for the care of the whole family (Cho 1997, 9). This same pattern is evident in many other countries where women were responsible for the nursing care of their household members, including Greece where, prior to Hippocrates' time, little attention was paid to nursing care as it seemed to be assumed that the role of women was to look after their own families.

Lanara (1981) suggests that nursing values were derived from classical Greece and the Byzantine Empire. The importance (1) of treating the patient as a whole person in giving care, and (2) of healing both body and soul, (3) of ensuring the patient and family are treated as individuals who participate in decisions about their care, (4) of supportive and compassionate care, (5) of personal and professional integrity, and (6) of involvement in society's problems in fighting against social and health evils, were emphasized. Fowler (2009) also adds the importance of appreciating non-Western bioethical issues so that we do not "miss the moral concerns patients from other religions and cultures identify" (403).

RELIGION, SPIRITUALITY, ETHICS, AND THE DEVELOPMENT OF NURSING

In Western countries there seems to be little doubt that Christianity had a major influence upon organized nursing. "A spiritual meaning became deeply attached to the care of the sick and suffering" (Donahue 1985, 95). Based upon Christian teachings of love and brotherhood, not only was society transformed but the development of nursing was based on altruism (Donahue 1985, 93). Caring for the sick allowed single women to acquire positions of usefulness and develop respected careers. The foundations of "nurses' calling" and of modern works of charity were laid and perpetuated in the early Christian Era of 1–50 A.D. (Donahue 1985, 101). Churches and their followers became involved in providing care in homes and in establishing early hospitals where religious deaconesses and other women (and some men) provided nursing care. In the modern era, when religious nursing orders renewed their activity in providing nursing care, the Sisters of Charity, one of the best known of these orders, was developed. In Canada, the influence of the French nursing sisters pre-dated Florence Nightingale's time. The Sisters must be acknowledged for their significant contributions to the thinking and values of nurses throughout hospitals and schools of nursing founded in the Catholic tradition (Ross-Kerr 1996).

Over the centuries the status of nursing rose and fell along with societal changes. Donahue documents details about the effects of feudalism, the Crusades, the development of military nursing orders, the rise of mendicant orders and secular nursing orders, as well as the effect of the Renaissance, Reformation, and the Industrial Revolution. Throughout these centuries disease epidemics plagued the Western world and nursing deteriorated along with the decay of early hospitals (Nutting and Dock 1974, 499–524). During the political, economic, industrial, and intellectual revolutions that followed, new directions were developing in medical science and both hospitals and nursing were reformed. Along with other social reforms there was public interest in improving the dire situation of nursing (as typified by Sarah Gamp, a nurse in England portrayed in the Dickens novel *Martin Chuzzlewit* [1844]). "This public concern resulted in the beginning of significant changes that directed steady reform in nursing" (Donahue 1985, 231–234).

The Deaconess Institute at Kaiserswerth, Germany, is credited with the regeneration of nursing. Established by Pastor Theodore Fliedner (1800–1884), this institute revived the role of deaconesses through the Protestant churches (Donahue 1985, 234). Florence Nightingale enrolled in the nursing program at Kaiserswerth in 1847 and "she spoke of the institute as her 'spiritual home'" (240). This Christian (Catholic and Protestant) influence on nursing in Canada has framed nurses' worldviews, including how we define health and moral responsibility in ways different from other religions and spiritual practices.

VALUES IN EARLY NURSING PRACTICE

In the late 1800s, Florence Nightingale was consulted by many hospitals in North America that wished to establish schools of nursing based on her model (Robb 1900; Woodham-Smith 1951). As hospitals grew in number across North America at the turn of the century, so did schools of nursing. These schools, however, differed in one important way from Nightingale's school—they were not financially independent from hospitals. Under the apprenticeship system, nursing students provided hospitals with nursing services, a system that hospital administrators and physicians recognized as "good business practice" and profitable (Ashley 1976). Among the values emphasized in early training schools were those of loyalty, acceptance of authority, and unselfishness. Loyalty to the hospital and to physicians was expected and students were instructed that their behaviour reflected on the reputation of the hospital. This placed nurses in a constant situation of others having "power over" their practice. Further, as Ashley noted, for decades the American public seemed unaware that in most hospitals, nursing services were provided by "partially trained, inexperienced, and unsupervised nurse students, not graduate, licensed nurses" (16).

Since hospitals were staffed by nursing students, graduates of nursing schools in Canada and the United States had to earn their living in private duty nursing practice. An individual who was ill was usually cared for at home by a physician and, if advised by the physician or requested by the family, by a private nurse. If hospitalization was necessary, the patient could hire a private nurse for "special" duty, although most could not afford special nurses and were cared for by students (Ellis 1927; Weir 1932).

As we note later in this chapter, nursing etiquette was frequently equated with nursing ethics. In private duty practice, the nurse worked closely with the physician, who often recommended her to his patients. From her obligations to the patient stemmed those duties "owed" to the physician. Together, the nurse and physician formed a team in the battle against disease and death (Byers 1922). The physician was "captain of the team," and the nurse's role was to observe the patient, to carry out the physician's orders, to ensure that the patient was as comfortable and contented as possible, and to report her observations and concerns to the physician when he visited. Any discord in this team was viewed as not being in the best interests of the patient—recovery would be jeopardized by any lack of confidence in the nurse or physician (Scovil 1917). In addition, an emphasis on etiquette was related to the 24-hour duty often required in the home, a situation in which the nurse must fit into family life while caring for her patient.

In this chapter we cannot do justice to the history of nursing in Canada, but we urge readers to be mindful of societal changes and events that had an effect on nursing practice and the image of nurses. Many nurse historians have recounted that history, for example, chapters in *On All Frontiers: Four Centuries of Canadian Nursing* (Bates, Dodd, and Rousseau 2005). The significant role nurses began to take in public health nursing, during World War I, the Halifax Explosion, and the Spanish flu epidemic are examples of events "that called for public service and courage on the part of Canadian nurses" (Lamb 1981, 8).

ALTRUISM AND NURSING ETHICS

By the 1920s, there was a growing concern that "materialism" was threatening traditional values, religion, and family life (Fairley 1923). Although nurses had long professed a belief in the need for self-sacrifice and altruism in nursing, during the early 1920s, some implied that contemporary life was so characterized by a concern with money and goods that ethics and the altruistic ideal could become a thing of the past within the profession (Canadian Association of Nursing Education 1924). The movement by private duty nurses to shorten their hours of duty while maintaining their daily fee rate generated fears that nursing was becoming commercialized, although nursing was supposed to be above "mere money getting" (Field 1923). In Canada, private duty nurses organized a section within the national association in the hope that official nursing support would help their cause and deal with public criticism. Over the decade of the 1920s, increasing unemployment among private duty nurses gave rise to growing sympathy for the plight of graduate nurses, suggestions for government-sponsored plans for care of the sick, and a decrease in the call for self-sacrifice in nursing (Lamb 1981).

Over time, hospitals became the primary place of employment for graduate nurses and whereas 60 percent of active nurses in Canada were engaged in self-employed private duty practice in 1930 (Weir 1932), more than 80 percent of nurses worked as employees in hospitals by 1970 (Canadian Nurses Association [CNA] 1971). The impact of the Depression and World War II led to developments in health and social policy in Canada: the growth of hospitals in the 1940s, publicly funded hospital insurance in the 1950s, and medicare in the 1960s, all of which had a profound effect on nursing. Following decades of continued effort by the profession to improve the education of nursing students, the practice of using nursing students to provide service ceased, and a major move of nursing education into systems of general education was underway by the late 1960s and early 1970s (Brown 1966; Ross-Kerr 2003). Similar reforms were also advocated in the United States. In Ashley's (1976) historical review of the development of nursing in the United States, she described how nursing education and practice had been systematically controlled by hospital administration and the medical profession. She argued that sexism and paternalism oppressed nurses and hampered the reform of hospitals and health care in the United States.

RESPONSES TO CONSTRAINTS ON ETHICAL PRACTICE

As nursing employment in hospitals became the norm, some of the traditional practices and values of nurses were challenged. One of these values was how to improve salaries and working conditions in a profession that had long emphasized service and personal sacrifice. In 1943, the Canadian Nurses Association (CNA) formed its first committee on labour relations following similar activities by several provincial associations (CNA 1968), and the national organization supported collective bargaining in nursing in 1944 (Lindabury 1968). However, in 1946, a CNA resolution affirmed that it was "opposed to any nurse going on strike at any time for any cause" (Lindabury 1968). Nevertheless, some provincial nursing associations that bargained collectively for nurses did not support such a "no-strike" policy, and services were withdrawn on a few occasions, albeit with great reluctance. By the mid-1960s, the salaries and working conditions of nurses were of widespread concern (MacLeod 1966). Although "many nurses still harboured reservations regarding the appropriateness of a profession participating in collective bargaining" (CNA 1968, 9–10), such sentiments gave way in both the United States and Canada, and nurses began to vote in support of strike action ("BC nurses vote" 1968; Lindabury 1968).

Moral Concerns in Nursing Practice

While the profession came to terms with collective bargaining, nurses continued to raise ethical concerns related to working conditions and institutional constraints in hospital nursing. In the 1960s, many nurses expressed concern about the "dehumanizing" aspects of hospitalization (McMurtry 1968). Hayter (1966), in an article on the meaning of "caring," emphasized the nurse-patient relationship and noted that "there is considerable guilt among nurses because they cannot give the kind of nursing care they would like to give" (31). The patient rights movement of the 1970s brought with it continuing concerns about depersonalized care in a health care system that seemed increasingly fragmented, specialized, and subject to cost constraints (MacLellan 1976; Marcus

1975). In general, the 1970s was a decade of protest by nurses about poor working conditions that affected their ability to provide the quality of care for which they felt accountable: an accountability emphasized in an era of standards development, quality assurance, and safety-to-practice programs in nursing ("Health Disciplines Act" 1975; "Quality assurance" 1977). Safe levels of staffing and quality of patient care were issues in a court case involving nurses in British Columbia (Hudson 1970), an arbitration board case in Sudbury ("Three Sudbury nurses" 1971), an arbitration board hearing in Toronto (Wahn 1979), and a year-long dispute at the Vancouver General Hospital during which several senior nursing administrators were fired. Inquiries were held into the firings, public protests by nurses were organized, the board of trustees was dismissed, and a public administrator was appointed, after which a new vice-president of nursing was also appointed ("Nurses fight" 1978; "Major changes" 1978). In a sociological analysis of the dispute, Lovell (1981) described the social organization of power in hospitals and how the "normative order" was challenged by nurses who believed that they were excluded from decision-making about nursing practice.

Nurses in Canada continued to express similar opinions in the 1980s, as described in Growe's (1991) book titled *Who Cares? The Crisis in Canadian Nursing*. The book describes strikes by nurses, the treatment of nurses during the Royal Commission of Inquiry into the deaths at the Hospital for Sick Children, and the shortage of nurses by the end of the decade, highlighting stories of nurses that reinforce the picture of hospitals as paternal and rigid bureaucracies. In the 1990s, nurses identified organizational factors that constrained their actions as moral agents, constraints that sometimes led to tragic consequences. In a particularly poignant example, operating room nurses in a pediatric cardiac program in Winnipeg used "proper channels" to report safety problems in the program during 1994, but without results. In the subsequent Pediatric Cardiac Surgery Inquest Report (Sinclair n.d.; Sibbald 1997) following the deaths of 12 young patients, Judge Sinclair identified how "serious and legitimate concerns" of nurses were dismissed and rejected and how this dismissal delayed recognition of serious problems in the pediatric cardiac surgery program.

Long-standing funding issues in health care in Canada and other Western countries intensified in the 1990s as governments sought to reduce debt. This focus led to cutbacks in health care and the layoff of nurses as hospitals closed large numbers of beds in Canada (Baumann et al. 2001). Reports of moral distress among nurses multiplied in all areas of health care but particularly in hospitals where the majority of nurses worked ("Managers must" 1997; CNA 2000). Storch (1999) suggested that nurses should work collectively to establish a "moral community" that is supportive of the moral concerns of nurses in the workplace. Varcoe and Rodney (2009) argued for the nursing profession to challenge resource allocation decisions at the societal level and to challenge blind acceptance of the emphasis on such corporate values as efficiency.

ETHICS IN NURSING EDUCATION

As a leader of education for nurses, Florence Nightingale recognized that if the "experiment" of a nursing school was to succeed, the behaviour of students of nursing must be above reproach. She emphasized the importance of character considerations in the selection of students, and each probationer was required to have a certificate of good character on admission. A monthly report on probationers included a "Moral Record" that addressed "punctuality, quietness, trustworthiness, personal neatness, cleanliness, ward management, and order" (Woodham-Smith 1951, 235). Training schools fulfilled their duty if they carefully selected candidates of good character; continued character formation through discipline and emphasis on obedience, loyalty, and respect for authority; and instilled the ideals of nursing as well as taught the etiquette required for successful practice. Nightingale's emphasis on the qualities that denoted "character" and on the ongoing character training of nursing students was reflected in nursing education and nursing ethics for many decades (Crawford 1926; Broadhurst 1917; Parsons 1916; Cadmus 1916; *American Journal of Nursing* [AJN] 1920). In the view of some, Nightingale's focus on forming character was interpreted by subsequent school superintendents in a way that led to indoctrination and an undue emphasis on discipline and etiquette (Brown 1966).

Over time, the education of nursing students with respect to nursing ethics fell under the broad rubric of Professional Adjustments—courses designed to socialize students into professional life and to transmit ethical values, principles, and philosophies (Densford and Everett 1946). The degree to which these courses addressed ethical principles and ethical issues in nursing likely varied widely across nursing schools; much of the course material was devoted to career success, residence life, democratic ideals, and professional organizations. A 1958 CNA course guide on the teaching of Professional Adjustments in nursing programs, a course in which "professional nursing problems" were to be addressed, made reference to the 1953 International Council of Nurses (ICN) Code. The guide suggested the "discussion of professional, moral and personal responsibilities, according to [the] philosophy of individual schools" (CNA 1958, 16). However, this suggested discussion was a very small aspect of the overall course, which focused more on relationships with patients, hospital, physicians, and the profession.

Although not the norm in writings about nursing ethics, some schools did include attention to ethical theories and ethical principles. By the 1950s, Catholic hospitals in Canada had adopted the Moral Code. *Ethical and Religious Directives for Catholic Hospitals* and textbooks designed for nursing students in Catholic hospitals discussed moral philosophy, moral reasoning, and civil and ecclesiastical law, as well as specific ethical issues such as euthanasia and abortion (Godin and O'Hanley 1957; McAllister 1955). In their textbook on ethics for nurses, Densford and Everett (1946), a nursing professor and a philosophy professor at an American university, discussed the "greatest-happiness principle," principles of morality, as well as issues of moral conflict in medicine and nursing.

During the 1970s and 1980s, nurse educators emphasized the importance of nurturing caring attitudes in nursing students (DuGas 1973; Mesolella 1974) and caring as a moral ideal of nursing. In the view of Bevis (1989), this ideal should infuse the curriculum, and Watson (1989), citing the "transformative thinking" of feminist writers, advocated a nursing curriculum model based on human caring and values. A second stream of influence with respect to ethics education came from bioethics, a field that Roy, Williams, and Dickens (1994) described as a much needed "growth industry." They noted that courses that focused on ethics in health care were offered by departments and faculties of philosophy, religious studies, medicine, and nursing. At the graduate level, nursing education drew from a growing literature addressing such topics as the claim to a distinct nursing ethics (Twomey 1989), the integration of nursing theory and nursing ethics (Yeo 1989), the concepts of power and caring in nursing (Falk Rafael 1996), moral distress (Corley 2002) and the development of a theory of nursing ethics (Fry 1989).

FROM CHARACTER TO AN ETHICS OF NURSING

As mentioned previously, in the earliest period of the development of nursing as a profession, the concept of "character" was central to nursing ethics. Character referred to the personal characteristics of the nurse that were required for nursing work, some of which were moral qualities and some of which were social qualities that led to success in nursing practice. Frequently mentioned characteristics included attentiveness to patients, vigilance, honesty, adaptability, patience, obedience and acceptance of authority, loyalty, unselfishness, tactfulness, devotion, and kindness (Broadhurst 1917; Crawford 1926; Dock 1893; Domville 1891; Robb 1900; Scovil 1917; Weeks-Shaw 1900). These qualities were considered to be those of the "good" nurse.

Moral conduct in nursing was considered to be largely dependent on character and the disposition to act in a certain manner. Within this view of morality, ideals were central concepts. The Christian ideal, the service ideal, and humanitarian ideals provided models that defined the sort of person whom the nurse should aspire to be (Potts 1921; Stewart 1918). Inspired by these ideals, the nurse would devote her (because at the time nurses were female) abilities to the individual in her care.

Isabel Hampton Robb (1900), a former superintendent of nurses and principal of the Training School for Nurses at John Hopkins Hospital in Baltimore, wrote in an early text on nursing ethics: "The rules of conduct adapted to the many diverse circumstances attending the nursing of the sick constitute *nursing ethics*" (14–15). She distinguished this from etiquette, which she viewed as important for nurses and as "the code of polite life," but she did not consider etiquette to have the same "moral weight" as ethics. Concerns of etiquette included appropriate dress and deportment, manners and expression, courtesy, and relationships with and respect for others ("A suggested code" 1926). Despite differing definitions, nursing ethics and nursing etiquette continued to be discussed together; the distinctions between the two were often unclear and seemed to have equal importance for some time. However, societal changes, such as the experience of women and nurses in World War I and the growing organization of the profession seemed to be consistent with a shift in focus from etiquette to ethics (Fraser 1925).

In the early 1930s in North America books on ethics for nurses, including the third edition of the book by a nurse educator, Aikens (1935), were published. Aikens' chapters are, in themselves, a testimony to what nurses once were taught and knew. For example, early in this text, she devotes a chapter to the importance of the nurse knowing herself, delving into psychology, self-analysis, and various character traits nurses should assess. From this discussion Aikens moves on to "poise of the soul" (a lecture on self-control and carriage of self), the conduct on duty, old-fashioned virtues (truthfulness, avoiding hasty judgments, loyalty, honesty, integrity), and the rights of others. In 1935 she also wrote about ethics and economy, tact and imagination, ethical phases of night duty, and ethics and everyday routine. In these latter three chapters, Aikens emphasizes the importance of imagination in seeing things from the patient's point of view, and relating to patients and their families and friends in a non-judgmental way. Her attention to ethics and the everyday routine is striking given our recent rediscovery in nursing of the importance of everyday ethics as differentiated from sensational issue-focused health ethics.

PROFESSIONAL OBLIGATIONS

The emphasis on the character of the individual nurse as a basis for nursing ethics gradually declined and the concept of the professional obligation of the nurse began to predominate. These changes in emphasis seemed to emerge from the experience of the growing profession and changes in society rather than from any formal ethical reflection and analysis. One of the notable changes over the time period was thinking about the relationship of nurses to physicians. Around the world, nurses who subscribed to the instruction received by generations of nursing students that they must be obedient to the physician's orders were severely shaken by the 1929 "Somera Case" involving a nurse in the Philippines who prepared an ordered drug that led to the death of a patient.[1] The nurse was sentenced to one year's imprisonment, despite testimony that this nurse "followed the rules which she had been taught" (Grennan 1930). Due to the intervention of the Philippine Nurses' Association, the International Council of Nurses, and women's groups, all of whom believed that the lower and higher court decisions were unjust, the nurse received a conditional pardon and was not imprisoned.

This case was influential in changing the view of the nurse as "subservient" (Grennan 1930). Nurse educators, who later referred to the case, taught students that there must be nurse "judgment on each order so far as her action in carrying it out is concerned, in that she is held responsible for any act which she knows would be dangerous for the patient" (Dietz 1950, 148). The organized profession began, into the 1960s, to emphasize an obligation to carry out doctors' orders "intelligently and loyally" ("Code of ethics" 1965), and nurses were not expected to give "blind obedience" to physicians (Pelley 1964). By the end of the 1960s, nurses in Canada preferred to refer to their obligations to physicians in terms of co-operation and teamwork (Lindabury 1967).

HUMAN RIGHTS AND NURSING ETHICS

The human rights movement of the 1960s led to a focus on patient rights in the 1970s, which had a profound effect on nursing ethics and health care ethics in general. Storch (1977; 1982) traces the rise of a consumer rights movement in the late 1960s and early 1970s, the growing sense of health as a right, and the emergence of the Patient's Bills of Rights in the United States and Canada ("Consumer rights" 1974; Medical Research Council 1978). This theme in health care focused on the legal rights of patients to be informed about treatment or to refuse treatment and was reflected in "contractual models of care" described by nurses (Curtin and Flaherty 1982; Ujhely 1973). The notion that patients were to be full partners on the health team was consistent with conceptual models of nursing that had emerged in the United States during the late 1960s and early 1970s (Orem 1971).

Tied to the notion of patient rights was the notion of patient advocacy, both reflecting the influence of legal concepts on nursing practice and nursing ethics (Jenny 1979). Adoption of the advocate role was viewed by some Canadian nurses as a natural extension of the traditional ethical obligation to protect patients from incompetent or unethical practice (Sklar 1979). Others believed that the role required a non-traditional and more active and assertive stance in view of the growth, rigidity, and complexity of health care bureaucracies ("Prepared to care" 1978). A number of nurses and others doubted that most nurses were in a position to advocate for patients, given their lack of power and employee status in health care settings (Sklar 1979; Storch 1977), and debate about the role and the ability of the nurse to be an advocate continues to the present day (Hewitt 2002; Peters 2008).

BIOTECHNOLOGY AND BIOETHICS

New developments in medical science and technology, from contraception[2] to resuscitation techniques, raised a host of ethical questions surrounding their use in health care. Developments in the transplantation of human organs and genetic manipulation had increased interest in medical ethics in the late 1960s and early 1970s (Ramsey 1970; Siminovitch, 1973), but by the mid-1970s, dramatic dilemmas, such as the Karen-Anne Quinlan case,[3] focused public attention on the ethical complexities of life-prolonging intervention in health care delivery (Branson et al. 1976). Changing social attitudes toward death and dying and reproductive technology fuelled re-examination of abortion and euthanasia. A federal Law Reform Commission was appointed to investigate and recommend legislation on such issues as euthanasia and the definition of death (Baudouin 1977). The 1970s saw the rise of "bioethics," a term that emerged as individuals from a wide variety of academic disciplines and professions began to examine "ethical issues posed by developments in the biological sciences, and their application to medical practice" (Roy, Williams, and Dickens 1994, 4).

New multidisciplinary organizations emerged in Canada that were devoted to the study of ethical issues in health care, and nurses participated actively in these. Philosophers, lawyers, nurses, and physicians began meeting at conferences to discuss bioethical issues (Davis, Hoffmaster, and Shorten 1977), and, subsequently, a number of bioethics institutes were established in various parts of the country (Katz 1980). Two groups, the Canadian Society for Medical Bioethics and the Canadian Society of Bioethics, were created in 1986. The first organization was composed of physicians, and the latter was composed of individuals from a wide range of disciplines and professions, such as nursing, law, theology, and philosophy. These groups joined to form a single organization, the Canadian Bioethics Society, in 1988 (Roy, Williams, and Dickens 1994).

During the 1980s and 1990s, nurses moved beyond consideration of legal obligations to explore moral obligations in two parallel, but different, streams of study. The first stream fell within the realm of moral philosophy, biomedical ethics, and, subsequently, bioethics. Nurses, as part of the larger community of those interested in ethics in health care, examined nursing ethics in terms of moral philosophy and how ethical concepts, principles, and classical ethical theory could guide nurses in their practice (Davis and Aroskar 1978). Beauchamp and Childress' (1983) book, *Principles of Biomedical Ethics,* had a major influence on discussions of nursing ethics (see Chapter 4).

NURSING PHILOSOPHY, FEMINIST ETHICS, AND NURSING ETHICS

The second way in which nurses examined nursing ethics had its roots in philosophic inquiry in nursing (Kikuchi 2003), nursing theory (Thorne 2003), and feminist ethics (Tong 1995; see also Chapter 3). Nurses engaged in a fundamental exploration of nursing values, the nature of the nurse-patient relationship, and the social role of nursing in society to consider what these meant for ethical nursing practice. Central to this inquiry was the concept of "caring," which received increasing attention in the 1970s, 1980s, and 1990s. Nurses had long considered themselves unique among health professionals in that their traditional focus was the "whole person" as an individual, rather than a limited interest in the disease, condition, or physical status (Murray 1970; Mussallem 1968). The word "care," as in nursing care, had always been used by nurses, but during the 1970s, this word seemed to take on special meaning. Although not clearly defined by all who used the word, caring seemed to signify a humanistic philosophy of nursing, and the term conveyed a concern for the individual person, commitment to the welfare of the patient, empathy and sensitivity to the patient's emotional state, human compassion, and a respect for human worth and dignity. As expressed by various nurses, caring was a capacity (Poole 1973), an attitude (Christo 1979), a quality in nursing (Flaherty 1977), a natural human quality (Roach 1976), and a "basic way of being in the world" (Benner and Wrubel 1989, xi).

Feminist scholarship from a variety of disciplines, such as Gilligan's (1982) work on women's moral development and Noddings' (1984) work on caring and the ethic of care, seemed to resonate with nurses (Crigger 2001; Fry 1989; Peter and Morgan 2001). Gilligan's empirical work found that women, when faced with a moral dilemma, tend to focus on relationships and the details of the situation and to seek solutions that maintain relationships. Noddings' ethic of care rejects the abstract rules of traditional ethics and requires an opening up to another person and acting on his or her behalf. This perspective seems to have influenced subsequent scholarship on relational ethics in nursing (MacDonald 2006) and virtue ethics (Begley 2006; see Chapters 4 and 5).

In the past 20 years, scholarship in nursing ethics has grown. Nurses have continued to explore nursing ethics through theory development (Corley 2002; Fry 1989; Peter and Morgan 2001), conceptual and moral analysis of phenomena (Carnevale 2009), and empirical study (Crigger 2001; Crowley 1989; Ellenchild Pinch and Spielman 1996). In reviewing the past two decades, Tschudin (2010) identified several themes in nursing ethics from her perspective as founding editor of the international journal *Nursing Ethics*. Over the past 18 years, Tschudin has noted an increasingly global approach to nursing ethics, a growth in empirical research, and a shift from principles to care ethics.

In the past 10 years, she has noted a move toward virtue ethics as a preferred theory and a better understanding of and an appreciation of ethics in practice.

ORGANIZATION OF THE PROFESSION AND CODES OF ETHICS

Within several decades of the development of nursing schools, leaders emerged who began to organize the profession. The first professional association, the British Nurses' Association, was established in 1888; an American Society of Superintendents of Training Schools, composed of Canadian and American superintendents, was formed in 1893; and the International Council of Nurses (ICN) was formed in 1899 (Mussallem 1992). From the earliest days of the organized profession, calls were made for the development of a code of ethics, but leaders recognized that such an undertaking would take time and would require the building of a consensus among nurses (Robb 1898).

Members of the Canadian National Association of Trained Nurses (CNATN) and the American Nurses Association (ANA) expressed interest in a code during the 1920s (Catton 1921; "A suggested code" 1926). ANA's draft showed some signs of a shift in the thinking about the ethical aspects of nursing, including the nurse-physician relationship and the obligations of the nurse. In this "suggested code," ideas of mutual respect, interdependence, and co-worker characterized the relationship. There were some indications that "vaunted professional etiquette" was out of date (Fraser 1925), as was traditional respect for authority and discipline. A Tentative Code (1940), drafted by a committee of ANA began with the statement that "Nursing is a profession" (1977). This draft document contained a requirement to respect the religious beliefs of others, but for the most part was similar in tone to traditional views of nursing ethics in its references to "high ideals" and "honesty, understanding, gentleness, and patience" (978).

Similarly, a draft Code of Ethics prepared by a committee of the Canadian Nurses Association in 1954 identified confidentiality, sympathy, understanding, and "the best in knowledge and skill" as obligations of the nurse to the patient. This draft code was not adopted, however, as the Canadian Nurses Association decided to adopt the ICN Code (CNA 1955).

During the 1950s, both the ANA ("What's in our code" 1952) and the ICN ("The ICN in Brazil" 1953) adopted codes of ethics that were almost identical and that departed considerably from earlier attempts to establish a code. First, these codes reflected the societal emphasis on human rights in that the preamble to these codes included a statement that nursing service was to be "unrestricted by consideration of nationality, race, creed, colour, politics or social status" (Tate 1977). Commentary on the code in the *American Journal of Nursing* made explicit reference to the Universal Declaration of Human Rights and the "intrinsic dignity and value of each human being" ("What's in our code" 1952, 1248). The one significant change in the 1965 ICN Code of Ethics was the inclusion of the Red Cross Principles that stressed impartiality and universality ("Code of ethics" 1965).

For the most part, nursing codes and their revisions during the 1950s and 1960s did not expand on the rights of patients and continued to highlight relationships with physicians, including prohibitions not to treat (except in emergencies), to sustain confidence in the physician, to "carry out the physician's orders intelligently and loyally, and to refuse to participate in unethical procedures" (CNA 1954; "Code of ethics" 1965). Pellegrino (1964), in a review of codes of ethics for physicians and for nurses in the United States, identified that these codes still contained a number of statements of etiquette and noted that "their violation may impair the dignity of the some of the goals of professions, but they do not by their nature involve usurpation of the human rights of the patient," and that the "ethical core" of codes related to the "rights of the patient as a person" (41).

Nursing organizations have adopted or revised codes of ethics since the 1970s, and these revisions changed codes considerably from those of the 1960s. The 1973 ICN Code included an explicit statement on the primacy of the nurse's responsibility to the patient—the obligation to respect the "beliefs, values, and customs of the individual"—and deleted specific reference to physicians. To all health workers, the nurse owed co-operative effort. The one remaining reference to personal conduct now carried the modifier, "when acting in a professional capacity." According to Bergman (1973), nursing students were key in arguing for changes to the code and rejecting any statement that suggested the subservience of nursing to medicine or outdated customs.[4]

For many years, both the Canadian Nurses Association and many of the provincial nursing organizations responsible for nursing legislation in Canada had adopted the ICN Code of Ethics as their guide to ethical conduct, including the revision of 1973. As the regulatory role of nursing organizations came to the fore, some provincial regulatory bodies in Canada developed their own standards of ethical conduct. The CNA adopted its own code in 1981, one that generated considerable controversy as it seemed to suggest to some nurses that participation in strikes was unethical. The subsequent CNA (1985) Code of Ethics for Nursing identified an obligation for nurses to take steps to protect patients in any job action (CNA 1985), an obligation that remained in subsequent revisions of the CNA Code (CNA 2002; 2008).

In addition to new and revised codes of ethics, the organized profession addressed specific ethical issues in policy statements and other publications. For example, the CNA, in a series of documents titled *Ethics in Practice*, addressed issues such as working with limited resources (CNA 2000), advance directives (1998), and quality practice environments (2010). These guides acknowledged the reality of moral constraint, moral distress, and moral uncertainty for nurses who worked in a health care system that often functions with government cost constraints, scarce resources, and staff shortages.

Summary

In summary, the emphasis in the early years of nursing was on character, ideals, and etiquette as the basis for ethical conduct. The emphasis on etiquette served to prepare graduates to go into independent private duty, away from the influence of the military discipline of the training school, where they would have to succeed in practice, not only in terms of their professional knowledge and skill, but also in terms of their relationships with patients, family members, and physicians. Gradually, the traditional ideals of self-sacrifice and service were challenged as private duty nurses attempted to improve their income and working hours. Access to affordable nursing services became an issue, and solutions emerged to the dilemma of providing affordable nursing services while offering adequate income to nurses.

The organized profession was still in its infancy, focusing on such issues as building nursing organizations, achieving registration, developing public health nursing, improving nursing education, and instituting a shorter working day. Although organizations recognized the importance of nursing ethics, early calls for, or drafts of, a code of ethics did not result in definitive statements on ethics from the nursing profession until the 1950s, and these moved away from a focus on the character of the nurse to a focus on the nurse's obligations and responsibilities as a professional. Gradually, the focus changed from who the nurse should *be* to what the nurse should *do*. Human rights and the dignity of the person began to receive emphasis, as well as a more frequent focus on the primacy of obligations to the patient. Although there was continued attention to relationships with physicians, obligations such as carrying out physicians' orders and not engaging in medical treatment were situational rather than blanket obligations. The early emphasis on etiquette, respect for authority, obedience to physicians' orders, and loyalty, all but disappeared by the end of the 1960s, a decade that was marked by considerable distrust of public institutions and social protest. The gradually developing opinion within the profession was that nurses were independent professionals who were required to use their judgment.

In conclusion, it is clear that since the beginning of "modern" nursing in the 1800s, nurses have believed that their role in society brought with it specific moral obligations. The emphasis shifted over time from the obligations of a nurse to physicians and those in authority to the nurse's obligations to the patient. The degree to which nursing, as a profession, has attended to ethical questions has varied from one time period to another. This level of attention has been influenced by developments in health care and by the broader concerns of society. What has been consistent over time is a sense of *ethical distress* related to the conditions under which nurses have worked, ranging from expectations of long hours for private duty nurses in the 1920s to the lack of an authoritative nursing voice in hospital bureaucracies and staff shortages in the 1990s. The last century and a half has culminated in a period of intense examination of ethics in nursing, a growing understanding of the moral dimension of nursing, and the beginnings of theory development in nursing ethics.

For Reflection

1. Do any of the issues in nursing ethics from the past resonate with your current experience in nursing?

2. How has your perception of nursing ethics changed during your career?

3. Has your view of nursing obligations been influenced by your work environment? By social issues and developments? By your professional organization?

Endnotes

1. The "Somera Case," as it was known, was reported in the *International Nursing Review* in 1930 following the nurse's conditional pardon and was referred to in subsequent nursing texts to underscore that nurses were as equally responsible as doctors and were not subservient to them.

2. The discovery of safe and reliable contraceptives also changed the role of women in society and impacted nurses and nursing.

3. Karen Ann Quinlan was a 21 year old who for reasons unknown ceased breathing in April 1975. She was hospitalized and placed on a respirator but remained comatose. Her family filed a petition to authorize discontinuation of extraordinary medical procedures. The New Jersey Superior Court ruled against the request but then reversed their decision in 1976 contingent upon an ethics committee concluding that there was no hope for her recovery. Karen was then withdrawn from the respirator but she continued to breath and was not declared dead until June 1986, after more than 10 years in a nursing home (Branson et al. 1976; Pence 1995).

4. According to Johnstone (1989), the nursing students who formally presented objections to "subservient" statements to both their national nursing association representatives and the ICN were Canadian, and, as a result, a clause in the code was deleted. There is continuing interest in ethics by nursing students—in the United States, the National Student Nurses' Association, Inc. (2001) has adopted a Code of Academic and Clinical Conduct.

References

A suggested code. Code of ethics presented for the consideration of the American Nurses' Association. 1926. *American Journal of Nursing, 26* (8), 597–601.

A tentative code. For the nursing profession. 1940. *American Journal of Nursing, 40* (9), 977–980.

Aikens, C.A. 1935. *Studies in ethics for nurses.* Philadelphia: W.B. Saunders Company.

American Journal of Nursing (AJN). 1920. The study of ethics in our schools of nursing. Paper presented at annual meeting of the CNA, 1919. *American Journal of Nursing, 20* (12), 988–989.

Ashley, J. 1976. *Hospitals, paternalism, and the role of the nurse.* New York: Teachers College Press.

Bates, C. Dodd, D., and Rousseau, N. (Eds.). 2005. *On all frontiers: Four centuries of Canadian nursing.* Ottawa: University of Ottawa Press.

Baumann, A., O'Brien-Pallas, L., Armstrong-Stassen, M., Blythe, J., Bourbonnais, R., Cameron, S., Irvine Doran, D., Kerr, M., McGillis Hall, L., Vezina, M., Butt, M., and Ryan, L. 2001. *Commitment and care: The benefits of a healthy workplace for nurses, their patients and the system.* Ottawa: Canadian Health Service Research Foundation.

Baudouin, J. 1977. Protection of life. *Canadian Nurse, 73* (6), 4.

BC nurses vote to strike. 1968. News. *Canadian Nurse, 64* (7), 7.

Beauchamp, T.L. and Childress, J.F. 1983. *Principles of biomedical ethics.* New York: Oxford University Press.

Begley, A.M. 2006. Facilitating the development of moral insight in practice: Teaching ethics and teaching virtue. *Nursing Philosophy, 7,* 257–265.

Benner, P. and Wrubel, J. 1989. *The primacy of caring. Stress and coping in health and illness.* Don Mills: Addison-Wesley.

Bergman, R. 1973. Ethics—concepts and practice. *International Nursing Review, 20* (5), 140–141, 152.

Bevis, E.O. 1989. The curriculum consequences: Aftermath of revolution. *Curriculum revolution: Reconceptualizing nursing education.* New York: National League for Nursing.

Branson, R., Casebeer, K., Levine, M.D., Oden, T.C., Ramsey, P., and Capron, A.M. 1976. The Quinlan decision: Five commentaries. *Hastings Center Report, 6* (1), 8–19.

Broadhurst, J. 1917. Ethics of nursing. *American Journal of Nursing, 17* (9), 792–797.

Brown, E.L. 1966. Nursing and patient care. In F. Davis (Ed.), *The nursing profession: Five sociological essays* (pp. 176–203). New York: Wiley.

Byers, W.G.M. 1922. The ideals of nursing. *Canadian Nurse, 18* (2), 85–90.

Cadmus, N.E. 1916. Ethics. *American Journal of Nursing, 16* (5), 411–416.

Canadian Association of Nursing Education. 1924. *Proceedings of the convention*, June 26–28, Hamilton, ON.

Canadian Nurses Association. 1954. *Report—Committee to draft a code of ethics.* Ottawa: Canadian Nurses Association.

Canadian Nurses Association. 1955. *Minutes of the Executive Committee meeting,* February 17–19. Ottawa: Canadian Nurses Association.

Canadian Nurses Association. 1958. Report of the special committee to study the teaching of professional adjustments in the basic programmes. Ottawa: Canadian Nurses Association.

Canadian Nurses Association. 1968. *The leaf and the lamp.* Ottawa: Canadian Nurses Association.

Canadian Nurses Association. 1971. *Countdown. Canadian nursing statistics.* Ottawa: Canadian Nurses Association.

Canadian Nurses Association. 1985. *Code of ethics for nursing.* Ottawa: Canadian Nurses Association.

Canadian Nurses Association. 1998. *Advance directives: The nurse's role.* Ottawa: Canadian Nurses Association.

Canadian Nurses Association. 2000. *Working with limited resources: Nurses' moral constraints.* Ottawa: Canadian Nurses Association.

Canadian Nurses Association. 2002. *Code of ethics for registered nurses.* Ottawa: Canadian Nurses Association.

Canadian Nurses Association. 2008. *Code of ethics for registered nurses.* Ottawa: Canadian Nurses Association.

Canadian Nurses Association. 2010. *Ethics, relationships and quality practice environments.* Ottawa: Canadian Nurses Association.

Carnevale, F.A. 2009. A conceptual and moral analysis of suffering. *Nursing Ethics, 16* (2), 173–183.

Catton, M.A. 1921. The question of a "Code of nursing ethics and etiquette" for Canadian nurses. *Canadian Nurse, 17* (9), 553–555.

Cho, H.S.M. 1997. *A Korean dream: Mo Im Kim's influence on Korean nursing, health care, and community.* Seoul: Hyunmun Publishing Co.

Christo, S. 1979. Too tired to care? Input. *Canadian Nurse, 75* (11), 6–7.

Code of ethics as applied to nursing. 1965. *International Nursing Review, 12* (6), 38–39.

Consumer rights in health care. 1974. *Canadian Consumer, 4* (2), 1–3.

Corley, M. 2002. Nurse moral distress: A proposed theory and research agenda. *Nursing Ethics, 9* (6), 636–650.

Crawford, B. 1926. How and what to teach in nursing ethics. *American Journal of Nursing, 26* (3), 211–215.

Crigger, N. 2001. Antecedents to engrossment in Noddings' theory of care. *Journal of Advanced Nursing, 35* (4), 616–623.

Crowley, M. 1989. Feminist pedagogy: Nurturing the ethical ideal. *Advances in Nursing Science, 11* (3), 53–61.

Curtin, L. and Flaherty, M.J. 1982. *Nursing ethics. Theories and pragmatics.* Bowie, MD: Prentice Hall.

Davis, A.J. and Aroskar, M.A. 1978. *Ethical dilemmas and nursing practice.* New York: Appleton-Century-Crofts.

Davis, J.W., Hoffmaster, B., and Shorten, S. (Eds.). 1977. *Contemporary issues in biomedical ethics.* Clifton, NJ: Humana Press.

Densford, K.J. and Everett, M.S. 1946. *Ethics for modern nurses. Professional adjustments I.* Philadelphia: Saunders.

Dietz, L.D. 1950. *Professional adjustments II* (3rd ed.). Philadelphia: Davis.

Dock, L.L. 1893. The relation of training schools to hospitals. In L. Petry (Ed.), *Nursing of the sick* (1949) (pp. 12–24). New York: McGraw-Hill.

Domville, E.J. 1891. *A manual for hospital nurses and others engaged in attending on the sick* (7th ed.). London: Churchill.

Donahue, M.P. 1985. *Nursing: The finest art.* Toronto: C.V. Mosby Company.

DuGas, B.W. 1973. Preparing tomorrow's practitioners. Innovations: A national view. In *National Conference on Nurses for Community Service,* November 13–16, 1973, Ottawa, (pp. 65–70). Ottawa: Canadian Nurses Association.

Ellenchild Pinch, W.J. and Spielman, M.L. 1996. Ethics in the neonatal intensive care unit: Parental perceptions at four years postdischarge. *Advances in Nursing Science, 19* (1), 72–85.

Ellis, B.L. 1927. Nursing education. *Canadian Nurse, 23* (9), 471–474.

Fairley, G.E. 1923. Report of the National Conference on Education and Citizenship. *Canadian Nurse, 19* (7), 414–421.

Falk Rafael, A.R. 1996. Power and caring: A dialectic in nursing. *Advances in Nursing Science, 19* (1), 3–17.

Field, C.C. 1923. Graduation address. Children's Hospital of Winnipeg, 1921. *Canadian Nurse, 19* (1), 14–17.

Flaherty, M.J. 1977. Accountability in health care practice: Ethical implications for nurses. In J. W. Davis, B. Hoffmaster, and S. Shorten (Eds.), *Contemporary issues in biomedical ethics* (pp. 267–276). Clifton, NJ: Humana Press.

Fowler, M.D. 2009. Religion, bioethics and nursing practice. *Nursing Ethics, 16* (4), 393–405.

Fraser, E.M. 1925. Nursing service in hospital wards. *Canadian Nurse, 21* (12), 639–641.

Fry, S.T. 1989. Toward a theory of nursing ethics. *Advances in Nursing Science, 11* (4), 9–22.

Gilligan, C. 1982. *In a different voice. Psychological theory and women's development.* Cambridge, MA: Harvard University Press.

Godin, E. and O'Hanley, J.P.E. 1957. *Hospital ethics. A commentary on the moral code of Catholic hospitals.* Bathurst, NB: Hotel Dieu Hospital.

Goodnow, M. 1942. *Nursing history in brief.* Philadephia: W.B. Saunders Company.

Grennan, E.M. 1930. The Somera case. *International Nursing Review, 5* (4), 325–333.

Growe, S.J. 1991. *Who cares? The crisis in Canadian nursing.* Toronto: McClelland & Stewart.

Hayter, J. 1966. What does "caring" really mean? *Canadian Nurse, 62* (10), 29–32.

Health Disciplines Act proclaimed in Ontario. 1975. News. *Canadian Nurse, 71* (9), 12.

Hewitt, J. 2002. A critical review of the arguments debating the role of the nurse advocate. *Journal of Advanced Nursing, 37* (5), 439–445.

Hudson, B. 1970. Timely and revealing. Letters. *Canadian Nurse, 66* (10), 4.

Jenny, J. 1979. Patient advocacy—Another role for nursing? *International Nursing Review, 26* (6), 176–181.

Katz, S. 1980. Life and death ethics. *Maclean's,* March 17, 45–47.

Kikuchi, J.F. (2003). Thinking philosophically in nursing. In J.C. Kerr and M.J. Wood (Eds.), *Canadian nursing. Issues and perspectives* (pp. 103–115). Toronto: Mosby.

Lamb, M. 1981. Nursing ethics in Canada: Two decades. Unpublished Master of Nursing thesis. University of Alberta, Edmonton.

Lanara, V.A. 1981. *Heroism as a nursing value. A philosophical perspective.* Athens, Greece: Sisterhood Evniki.

Lindabury, V.A. 1967. Editorial. *Canadian Nurse, 63* (9), 3.

Lindabury, V.A. 1968. Editorial. Withdrawal of service—A dilemma for nursing. *Canadian Nurse, 64* (7), 29.

Lovell, V. 1981. *"I care that VGH nurses care!" A case study and sociological analysis of nursing's influence on the health care system.* Vancouver: In Touch Publications.

MacDonald, H. 2006. Relational ethics and advocacy in nursing: literature review. *Journal of Advanced Nursing, 57* (2), 119–126.

MacLellan, B. 1976. Matthew my son: Prepared childbirth at the general. *Canadian Nurse, 72* (3), 38–39.

MacLeod, A.I. 1966. President's address. CNA 33rd general meeting. *Canadian Nurse, 63* (8), 19–22.

Major changes at Vancouver General Hospital. 1978. *RNABC News, 10* (7), 3–5.

Managers must help nurses beat moral distress. 1997. *Canadian Nursing Management, 115* (December), 3.

Marcus, C. 1975. Out of the mouths of patients. *Canadian Nurse, 62* (11), 16–17.

McAllister, J.B. 1955. *Ethics. With special application to the medical and nursing professions.* (2nd ed.). Philadelphia: Saunders.

McMurtry, D. 1968. A life without dignity. *Canadian Nurse, 64* (8), 51–52.

Medical Research Council. 1978. *Ethical considerations in research involving human subjects.* Report No. 6. Ottawa: Supply & Services Canada.

Mesolella, D.W. 1974. Caring begins in the teacher–student relationship. *Canadian Nurse, 70* (12), 15–16.

Murray, V.V. 1970. *Nursing in Ontario. A study for the Committee on the Healing Arts.* Toronto: Queen's Printer.

Mussallem, H.K. 1968. The changing role of the nurse. *Canadian Nurse, 64* (11), 35–37.

Mussallem, H.K. 1992. Professional nurses' associations. In A.J. Baumgart and J. Larsen (Eds.), *Canadian nursing faces the future* (2nd ed.; pp. 495–517). Toronto: Mosby.

Noddings, N. 1984. *Caring: A feminine approach to ethics and moral education.* Los Angeles: University of California Press.

Nurses fight for better care. 1978. *RNABC News, 10* (4), 3–7.

Nutting, M.A. and Dock, L. 1974. (Reprint). *A history of nursing,* Vol. 1. Buffalo, NY: The Heritage Press.

Orem, D. 1971. *Nursing: Concepts of practice.* Scarborough: McGraw-Hill.

Parsons, S.E. 1916. Ethics—the probationer. *American Journal of Nursing, 16* (10), 975–980.

Pellegrino, E.D. 1964. Ethical considerations in the practice of medicine and nursing. In American Nurses Association and American Medical Association (Eds.), *Medical and nursing practice in a changing world*, Proceedings of the First National Conference on Nurses and Physicians (pp. 39–48). Williamsburg, VA: American Medical Association.

Pelley, T. 1964. *Nursing. Its history, trends, philosophy, ethics and ethos.* Philadelphia: Saunders.

Pence, G.E. 1995. *Classic cases in medical ethics* (2nd ed.). New York: McGraw Hill Inc.

Peter, E. and Morgan, K.P. 2001. Explorations of a trust approach for nursing ethics. *Nursing Inquiry, 8,* 3–10.

Peters, E. 2008. Seeing our way through the responsibility-vs-endeavour conundrum: The Code of Ethics as both product and process. Guest Column. *Nursing Leadership, 21* (2), 28–31.

Poole, P.E. 1973. Nurse, please show me that you care. *Canadian Nurse, 66* (2), 25–27.

Potts, F.J. 1921. Nursing ethics. *Canadian Nurse, 17*(4), 222–224.

"Prepared to care," Alberta nurses kick off province-wide campaign. (1978). News. *Canadian Nurse, 74*(7), 26.

Quality assurance off to a flying start. (1977). News. *Canadian Nurse, 73* (8), 12.

Ramsey, P. 1970. *The patient as person*. New Haven: Yale.

Roach, M.S. 1976. A framework for the nursing curriculum at St. Francis Xavier University. *Nursing Papers, 7* (4), 23–27.

Robb, I.H. 1898. The spirit of the associated alumnae. In L. Flanagan (Ed.). 1976. *One strong voice. The story of the ANA*. (pp. 301–331). Kansas City: American Nurses Association.

Robb, I.H. 1900. *Nursing ethics. For hospitals and private use*. Cleveland: E.G. Koeckert.

Ross-Kerr, J.C. 1996. Nursing in Canada from 1760 to the present: The transition to modern nursing. In J.C. Ross-Kerr and J. MacPhail (Eds.), *Canadian nursing: Issues and perspectives* (3rd ed.; pp. 11–22). Toronto: Mosby.

Ross-Kerr, J.C. 2003. The origins of nursing education in Canada: The emergence and growth of diploma programs. In J.C. Ross-Kerr and M.J. Wood (Eds.), *Canadian nursing. Issues and perspectives* (4th ed.; pp. 330–348). Toronto: Mosby.

Roy, D.J., Williams, J.R., and Dickens, B.M. 1994. *Bioethics in Canada*. Scarborough: Prentice Hall.

Scovil, E.R. 1917. The ethics of nursing. *Canadian Nurse, 13* (8), 462–472.

Sibbald, B. 1997. A right to be heard. *Canadian Nurse, 93* (10), 22–30.

Siminovitch, L. 1973. Genetic manipulation: Now is the time to consider. *Canadian Nurse, 69* (11), 30–34.

Sinclair, C.M. n.d. The report of the Manitoba Pediatric Cardiac Surgery Inquest: An inquiry into twelve deaths at the Winnipeg Health Sciences Centre in 1994. Winnipeg: Provincial Court of Manitoba.

Sklar, C. 1979. Patient's advocate—a new role for the nurse? *Canadian Nurse, 75* (6), 39–41.

Stewart, I.M. 1918. How can we help to improve our teaching in nursing schools? *Canadian Nurse, 14* (11), 1393–1399.

Storch, J.L. 1977. *Consumer rights and nursing*. Edmonton: Masters in Nursing Research Trust Fund, University of Alberta.

Storch, J. 1982. *Patients' right: Ethical and legal issues in health care and nursing*. Toronto: McGraw-Hill Ryerson.

Storch, J. 1999. Ethical dimensions of leadership. In J.M. Hibberd and D.L. Smith (Eds.), *Nursing management in Canada* (2nd ed.; pp. 351–367). Toronto: Saunders.

Tate, B.L. 1977. *The nurse's dilemma. Ethical considerations in nursing practice*. Geneva: ICN.

The I.C.N. in Brazil. 1953. *Canadian Nurse, 49* (9), 687.

Thorne, S. 2003. Theoretical issues in nursing. In J.C. Kerr and M.J. Wood (Eds.), *Canadian nursing. Issues and perspectives* (pp. 116–134). Toronto: Mosby.

Three Sudbury nurses win hospital settlement after 13 months' fight. 1971. News. *Canadian Nurse, 67* (9), 14, 16.

Tong, R. 1995. What's distinctive about feminist bioethics? In F. Baylis, J. Downie, B. Freedman, B. Hoffmaster, and S. Sherwin (Eds.), *Health care ethics in Canada* (pp. 22–30). Toronto: Harcourt Brace.

Tschudin, V. 2010. Nursing ethics: The last decade. *Nursing Ethics, 17* (1), 127–131.

Twomey, J.G. 1989. Analysis of the claim to distinct nursing ethics: Normative and non-normative approaches. *Advances in Nursing Science, 11* (3), 25–32.

Ujhely, G.B. 1973. The patient as equal partner. *Canadian Nurse, 69* (6), 21–23.

Varcoe, C. and Rodney, P. 2009. Constrained agency: The social structure of nurses' work. In B.S. Bolaria and H. Dickinson (Eds.), *Health, illness and health care in Canada* (4th ed.; pp. 122–151). Toronto: Nelson Education.

Wahn, E.V. 1979. The dilemma of the disobedient nurse. *Health Care in Canada, 21* (2), 43–44, 46.

Watson, J. 1989. Transformative thinking and a caring curriculum. In E.O. Bevis and J. Watson (Eds.), *Toward a caring curriculum: A new pedagogy for nursing.* (pp. 51–60). New York: National League for Nursing.

Weir, G.M. 1932. *Survey of nursing education in Canada.* Toronto: University of Toronto Press.

Weeks-Shaw, C.S. 1900. *Text-book of nursing. For the use of training schools, families, and private students* (2nd ed.). New York: Appleton and Company.

What's in our code? 1952. *American Journal of Nursing, 52* (10), 1246–1247.

Woodham-Smith, C. 1951. *Florence Nightingale.* Toronto: McGraw-Hill.

Yeo, M. 1989. Integration of nursing theory and nursing ethics. *Advances in Nursing Science, 11* (3), 33–42.

CHAPTER 3

Philosophical Contributions to Nursing Ethics

Barbara Pesut and Joy L. Johnson

Our leaders of tomorrow must be able to draw upon every tool available to them to support ethical nursing practice; one such tool is philosophy.

Philosophy has been described as "everybody's business." As humans it is in our nature to try to make sense of our world, and to ask questions about the meaning of life and our existence. When we wonder about what it means to be a good person, whether we have free will, or how language is possible, we are engaged in philosophical thinking. These types of questions have generated wonder for thousands of years.

To conduct a philosophic study, one relies on one's natural capacities to think and reason about the world in which we live. This capacity is captured in Plato's writings about Socrates who philosophized by simply asking questions of the citizens of Athens. In answering Socrates' questions the citizens were led to logical and justified conclusions by considering their own experiences in the world. The practice of philosophizing involves exploring ideas and thinking through possible arguments for and against different positions. **Argumentation** is a key instrument of philosophy, and involves providing logical reasons or evidence in support or denial of a particular position.

In drawing distinctions between philosophy and other realms of inquiry, Nagel (1987) maintains that the main concern of philosophy is to question and understand common ideas that many of us take for granted. He illustrates the distinction between philosophy and other forms of inquiry by pointing out that while an historian might investigate past events, a philosopher would ask, "What is time?" Similarly, while anyone might ask a question, such as whether it is wrong to conceal the truth about a diagnosis from a patient, a philosopher would consider what makes an action right or wrong. The aim of this type of inquiry is to push our thinking and understanding of a matter, and to deepen our insights. Philosophy is also a frontier in that the questions that are considered by philosophers are seemingly limitless. The more we know, the more we are inspired to ponder what remains unknown.

Nursing philosophy is just beginning to receive the attention it deserves. In this chapter we consider the ways in which philosophy can contribute to the evolution of nursing ethics. We begin by examining what we mean by nursing philosophy, the types of philosophical questions that are of concern to nurses and the relationship of nursing theories to nursing philosophy. We briefly examine how the world of philosophy has contributed to the realm of nursing ethics. We then consider the boundaries between nursing science and nursing ethics and reflect on the challenge of finding a common nursing ontology and ethic. The chapter closes with an examination of some of the unresolved philosophical issues facing the field of nursing ethics—issues that other authors in this book will take up in various ways. All nurses can benefit from becoming more strongly grounded in philosophy and learning ways to use philosophic approaches to deepen their understanding of the nurse's world. Our leaders of tomorrow must be able to draw upon every tool available to them to support ethical nursing practice; one such tool is philosophy.

WHAT IS NURSING PHILOSOPHY?

Many nurses go about their work without questioning why it is that they do the things they do. Nursing is a practice profession, and so it is appropriate that we focus on accomplishing tasks and completing nursing actions. While we would not accomplish our goals in nursing practice if we were forever questioning the very essence of nursing, it is highly appropriate that we, on occasion, step back and consider philosophic questions related to nursing. Just like the questions that philosophy addresses, nursing philosophy is directed toward considering "big" questions such as, "What is the goal of nursing?" "What ought nurses to do when faced with difficult choices?" And, "How can we distinguish nursing from other professional practices such as medicine?" Other professions such as medicine and law similarly struggle to understand the nature of their work and objectives they should legitimately direct their efforts toward.

Nursing has an impressive philosophic legacy. Kikuchi and Simmons (1994) pointed out, "If the study of philosophical thought in nursing were to be undertaken, there would be no shortage of materials. . . . Nurses have reflected upon, and continue to reflect upon, the nature of their work and they continue to put their thoughts in writing, as a 'philosophy of nursing'" (1). Kikuchi and Simmons deliberately placed the term "philosophy of nursing" in quotation marks because until lately much of nursing scholarship, although philosophic in nature, was not recognized as philosophic writing. An excellent case in point can be found in the writings of Florence Nightingale, a well-known scholar of the 1800s. In writings such as *Notes on Nursing: What It Is and What It Is Not* and *Sick Nursing and Health Nursing*, Nightingale applied logic and reasoning to consider the nature of nursing. She contrasted nursing to other forms of work, and used her own experience to reason through possible solutions to problems such as determining "what nursing is, and what it is not." (See also Chapter 2 in this book.)

Beginning in the 1970s, several scholars, who became known as the "nursing theorists," developed conceptual frameworks for nursing practice. Numbered among these works are those by Dorothea Orem (1991), Martha Rogers (1970), and Rosemarie Parse (1981). The conceptualizations of nursing proposed in their works were developed to direct nursing practice and research by addressing questions such as "What is it good to do and seek in nursing?" Although some might reject the idea of classifying these works as philosophic, they address questions that are philosophic in nature and appear to employ the methods of philosophy (i.e., reason and logic). As nursing theorists sought to define what have been referred to as the meta-domains of nursing (i.e., person, health, and the environment) they were asking the same questions that philosophers have asked for centuries. **Philosophies of nursing** are aimed at systematically articulating through the methods of philosophy the nature, scope, and object of nursing. The term **"philosophy in nursing"** or **"nursing philosophy"** connotes the activity of philosophizing that focuses on questions relevant to nursing, of which philosophies of nursing are one aspect.

Since the 1990s, nursing scholars have more fully embraced the role and contribution of philosophy. Conferences have been held and books and journal articles have been published that address nursing philosophic issues. Centres for the study of nursing philosophy have been established, and a journal entitled *Nursing Philosophy* has been launched. These developments attest to the emergent field of nursing philosophy. With increasing frequency nurses are recognizing that science is unable to answer many of the important questions facing nursing, and are consequently turning to philosophy.

Nurses, whose works are grounded in Western philosophic traditions, have tended to focus their philosophic inquiries on three types of questions: *ontological* (concerning what is), *epistemological* (concerning how we know), and *moral* (concerning what we ought to do and seek). Examples of ontological questions are, "What is the nature of nursing?" and "What is the essence of the nurse–patient relationship?" Examples of epistemological questions are, "What is the nature of nursing knowledge?" "What is the type of evidence nurses need in their practice?" and "How can scientific findings be applied in particular situations?" Finally, examples of moral questions that nurses have addressed include, "What are nurses' obligations in relation to end-of-life decision-making?" "How should a nurse deal with matters of privacy and privilege?" and "How ought nurses ensure that their care is directed toward the needs of patients and not to the institutional system for which they work?" Ontological, epistemological, and moral questions in nursing are interconnected and reciprocal. For example, to understand what nursing knowledge is we must first understand what nursing is. If we are to grapple with what a good action is for a nurse we must understand the nature of nursing as well as the nature of goodness. Likewise, ontological questions about the nature of nursing are influenced by what we believe to be good nursing and the knowledge that is required to nurse well. As discussed earlier, philosophizing helps us to probe our common conceptions of nursing and to deepen our understanding of the problems facing nursing.

Much of the philosophical writing in nursing has been aimed at considering how the works of philosophers such as Kant, Merleau-Ponty, and Foucault are relevant to nursing. These questions can be thought of as *second order questions*, and while important, solely focusing on this type of question has its limitations. Knowledge of the *first order* is knowledge about reality; knowledge of the second order is knowledge about knowledge itself. It follows that in philosophy, first order questions are metaphysical or ontological in nature. These are questions about that which is or happens, or about what we should do or seek, such as, 'What is the nature of nursing?' 'What is the essence of the nurse-patient relationship?' and "What are the essential values that underlie nursing practice?" In contrast, second order questions are about our first order knowledge. Second order philosophic knowledge allows philosophy to be critical of its own concepts and language and to examine its own knowledge. Examples of second order questions include "What are the issues and controversies inherent in the ways that the art of nursing has been conceptualized by nursing scholars?" and "What are the limitations inherent in Parse's (1981) conception of nursing?" In modern philosophy we have seen an emphasis on second order questions. Thus, we see more philosophers concerning themselves with the limitations of our knowledge of the world than with knowledge of the world itself. *We have spent considerable time accounting for the nature of nursing knowledge and relatively little effort considering the nature of nursing as nursing.* This is concerning because an exclusive focus on questions about how or what we know is ultimately nihilistic in that it keeps a discipline from considering substantive questions necessary to push the frontiers of knowledge forward.

We need to philosophize about nursing. If we do not engage in this work, the nature of nursing work will be determined by whatever forces are the strongest, be they political, administrative, or the opinions of other health professionals. If we are unable to determine what nursing is, we will be unable to defend its borders, or the interventions that we believe are required to achieve nursing goals. Philosophy also holds implications for our ethical actions as nurses. If nurses cannot articulate what it means to nurse well, they will be unable to make judgments about whether nurses have conducted themselves in ways that are consistent with an appropriate view of nursing. This type of work is difficult and will not easily yield clear answers; the aim of this work is to push our thinking and understanding about nursing, and to deepen our insights.

While there has been much debate among nurses about the nature of nursing and the type of knowledge required for nursing practice, there is wide agreement that nursing is a moral endeavour. Nurses have vigorously pursued answers to questions regarding the moral realm of nursing. One approach used in this pursuit has involved drawing on knowledge from the realm of ethics and philosophy to help address nursing's moral issues. Some of these philosophic influences are considered in the following section.

PHILOSOPHICAL INFLUENCES ON NURSING ETHICS

As demonstrated in the table of contents of this text, the branch of philosophic work known as nursing ethics covers a wide variety of topics and concerns. All of the chapters in this text are influenced by philosophical assumptions related to what nursing is, what is knowable, and what is ethical. There is no agreement about what these assumptions are or should be, and so to examine any given conclusion one must consider the position on which the claim is based. A few examples can help to illustrate this point. In her paper on the ethics of care, Bowden (2000) draws on feminist philosophy to argue against considering "ethics in a vacuum." Feminist philosophy's concern with the subjectivity of experience and the ways that political and institutional structures shape experience inform her position (see also Chapter 5). In contrast, in his paper on the ethics of care Paley (2002) draws on a Kantian perspective (derived from the work of Emanuel Kant) and posits that Kant's work adequately accounts for the particularity of context and at the same time locates ethics in a fuller and universal account of moral conduct and moral character. While both of these papers address the ethics of care, each author is informed by different perspectives and draws different conclusions.

Nurses have drawn from a variety of philosophic works in their consideration of ethical questions (Hodkinson 2008; Lundqvist and Nilstun 2009). One need only to scan the reference lists of papers related to ethical issues to see the variety of philosophic works that have been relied upon by nursing scholars in their consideration of moral issues in nursing. In general, nursing scholars have used these works to help position themselves and to provide context for the assumptions guiding an analysis, or they have applied key aspects of a philosopher's work to help shed light on problems or concerns. The philosophic works nurses have used can be roughly divided into a variety of schools or perspectives related to ontological positions such as **critical realism** (a position that emphasizes that our understanding of the world comes from an analysis of the world itself), **pragmatism** (a position that emphasizes that our understanding of the world should arise from an understanding of what works or is reasonable), **existentialism** (a position that emphasizes that our understanding of the world is subjective and emerges from a struggle with personal concerns and projects), and **postmodernism** (a position that emphasizes that our understanding of the world is constructed through social and political structures and that accordingly meta-theories are to be rejected). There are of course numerous other perspectives that nurses draw on and an attempt to classify them is beyond the scope of this chapter.[1]

Nurses have drawn heavily upon academic philosophy to address nursing ethics. However, some have suggested that nursing ethics has not received the attention it deserves, perhaps because historically good nursing practice was defined by nurses' behaviours and scientific principles (Andrist, Nicholoas, and Wolf 2006). In the next part of this chapter we will turn to looking at the important relationship between nursing ethics and nursing science.

THE CONTESTED BOUNDARIES OF NURSING ETHICS AND NURSING SCIENCE

Nursing ethics and nursing science have often been thought of as distinct domains. From this perspective, whereas philosophy (of which ethics is a part) is concerned with broad questions about the nature of the world, science is concerned with questions that can only be answered through the application of specialized methods. Whereas scientific inquiry relies on the collection of data to answer questions, philosophical inquiry typically relies on reason and logic and "everyday" knowledge of the world. Kikuchi (1992) pointed out that nurses have gotten themselves into a muddle by trying to answer philosophical questions with scientific methods. Science's investigative, interviewing, and measurement tools will not enable us to answer questions such as what nurses ought to do, or what justice is. Similarly, Reed and Ground (1997) pointed out, "There are questions which scientists can and do ask themselves but which, purely as scientists, cannot be answered by them. Typically ethical questions are of this form" (65).

However, the distinction between nursing science and nursing ethics is not always so clear. The idea that they are different domains of knowledge arose out of unique theoretical developments within nursing (Risjord 2010). Early debates in nursing theory surrounded the differences between facts and values, between scientific and ethical theories. Nurses endeavoured to identify and isolate the types of knowledge guiding nursing practice. Philosophic nursing pioneers such as Barbara Carper (1978) theorized the types of knowledge needed for practice. She proposed four types of knowledge: *esthetic*, *personal*, *empirical*, and *moral*. Although Carper's work was groundbreaking, the idea of distinct domains of knowledge is problematic. These "patterns of knowing" are assumed to be distinct. However, how one might validate these different forms of knowing or integrate them in practice situations has not been well developed (Risjord 2010). Thinking of science and ethics as different forms of knowing and inquiry also ignores the fact that science and ethics are highly interdependent intellectual endeavours. How we reason about the world, even about what we think is good and right to do, is largely shaped by our empirical experiences in the world.

In essence, the same movement away from binary thinking that has shaped much of nursing's theoretical thinking (Thorne et al. 2004) is also occurring within the boundaries of nursing science and nursing ethics. The process of "doing" nursing science and nursing ethics are complementary. We might philosophize about what is good and right to do but as part of our accountability to professional knowledge we test those assumptions empirically (Porter 2010). Likewise, the large number of empirical studies that highlight the ethical dilemmas faced by nurses and provide data about nurses' "everyday experiences" provide rich ground for philosophizing. Empirical methods that use a critical social science perspective have similarities with philosophic inquiry. Both focus on human experience, adopt a critical lens, and seek to determine what is good and right to do (Pesut and Johnson 2008). This movement of integration between philosophy and empirics is also reflected in other disciplines. Constructivist methodologies are attempting to reunite the social sciences with moral philosophy (Schwandt 1990). Ethicists are calling for the use of the empirical methods such as ethnography as a way to contextualize and provide a deeper understanding of ethical problems (Hoffmaster 1992; Singer, Pellegrino, and Siegler 2001; see also Chapter 5).

The debate between fact and value in nursing has now largely been replaced by the acceptance that nursing is a moral practice. Unlike basic sciences where facts can be considered independently of how those facts are used, the best scientific evidence and the moral good must be integrated in a practice discipline. However, how we approach that integration is particularly important from an ethical perspective. In the next part of the chapter we will turn to considering the challenges of trying to find unity in nursing ontology and nursing ethics.

CHALLENGES OF UNITY IN NURSING ONTOLOGY AND NURSING ETHICS

The philosophic position one holds is based on assumptions about the nature of the world and the nature of knowledge and therefore has implications for the claims one makes about nursing, and the conclusions one draws about what might be morally good or ethical. In this way, nursing ontology (ideas about the nature, object, and scope of the discipline) and nursing ethics are interdependent. For example, McCarthy (2010) illustrated how changing understandings of persons and the environment have created significant moral instability in nursing. When personhood was believed to be stable, individuals as moral agents were capable of making choices in accordance with law, nature, or reason. However, when ideas shifted to personhood as being intersubjectively and contextually constituted, confidence in moral nature and reason were less certain. Similarly, the way we think about what nursing is influences how we think about "good" nursing. For example, Liaschenko and Peter (2004) traced the historical understandings of nursing from a vocation to a profession to a practice, illustrating how the ethical focus has shifted from external principles and codes (whether religious or professional) to a view that every action of the nurse is inherently a moral endeavour (see also Chapter 9). This perspective has fostered a renewed interest in virtue ethics where the character of the nurse once again becomes central to ethical practice.

However, this type of philosophic thinking, where nurses speculate about the nature of the world in the context of nursing practice, has resulted in somewhat of an ethical dilemma for the discipline. The dilemma arises when nursing theorists suggest that there should be a unified ontology of the discipline based in broad philosophic claims about the nature of the world (Pesut 2009). Over the history of nursing's theoretical thinking, some nurses have argued that it is essential to have a common ontology to build disciplinary knowledge. You will recall from earlier in the chapter that part of nursing's theoretical heritage has been the building of nursing models that make claims about health, persons, and the environment. These claims are not morally neutral; they contain many value commitments (see also Yeo 1989). Indeed, Risjord (2010) has referred to health as a "thick moral concept," meaning that there are many moral assumptions upon which the idea of health is based. Yet, rarely are the underlying moral assumptions of these claims articulated.

The ethical problem arises when we assume these philosophies are value neutral and propose that one set of beliefs about the world should be the basis for nursing's ontology. Indeed, using philosophy to establish a single "truth" about the world is pragmatically problematic. Philosophy seeks to answer the big questions such as the meaning of persons and the nature of the universe. The philosophic answers that can be considered are representative of the diversity inherent in our world. This is not necessarily a negative outcome. Indeed, as is argued in other chapters of this text (particularly Chapters 5 and 13), one might claim that the power of philosophy lies in its ability to answer questions from multiple angles. This is not to suggest that there are no universally held values. Rather, this is to point out the difficulties inherent in establishing a universally held ontology of nursing, if that ontology is based upon metaphysical claims that may not be commonly shared.

Eastern and Western philosophy are important aspects of this diversity. The majority of philosophers' works nurses have drawn upon have emanated from the West. Eastern philosophy is a frontier that has been largely unexplored by nurses. There is an awakening interest among nurses in perspectives drawn from the East that challenge foundationalist approaches adhered to by Western philosophers. For example, in her dissertation Bruce (2002) explores the notion of living with dying. She draws on a Buddhist perspective to deepen our understanding of notions of impermanence and to challenge our need for certainty and solidity. Rather than being consumed with doing for and knowing that, she prompts us to consider how we might mindfully be with a person and acknowledge the impermanence of being. Her approach has profound ethical implications for how nurses might provide care in the midst of suffering. Rodgers and Yen (2002) also claim that the Eastern philosophic perspectives have a great deal to offer nursing and suggest that given the growing globalization that surrounds us, nurses need to "empty their cups" and ponder different approaches to considering the discipline. We cannot afford to adopt a single ontology for the discipline if it fails to respect these diverse ideas. (See also Chapter 5 for a discussion of how Buddhist and Aboriginal perspectives, for example, can enrich ethical theorizing.)

Spirituality as a Unifying Idea for Nursing Ontology and Ethics

As nursing sought for a united ontology and ethic, two ideas gained immense popularity as a solution: caring and spirituality. Doing nursing philosophy entails trying to reason about why certain ideas become popular, considering the assumptions upon which they rest, and imagining the implications they hold for nursing thought and action. The idea of caring as an ethic for nursing arose from the influence of feminist ethics. Feminist scholars such as Carol Gilligan (1982) and Nell Noddings (1984) provided rich theoretical insights for how the being and doing of nursing work could be united within an ethic of care. Chapters 5, 7, and 8 in this book look at *relational* forms of ethics—which have been influenced by care theory—in more detail. What we want to reflect on here is the role that the idea of spirituality has played more recently in attempting to unite nursing ontology and ethics.

Spirituality (as opposed to religion) first became visible in the nursing literature in the 1980s and has since gained enormous popularity. Definitions of spirituality in nursing literature typically characterize it as separate from religion and link it to ideas such as meaning, energy, harmony, connectedness, mysteriousness, and transcendence (Chiu et al. 2004; see also Simington 2004). *Inherent in these ideas are assumptions of what constitutes ethical nursing practice.* For example, some theorists who have placed spirituality as central to nursing practice assume that nurses practice within a somewhat mysterious environment where principles of cause and effect do not always hold true (Parse 1998; Parse 2007; Watson 2005). Therefore, it is important to focus more upon individual choice regarding quality of life than normative (values based) states of health. Good care within that environment promotes meaning, harmony, connectedness, and a sense of transcendence. Considerations of spirituality in the context of nursing diagnoses have a long list of interventions and outcomes that nurses focus on as part of good practice. Pesut's (2006; 2008a; 2008c) philosophic work examined the major assumptions underlying definitions of spirituality within nursing literature. What was revealing in this work was how these definitions were implicitly grounded within quite different philosophic and religious views of the world and that these views had important, but often unarticulated, implications for nursing ontology, epistemology, and ethics.

It is interesting to ponder the relationship between caring and spirituality in nursing theory. One of the major critiques of caring as an ethical foundation for the profession is that it is essentially ungrounded—meaning that it fails to have normative ethical standards about how one should care (Allmark 1995). One might argue that at least some of the recent popularity around spirituality has been an attempt to ground caring. For example, Jean Watson's (2005) popular theory of "Caring Science as Sacred Science" grounds caring within the sacred. By including the sacred as grounding for caring it provides a normative frame of reference toward which good nursing care should be directed (i.e., meaning, harmony, connection). It is also interesting to note that the grounding occurs within an idea of individualized spirituality as opposed to institutional religion. This would more adequately reflect nursing's commitment to a feminist caring ethic as opposed to the religious ethic that was profoundly influential in early nursing. The challenge of course is that not all individuals believe in the existence of spirituality or the way that spirituality is defined in nursing literature. This is yet another example of how trying to adopt a common ontology (i.e., accepting that nursing practice is spiritual practice) may be ethically problematic in a diverse society. The spirituality in nursing discourse has produced healthy debate in the nursing philosophy literature (Betts and Smith-Betts 2009; Leget 2008; Paley 2008; 2010; Pesut 2008b). This type of debate helps to ensure that diverse ideas will be represented in our theoretical thinking, which will in turn ensure that "good" nursing will take into account the diverse contexts within which practice occurs.

UNRESOLVED ETHICAL NURSING ISSUES

There remain several unresolved philosophical issues in the field of nursing ethics that present significant challenges for the profession. In the following sections we highlight some of these issues and discuss why they are significant. These issues concern the role of ethical principles in nursing, the question of whether nursing has a unique ethical perspective, and issues related to what constitutes good, or artful, nursing practice.

The Role of Ethical Principles in Nursing

One issue concerns whether there are universal ethical principles—that is, principles about what constitutes good action that hold across time, place, and person. This is a central issue that has implications for nursing ethics as well as other forms of ethics. Do we believe that there can be a code of ethics that can be applied to all nurses in all situations, or do we acknowledge that there are always contingencies that must be taken into consideration? Can both positions be accommodated? Austin (2001) raised this issue when she asked, "Can we conceive of a macro-ethic that could guide our moral actions in a global community?" (11). Likewise, Gallagher (2010) cautioned against the assumption that nurses from other countries would necessarily value a humanistic or social justice perspective. Writers such as Gadow (2000) who are grounded in a postmodern perspective—a position that holds that knowledge is socially constructed and must be subjected to systematic deconstruction to reveal the ways in which it is partial—raise serious concerns about the very possibility of ethical principles. Others have suggested that rather than taking a principle-based approach to ensuring good practice we should consider the virtues necessary to nurse well. If we are to endorse and use ethical guidelines and moral codes, we must come to a common understanding of what they are and how they should be used. If they are not possible, or useful, we need to acknowledge this and determine how we might ensure that nursing practice is moral.

If one holds that such principles are possible how ought they to be derived? Possible responses are that principles ought to be derived from social consensus, or from a notion of goodness that is grounded in an understanding of the nature of humans, or from some other approach. Depending on how one views the nature of the world and human beings, one would adopt different answers to this important question. This issue has been debated by moral philosophers for centuries. It is important to recognize that while it will likely remain unresolved, the perspective one takes has implications for the ways in which we might assess moral conduct in nursing practice.

The Uniqueness of Nursing's Ethical Perspective

An important matter raised in an editorial by Carnevale (2002) concerns whether nursing has its own unique ethical perspective and is responsible for deriving ethical principles unique to nursing, or whether nursing's ethical perspectives should be drawn from the field of moral philosophy. Kikuchi (1992) suggested that while the field of moral philosophy addresses questions related to what is good to do and seek as humans, *nurses* are responsible for considering what it is we ought to do and seek as nurses.

Currently, there is considerable scholarly work being conducted to clarify nursing's unique ethical perspective. Scott (2000), for example, argued that any theory of ethics that denies the moral significance of the emotions would be problematic for nursing. Her approach brings us closer to understanding the essential elements of an ethics of nursing, but does not fully address what else is required. Grace (2001), on the other hand, examined "advocacy" as an ideal ethic for nursing practice, and concludes that a broad sense of advocacy that encompasses both individual and societal needs is appropriate for the practice of nursing. Peter and Liaschenko (2004) pointed out that at least some of the search for a common ethic has been located within the assumption of nursing's proximity to patients, that is the idea that nurses hold a unique closeness in relation to patients. This idea, which places nurses in a position of advocacy, has also resulted in moral distress and ambiguity. They recommend "moving others closer to the bedside" as a means to alleviating this state (218). As the quest for an ethical perspective for nursing carries on we can anticipate that philosophic work such as this will continue. Indeed, many of the subsequent chapters in this book are taking up the quest. These types of analyses will help to push the frontiers of nursing ethics forward by broadening our understanding of moral conduct in nursing practice.

THE NATURE OF GOOD NURSING PRACTICE

Ethics is concerned with ensuring that our actions are morally good. When we think about good nursing practice, we often think about the required skills and values. The ability to nurse well is frequently referred to as "the art of nursing." An important question that has arisen in relation to nursing ethics is the relationship between nursing art and nursing ethics. While there is much disagreement about what it takes to be an artful nurse, there is growing acceptance of the idea that nursing art is by nature a moral art.

ETHICS IN PRACTICE 3-1

The Artful Nurse

A nurse is observed caring for a post-surgical patient. She assesses the client comprehensively and plans the care she will provide for the day. She anticipates all of the patient's post-surgical needs, providing pain medication when it is required, encour-aging deep breathing and coughing, speaking with the patient and family and preparing them for discharge. The nurse appears to be very knowledgeable and has tremendous skill and efficiency. Toward the end of her shift she strongly encourages the patient to sit in a chair, knowing this would be good for the patient. The patient is tired, scared, and unwilling to cooperate. The nurse persists and eventually, with the help of another nurse, easily transfers the patient

into a chair. The nurse is pleased that all the goals she set for the patient have been accomplished. The patient is clean, the dressing is changed, and the bedside is tidy. Is this an artful nurse?

On first blush we might consider the nurse in Ethics in Practice 3-1 to be artful. But is skill in assessing and caring for a patient enough? The art of the nurse involves more than the skill and cunning required to make something occur. The nurse in the above scenario selected a course of action that was scientifically sound, and ignored the will of the patient. Unlike "artisans" who make things, nurses deal with human beings, and so in addition to having specific skills we expect nurses to comport themselves in particular ways. Not only must a nurse know what to do, she or he also must choose appropriately among means to decide the best course of action.

The question of the relationship between morality and art has long been a subject of debate among philosophers. Oscar Wilde summed up one position of this argument with the statement, "The fact of a man being a poisoner is nothing against his prose" (cited in Maritain 1959, 81). With this statement, Wilde implied that the world of art and morality are two entirely autonomous worlds. The fine artist (painter, poet, etc.) does not pursue a moral good, but rather the good of the work. A good writer need not be a good person and good art is judged on its artistic merit alone not moral grounds. The same cannot be said for the art of nursing. *A nurse may be technically competent and knowledgeable, yet if she or he does not make moral choices in the performance of nursing care she or he is not artful.* According to this view, artful nursing is inextricably intertwined with human life and achievement of particular human ends. Leah Curtin (1979), a pioneering nursing ethicist, summed this notion up:

> The end or purpose of nursing is the welfare of other human beings. This end is not a scientific end, but rather a moral end. That is, it involves the seeking of good and it involves our relationship with other human beings. The science that we learn, the technological skills that we develop are shaped and designed by that moral end—much as an artist using a brush. Therefore, nursing is a moral art. (2)

It is even in the smallest of actions that the nurse expresses the values to which she or he is personally committed. Almost every moment a nurse is confronted with the need to choose between a great and lesser good (Lanara 1981). Accordingly, all nursing acts, to the extent that they are voluntary and affect human lives, are subject to moral judgment. Whereas the technician uses techniques that are evaluated by efficiency, "the professional makes decisions which are evaluated by the good" (Bishop and Scudder 1990, 69).

Although there is emerging agreement that nursing art involves practicing in such a way that **a moral good**, or objective that is good for a person and ethically defensible is realized, there is little agreement about how this is best accomplished, or what constitutes the good. Some authors, such as Beckstrand (1978), have suggested that moral practice can be achieved through the application of moral theory. Nurses need to simply apply ethical theory in their clinical reasoning processes. As discussed earlier, the problem with this approach is that it fails to accommodate the idiosyncrasies of a particular situation. In contrast, authors such as Gadow (1985) suggested that moral nursing practice can only be achieved when nurses enter into subjective caring relationships in which both the patient's and the nurse's values are considered. The moral good is thus achieved intersubjectively, between the nurse and the patient. In contrast, Benner (1991) took the position that nurses learn skilful ethical comportment over time as they participate in their practices and gain a sense of what it means to be "better" or "worse." *An unresolved issue inherent in these positions is the question of whether a nurse's sense of what is morally good is **subjective,** arising from a personal sense of what is right, or whether there is some form of **objective** or external criterion with which to judge what is good.* When a nurse chooses a course of action because she or he has a sense that it is a good course of action, or when a nurse and patient together choose a course of action, does this inherently make the action good? It would seem that neither the blind application of moral principles nor the nurse's personal sense of what is good is enough to ensure an action is morally good. The answer to this issue may indeed lie in the melding of principles and perception so that the nurse carefully determines a correct course of action.

The notion of the good also applies to the realm of nursing leadership and administration. In these situations it is easy for nurses to lose sight of the good they are attempting to serve. What is "good" for the economic efficiency of a hospital is not necessarily "good" for patients; similarly what is good for nurses is not always good for patients. Aristotle conceived of **politics** as a realm of philosophy related to ethics. While ethics is concerned with what is good for individuals, politics focuses on what is good for groups of humans, specifically the types of organizations that most benefit human beings (see also Chapter 18). The moral art of nursing administration, or nursing leadership, is perhaps one of the least developed areas in nursing philosophy and is deserving of attention. What is the good that nursing administrators serve? What types of skills and virtues do artful nursing administrators require?

The Virtues of the Good Nurse

As has been discussed earlier in this chapter there is growing recognition that moral practice cannot simply be achieved by applying ethical principles to complex situations. With the acknowledgment of the limitations of principle-driven approaches there has been increasing attention focused on determining alternative approaches (see also Chapters 4, 5 and 18). Virtue-based approaches to moral practice are being increasingly considered as alternatives. Sellman (2000), for example, applied MacIntyre's (1984) notion of virtue in considering the nature of nursing practice. This approach seeks to understand the **virtues** or habits of good operation that are required for moral practice. Instead of considering the principles that need to be applied for a moral practice, a virtue-based approach considers the virtues nurses require to be moral in their practice. The challenge this latter approach presents is for us to identify the virtues necessary to the practice of nursing.

Most would agree that the possession of skill and knowledge are necessary conditions for the moral conduct of nursing practice. It is hard to imagine a situation where incompetent nurses can morally conduct themselves in nursing practice; their lack of competency would not enable them to achieve desired goals. In identifying one's self as a professional, one is claiming a certain level of competence. The license to practice nursing does not include permission to practice poorly. The moral responsibility of the nurse involves a commitment not only to nurse a patient competently, but also to "sustain excellent practice in the face of unreasonable demands and lack of appreciation on the part of patients" (Bishop and Scudder 1987, 37). The good nurse must not only be competent, but must consistently demonstrate competence in her or his practice, no matter how arduous the circumstances. Pask (2001) emphasized this point, describing how nurses can feel challenged when "times get hard and they struggle to turn from their own suffering, to focus instead upon the needs of their patients" (45).

As suggested in Ethics in Practice 3-2, the other virtues that are required by nurses are moral virtues, or characteristics that ensure a nurse makes good choices in her or his practice.

ETHICS IN PRACTICE 3-2

Nursing in Difficult Conditions

It is three o'clock in the morning. The nursing unit is short-staffed and all the nurses have been inordinately busy. There are several patients who are very ill and who require regular monitoring. The nursing staff are tired and have missed all their rest breaks. The patient in Room 200, not the sickest of the patients, has been "on the call bell all night." Every time one of the nurses makes the trek down the hall, it is for some minor request or complaint. There is finally a lull and everyone has a chance to sit down, and the call bell goes on again. How will the character of the nurse who answers the call influence this situation?

Bishop and Scudder (1990) maintained that it is the possession of certain moral virtues that enables a nurse to nurse artfully. Philosophers have long considered the nature of virtue; is it a natural propensity or can it be cultivated? Most agree that it can be developed. Similarly, in nursing, while there is a sense that nurses must by nature be ethical, there is also a sense that the ability to comport oneself in difficult situations can be developed over time. Pask (2001), for example, suggested that it is "through the conscious training of their habitual responses, that a nurse comes disposed to respond, and to act with compassion" (51). What enables a nurse to act morally under difficult situations?

Since the time of Florence Nightingale nurses have discussed the virtues required to nurse artfully. Numbered among the primary virtues are charity, love, and compassion. In recent years caring has been upheld as the virtue that drives artful nursing. Benner and Wrubel (1989) suggested that the same act done in a caring and uncaring way may have different effects, and only the nurse who cares will notice small differences in their patients' behaviours and create unique solutions to patients' needs. Jaegar (2001) suggested that moral sensitivity is the key capacity or virtue that must be fully developed by nurses. She maintains that being able to place oneself in another's position is not enough. One must be able to be open to the possibility that one does not share the same moral framework with the other person. Moral sensitivity is the capacity to be sensitive to these differences (see also Nortvedt 2004). Her concern is that in today's environment health care workers are in danger of losing their moral sensitivity and that moral theories describe too abstractly what it means to respect another person. Her claim is that the cultivation of moral sensitivity is an antidote to administrative policies that rely on the formulaic application of traditional moral theories.

Often educators and administrators are focused on ensuring that nurses have skills and competencies. In addition to possessing these skills nurses need to consistently use these competencies in an ethical manner. What virtues do nurses require? And how might nursing educators and administrators help to cultivate those virtues in the nurses they educate and supervise? Must a nurse possess these virtues innately or can they be taught? What institutional factors need to be in place to support nurses to develop and use their virtues? These are important questions that require our urgent attention in that answers to these questions have the potential to help us to assist nurses to develop the capacity to consistently respond to the challenges they face in an ethical manner. Such questions are taken up in various forms in all the chapters of this book.

Summary

Philosophical contributions to nursing ethics are multifaceted. While the works of non-nursing philosophers provide valuable insights that can help to inform nursing ethics, these contributions cannot be simply applied to nursing situations and will not resolve nursing's fundamental ethical issues. Philosophical work focused specifically on nursing can help to answer questions related to the nature of nursing and the nurse–patient relationship and provide valuable direction for the development of nursing ethics. The mandate to develop nursing philosophy cannot be relegated solely to nursing scholars—to do so is to condemn nursing philosophy to obscurity. If nursing philosophy is to be relevant it must also be based on contributions and insights of clinicians, researchers, educators, administrators, and policy makers. This chapter has raised a number of philosophical questions related to nursing ethics that remain unanswered. In addition to considering the questions posed below, we encourage readers to consider the questions raised in the chapter and to attempt to formulate sound responses. Philosophy is, after all, every nurse's business.

For Reflection

1. Consider any one of the chapters in this text. What philosophical assumptions underlie the author's arguments? Are these assumptions implicit or explicit?

2. What do you contend is the nature, scope, and goal of nursing? What implications does your position have for ethical nursing practice?

3. How might "good" nursing practice differ between a perspective of persons as autonomous moral agents and persons as morally constructed by their environment?

4. What are the implications of using ideas such as caring and spirituality to "ground" nursing ethics?

5. Can a nursing leader be a good leader without a firm understanding of the nature of nursing?

6. Consider the practice of a nurse who you consider to have demonstrated the finest attributes of nursing art. What are the virtues required by nursing, and how can they be cultivated?

7. What are the most important questions facing nursing ethics? How can these issues be resolved?

Endnote

1. Readers may find it useful to look at various sources linking ontology, epistemology, and methodology with paradigms of inquiry. See, for example, Denzin and Lincoln (2005) and Guba and Lincoln (2005).

References

Allmark, P. 1995. Can there be an ethics of care? *Journal of Medical Ethics, 21*, 19–24.

Andrist, L.C., Nicholoas, P.K., and Wolf, K. 2006. *A history of nursing ideas*. Mississauga, ON: Jones and Bartlett.

Austin, W. 2001. Nursing ethics in an era of globalization. *Advances in Nursing Science, 24* (2), 1–18.

Beckstrand, J. 1978. The notion of a practice theory and the relationship of scientific and ethical knowledge to practice. *Research in Nursing and Health, 1*, 131–136.

Benner, P. 1991. The role of experience, narrative, and community in skilled ethical comportment. *Advances in Nursing Science, 14* (3), 13–28.

Benner, P. and Wrubel, J. 1989. *The primacy of caring: Stress and coping in health and illness*. Menlo Park, CA: Addison Wesley.

Betts, C.E. and Smith-Betts, A.F.J. 2009. Scientism and the medicalization of extistential distress: A reply to John Paley. *Nursing Philosophy, 10*, 137–141.

Bishop, A.H. and Scudder, J.R. Jr. 1987. Nursing ethics in an age of controversy. *Advances in Nursing Science, 9* (3), 34–43.

Bishop, A.H. and Scudder, J.R. Jr. 1990. *The practical, moral, and personal sense of nursing: A phenomenological philosophy of practice*. Albany, NY: State University of New York Press.

Bowden, P. 2000. An "ethic of care" in clinical settings: Encompassing "feminine" and "feminist" perspectives. *Nursing Philosophy, 1*, 36–49.

Bruce, W.A. 2002. Abiding in liminal space(s): Inscribing mindful living/dying with(in) end-of-life care. Unpublished doctoral dissertation. Vancouver, BC: University of British Columbia.

Carnevale, F. 2002. Betwixt and between: Searching for nursing's moral foundation. *Canadian Journal of Nursing Research, 34* (2), 5–8.

Carper, B.A. 1978. Fundamental patterns of knowing in nursing, *Advances in Nursing Science, 1*, 13–23.

Chiu, L., Emblen, J.D., Van Hofwegen, L., Sawatzky, R., and Meyerhoff, H. 2004. An integrative review of the concept of spirituality in the health sciences. *Western Journal of Nursing Research, 26* (4), 405–428.

Curtin, L.L. 1979. The nurse as advocate: A philosophical foundation for nursing. *Advances in Nursing Science, 1* (3), 1–10.

Denzin, N.K. and Lincoln, Y.S. 2005. Paradigms and perspectives in contention. In N.K. Denzin and Y.S. Lincoln (Eds). *The Sage handbook of qualitative research* (3rd ed.; pp. 183–190). Thousand Oaks, CA: Sage.

Gadow, S. 1985. Nurse and patient: The caring relationship. In A.H. Bishop and J.R. Scudder Jr. (Eds.), *Caring, curing, coping: Nurse physician, patient relationships* (pp. 31–43). Tuscaloosa, AL: University of Alabama Press.

Gadow, S. 2000. Philosophy as falling: Aiming for grace. *Nursing Philosophy, 1,* 89–97.

Gallagher, A. 2010. Editorial: The ethics of mutuality. *Nursing Ethics, 17* (5), 539–540.

Gilligan, C. 1982. *In a different voice.* Cambridge, MA: Harvard University Press.

Grace, P.J. 2001. Professional advocacy: Widening the scope of accountability. *Nursing Philosophy, 2,* 151–162.

Guba, E.G. and Lincoln, Y.S. 2005. Paradigmatic controversies, contradictions and emerging confluences. In N.K. Denzin and Y.S. Lincoln (Eds). *The Sage handbook of qualitative research* (3rd ed.; pp. 191–215). Thousand Oaks, CA: Sage.

Hodkinson, K. 2008. How should a nurse approach truth-telling? A virtue ethics perspective. *Nursing Philosophy, 9* (4), 248–256.

Hoffmaster, B. 1992. Can ethnography save the life of medical ethics? *Social Science and Medicine, 35,* 1421–1431.

Jaeger, S.M. 2001. Teaching health care ethics: The importance of moral sensitivity for moral reasoning. *Nursing Philosophy, 2,* 131–142.

Kikuchi, J. 1992. Nursing questions that science cannot answer. In J. Kikuchi and H. Simmons (Eds.), *Philosophic inquiry in nursing* (pp. 26–37). Thousand Oaks, CA: Sage.

Kikuchi, J. and Simmons, H. 1994. *Developing a philosophy of nursing.* Thousand Oaks, CA: Sage.

Lanara, V. 1981. *Heroism as a nursing value: A philosophical perspective.* Athens: Sisterhood Evniki.

Leget, C. 2008. Spirituality and nursing: Why be reductionistic? A response to John Paley. *Nursing Philosophy, 9* (4), 277–278.

Liaschenko, J. and Peter, E. 2004. Nursing ethics and conceptualizations of nursing: Profession, practice and work. *Journal of Advanced Nursing, 46* (5), 488–493.

Lundqvist, A. and Nilstun, T. 2009. Nodding's caring ethics theory applied in a paediatric setting. *Nursing Philosophy, 10* (2), 113–123.

MacIntyre, A. 1984. *After virtue* (2nd ed.). Notre Dame, ID: University of Notre Dame Press.

Maritain, J. 1959. Art as a virtue of the practical intellect. In M. Weitz (Ed.), *Problems in aesthetics: An introductory book of readings* (pp. 76–92). New York: Macmillan.

McCarthy, J. 2010. Moral instability: The upsides for nursing practice. *Nursing Philosophy, 11* (2), 127–135.

Nagel, T. 1987. *What does it all mean? A very short introduction to philosophy.* Oxford, UK: Oxford University Press.

Nortvedt, P. 2004. Emotions and ethics. In J. Storch, P. Rodney, and R. Starzomski (Eds.), *Toward a moral horizon: Nursing ethics for leadership and practice* (pp. 447–464). Toronto: Pearson-Prentice Hall.

Noddings, N. 1984. *Caring: A feminist approach to ethics and moral education.* Berkeley, CA: University of California Press.

Orem, D. 1991. *Nursing concepts of practice* (4ᵗʰ ed.). St. Louis, MO: Mosby Year Book.

Paley, J. 2002. Virtue of autonomy: The Kantian ethics of care. *Nursing Philosophy, 3,* 133–143.

Paley, J. 2008. Spirituality in nursing: A reductionist approach. *Nursing Philosophy, 9* (1), 3–18.

Paley, J. 2010. Spirituality and reductionism: Three replies. *Nursing Philosophy, 11* (3), 178–190.

Parse, R.R. 1981. *Man-living-health: A theory of nursing.* New York: John Wiley and Sons.

Parse, R.R. 1998. *The human becoming school of thought: A perspective for nurses and other health professionals.* Thousand Oaks, CA: Sage.

Parse, R.R. 2007. The human becoming school of thought in 2050. *Nursing Science Quarterly, 20,* 308–311.

Pask, E.J. 2001. Nursing responsibility and conditions of practice: Are we justified in holding nurses responsible for their behaviour in situations of patient care? *Nursing Philosophy, 2,* 45–52.

Pesut, B. 2006. Fundamental or foundational obligation: Problematizing the ethical call to spiritual care. *Advances in Nursing Science, 29* (2), 125–133.

Pesut, B. 2008a. A conversation on diverse perspectives of spirituality in nursing literature. *Nursing Philosophy, 9,* 98–109.

Pesut, B. 2008b. A reply to spirituality and nursing: A reductionist approach by John Paley. *Nursing Philosophy, 9,* 131–137.

Pesut, B. 2008c. Spirituality and spiritual care in Nursing Fundamentals textbooks. *Journal of Nursing Education, 47* (4), 167–173.

Pesut, B. 2009. Ontologies of nursing in an age of spiritual pluralism: Closed or open worldview. *Nursing Philosophy, 11,* 15–23.

Pesut, B. and Johnson, J. 2008. Reinstating the "Queen": Understanding philosophical inquiry in Nursing. *Journal of Advanced Nursing, 61* (1), 115–121.

Peter, E. and Liaschenko, J. 2004. Perils of promimity: A spatiotemporal analysis of moral distress and moral ambiguity. *Nursing Inquiry, 11* (4), 218–225.

Porter, S. 2010. Fundamental patterns of knowing in nursing: The challenge of evidence-based practice. *Advances in Nursing Science, 33* (1), 3–14.

Reed, J. and Ground, I. 1997. *Philosophy for nursing.* London: Arnold.

Risjord, M. 2010. *Nursing knowledge: Science, practice and philosophy.* Oxford, UK: Wiley-Blackwell.

Rodgers, B.L. and Yen, W. 2002. Re-thinking nursing science through the understanding of Buddhism. *Nursing Philosophy*, *3*, 213–221.

Rogers, M.E. 1970. *An introduction to the theoretical basis of nursing.* Philadelphia: F.A. Davis.

Schwandt, T.R. 1990. Paths to inquiry in the social sciences: scientific, constructivist, and critical theory methodologies. In E. Guba (Ed.), *The paradigm dialogue* (pp. 258–276). Newbury Park, CA: Sage.

Scott, P.A. 2000. Emotion, moral perception, and nursing practice. *Nursing Philosophy, 1*, 123–133.

Sellman, D. 2000. Alasdair MacIntyre and the professional practice of nursing. *Nursing Philosophy, 1*, 26–33.

Singer, P.A., Pellegrino, E.D., and Siegler, M. 2001. Clinical ethics revisited. *BMC Medical Ethics, 2* (1). Available at http://www.biomedcentral.com/1472-6939/2002/2001.

Simington, J.A. 2004. Ethics for an evolving spirituality. In J. Storch, P. Rodney, and R. Starzomski (Eds.), *Toward a moral horizon: Nursing ethics for leadership and practice* (pp. 465–484). Toronto: Pearson-Prentice Hall.

Thorne, S., Henderson, A., McPherson, G., and Pesut, B. 2004. The problematic allure of the binary in nursing theoretical discourse. *Nursing Philosophy, 5*, 208–215.

Watson, J. 2005. *Caring science as sacred science.* Philadelphia: FA Davis.

Yeo, M. 1989. Integration of nursing theory and nursing ethics. *Advances in Nursing Science, 11* (3), 33–42.

CHAPTER 4

Our Theoretical Landscape: A Brief History of Health Care Ethics

Patricia Rodney, Michael Burgess, J. Craig Phillips, Gladys McPherson, and Helen Brown

The Socratic injunction "know thyself" names the task at the entrance to the moral life. Through our upbringing and acculturation . . . we acquire numerous beliefs about right and wrong and good and bad. Beliefs thus acquired are deeply constitutive of who we are as adults, and may manifest themselves in our actions without our ever having reflected upon them. . . . The choice of the ethical life as expressed in the injunction "know thyself" commits one to bringing such unreflected beliefs to light and, having clarified them, to explicitly and responsibly embrace, reject, or modify them. (Yeo 2010a, 21)

The challenge that Canadian philosopher Michael Yeo has articulated above applies to every one of us who practises in nursing and other health care professions. And it applies to ethical inquiry in each of our disciplines. Thus, a central tenet of this text is that ethical practice requires thoughtful scrutiny of the beliefs and values that underpin our adoption of ethical theories and our ethical theorizing. Ethical practice demands that we understand the sources of the theories that guide us, including the assumptions that are embedded in them, and how that theory is evolving. Most importantly, we must carefully consider how we might use—and shape—ethical theory to improve the practice of nurses and other health care professionals toward the goal of fostering the health and well-being of patients, families, and communities. In other words, our adoption and development of ethical theory should be thoughtful and conscious, and our theorizing (or application of theory) should involve processes of critical reflection. Pesut and Johnson situated such processes in relation to nursing theorizing in Chapter 3. In this chapter we address theory and theorizing as it has evolved in health care ethics more broadly.

More specifically, it is our intent to provide an orientation to the development of health care ethics, including an overview of its history and theoretical underpinnings, and to describe some of the challenges we face in contemporary health care ethics. We will also link this orientation to related thinking about human rights, as a rights focus is gaining prominence as a means of addressing local and global inequities in health and health care (Macklin 2008). While we lay out our understandings, we will be endeavouring to highlight the strengths and limitations of traditional approaches to health care ethics as guides to thinking in ethically troubling situations. We will close this chapter by considering what it is that health care providers need from ethical theory. In Chapter 5, we sketch out some of the newer theoretical possibilities opened up by cultural, feminist, Aboriginal, and relational writings in health care ethics (we consider all four to be large and internally diverse subsets of contextualist ethics). Later, we explore the implications for applications in ethical practice in health care (Chapter 13) as well as organizational ethics and health/health care policy (Chapter 18).

Throughout this text we are not embarking on a process of delineating the best or correct approach to ethical theory or theorizing. Rather, our intent is to demonstrate some of the various forms and possibilities of ethical theories and the implications of their application. Ultimately, the ethical theory we and other authors in this text draw on will "look more like a tapestry composed of threads of many different hues than one woven in a single color" (Fraser and Nicholson 1990, 35).

A BRIEF HISTORY OF HEALTH CARE ETHICS

Ethical theorizing has been a significant undertaking in Western as well as Eastern and Aboriginal societies throughout the ages. In Western society, philosophers have been engaged in dialogue about what has been described as the "ultimate task of morality"— that is, to find out "how best to live" (Hadot 1995) or how to lead the "good life" and enjoy well-being (Pojman 2001). Ethics has been popularly used as a generic term referring to ". . . various ways of understanding and examining the moral life" (Beauchamp and Childress 1994, 4). Indeed, ethics has been the subject of rigorous philosophical debates in Western philosophy for almost 2500 years (Meilaender 1995; Pojman 2001). Despite the controversy about the task and methods of ethics, the works of the influential ancient Greek philosophers (namely Socrates, Plato, and Aristotle) firmly established ethics as a branch of philosophical inquiry which sought ". . . dispassionate and rational clarification and justification of the basic assumptions and beliefs that people hold about what is to be considered morally acceptable and morally unacceptable behavior" (Johnstone 1999, 42). Over time, the application of ethics to health care has been greatly influenced by the historical evolution of philosophy and ethics as well as theology.

Some Modern Ethical Theories and Approaches

The history of Western ethics over the last few centuries has focused largely on metaethics (Winkler 1996). The objective of this theoretical enterprise is the working out of general theories that account for accepted moral judgments and assist in determining correct moral action in controversial circumstances. Most popular of these theories are versions of Immanuel Kant's deontology or duty-based ethics, John Stuart Mill's utilitarianism or consequentialist ethics, and John Rawls' contractarian approach[1] (Arras, Steinbock, and London 1999; Keatings and Smith 2010; Yeo 2010b).

Deontology Philosophical writing has always used examples to illustrate the adequacy of ethical theory in elucidating right- or wrong-making characteristics. For example, one version of Kant's categorical imperative, "Always act in a manner that in so doing you can will that your action become a universal principle," is typically used to explain why lying is immoral even when the consequences are better than that of telling the truth. This aspect of Kant's theory is often referred to as "universalizability." But the generalization can be limited by including very specific descriptions of the situation. For example, a health care provider might contemplate lying to an irreversibly ill person to allow her to fulfill her cherished plans for a long vacation. In this instance, if we hold truth-telling as a categorical imperative, ethical behaviour would not accommodate lying unless we can arrive at a more sophisticated categorical ethical principle. Universalizing the principle that lying in this example is defensible might yield a rule like "Always lie to a patient who is dying if the truth will not provide any advantage and the lie may result in considerable benefit." Of course, such generalizations can lead to difficulties in practice.

Utilitarianism In contrast to Kant's deontological perspective, utilitarianism assesses the morality of actions or policies based on their effects or consequences. The good and bad effects anticipated for each alternative action or policy must be compared. The morally required or "ethical" action or policy is that which produces the best outcomes. Some utilitarians use the standards of happiness and unhappiness to assess whether consequences are good or bad, while others judge consequences in terms of whether they produce pleasure or pain. It is also important to note that, in weighing consequences, most utilitarian theories demand that all persons affected by the action or policy are considered, whether taxpayers or bereaved relatives.

Contractarianism Contractarianism stands in opposition to utilitarianism, suggesting that the pursuit of happiness or pleasure is not the ultimate good and cannot be used as justification for means that impose unfair disadvantages on certain societal groups. This view is most often associated with the work of the American theorist John Rawls (1971), who articulated the notion of a *social contract*:

> [that] derives, from a strictly hypothetical and non-historical original position, the conclusion that, as a matter of (social) justice no one, or rather no group, has any business to be any better off than anyone else, or than any other group; save in so far as their being in this happier position is indirectly to the benefit of (not all those who are worse off but only) the least-advantaged group. (Flew 1979, 299)[2]

It other words, while happiness or pleasure may be an unintended consequence of ethically justifiable action, it should not be taken as the primary rationale for determining how we ought to act. Rawls' intent was to work towards a fair process for the distribution of societal goods such that the least well off in a society were protected. The current Canadian health insurance program reflects, at least to some extent, the results of this type of thinking (see also Chapter 12).

Interim Summary In summary, while deontology, utilitarianism, and contractarianism were just three of the theoretical perspectives addressed by early modern ethical theory, they were some of the most influential on the development of bioethics. They remain important because of the significant influence they have had—and continue to have—on thinking about how health care services ought to be distributed, and about the nature of professional–patient relationships. In other words, these theories have become entrenched in the more recently developed field of bioethics. Other early influences on the development of bioethics came from theology and law (Arras, Steinbock, and London 1999; Furrow 2009; Hoffmaster 1999; Roy, Williams, and Dickens 1994). Theology had a particularly strong early influence, especially in terms of virtue theory and natural law. Many early anthologies in bioethics therefore included some version of both.

Virtue Theory This theory has been strongly influenced by Aristotle and Aquinas and has a significant theological heritage. It is not a single moral theory, but, rather, a "family of moral theories that are specially concerned with or that give special priority to the role of virtues in the moral life" (Arras, Steinbock, and London 1999, 30). Johnstone (2004) notes that virtue theory fell out of favour in our early modern era, but is experiencing a resurgence of interest. Alisdair MacIntyre is an important contemporary theorist on virtue ethics. He describes virtues as consistent dispositions manifested in varying kinds of situations, aimed at the pursuit of ethical goods and expressed in a consistent narrative of self (MacIntyre 1987). The traditional virtues of health professionals have been proposed to derive from health care relationships (Johnstone 2004; Pellegrino 2001) and are frequently claimed to include compassion, discernment, trustworthiness, and integrity (although the virtues displayed vary depending on the nature of the relationships) (Beauchamp and Childress, 1994). Virtues are embedded in both professional roles and practices and embody social expectations as well as professional standards and internal ideals.[3]

Interestingly, MacIntyre (1987/1984) links virtues to the living traditions of institutions such as universities and hospitals, claiming that

> Lack of justice, lack of truthfulness, lack of courage, lack of the relevant intellectual virtues—these corrupt traditions. . . . [A]n adequate sense of tradition manifests itself in a grasp of those future possibilities which the past has made available to the present. (587)

We will have more to say about virtue theory as applied to health care organizations in Chapter 18.

Natural Law This is also a theoretical approach that arose from theology, and consists of

> A set of codes (rules, precepts) (a) intended by nature and grounded in some "higher" or "transcendent" reality, (b) which prescribes what should or should not be done, (c) which is universally binding upon all humans, and (d) which can be found by a rational examination of nature. (Angeles 1981, 150)

In secular health care ethics work today, natural law has more of an historical than contemporary influence. *Secular law* as jurisprudence has positivist roots that articulate complex systems of rules and responsibility (Flew 1979,197–198). Secular law furnishes "a rich source of seminal cases, about matters such as refusal of treatment, the termination of life, and surrogate motherhood . . ." (Hoffmaster 1999, 139–140). Although the law has had an effect that was "overwhelmingly reactive in nature", together with theology and liberal political ideology it helped to entrench human rights in early bioethics (Hoffmaster 1999, 140; see also Furrow 2009).

Human Rights A right is a justified claim or an entitlement (Sim 1995). Rights can be understood as constraining more powerful individuals from overriding certain interests of less powerful individuals. There are many views about what constitutes rights, how rights are claimed, and the power of rights.[4] Human rights and legal theorists encourage the advancement of human rights through a mechanism of progressive realization that allows for states or nations to set benchmarks and actively work toward achievement of them (Clapham 2007). This regime of progressive realization is often contentious because of the fiscal and resource constraints of many states or nations. A right to health care is not so much based on some notion of what is essential to be respected as a person, as on what is fair treatment in a society with a particular set of medical and economic resources.

It is important to note that human rights approaches are now being increasingly advocated for addressing complex social and medical challenges such as HIV disease (UNAIDS 2008a; UNAIDS 2008b). Although these rights approaches hold great hope, they require exploration of their strengths and limitations (Austin 2001/2003). For example, a human rights approach to HIV requires thoughtful consideration of the competing needs of persons living with HIV and the social contextual constraints that contribute to full realization of human rights approaches to HIV for all persons in a given jurisdiction.

Current understandings of *international* human rights provide for the protection of basic needs to sustain human life and dignity (United Nations 1948; Office of the United Nations High Commissioner on Human Rights 1966a). It is critical to understand that recognizing limitations to a state's (or nation's) ability to meet every need of persons within its geographic boundaries does not preclude the state from its international obligation to establish policies to bring about the progressive realization of human rights for all (UNAIDS 2008a; 2008b). We need sufficient understanding of human rights approaches to support global strategies respectful of human dignity, particularly in situations such as the criminalization of HIV transmission (UNAIDS 2008a).

Concluding Summary What our brief sketch above has shown is that utilitarianism, deontology, contractarianism, virtue theory, natural law, secular law, and rights theory contributed a great deal to the development of early bioethics and continue to influence health care ethics today. Students in philosophy and early bioethics learned the various theories and engaged in the critique of them from alternative perspectives. Although philosophers often argued for the superiority of a particular theory, more generally the field— particularly in its early days—could reasonably be characterized as one of competition between incommensurable moral theories. In other words, adherence to one perspective necessarily required that one held the position that other theories were, at best, misguided. In the meanwhile, it is interesting to note that one feature of our recent historical trajectory is a growing re-emphasis of the importance of virtues and human rights, at least in part as a response to widening social inequities from local through to global contexts.

Early History and Traditions of Bioethics

As the medical ethical historian Jonsen (1997) noted, "the work of healing, from time immemorial and in all cultures, has been wrapped in moral and religious meanings" (3). However, the biotechnological advances throughout the 1950s and 1960s, as well as post-World War II concerns about Holocaust medical experimentation, generated new problems that resulted in the birth of a new discipline—bioethics (Arras, Steinbock, and London 1999; Caplan 2009; Evans 2000; Jonsen 1997; Pellegrino 1993; Roy, Williams, and Dickens 1994; Yeo 2010a). Bioethics emerged in response to grave and sometime unanswerable questions that resulted from the use and institutionalization of new technologies of science—uses that could lead to immense good or unspeakable harm. The Nuremberg trials and related concerns about human experimentation (United Nations War Crimes Commission 1947–1949), along with other discoveries including publication of reports of blatant ethical misconduct in research involving human subjects (Beecher 1959; 1966), resulted in widespread fear about the clear dangers of unrestricted and unpoliced use of technology (see also Chapter 14). The resultant distrust of professionals and institutions was also manifested in the "anti-establishment" movement of the 1960s and was evident in the considerable attention given to iatrogenic effects of medical treatments. An early project of bioethics—one that soon became known as the *doctrine of informed consent* (discussed in more detail in Exhibit 4-2)—was initially intended to assure that human participants in medical research projects were truly voluntary. With the acceptance that informed consent was an essential element of medical treatment and the participation in research, the cultural authority of physicians and medical institutions, although far from undermined, came under critical assessment. These events also resulted in codification of international legal instruments to set minimal standards for fundamental human rights (Office of the United Nations High Commissioner on Human Rights 1966a; 1966b; United Nations 1948).

Early bioethical issues such as the problem of informed consent were articulated as problems through the early modern discourse we described above. *However, practitioners' intuitive responses about right actions or policies began to challenge the primacy of the philosophical theories.* In this emerging world of biomedical technology and its associated ethical complexities, the offerings of philosophers seemed relatively humble. At the same time, theologically inclined theorists (who gained prominence in early bioethics work) were more concerned with practical problems individuals faced as they endeavoured to provide members of their faith with the means to reconcile their beliefs with ethical problems and to act in a manner consistent with their religious commitments. These changes in focus marked a shift from the use of health care examples in philosophical discourse to illustrate metatheoretical concepts to what we now know as bioethics—the topical discussion of health care issues from theoretical perspectives. Interestingly, theological contributions to bioethics are also evident in human rights discourses and includes contributions from liberation theology.[5]

Initial efforts in bioethics proposed internally consistent, systematic approaches to ethical issues in health care. Although some philosophers maintained their commitment to particular ethical theories, many others seemed to abandon the search for unifying and justifying metaethical foundations. Instead, they focused on developing theories of bioethics that made sense of specific moral intuitions about health, health care, doctor–patient relationships, patient values, and social values. The result was a proliferation of bioethics texts, commencing in the late 1970s and early 1980s. The primary focus was on the theoretical support for agreement about what constituted the ethical elements of the problem. All of these texts shared a selective use of ethical theories to argue for the reasonableness of their claims that certain values were moral values and important (e.g., autonomy). Concepts developed to explain shared moral intuitions were used to provide guidance in the more controversial examples. While different positions were held on moral issues such as abortion, positions were not usually presented as strictly deduced from one specific moral theory. Many of the advances in bioethics were tied to cross-cutting conceptual analyses that clarified moral issues. Jane English's (1975) discussion of a self-defense argument for abortion and James Rachels' (1975) attack on the distinction between active and passive euthanasia stand as important examples of these early conceptual advances.

Corresponding with the growth of bioethics was the growth of health professionals' interest in bioethics. Physicians, lawyers, nurses, chaplains, and a variety of other health-related professionals, as well as patients, administrators, and politicians, became interested in the concepts developed by those involved in bioethics. They were primarily interested in the concepts as tools to assist in the resolution of specific cases and policy issues. Collaboration between physicians and philosophers or theologians resulted in finer-tuned presentations of clinical and personal details in specific ethical problems, clarifying the range and specific justification for practices and policies. Bioethics became a practice and academic discipline that was interdisciplinary in nature and was located in the institutions of health care, education, law, and policy. It is now a unique and substantial domain of applied ethics (see Exhibit 4-1).

EXHIBIT 4-1

Classifications and Terminology

Ethics is a branch of philosophy.[6] In orienting to the field of ethics, it is important to note that, as generally understood, the major divisions of ethics as a discipline include descriptive ethics, normative ethics, and metaethics (Yeo 2010a). *Descriptive ethics* focuses on factual descriptions of moral behaviour and belief systems or beliefs; *normative ethics* focuses on the formulation and defense of basic principles, values, virtues, and ideals governing moral behaviour[7], and *metaethics* focuses on an analysis of meaning, justification, and inferences of moral terms, concepts, and statements (Hoffmaster 2001). *Applied ethics* focuses on problems associated with specific practice contexts (Fisher 2009, 4). Whereas the term "ethics" usually refers to any of the above as a formal field of inquiry, "morality" usually refers to personal attributes and actions, though the two terms are often used interchangeably. As distinguished from ethical theory, *moral*

theory has been influenced by the field of developmental psychology—the study of at what point and under what circumstances individuals develop the capacities to act according to acceptable standards (see, for example, Flanagan 1991). This is important because these origins colour prevailing beliefs about how persons act morally, a topic that we will elaborate on in later chapters, particularly Chapter 9.

The terms "bioethics," "biomedical ethics," "medical ethics," "clinical ethics," and "health care ethics" are also often used interchangeably in common parlance. Our own preference is to use the term *health care ethics* (instead of "bioethics," "biomedical ethics," or "clinical ethics") to refer to the field of applied ethics that addresses ethical concerns affecting the health care system—concerns experienced by patients, families, health care professionals/providers, health care organizations, and society as a whole

(Rodney 1997). Within health care ethics, there are concerns particular to the sciences of biomedicine (for instance, debates about cloning), concerns that are particular to each of the professions (medical ethics, nursing ethics, pharmacy ethics, and so on, all of which are also related to professional ethics), and concerns that are particular to organiza-tions (which are also related to business ethics).[8] When we use the term "bioethics" in this chapter, we will be referring to the more traditional (circumscribed) study of health care ethics that occurred early in the development of the discipline and continues to some extent today. Otherwise, our preferred term will be "health care ethics."

The Principles of Bioethics

Introduction As bioethics became established in the late 1970s and early 1980s, *practitioners and theorists sought an approach that would preserve the wisdom found in the ethical theories but would not demand the restrictions created by commitment to any one specific theory.* They also sought an approach that would focus more strongly on particular situations. Ethical principles offered great promise here. An ethical principle was seen as "an essential norm in a system of thought or belief, forming a basis of moral reasoning in that system" (Beauchamp 1996, 81). "Principlism" was the belief that some set of principles could be arrived at from multiple ethical theories that would be useful in concrete applications. The search for and application of these principles consumed bioethicists throughout the last quarter of the twentieth century. Moreover, there was a strong related interest on the part of government policy-makers. American groups such as the National Commission for the Protection of Human Subjects of Biomedical and Behavioral Research (in the 1970s) and the President's Commission for the Study of Ethical Problems in Medicine and Biomedical and Behavioral Science (in the 1980s) established principles that were used to justify policy positions and were applied in health care related decision making (Evans 2000).

The most often-cited work articulating ethical principles is Beauchamp and Childress' *Principles of Bioethics*, a detailed explication of which was presented in the fourth edition of their book (1994; see also Beauchamp and Childress 2008). Building on the work of the philosopher W. D. Ross, Beauchamp and Childress chose four *prima facie* principles especially appropriate for bioethics and relevant to human rights: autonomy, beneficence, nonmaleficence, and justice (Pellegrino 1993, 1160). As the medical ethicist Edmund Pellegrino (1993) explained, this "tetrad of principles had the advantage of being compatible with deontological and consequentalist theories and even with some aspects of virtue theory" (1160). Beauchamp and Childress' work was theoretically rich enough to be the object of philosophical study and adequately non-technical to encourage study by health care professionals interested in bioethics. Principle-oriented bioethics evolved into the rational, objective, and impartial application of the four ethical principles in bioethical theory and moral development theory (Arras, Steinbock, and London 1999; Tong 1997; Yeo 2010b).

Autonomy The principle of autonomy became central to the work of Beauchamp and Childress (1994), within the American commissions we cited above, and, subsequently, within bioethics in general (Arras, Steinbock, and London 1999; Tong 1997). Autonomy can be understood as an observation about human nature and morality, with an ethical imperative drawn from it. The observation about human nature is that human beings *have the ability to act voluntarily, based on information*. Evidence of human autonomy can be found in the moral experience of guilt, blame, or shame—emotions that are contingent on a belief that in a particular instance we could have acted otherwise. That we believe we would have behaved differently if we knew then what we know now is further evidence of our belief in autonomy. The observation about morality is that it makes sense to hold people morally responsible for their actions only if they actually *could* have chosen to act differently (i.e., were autonomous). Coercion and incorrect belief are reasonable moral excuses because they qualify this sense of autonomy.

It is important to note that the *doctrine of informed* consent (discussed further in Exhibit 4-2) is rooted in the principle of autonomy (Arras, Steinbock, and London 1999; Hoffmaster 1999; Tong 1997). The ethical imperative is that autonomy, as the element of human nature that makes morality possible, should be protected. Tristam Engelhardt Jr. (1986) described this form of argument about autonomy as a requirement of morality per se and therefore as a side-constraint on all theories. The principle of autonomy is also an essential element to human rights approaches to health. For individuals to claim—and fully realize—their fundamental human rights, they must be able to autonomously act to engage with their rights and the responsibility that accompanies each human right.

Beneficence and Nonmaleficence The principles of beneficence and nonmaleficence are sometimes combined under the former term, and, at other times, considered to be different from one another. In bioethics, these two principles may be used in either a Kantian or a utilitarian manner (Arras, Steinbock, and London 1999; Tong 1997; see also Yeo and Moorhouse 2010). In early bioethics—and in some more recent writings—there is a definite utilitarian flavour to the use of "beneficence" and "nonmaleficence," in that every act or option is subject to a harm–benefit analysis. This may be partially due to the nature of medical practice, in which patient benefit is sought, but only by actions that are less harmful than beneficial. This has been characterized in ethics or philosophy of medicine as *primum non nocere*. On the other hand, a Kantian influence can be discerned when beneficence, or promoting benefit to other persons, is considered "weaker" than duties to avoid harm, such as nonmaleficence.

The implementation of the principle of autonomy together with beneficence and nonmaleficence can be illustrated by considering appropriate moral practice in delivering health care services. First, it is the duty of health care professionals to evaluate specific interventions to determine whether they are more beneficial than harmful when applied to the relevant population (i.e., to those with a similar clinical condition). Similarly, the principles of beneficence and nonmaleficence are embodied in the clinical judgment of whether individual patients are at heightened risk or are likely to benefit (e.g., contraindications). But even with the scrupulous application of beneficence and nonmaleficence, patients' autonomy must be respected. *In more Kantian terms, patients are not to be treated simply as means to the end of their health, but as ends in themselves.* This requires that persons who will be recipients of health care services themselves evaluate the options and possible harms and benefits, and that they choose how to be treated. This additional requirement, labelled the "doctrine of informed consent," is an attempt to balance health care professionals' endeavours to benefit patients with patients' expression of informed choice. This is the challenge that all health care professionals face—negotiating between the tension created by competing perspectives on "the good" in general situations and applying these in particular moments of practice with particular persons (see Exhibit 4-2).

EXHIBIT 4-2

Informed Consent

One of the central values of the Canadian Nurses Association's (2008) *Code of Ethics for Registered Nurses* is to promote and respect informed decision making (11–12). This value is based on respect for individual autonomy—respect that all health care professions ascribe to in their codes of ethics. A key means of operationalizing this respect is through the process of informed consent for options for treatment and care. Patients need to be able to understand information as it is provided, to evaluate the information and their own concerns, and to consider continuing commitment or withdrawal of consent. And nurses have an obligation to ensure that the entire process is voluntary, informed, respectful, and supportive.[9]

It is important to note that health care professionals can play a significant role in the gatekeeping of information and services. *Consent will often be only as informed as the health care professional allows,* since options may be omitted, risks or benefits may be emphasized or minimized, and professional opinions may carry considerable persuasive weight. For example, alternative forms of health care or options that a health care professional considers inappropriate may not be disclosed. Further, patient autonomy has never, in the complex version of principles of bioethics, been given full authority—a request for service that a health professional considers harmful and without justifying benefit does not establish an obligation to provide the service. Decision making is supposed to be done collaboratively between (ideally) reflective and active patients and professionals who provide the information and expertise to assist in the interpretation of the choices the patient faces (see also Chapter 13). But collaborative decision making also recognizes that the wishes of a patient do not authorize access to health care resources independent of the assessment of a health care professional that the service is helpful and without undue risk. Individual patients are expected to make the right decisions for themselves if they are logical and if they are given the right information, and if they fail to do so, the professional (usually the physician) intervenes. If they are judged not competent, an individual proxy (substitute) decision maker is appointed (see also Chapter 14).

Informed consent *should be* a reflection of continuing communication, collaboration, and commitment. Rather than being a one-time evaluation of information and a decision about how to proceed, the emphasis *should* be on a *relationship* in which the health professional provides new information about effectiveness and risks, encourages patients to reflect on and express their interests, and takes action to make options available (see also Chapter 5 as well as Moorhouse, Yeo and Rodney 2010).

The emphasis on continuing communication, collaboration, and commitment, and the delineation of the professional–patient relationship (including boundaries) in the above conceptualization of informed consent are useful in clinical practice. *However, the emphasis in the traditional bioethical approach is on the role of the health care professional in relation to individual, rational patients.* This leaves us with little insight into the role of emotion, conflict, or power imbalances in patient–professional relationships (Hoffmaster 2001; Rodney et al. 2002; Sherwin 1992; 1998; Wolf 1994a; see also Chapter 8). It also leaves us with little insight into the role of family or community in decision making (Burgess et al. 1999; Nelson 1998; Robinson 2011.). We will say more about these limitations as we close this chapter and in Chapter 5.

Justice This fourth principle is best known as a basis to argue for a right to health care (Daniels 1985; Rawls 1971; 1993; Yeo, Rodney, Moorhouse and Khan 2010). However, over the history of bioethics, justice has been the most poorly operationalized ethical principle (Aroskar 1992; Bekemeier and Butterfield 2005; Daniels 1996; Reimer-Kirkham and Browne 2006), and, in our current sociopolitical era, it is under the most threat (Anderson et al. 2009; Daniels, Kennedy, and Kawachi 2004; Sen 2009).[10] As will be shown in subsequent chapters in this book (particularly Chapters 12, 18 and 21), patients, families, communities, and health care providers currently face deep and disturbing questions about justice in health care delivery, so we will offer some elaboration here on this fourth principle. Indeed, it is more than a principle—it is also a theory and is closely tied to political philosophy. While we cannot elaborate on political philosophy here,[11] we can say more about the theory that underlies justice.

Justice, and in particular *distributive justice*, is an attempt to decide how to be fair in the distribution of resources. Justice is also used to provide other reasons to limit patient "demands" for treatments. Some treatments are inadequately beneficial to justify resource dedication. On the other hand, beneficial treatments may be too expensive to meet the full demand without unacceptable loss of other important opportunities. The use of available evidence to guide health policy holds promise for the improvement of health status for many persons and includes interventions to address determinants of health and the rational use of health-related goods and services.

Philosophical discussions that enrich the use of justice in bioethics are broad, and can be divided in two manners. *One split is between* **procedural** *and* **substantive** *rules of justice*. References to "due process" and lotteries or "first come–first served" maxims are examples of procedural rules of justice. John Rawls' (1971) mechanism of the "veil of ignorance" is an example of a procedural approach to determining justice in policy.[12] Substantive approaches to justice attempt to make a strong case for particular rules of distribution that are fair, such as "to each according to ability" or "to each according to need." Rawls' (1971) view of justice is based on a sophisticated form of a substantive rule that accepts as just rational self-interest arrived at through a process of reflective equilibrium.[13] Norman Daniels (1985) extends Rawls' work to health care, articulating a view of justice based on human needs and fair equality of opportunity.

The second way of splitting the discussion of justice in bioethics *is by types of resources being allocated*. These discussions typically divide considerations of justice into three levels: micro-, meso-, and macro-allocation (Kluge 1992; Yeo 1993; Yeo, Rodney, Moorhouse and Khan 2010). **Macro-allocation** is usually characterized as the division of societal resources into various types of services to benefit the population. The central question is how much to invest in each of the different ways to address the public's interests. The issue may be whether education and health care should receive similar or different levels of funding (or reductions). This decision making is typically governmental. Proposals and commentaries for health care reform based on claims about citizens' rights to health or health care are also examples of macro-allocation. More recent efforts by health care economists, human rights advocates, and a growing number of ethicists emphasize that the goal of health care should be to improve the population's health (see, for example, Daniels et al. 2004; Farmer 2003; Marmot 2004; and Sen 2009; see also Chapters 12 and 20). They claim that determinants of health are more effective approaches to improving population health and to narrowing the gap of health between economic groups and between different countries (see also World Health Organization 2008a; 2008b). As we will discuss further in Chapter 5 in relation to *social* justice, these efforts to determine a fair distribution of societal resources to health care are themselves embedded in claims about the role of health care in society. For example, Daniels (1985) claims that the moral goal of access to health care is to promote equality of opportunity, and secondarily to compensate for irreversible loss of opportunity.

Meso-allocation is typically the division of a health care budget among various health care services. This decision making can be governmental, regional, or institutional. Some meso-allocation policies come from professional bodies, or from departments of health care professionals within institutions (e.g., policy decisions about whether to perform genetic testing for sex-determination or cleft palate). The type of meso-allocation closest to macro-allocation is focused on determining what services to include in a publicly funded health care system (see also Chapters 12 and 19). More specific policies regarding criteria for patients who are eligible for specific services such as transplants, other surgical techniques, and expensive diagnostic imaging are also meso-allocation decisions. Most of these policies operate implicitly on a *material principle* of justice of "to each according to need," whereby it is not unjust to deny access to a service from which one cannot benefit. This principle is inadequate to eliminate scarcity, because there are genuine shortages (e.g., of organs), and because there may be a lack of will or ability to dedicate adequate resources at the macro level to cover all services that genuinely meet need. Further, justice according to need distributes knowledge and technologies reactively once they have been developed, not proactively in anticipation of need. Nonetheless, justice according to need can serve as a basis to assign health priorities based on population health research (see also Chapters 18 and 20).

Given the above, the material principle of meso-allocation is typically supplemented with some sort of *procedural principle* that allows persons of similar need (i.e., those who stand a roughly equal chance of benefitting from the service if they receive it) to have an equal chance of getting the service. This may be first come–first served, or a lottery. In a situation in Oregon a number of years ago when public dialogue took place about how to allocate resources at a state level, there was an attempt to construct a community-wide ranking of the importance of the services and a cutoff point on the list based on an estimate of what the state could afford to fund from a set budget (Hadorn 1992; Starzomski 1997; see also Daniels and Sabin 2008). Neither approach is adequate. Better procedural principles for just meso-allocation decision making are urgently needed in today's era of regionalization of health care services, and more comprehensive public participation in meso-allocation decision making is crucial (see also Chapters 18 and 21).

Daniels and a number of colleagues have been pursuing the operationalization of "accountability for reasonableness" in an attempt to work towards better procedural principles (Daniels and Sabin 1997; 2008; Martin, Abelson, and Singer 2002). The conditions for accountability for reasonableness include *relevance* (based on sound evidence, reasons, and principles), *publicity* (public accessibility), *appeals* (a mechanism for challenges and dispute resolution), and *enforcement* (voluntary or public regulation) (Martin, Ableson, and Singer 2002, 223; see also McDonald's "An Ethical Framework for Making Allocation Decisions" in Appendix C).

Micro-allocation is the distribution of services to individual patients. The primary decision is professional determination of whether the individual would benefit from a service, and whether the person wants the service. Individual health care professionals or health care teams typically make micro-allocation decisions. However, concerns about economic pressures sometimes motivate micro-allocation decisions that are more appropriately determined as meso-allocation issues. For instance, an expensive treatment might not be offered to a particular patient who, although she would benefit, does not have a supportive family or does not speak English or is seen as having "caused" her own problem (see also Chapter 21). It is important to note that there is a danger that health care professionals will violate their ethical obligations if they try to save program costs (meso-allocation) through such ad hoc rationing at the micro level (Pellegrino 1993; Starzomski and Rodney 1997; Yeo, Rodney, Moorhouse and Khan 2010). This is a real danger in today's era of escalating cost constraint (Caulfield 2002; Mohr and Mahon 1996; Rodney and Varcoe in press). The use of individual ethical decision-making models can help health care providers to work toward more just decision making at the micro level (see also Chapter 13 of this text and McDonald's "An Ethical Decision-Making Framework for Individuals" in Appendix B).

Summary The principles of bioethics as described above have enabled a diverse set of professionals and academics as well as some community members and advocacy groups to find a language with which to discuss problematic health care situations. They provided some needed clarity in ethical debates, furnishing "an orderly way to 'work up' an ethical problem," leading to "fairly specific action guidelines," and avoiding "direct confrontation with the intractably divisive issues of abortion, euthanasia, and a host of other issues on which agreement seemed impossible" (Pellegrino 1993, 1160). Organizing the information about a case or information relevant to a policy around ethical principles has often encouraged discussion about the goals of treatment and the involvement of patients and family to assess goals, benefits, and harms from their particular perspectives. However, as we have indicated in our analysis so far (and will expand on in the section below and in Chapter 5), this traditional approach does not help us to understand and to deal with the personal, social, and cultural aspects of health as well as the complex sociopolitical climates in which health care is delivered and in which resources for health are embedded. In philosophical terms, we see the principles as necessary but not sufficient.

A CONFLICTED LANDSCAPE? CHALLENGES IN THEORY AND APPLICATION IN HEALTH CARE ETHICS

Critiques

Human Rights As we argued earlier in this chapter, the re-emergence of a human rights emphasis to support equitable access to the resources for health and health care is promising. However, a remaining challenge with international legal frameworks for human rights is a lack of enforcement mechanisms for many macro-level treaties. At the same time, justice at the macro-allocation level has always presented a problem of resources and lost opportunity costs for highly differentiated needs. The problem of establishing the strength of justice claims across diverse ways to meet needs will likely remain challenging and subject to opportunities presented by the trajectories of technologies as well as strong vested interests in competition with each other.

Notwithstanding the challenges we have noted above, in future work it will be important to further consider the reciprocal relationship between law and ethics—especially in human rights discourses—such that each contributes to the advancement of the other. This kind of discourse must include a full exploration of the interrelationships between ethics, morals, values, and the laws of human rights (Weissner and Willard 1999). Overall, there is a need for better articulation of the role of human rights law and human rights approaches to health care challenges. Such an integration of human rights and ethics approaches may bring about the realization of more just outcomes where health outcomes and human dignity would be the ultimate goal. In Chapter 18 on organizational ethics and health/health care policy and Chapter 21 on challenging inequities, we explore this problem in our local Canadian context further and point toward some solutions.

Ethical Principles Although the principle-oriented approach to health care ethics has been widely accepted, over the past two decades or so there have been serious concerns raised about its adequacy. It is important to note that some of the concerns may be related to how the principles have been used in practice rather than theoretical limitations in the principles themselves (Levi 1996; Pellegrino 1993; Yeo 2010b).[14] In the hands of busy clinicians, educators, and even ethicists, there has been a tendency to employ them in a non-contextual and reductionist manner. For instance, in applying the principle of autonomy to a dying patient's request not to have his family told of his prognosis, the discussion might quickly centre around whether he was competent, informed, and unconstrained, with little exploration of the meaning behind his request, his understanding of his own and his family's grief processes, the values he held about his family's well-being, and so on. The principle of autonomy, despite its rich theoretical traditions, can too easily be reduced to binary equations (competent/incompetent; informed/uninformed; constrained/ unconstrained) if not handled with careful reflection and good clinical insight.

Even given that many of the problems with bioethical principles may have to do with how they are used rather than with the theory underlying principles, there remain a number of problems with using principlism as the sole basis for work in health care ethics. It appears that there is a lack of consensus about the nature of fundamental ethical principles, and that ethical principles are not easily prioritized or applied to concrete moral situations (Ackerman 1983, 170–173). Principle-oriented ethics has been criticized for relying on ethical principles to the exclusion of other variables known to influence ethical practice, for not reflecting the breadth and diversity of concepts available in the general ethics literature, and for fostering a prescriptive, formal approach by which principles are applied in a process-dominated manner (Penticuff 1991, 236–240; see also Baker 2009 and De Vries 2004). The sources of theory and the processes of theorizing are thus both being held up for scrutiny.

One area of critique comes (directly and indirectly) from virtue-based discourses. Beauchamp and Childress (1994) themselves acknowledge that ". . . morality includes more than obligation" (452). They suggest that morality is a combination of the character traits of persons who make judgments as well as the obligations expressed in principles and rules. In this way, both virtue-based and principle-based approaches are required to describe the ethical obligations, ideals, "reliable character," and "moral good sense" in professional–patient relationships (Pellegrino 2001; Pellegrino, Veatch, and Langan 1991; Sellman 2000; 2006). Megan-Jane Johnstone (2004) goes further, claiming that virtue ethics have been revitalized in response to dissatisfaction with dominant mainstream theories' ability to provide an adequate account of the "moral life." *In our view, virtue-based accounts of morality are a useful supplement to principlism.* They help to overcome the tendency for bioethical principles to place an undue emphasis on the moral minimum of obligations while largely ignoring characters and personal dispositions for their influence on moral deliberation and action (see also Chapter 9).

A second area of critique comes from *discourses about culture.* The principle-based approach has been criticized as "culturally specific and intellectually problematic" in terms of its "uncritical emphasis . . . on the individual and his or her rights (as opposed to the web of human relationships that engender mutual obligations and interdependence), the techniques of rational abstraction that uproot issues from their concrete human reality, and the assumption that these techniques and values have universal applicability" (Weisz 1990, 3; see also Geertz 2000 and De Vries 2004). What this means is that health care ethics has not, historically, attended very well to diverse human meanings related to culture. And it has certainly not been terribly reflective about the cultural inheritance it has received from biomedicine, liberal individualism, and a variety of other sources. We will have more to say about these areas of critique in Chapters 5 and 18.

Thirdly, *feminist theorists* have made significant contributions to the critique—and reformulation of—theory and theorizing in health care ethics. Feminists have warned for some time now that health care ethics "has been strong on proclaiming individual autonomy to choose, but weak on insisting on access to health care and the creation of choices for those who have few" (Wolf 1994b, 402; see also Peter 2011). Feminists have also warned that the rational, non-contextual application of ethical principles misses the subtle and pervasive power dynamics that infuse patient/family/provider relationships within hierarchical institutions. Once again, in Chapter 5 we will have more to say about this area of critique and the subsequent contextual (cultural, feminist, Aboriginal, and relational) theorizing in ethics that is now beginning to flourish.

A Peace Proposal: Integrating New Approaches to Theorizing in Health Care Ethics

Where do these critiques leave us in our pursuit of ethical theory and theorizing for practice in nursing and other health care disciplines? Put simply, we contend that no one theoretical schema—whether metaethical theories, ethical principles, virtues, or even cross-cultural or feminist theory—can furnish everything we need to inform the study and practice of health care ethics. As Arras, Steinbock, and London (1999) have argued, we ought not to "view the various theoretical alternatives as mutually exclusive claims to moral truth. Instead, we should view them as important but partial contributions to a comprehensive, although necessarily fragmented, moral vision" (9).[15] This is still a fairly recent development in the way that theory is developed and used in health care ethics. As we indicated at the outset of this chapter, the early history of work in ethics was such that adherence to one perspective necessarily required that one held the position that other theories were, at best, misguided. We believe that the growing call from theorists to work with more than one form of theory marks a significant shift and offers great promise. Indeed, the premise of this entire text is that we ought to consciously explore, develop, and apply the insights of theorists from various perspectives arising in philosophy, nursing, medicine, law, psychology, the social sciences, political sciences, cultural studies, and other related fields.

It is important to be clear that we are not arguing for the ad hoc and potentially sloppy development and application of theory. Rather, *we are arguing for the use of a broad range of theory that best serves the ethical practice of nurses and other health care providers and best informs ethical health care policy work.* This requires understanding the history, strengths, and challenges of whatever theory we work with, and it necessitates reconciling tensions between various forms of theory (McGee 2003). As will be argued in the next chapter, for instance, we will want to hold on to the protection of individual rights that the ethical principle of autonomy offers, but also broaden autonomy to encompass contextual concerns (Baylis et al. 2008; Burgess 1999; Sherwin 1998). *How* to manage a coherent and effective traverse of such a variety of perspectives is not yet entirely clear, but, fortunately, a growing number of theorists such as Daniels are working on it.

In an insightful (and entertaining) chapter that tackles the current controversies in the use of theory in health care ethics, Daniels (1996) created a Tolkien-esque metaphor of a war between three kingdoms (see Exhibit 4-3).

EXHIBIT 4-3

A War between Kingdoms (Based on Daniels 1996)

The Uplanders—Theorists who subscribe to grand theories such as deontology
The Middle Kingdom—Principlists who subscribe to mid-range ethical principles

The Lowlanders—Contextualists (for instance, feminists and cultural theorists) who prefer to rely on experiential knowledge

---

Daniels' (1996) metaphor provides an historical exploration of the problems and interactions among the levels. He subsequently draws up a "peace proposal" for the three kingdoms. The first declaration in his peace proposal is "There is not one kind of ethical problem, but there are many kinds, and different problems require somewhat different approaches" (Daniels 1996, 112).

The application of Daniels' peace proposal relies on his adaptation of Rawls' (1971) concept of reflective equilibrium. Daniels articulates a notion of *"wide reflective equilibrium,"* which "seeks coherence among three divisions of moral thought" (Winkler 1996, 64)—that is, between the three kingdoms. More specifically:

> The method of wide reflective equilibrium . . . seeks coherence among three divisions of moral thought: our considered moral judgements, a set of principles designed to rationalize and order these judgements, and a set of relevant background theories or understandings about subjects such as human nature and psychology, the workings of the law and procedural justice, conditions for social stability and change, and the socio-economic structure of society. (Winkler 1996, 64)

Summary

As we said at the outset of this chapter, our adoption and development of ethical theory should be thoughtful and conscious, and our theorizing should involve processes of critical reflection. In closing, we agree with Daniels and Winkler that we need to adopt and continue to refine theory from all three kingdoms. And we agree that our theorizing can benefit from processes such as wide reflective equilibrium. In Chapter 5 we will continue to explore both of these conclusions.

For Reflection

1. Through what stages has health care ethics theorizing evolved, and what have some of the challenges been at the various stages?

2. How might the values embedded in utilitarian theory differ from deontological theory?

3. One of the challenges in using principle-based ethics is that strategies to support one principle might threaten another. Can you think of clinical situations in which supporting autonomy might threaten beneficence?

4. Given that justice is the least understood and the most badly operationalized principle, what are the implications for policy related to distribution of resources?

5. Think about Daniels' (1996) claim that "There is not one kind of ethical problem but there are many kinds, and different problems require somewhat different approaches" (112). Can you list some of the different kinds of ethical problems you encounter in your practice? You may find it helpful to distinguish between problems that you encounter at the micro, meso, and macro levels.

Endnotes

1. In everyday language, utilitarianism can be thought of as "the end justifies the means," and deontology can be thought of as "do unto others as you would have them do unto you." Contractarianism focuses more on fair process. See also Keatings and Smith (2010) and Yeo (2010b) for further elaboration on the complexities of ethical theories.

2. Rawls' social contractarianism has been described as Kantian because people are to be valued as ends in themselves in his theory—in other words, people are not to be used as the means to others' ends (Arras, Steinbock, and London 1999, 17–19). The late Rawls continued his work on contractarianism

and his related theory of justice after the publication of his influential *A Theory of Justice* (1971), working toward an understanding of "justice as fairness as a form of political liberalism" (1993, xxix). See also Sen (2009) for a recent analysis and extension of Rawls' theorizing.

3. See Kihlbom (2000) for an interesting analysis of a particularist version of virtue ethics, Sellman (2000; 2006) for an application of virtue ethics to nursing, and Holland (2010) for a critique of a virtue ethics approach to nursing.

4. See, for example, Sumner (1989) for comprehensive overviews of rights and Daniels (1985, 4–9) for a discussion of rights to health care. The Canadian HIV/AIDS Legal Network (2009/2004) has also published an informative document on human rights, privacy, public policy, and law. Johnstone (2004) and Austin (2001/2003) provide further analyses and applications of rights approaches in nursing ethics.

5. Major theological organizations have established human rights documents, including the *Cairo Declaration on Human Rights in Islam* (United Nations 1990) and *Dignitatis Humanae* (Vatican 1965), the latter of which is the Roman Catholic Church's seminal document recognizing the importance of human rights on a global scale.

6. The other fields include epistemology, ontology (or metaphysics), logic, and aesthetics.

7. In philosophy, "normative" has to do with questions of value. However, within the social sciences, the word holds a somewhat different meaning—normative implies what is standard, and hence "normal."

8. This is by no means a well-standardized nomenclature, and several of the fields overlap. Many theorists see health care ethics (or bioethics), business ethics, and professional ethics as subsets of the larger field of applied ethics. It is worth noting that Roy, Williams, and Dickens (1994) warned that the concept of applied ethics itself is problematic, that by definition ethics *is* application—a guide to how humans ought to act in relation to one another.

9. Readers are encouraged to familiarize themselves with the practice guidelines for informed consent within their own professional and geographic locations. For nurses in Canada, the Canadian Nurses Association (2008) *Code of Ethics for Registered Nurses* provides significant guidance, and provinces have related practice standards about how informed consent should be operationalized (see, for example, the College of Registered Nurses of BC [2011] *Practice Standard: Consent for Registered Nurses and Nurse Practitioners* at https://www.crnbc.ca/Standards/Lists/Standard Resources/359ConsentPracStd.pdf.) Further, Chapter 6 in Keatings and Smith (2010) provides a comprehensive overview of the ethical and legal foundations of and practices to promote informed consent. And Chapter 6 in Oberle and Raffin Bouchal (2009) provides a thorough and insightful discussion of how nurses can promote informed decision making. See also Williams (2008) for a bioethical analysis of consent and its application.

10. One of the major challenges of justice claims is that they are complicated, involving a wider cast of persons than most other principles, and the duties that follow include commitments of resources from identifiable persons or institutions.

11. Political philosophy is an important field of study that can shed light on many of the justice problems we face in health care ethics. It covers theories such as utilitarianism, liberal equality, libertarianism, Marxism, communitarianism, and feminism (Jaggar 1988; Kymlicka 1990), as well as theories related to multiculturalism (Farrelly 2004; Kymlicka 1995; Taylor 1992). We will say more about political philosophy in Chapter 18.

12. The *veil of ignorance* is a hypothetical procedure in which individuals make decisions about fair allocation of resources in a society. Their decisions are based on a general knowledge of human society, political affairs, economic theory, and so on, but *not* on knowledge of the particular circumstances of

their own society, or on what their particular position will be (Rawls 1971, 136–150). Because the individuals engaging in this procedure are rational and do not know how vulnerable their particular position might be, they will, Rawls (1971) argues, "prefer more primary social goods than less" (142).

13. Rawls' theory of justice (1971) is based on two components. One "proposes a criterion of justice that ranks feasible alternative basic structures by the minimum representative lifetime share of social primary goods each of them tends to generate" (Pogge 1989, 109). The second component "imposes two requirements upon the social and economic inequalities an institutional scheme may generate: the *opportunity principle* and the *difference principle* [emphases in original]" (Pogge 1989, 161). In the opportunity principle Rawls argues that there must be equality of opportunity, and in the difference principle he argues that the distribution of goods should benefit the least well off (Pogge 1989, 161–165). In other words, both principles put limits on rational self-interest such that the worst off in society are advantaged. The process of reflective equilibrium is "the study of principles which govern actions shaped by self-examination. . . . A knowledge of these principles may suggest further reflections that lead us to revise our judgements" (Rawls 1971, 48–49). Thus, reflective equilibrium suggests that our moral judgments can be influenced by theory. See Sen (2009) for a recent theory of justice that is based in part on Rawls' work. Sen's focus is on the role of public reason in establishing what can make societies less unjust.

14. In a chapter responding to various critiques of principlism, Beauchamp (1996) explains that he believes "that a misunderstanding of principles and a misleading account of the theories that are under attack appear in many of these criticisms" (80). He goes on to explain that he is using a *prima facie* rather than a robust conception of principles. This means that principles are "exceptionable and nonfoundational" and we are therefore "free to view every moral conclusion supported by a principle and every principle itself as subject to rejoinder, refutation, and reformulation" (85).

15. Susan Wolf (1994b) calls this approach the rise of *pragmatism*. See Rorty (1999), Bernstein (1991), and McGee (2003) for thoughtful discussions of pragmatism and ethics. See also Hartick Doane and Varcoe (2005) for a thoughtful discussion of pragmatism and ethical nursing practice.

References

Ackerman, T.F. 1983. Experimentalism in bioethics research. *Journal of Medicine and Philosophy, 8* (3), 169–180.

Anderson, J.M., Rodney, P., Reimer-Kirkham, S., Browne, A.J., Khan, K.B., and Lynam, M.J. 2009. Inequities in health and healthcare viewed through the ethical lens of critical social justice: Contextual knowledge for the global priorities ahead. *Advances in Nursing Science, 32* (4), 282–294.

Angeles, P.A. 1981. *Dictionary of philosophy*. New York: Barnes & Noble Books.

Aroskar, M.A. 1992. Ethical foundations in nursing for broad health care access. *Scholarly Inquiry for Nursing Practice, 6* (3), 201–205.

Arras, J.D., Steinbock, B., and London, A.J. 1999. Moral reasoning in the medical context. In J.D. Arras and B. Steinbock (Eds.), *Ethical issues in modern medicine* (5th ed.; pp. 1–40). Mountain View, CA: Mayfield.

Austin, W. 2003. Using the human rights paradigm in health ethics: The problems and the possibilities. In V. Tschudin (Ed.), *Approaches to ethics: Nursing beyond boundaries* (pp. 105–114) Edinburgh: Butterworth Heinmann. (Reprinted from *Nursing Ethics* 2001; *8* [13], 183–195.)

Baker, R. 2009. The ethics of bioethics. In V. Ravitsky, A. Fiester, and A.L. Caplan (Eds.), *The Penn Centre guide to bioethics* (pp. 9–20). New York: Springer Publishing.

Baylis, F., Kenny, N.P., and Sherwin, S. 2008. A relational account of public health ethics. *Public Health Ethics, 1* (3), 196–209.

Beauchamp, T.L. 1996. The role of principles in practical ethics. In L.W. Sumner and J. Boyle (Eds.), *Philosophical perspectives on bioethics* (pp. 79–95). Toronto: University of Toronto Press.

Beauchamp, T.L. and Childress, J.F. 1994. *Principles of biomedical ethics* (4th ed.). New York: Oxford University Press.

Beauchamp, T.L. and Childress, J.F. 2008. *Principles of biomedical ethics* (6th ed.). New York: Oxford University Press.

Beecher, H.K. 1959. *Experimentation in man*. Illinois: Charles C. Thomas.

Beecher, H.K. 1966. Ethics and clinical research. *New England Journal of Medicine, 274*, 1354–1360.

Bekemeier, B. and Butterfield, P. 2005. Unreconciled inconsistencies: A critical review of the concept of social justice in 3 national nursing documents. *Advances in Nursing Science, 28* (2), 152–162.

Bernstein, R.J. 1991. *The new constellation: The ethical–political horizons of modernity/ postmodernity*. Cambridge, MA: MIT Press.

Burgess, M. 1999. Introduction: Part III: Ethical issues in the delivery of health care services. In H. Coward and P. Ratanakul (Eds.), *A cross-cultural dialogue on health care ethics* (pp.157–159). Waterloo, ON: Wilfrid Laurier University Press.

Burgess, M., Stephenson, P., Ratanakul, P., and Suwonnakote, K. 1999. End-of-life decisions: Clinical decisions about dying and perspectives on life and death. In H. Coward and P. Ratanakul (Eds.), *A cross-cultural dialogue on health care ethics* (pp. 190–206). Waterloo, ON: Wilfrid Laurier University Press.

Canadian HIV/AIDS Legal Network. 2009. 3.2 Privacy and confidentiality: Privacy: Human rights, public policy, and law. In J. Fisher (Ed.), *Biomedical ethics: A Canadian focus* (pp. 80–94). Don Mills, ON: Oxford University Press. (Reprinted from Canadian HIV/AIDS Legal Network. 2004. *Privacy protection and the disclosure of health information: Legal issues for people living with HIV/AIDS in Canada*, www.aidslaw.ca/publications/interfaces/download File.php?ref=189.)

Canadian Nurses Association. 2008. *Code of ethics for registered nurses*. Ottawa, ON: Authors.

Caplan, A.L. 2009. The birth and evolution of bioethics. In V. Ravitsky, A. Fiester, and A.L. Caplan (Eds.), *The Penn Centre guide to bioethics* (pp. 3–7). New York: Springer Publishing.

Caulfield, T.A. 2002. Malpractice in the age of health care reform. In T.A. Caulfield and B. von Tigerstrom (Eds.), *Health care reform & the law in Canada: Meeting the challenge* (pp. 11–36). Edmonton: University of Alberta Press.

Clapham, A. 2007. *Human rights: A very short introduction*. Oxford: Oxford University Press.

College of Registered Nurses of British Columbia. 2011. *Practice standard: Consent for registered nurses and nurse practitioners*. Vancouver, BC: Authors.

Daniels, N. 1985. *Just health care*. New York: Cambridge University Press.

Daniels, N. 1996. Wide reflective equilibrium in practice. In L.W. Sumner and J. Boyle (Eds.), *Philosophical perspectives on bioethics* (pp. 96–114). Toronto: University of Toronto Press.

Daniels, N., Kennedy, B., and Kawachi, I. 2004. Health and inequality, or, why justice is good for our health. In S. Anand, F. Peter, & A. Sen (Eds.), *Public health, ethics, and equity* (pp. 63–91). Oxford: Oxford University Press.

Daniels, N. and Sabin, J.E. 1997. Limits to health care: Fair procedure, democratic deliberation and the legitimacy problem for insurers. *Philosophy and Public Affairs 26,* 303–350.

Daniels, N. and Sabin, J.E. 2008. Accountability for reasonableness: An update. *British Medical Journal, 337,* a1850.

De Vries, R. 2004. How can we help? From "sociology in" to "sociology of" bioethics. *Journal of Law, Medicine & Ethics, 32,* 279–292.

Engelhardt, H.T. Jr. 1986. *The foundations of bioethics* (2nd ed.). New York: Oxford University Press.

English, J. 1975. Abortion and the concept of a person. *Canadian Journal of Philosophy, 5* (2), 233–234.

Evans, J.H. 2000. A sociological account of the growth of principlism. *Hastings Center Report, 30* (5), 31–38.

Farmer, P. 2003. *Pathologies of power: Health, human rights, and the new war on the poor.* Berkeley: University of California Press.

Farrelly, C. 2004. Introduction: Part seven: Multiculturalism. In C. Farrelly (Ed.), *Contemporary political theory: A reader* (pp. 263–267). London: Sage Publications.

Fisher, J. 2009. Morality and ethics. In J. Fisher (Ed.), *Biomedical ethics: A Canadian focus* (pp. 1–21). Don Mills, ON: Oxford University Press.

Flanagan, O. 1991. *Varieties of moral personality: Ethics and psychological realism.* Cambridge, MA: Harvard University Press.

Flew, A. (Ed.). 1979. *A dictionary of philosophy* (2nd ed.). New York: St. Martin's Press.

Fraser, N. and Nicholson, L.J. 1990. Social criticism without philosophy: An encounter between feminism and postmodernism. In L.J. Nicholson (Ed.), *Feminism/postmodernism* (pp. 19–38). New York: Routledge.

Furrow, B.R. 2009. Health law and bioethics. In V. Ravitsky, A. Fiester, and A.L. Caplan (Eds.), *The Penn Centre guide to bioethics* (pp. 35–45). New York: Springer Publishing.

Geertz, C. 2000. *Available light: Anthropological reflections on philosophical topics.* Princeton, NJ: Princeton University Press.

Hadorn, D. 1992. The problem of discrimination in health care priority setting. *Journal of the American Medical Association, 268* (11), 1454–1459.

Hadot, P. 1995. *Philosophy as a way of life: Spiritual experience from Socrates to Foucault.* New York: Blackwell.

Hartrick Doane, G., and Varcoe, C. 2005. Toward compassionate action: Pragmatism and the inseparability of theory/practice. *Advances in Nursing Science, 28* (1), 81–90.

Hoffmaster, B. 1999. Secular health care ethics. In H. Coward and P. Ratanakul (Eds.), *A cross-cultural dialogue on health care ethics* (pp. 139–145). Waterloo, ON: Wilfrid Laurier University Press.

Hoffmaster, B. 2001. Introduction. In B. Hoffmaster (Ed.), *Bioethics in social context* (pp. 1–11). Philadelphia: Temple University Press.

Holland, S. 2010. Scepticism about the virtue ethics approach to nursing ethics. *Nursing Philosophy, 11* (3), 151–158.

Jaggar, A.M. 1988. *Feminist politics and human nature*. Totowa, NJ: Rowman and Littlefield.

Jonsen, A.R. 1997. Introduction to the history of bioethics. In N.S. Jecker, A.R. Jonsen, and R.A. Pearlman (Eds.), *Bioethics: An introduction to the history, methods, and practice* (pp. 3–11). Boston: Jones and Bartlett.

Johnstone, M.J. 1999. *Bioethics: A nursing perspective* (3rd ed.). Sydney: Harcourt Australia.

Johnstone, M.J. 2004. *Bioethics: A nursing perspective* (4th ed.). Sydney: Churchill Livingstone.

Keatings, M. and Smith, O. 2010. *Ethical and legal issues in Canadian nursing* (3rd ed.). Toronto, ON: Mosby Elsevier.

Kihlbom, U. 2000. Guidance and justification in particularistic ethics. *Bioethics, 14* (4) 287–309.

Kluge, E.H.W. 1992. *Biomedical ethics in a Canadian context*. Scarborough, ON: Prentice-Hall.

Kymlicka, W. 1990. *Contemporary political philosophy: An introduction*. Oxford: Clarendon Press.

Kymlicka, W. 1995. *Multicultural citizenship: A liberal theory of minority rights*. Oxford: Clarendon Press.

Levi, B.H. 1996. Four approaches to doing ethics. *The Journal of Medicine and Philosophy, 21*, 7–39.

MacIntyre, A. 1987. The virtues, the unity of a human life, and the concept of a tradition. In G. Sher (Ed.), *Moral philosophy: Selected readings* (pp. 574–589). San Diego: Harcourt Brace Jovanovich.

Macklin, R. 2008. Global justice, human rights, and health. In R.M. Green, A. Donovan, and S.A. Jauss (Eds.), *Global bioethics: Issues of conscience for the twenty-first century* (pp. 141–160). Oxford: Clarendon Press.

Marmot, M. 2004. Social causes of social inequalities in health. In S. Anand, F. Peter, and A. Sen (Eds.), *Public health, ethics, and equity* (pp. 37–61). Oxford: Oxford University Press.

Martin, D., Abelson, J., and Singer, P. 2002. Participation in health care priority-setting through the eyes of the participants. *Journal of Health Services Research & Policy, 7* (4), 222–229.

McGee, G. 2003. Preface to the second edition. In G. McGee (Ed.), *Pragmatic bioethics* (pp. xi–xvi). Cambridge: MIT Press.

Meilaender, G.C. 1995. *Body, soul, and bioethics*. Notre Dame: University of Notre Dame Press.

Mohr, W.K. and Mahon, M.M. 1996. Dirty hands: The underside of marketplace health care. *Advances in Nursing Science, 19* (1), 28–37.

Moorhouse, A., Yeo, M., and Rodney, P. (2010). Autonomy. In M. Yeo, A. Moorhouse, P. Khan, and P. Rodney (Eds.), *Concepts and cases in nursing ethics* (3rd ed.; pp. 143–179). Peterborough, ON: Broadview Press.

Nelson, J.L. 1998. Death, medicine, and the moral significance of family decision making. In J.F. Monagle and D.C. Thomasma (Eds.), *Health care ethics: Critical issues for the 21st century* (pp. 288–294). Gaithersburg, MD: Aspen.

Oberle, K. and Raffin Bouchal, S. 2009. *Ethics in Canadian nursing practice: Navigating the journey.* Toronto: Pearson Prentice Hall.

Office of the United Nations High Commissioner on Human Rights. 1966a. *International Covenant on Economic, Social, and Cultural Rights* [ICESCR]. Geneva: Author.

Office of the United Nations High Commissioner on Human Rights. 1966b. *International Covenant on Civil and Political Rights* [ICCPR]. Geneva: Author.

Pellegrino, E.D., Veatch, R.M., and Langan, J.P. 1991. Preface. In E.D. Pellegrino, R.M. Veatch, and J.P. Langan (Eds.), *Ethics, trust, and the professions: Philosophical and cultural aspects* (pp. vii–ix). Washington, DC: Georgetown University Press.

Pellegrino, E.D. 1993. The metamorphosis of medical ethics: A 30-year retrospective. *Journal of the American Medical Association, 269* (9), 1158–1162.

Pellegrino, E.D. 2001. The internal morality of clinical medicine: A paradigm for the ethics of the helping and healing professions. *Journal of Medicine and Philosophy, 26* (6), 559–579.

Penticuff, J.H. 1991. Conceptual issues in nursing ethics research. *Journal of Medicine and Philosophy, 16* (3), 235–258.

Peter, E. 2011. Fostering social justice: The possibilities of a socially connected model of moral agency. *Canadian Journal of Nursing Research, 43* (2), 11–17.

Pogge, T.W. 1989. *Realizing Rawls.* Ithaca: Cornell University Press.

Pojman, L.P. 2001. *Ethics: Discovering right and wrong.* Toronto, ON: Wadsworth.

Rachels, J. 1975. Active and passive euthanasia. *New England Journal of Medicine, 292*, 78–80.

Rawls, J. 1971. *A theory of justice.* Cambridge, MA: Harvard University Press.

Rawls, J. 1993. *Political liberalism.* New York: Columbia University Press.

Reimer Kirkham, S. and Browne, A.J. 2006. Toward a critical theoretical interpretation of social justice discourses in nursing. *Advances in Nursing Science, 29* (4), 324–339.

Robinson, C.A. 2011. Advance care planning: Re-visioning our ethical approach. *Canadian Journal of Nursing Research, 43* (2), 18–37.

Rodney, P.A. 1997. *Towards connectedness and trust: Nurses' enactment of their moral agency within an organizational context.* Unpublished doctoral dissertation, University of British Columbia, Vancouver.

Rodney, P. and Varcoe, C. in press. Constrained agency: The social structure of nurses' work. In F. Baylis, J. Downie, B. Hoffmaster, and S. Sherwin (Eds.), *Health care ethics in Canada* (3rd ed.). Toronto, ON: Nelson. (Revised version of Varcoe C. and Rodney P. 2009. Constrained agency: the social structure of nurses' work. In B.S. Bolaria and H.D. Dickinson [Eds.], *Health, illness, and health care in Canada* [4th ed; pp. 122–151]. Toronto, ON: Nelson Education.)

Rodney, P., Varcoe, C., Storch, J.L., McPherson, G., Mahoney, K., Brown, H., Pauly, B., Hartrick Doane, G., and Starzomski, R. 2002. Navigating toward a moral horizon: A multi-site qualitative study of nurses' enactment of ethical practice. *Canadian Journal of Nursing Research, 34* (3), 75–102.

Rorty, R. 1999. *Philosophy and social hope*. London: Penguin.

Roy, D.J., Williams, J.R., and Dickens, B.M. 1994. *Bioethics in Canada*. Scarborough: Prentice-Hall.

Sellman, D. 2000. Alasdair MacIntyre and the professional practice of nursing. *Nursing Philosophy, 1*, 26–33.

Sellman, D. 2006. The importance of being trustworthy. *Nursing Ethics, 13* (2), 105–115.

Sen, A. 2009. *The idea of justice*. Cambridge: The Belknap Press.

Sherwin, S. 1992. *No longer patient: Feminist ethics & health care*. Philadelphia: Temple University Press.

Sherwin, S. 1998. A relational approach to autonomy in health care. In S. Sherwin et al. (Eds.), *The politics of women's health* (pp. 19–47). Philadelphia: Temple University Press.

Sim, J. 1995. Moral rights and the ethics of nursing. *Nursing Ethics, 2* (1), 31–40.

Starzomski, R.C. 1997. *Resource allocation for solid organ transplantation: Toward public and health care provider dialogue*. Unpublished doctoral dissertation, University of British Columbia, Vancouver.

Starzomski, R. and Rodney, P. 1997. Nursing inquiry for the common good. In S.E. Thorne and V. E. Hayes (Eds.), *Nursing praxis: Knowledge and action*. (pp. 219–236). Thousand Oaks: Sage.

Sumner, L.W. 1989. *The moral foundation of rights*. Toronto: University of Toronto Press.

Taylor, C. (with A. Gutmann, S.C. Rockefeller, M. Walzer, and S. Wolf). 1992. *Multiculturalism and "the politics of recognition."* Princeton: Princeton University Press.

Tong, R. 1997. *Feminist approaches to bioethics: Theoretical reflections and practical applications*. Boulder, CO: Westview.

United Nations. 1948. *Universal declaration of human rights*. Geneva: Author.

United Nations. 1990. *Cairo declaration on human rights in Islam*. (U.N. GAOR, World Conf. on Human Rights [English translation]). Geneva: Authors.

UNAIDS. 2008a. *Policy brief: Criminalization of HIV transmission*. Geneva: Author.

UNAIDS. 2008b. *Report on the global HIV/AIDS epidemic 2008*. Geneva: Author.

United Nations War Crimes Commission. 1947–1949. *Law Reports of Trials of War Criminals: Selected and prepared by the United Nations War Crimes Commission: 1947–1949*. Geneva: Author.

Vatican. 1965. *Declaration on religious freedom: Dignitatis humanae on the right of the person and of communities to social and civil freedom in matters religious promulgated by His Holiness Pope Paul VI*. Rome: Author.

Weissner, S. and Willard, A.J. 1999. Policy-oriented jurisprudence. *German Yearbook of International Law, 44*, 96–112.

Weisz, G. 1990. Introduction. In G. Weisz (Ed.), *Social science perspectives on medical ethics* (pp. 3–15). Philadelphia: University of Pennsylvania Press.

Williams J.R. 2008. Consent. In P.A. Singer and A.M. Viens (Eds.), *The Cambridge textbook of bioethics* (pp. 11–16). Cambridge: Cambridge University Press.

Winkler, E. 1996. Moral philosophy and bioethics: Contextualism versus the paradigm theory. In L.W. Sumner and J. Boyle (Eds.), *Philosophical perspectives on bioethics* (pp. 50–78). Toronto: University of Toronto Press.

Wolf, S.M. 1994a. Health care reform and the future of physician ethics. *Hastings Center Report, 24* (2), 28–41.

Wolf, S.M. 1994b. Shifting paradigms in bioethics and health law: The rise of a new pragmatism. *American Journal of Law & Medicine, 20* (4), 395–415.

World Health Organization. 2008a. *Closing the gap in a generation: Health equity through action on the social determinants of health.* (Final Report of the Commission on Social Determinants of Health). Geneva: Authors.

World Health Organization. 2008b. *World Health Report 2008: Primary health care: Now more than ever.* Geneva: Authors.

Yeo, M. 1993. *Ethics and economics in health care resource allocation.* Ottawa: Queen's-University of Ottawa Economic Projects.

Yeo, M. 2010a. Introduction. In M. Yeo, A. Moorhouse, P. Khan, and P. Rodney (Eds.), *Concepts and cases in nursing ethics* (3rd ed.; pp. 11–36). Peterborough, ON: Broadview Press.

Yeo, M. 2010b. A primer in ethical theory. In M. Yeo, A. Moorhouse, P. Khan, and P. Rodney (Eds.), *Concepts and cases in nursing ethics* (3rd ed.; pp. 37–72). Peterborough, ON: Broadview Press.

Yeo, M. and Moorhouse, A. 2010. Beneficence. In M. Yeo, A. Moorhouse, P. Khan, and P. Rodney (Eds.), *Concepts and cases in nursing ethics* (3rd ed.; pp. 103–114). Peterborough, ON: Broadview Press.

Yeo, M., Rodney, P., Moorhouse, A., and Khan, P. 2010. Justice. In M. Yeo, A. Moorhouse, P. Khan, and P. Rodney (Eds.), *Concepts and cases in nursing ethics* (3rd ed.; pp. 293–316). Peterborough, ON: Broadview Press.

CHAPTER 5

Our Theoretical Landscape: Complementary Approaches to Health Care Ethics

Patricia Rodney, Michael Burgess, Bernadette M. Pauly, and J. Craig Phillips

Most ethical problem solving cannot . . . be either top down or bottom up but must be multifaceted and responsive to the demands of both context and theory. (Daniels 1996, 112)

While biomedicine has made great strides in understanding and treating a host of medical problems, and traditional bioethical theory has helped to promote respect for patients as self-determining persons, much more needs to be done. In particular, within ethics, nursing, and other health care professions we need to better understand and address the personal, social, and cultural aspects of health as well as the complex sociopolitical climates in which health care is delivered and in which resources for health are embedded. Such an understanding is necessary if we are to foster ethical practice and policy at all levels—from local through to global (Hoffmaster 2001; Sherwin 1998; 2011; Tong 1997). This entire text is constructed to help nurses as well as others involved in health care ethics to take up the challenge. And this chapter is meant to point to some complementary sources of contextual theory that can help. In particular, we sketch out some of the newer theoretical possibilities opened up by cultural, feminist, and relational writings in health care ethics.

CONTEXTUAL ETHICAL INQUIRY

In Chapter 4 we argued that our adoption and development of ethical theory should be thoughtful and conscious, and that our theorizing should involve processes of critical reflection. We agreed with the ethicists Norman Daniels (1996) and Earl Winkler (1993; 1996) that we need to take up and continue to refine ethical theory/insights from three different levels: (1) general theories (such as utilitarianism, deontology, and contractarianism); (2) mid-range ethical principles (autonomy, beneficence, non-maleficence, and justice); and (3) contextual (experiential or case) knowledge. And we agreed that our theorizing can benefit from processes such as wide reflective equilibrium.[1] The complementary approaches we explore in this chapter fall primarily in the third level—contextualism.

Winkler (1993) defines contextualism as

the idea, roughly, that moral problems must be resolved within concrete circumstances, in all their interpretive complexity, by appeal to relevant historical and cultural traditions, with reference to critical institutional and professional norms and virtues, and by utilizing the primary method of comparative case analysis. (344)[2]

The essential feature to understand about contextualism is that it "moves from the bottom up" (Winkler 1996, 52). In other words, it is an inductive approach to ethical theorizing. *We believe that it is most useful to think of contextualism as a lens through which we notice moral aspects that a different theoretical lens might tend to miss or distort.* As Margaret Urban Walker (2003) puts it:

> When context is ignored or effaced in theorizing, what we get is irrelevant or bad theory: theory that does not connect with life; theory that distorts, rather than reveals and clarifies its subject matter; theory that becomes a pastime and even a competitive game for theory-makers independently of whether the theory enhances our understanding of its subject matter. (xiii)

This does not mean that the distinction between context and theory is a "real" distinction—both intend to describe and appraise the moral components of life, and often overlap. The various forms of contextualist ethics include (but are not limited to) a revival of casuistry, the call for an inductivism based on empirical information or ethnography, interest in narrative bioethics, the articulation of care-based ethics, and relational ethics (Gadow 1999; Wolf 1994, 400).[3] Overall, we find that a contextual approach illuminates social, political, and historical factors that shape differences among individuals and groups along lines of ethnicity, gender, class, sexual orientation, and so forth. A contextual approach highlights how social location within a broader context is important. In so doing, it helps us to better appreciate how individual agents are situated within—and also influence—larger sociopolitical structures (Sewell 1992).

In advocating contextualism, it is important to note that we are *not* subscribing to or promoting relativism. That is, we do not believe that looking to attend to a diversity of experiences and contexts commits us to *cultural relativism* ("anything goes if it is particular to a culture") or *ethical relativism* ("ethical values are just individual preferences").[4] In our postmodern era when we are no longer convinced that there are absolute truths (Crotty 1998) it is nonetheless possible to look for values-based direction for action (Bernstein 2001; Geertz 2000; Rorty 1999; Squires 1993). As the anthropologist Clifford Geertz (2000) puts it, "the answers to our most general questions—why? how? what? whither?—to the degree they have answers, are to be found in the fine detail of lived life" (xi).

Contextual ethical inquiry seeks to gather subjective as well as objective data about the real world in which ethical theory is to be implemented and ethical action takes place. In other words, contextualism draws our attention to particular people and particular relationships in particular contexts. While contextualism requires that specific ethical judgments are based on the relevant details of specific situations, it also benefits from and generates more general insight on what counts as ethically relevant details across situations. This situation-specific relevance of contextualism is distinct from the stronger claim of ethical relativism that all ethical judgments are only situation-specific expressions of approval or disapproval. This is why we believe that the ability to draw on all three levels of ethical thought (general theories, mid-range ethical principles, and contextual knowledge) is so important (see also McCarthy 2006 and Yeo 2010). Theories and principles propose at least provisional general standards, while contextual insights help us to be more sensitive to nuance, personal meaning, social location, and the influence of context as we move toward the implementation of such standards. For example, let us consider how best to support a dying child and her grieving parents. We would want to understand her parents' social location and the resources they had available to deal with their grief (contextual features of the family), and we would also want to prevent the suffering of the child and engage her in decision-making as much as possible, based on her unique wishes and capacities (actions based on beneficence, nonmaleficence, and autonomy as well as individual features of the child).

In what follows in this chapter we will explore how cultural, feminist, Aboriginal, and relational ethics—which we treat as large and internally diverse subsets of contextualist ethics—direct our attention to concerns about the particular. All four subsets rely on inductive approaches that seek to illuminate the socio-political historical context in which individuals are located. Later, in Chapter 11, Marck widens the analysis we offer here to include ecological theory. Then in Chapter 18 we move to a more explicit analysis of how concerns about the socio-political context lead to considerations of organizational ethics and ethical policy for health/health care.

The complementary approaches we explore in this chapter help us to identify and integrate contextual features into our ethical analysis, and, subsequently, into our ethical practice. The approaches we explore in this chapter are fruitful, as each illuminate somewhat different contextual features. There are other approaches that are also capable of generating important insights for work in health care ethics. For instance, ethnography, critical social sciences, and economic analyses serve similar purposes. They can greatly enrich the approaches we discuss in this chapter.[5] Many of the various forms of contextualism will be elaborated on in more detail later in the text. For instance, Nisker will explore the use of narrative-based ethics in Chapter 6, and Bergum as well as Hartrick Doane and Varcoe will explore relational ethics in Chapters 7 and 8 respectively. What these chapters share is the insight that moral problems ought to be addressed within real and concrete contexts and circumstances.

Cultural Terrain

Critiques

Theorists and practitioners interested in ethics from the lens of culture have told us that Western medicine is not neutral but, rather, "modern Western medicine is itself a culture alongside the other cultures" (Coward and Ratankul 1999, 3). Traditional ethical theories such as utilitarianism, Kantian ethics, social contract theory, libertarianism, or other human rights–based theories reflect the cultural values and beliefs of the Western world and are dominated by European and American influences and infused with an inherent cultural ethnocentricity (Coward and Ratankul 1999; Fox 1990; Fox and Swazey 2008; Kleinman 1995). As one theorist has observed,

> In their analyses of complex situations, ethicists often appear grandly oblivious to the social and cultural context in which these occur, and indeed to empirical referents of any sort. Nor do they seem very conscious of the cultural specificity of many of the values and procedures they utilize when making ethical judgements. (Weisz 1990, 3; see also De Vries 2004)

Although there has been significant progress since Weisz (1990) delivered his sting-
ing critique, in Western health care and health care ethics we have tended to treat culture as being relevant only when we encounter people from "other" ethnic groups,
forgetting that everyone, including those of us who have white skin and speak English,
come from an ethnic background (Coward and Ratanakul 1999). Even so, culture is
much more than just ethnicity. It includes individualized as well as shared values and
beliefs. A richer notion of culture is that of "shared meaning systems" (Shweder 1984, 1)
that are fundamental to individuals' understandings of "what selfhood is" (Geertz 1984,
126; see also Coward and Ratanakul 1999; Geertz 2000). Our conceptualization of
culture ought to be inclusive of understandings of differences in gender, sexual orientation, ethnicity, race, and class. Culture is not static, but is fluid and evolves over
time. Thus, our conceptualization of culture ought to recognize that "definitions and
meanings of ethnicity and race are social constructions that shift constantly, reflecting
the changing dynamics of gender, race/ethnic, and class relations over time" (Ng 1993,
227; see also Bhabha 1994; Varcoe, Pauly, and Laliberté in press; and Chapter 13). In
other words, conceptualizations of culture must include historical origins as well as
evolving practices and relationships. Finally, culture permeates everything we do:
"[C]ulture is a process occurring between people(s) . . . the transmission and creation of
both illness and health care are also cultural processes" (Stephenson 1999, 84). *This
means that all of us involved in health care delivery and/or health care ethics come from
our own disciplinary, specialty, and organizational orientations, as well as from our
own background of personal, familial, and community values and beliefs.* Indeed, nursing as a profession has its own complex and varied culture[6], as do the other health care
professions. Culture therefore operates in health care at all levels—from individual values, beliefs, and meanings, to group norms and practices, to organizational patterns and
societal ideologies (see Chapter 18 for an exploration of societal ideologies).

The understandings of culture we have articulated above have, historically, not been
well operationalized in Western health care or Western health care ethics. There is evidence of a lack of sensitivity to social and cultural contexts, and evidence of the effects
of what happens when Western biomedicine dominates non-Western and traditional or
aboriginal cultures. Within the West, despite our liberal ideology, there are serious social
inequities based on attributes such as gender, sexual orientation, ethnicity, race, and
class. When people who are recent immigrants, people of Aboriginal ancestry, people
who are impoverished, women, youth, people who struggle with substance use, the
chronically ill, the aged, those with a non-heterosexual orientation, and any others who
are marginalized because of how they are stigmatized by society try to access the Western health care system, they frequently confront communication barriers and conflicts in
ideology, if not outright discrimination (Anderson et al. 2009; Canales 2010; Dodds
2005; Pauly 2008a; Peternelj-Taylor 2004; Thorne, Bultz, and Baile 2005; Tait 2008;
Tarlier, Browne, and Johnson 2007). In the situation of Western health care in Canada
for Aboriginal cultures,[7] there has been little opportunity for Aboriginal Canadians to
engage in informed or participatory relationships with health care providers (Browne et
al. 2011). In fact, Western health care delivery systems and other social systems (such as
the residential schools that existed until a few decades ago) have disrupted the Aboriginal communities and systems of care that sustained people in more traditional times

(Browne, Smye, and Varcoe 2005; Ermine 2007; Report of the Royal Commission on Aboriginal People 1996a; 1996b; 1996c).[8] Western health care and health care ethics have been increasingly influenced by the evolution of a global corporate culture in which capital flows around the world largely to serve the interests of an economically dominant elite (Coburn 2010; Rodney and Varcoe in press; Saul 2005; 2008).[9] The consequences for fiscally constrained health, educational, and social services have been serious, and include progressively widening inequities in the resources for health and health care (Austin 2011; Coburn 2010; Commission on the Future of Health Care in Canada 2002; Myrick 2004; Rodney and Varcoe in press; Stein 2001; Storch 2010).[10] Thus, when Western health care is exported to other cultures, the results can be problematic. Education of health care professionals and the adoption of health care technology to other countries are often accompanied by implicit or explicit instruction in Western notions of health and health care ethics (Coward and Ratanakul 1999; Fox and Swazey 2008; Frenk et al. 2010). Overall, there is a certain ethnocentrism in Western health care ethics that devalues the contribution of other cultures to the process of ethical reflection and decision-making (Burgess 1999a; 1999b; De Vries 2004). While the historical concern in Western health care ethics to avoid ethical relativism is understandable, there has not been enough room left to negotiate between different meanings or to understand the influence of different contexts.[11]

Let us illustrate with an example. Ethics in Practice 5-1 comes from a focus group interview with nurses practicing in an emergency department. The nurse we have quoted was participating in a qualitative study of nurses' ethical practice. In this research transcript segment, she tells a story of an encounter that has left her troubled.

ETHICS IN PRACTICE 5-1

An Emergency Nurse's Story

There was a man not too long ago, his wife was miscarrying, and she didn't speak English, right—only he spoke English—so the surgeon explains [what is wrong with her and the proposed surgery] and the man is standing there supposedly translating to the woman. So I say to him, "She's going to sign the consent, ask her what she understands about it." He replied, "Doctor is going to fix it and make the baby okay." Because that's what he told her. So I say to the man, "She doesn't understand." He replied, "Yes, that's what I want her to know." So, he wasn't too pleased with me because I got the Interpreter Services to come and explain to her because she's signing a legal consent so that she understands what's going to happen to her. The man was so pissed off at me because he would tell her later in his own time that the baby was gone . . . or maybe not. (Adapted from Storch et al. 2001)

Our intent in citing the situation in Ethics in Practice 5-1 is not to judge whether the nurse's actions were right or wrong, or to label the nurse as praiseworthy or blameworthy. Rather, in this chapter we want to use the emergency nurse's story to shed light on some of the practical challenges of health care ethics, and to illustrate the promise of some of the insights that cultural, feminist, organizational, and political perspectives can bring. We will therefore reflect on Ethics in Practice 5-1 at various points throughout the rest of the chapter.

For a start, on the face of it, the emergency nurse's story tells of her attempt to protect the patient's autonomy and uphold her right to informed consent.[12] These are important goals and, indeed, are enshrined in the code of ethics that directs the nurse's practice (Canadian Nurses Association 2008). However, the nurse has apparently focused on the patient in isolation from (in fact, in opposition to) her husband and possibly the rest of the patient's family.[13] As we indicated in Chapter 4, this kind of individualistic approach to autonomy has been part of the philosophical, legal, and political heritage of traditional bioethics. This does not make the nurse's worry about autonomy incorrect. But it does mean that there were other morally relevant features in the situation that she presumably overlooked. Morally relevant features are often rendered invisible by a limited clinical and ethical focus.[14]

The patient and husband portrayed in Ethics in Practice 5-1 came from an ethnic background different from the nurse's and from the majority of other health care providers in the emergency department, and they were not fluent in English. Regardless of their ethnic background, it would have been important to find out more about how the husband was making sense of the situation, and the personal meaning that he and his wife held about what she was going through. As well, it would have been important to try to understand their social location—such as being immigrants or refugees, being poor or disadvantaged in other ways. If the husband had a particular belief about protecting his family, it would have been important to find out more about that. *Such beliefs may or may not have been linked to his ethnic identity—it would have been crucial to avoid stereotyping him on the basis of language fluency, race, or any other characteristic.* Questions such as how he and his wife liked to make decisions in the family and what was important to him and his wife in this pregnancy would have been helpful (see also Chapter 13). And more use of the hospital's interpreter services could have assisted the nurse to better understand the wife's perspectives more directly. The nurse may have, in the end, made the same disclosure to the patient based on her concerns about autonomy, but she and the rest of the health care team would have *also* been better able to help the husband to understand and participate in the decision as much as possible. Instead, the husband was likely left feeling angry and betrayed, which would not help him to support his wife or help them both to deal with their grief.

The story recounted by the nurse in Ethics in Practice 5-1 also says something about *the culture of health care*. As a result of the global corporate culture we have sketched out above, health care delivery in general—and emergency departments in particular (Rodney et al. 2006; Sanders, Pattison, and Hurwitz 2011)—are operating under a pervasive *ideology of scarcity* that rewards quick problem solving and efficient processing (Rodney and Varcoe in press; Varcoe 2001). The nurse had a legitimate concern about the patient's informed consent, but little time to more fully explore that concern. Indeed, she was almost certainly facing a backlog of other patients waiting for the patient's bed. The structure of work in the emergency department—including the expectations of her colleagues to clear the patient out to surgery quickly—militated against the nurse's ability to spend more time with the patient and the patient's husband even though she had access to (at least some) interpreter services. This is not to absolve the nurse of her responsibility to try to work more with the patient and the patient's husband and/or to bring in other resources. But it is to say that the culture of the emergency department she was operating in made it difficult. She was left with protecting the patient's right to informed consent as her default position.

As Ethics in Practice 5-1 illustrates, the application of Western health care ethics to *all* cultures, and especially non-Western and traditional or Aboriginal cultures, needs critical examination. In the Western conception, a person has a bounded, unique, more or less integrated motivational and cognitive universe—a dynamic centre of awareness, emotion, judgment, and action supposedly organized into a distinctive whole. This whole is understood in isolation from other such wholes and in isolation from its social and natural background. Yet focusing on isolated individuals is a rather peculiar idea within the context of many of the world's cultures. Understanding others demands recognizing our individualistic orientation, and seeing others' experiences within the framework of their own ideas of selfhood (Coward and Ratanakul 1999; Fox and Swazey 2008; Geertz 1984, 126; 2000).

Possibilities

While the traditions of Western ethics have made considerable contributions (such as in the area of human rights), *cultural imperialism*[15] remains a serious challenge. The moral issue is that we have not recognized the worth of other cultures as resources for our ethical theory and theorizing (Ermine 2007; Jameton 1990; Taylor 1992). This occurs at least in part because *we have failed to recognize the role of our own culture in our theories and judgments.* Taylor (1992) has suggested that we need to begin the study of any other culture with the presumption that "we owe equal respect to all cultures" (66). One major implication is that we ought to respect the contributions that the wisdom of various cultures can offer to Western health care ethics. If the culture of Western health care is to improve, we will need to have a richer composite of ethical approaches—as Daniels (1996) has articulated, theory and theorizing from general ethical theories, mid-range principles, and contextual approaches.

There is an opportunity here for us to draw on theories and traditions from various cultures for cross-cultural dialogue on the nature of ethics and the goals of health and health care. For example, Aboriginal belief systems in Canada are, in general, based on a notion of a balanced universe made up of energy fields, where the world, the environment, the community, the family, and the self are interwoven and move in harmony together (Ermine 2007). Thus, the four components of body, mind, emotion, and spirit are interwoven and are believed to be balanced in health and imbalanced in disease (Shestowsky 1993, 7). Given the current critiques of the Western focus on isolated individuals, our development and use of ethical theory could be enriched by Aboriginal understandings of the need for balance and harmony between the self, the land, and the universe (Ellerby 2008; Willms et al. 1992).[16] Turning to another example, Western health care ethics could also be enriched by the Buddhist notion of compassion. Compassion is

> a central moral ideal in Buddhism. . . . [I]t is a universal and dispassionate love conjoined with knowledge. It radiates in the mind as a result of the recognition of human vulnerability to pain and suffering and the realization of the illusory nature of the Ego or the "I" that begets all form of self-seeking desires. (Ratanakul 1999, 122)

The Buddhist definition of compassion could contribute substantially to current Western discussions of ethics because of its acknowledgement of human vulnerability and its critique of self-interest (see also Keown 2008).

Drawing on the wisdom of Aboriginal and Buddhist perspectives, then, in Ethics in Practice 5-1 we could come to a recognition that the woman, her fetus, and her husband are part of an extended and integrated family, community, and geographic place that will have significant meaning to the woman and her family. Compassion extended toward her and her family would go beyond fulfilling duties related to achieving informed consent or "clearing a bed in the emergency department" and would more fully encompass the moral ideals to which we aspire in balancing or attention to individual rights and the social location of others. As well, we could look at the nurse's social location to be sure that we are not overly harsh in our judgment of her actions, recognizing the web of relationships she is responding to in her complex environment, including the needs of other patients, colleagues, and the emergency department in addition to her own expertise, education, and personal experiences (see also Chapters 9, 10, and 11).

Since morality is acted out in a cultural context, it is critical to try to engage in a dialogue with others about their cultural beliefs and practices before we pass judgment or implement decisions (see also Chapter 13). We therefore need to acquire the knowledge and skills required to create the opportunity and space for enhanced intercultural exchange and understanding. In the situation in Ethics in Practice 5-1, for instance, we need to know more about *how* to approach the patient and her husband with questions about the patterns of decision-making in their family and about what was important to them in this pregnancy. Fortunately, as we have indicated above, there is a growing body of work by Western health care professionals and ethicists aiming at just this kind of knowledge and skill. Moreover, there is an increasing array of theoretical, policy, and practice literature available that is written by individuals from a variety of ethnocultural groups. Such literature can enhance cultural understandings as well as the ongoing development of theory and theorizing in health care ethics.

Feminist Terrain

Some of the strongest challenges to the disciplinary history and the traditional theoretical focus of bioethics have been raised by feminist ethicists. Feminist ethics offers an alternate view of contemporary ethical issues and traditional ethical theory. Jagger (1991) has noted, "The two parallel strands of feminist ethical work—the attention to contemporary ethical issues on the one hand and the criticism of traditional ethical theory on the other—together gave rise to the term 'feminist ethics,' which came into general use in the late 1970s and early 1980s" (81). Initially, feminist ethics brought the perspective of women's experience into the field of health care ethics and a belief that theory should be based on women's life experience (Sherwin 1992; Warren 1989). While the early focus in feminist health care ethics was on reproductive issues, since then feminist ethics has taken on a wider range of issues, not just those that have to do with women's reproductive capacities (Wolf 1994, 404–405).[17] The gender attentiveness of feminist ethics highlights the limitations of the first two levels of theory (general theories and principles), which are not sensitive enough to context and individual particularities (Wolf 1994, 405).

A primary contribution of feminist ethics is the examination of a wider variety of ethical issues than in traditional bioethics, especially those issues related to gender bias and sexism in health care delivery (Liaschenko and Peter 2003; Sherwin 1992; Wolf 1994). An important shift over the past three decades in feminist theory and feminist ethics has been the recognition that the experiences of all women are not the same, and that factors such as race, class, and resources have an important impact on experience (Anderson et al. 2009; Lebacqz 1991; Reimer-Kirkham and Anderson 2010).

The Canadian ethicist Susan Sherwin has been an important contemporary voice in feminist ethics. She has further expanded the scope of feminist ethics to address issues of oppression and power inequities more broadly. In her early book, *No Longer Patient: Feminist Ethics and Health Care* (1992), she described the intent of feminist approaches to health care ethics as follows:

> Feminism expands the scope of bioethics, for it proposes that additional considerations be raised in the ethical evaluation of specific practices: it demands that we consider the role of each action or practice with respect to the general structures of oppression in society. Thus medical and other health care practices should be reviewed not just with regard to their effects on the patients who are directly involved but also with respect to the patterns of discrimination, exploitation, and dominance that surround them. . . . In addition, feminism encourages us to explore the place of medicine itself in society. (4–5)

Feminism explicitly raises issues such as the inequality and unequal treatment of women and others in health care (both patients and workers), discrimination on the basis of sexual orientation or (dis)ability or other personal attributes, sexist occupational roles in which gender roles of caring are assigned to female workers, job-related stress, and conflicts in relationships. *Embedded within these issues is the claim that ethical analysis requires attention to power in health care settings*—"who has it, how it works, and how to fix the current inequities" (Wolf 1994, 406). An additional claim made by feminist ethics is that "analysis of power and morality cannot proceed without careful attention to context and difference" (406). Feminist theory draws attention to the quality of relationships—particularly the power in those relationships—at individual, organizational, and societal levels. And in Sherwin's recent work (2011) she warns us that the societal power relationships within and between nations need more attention if we are to address the serious and growing inequities in access to resources for health and health care locally and globally.

A number of applications of feminist ethics appear later in this text, particularly in Chapter 9 (on nurses' moral agency), Chapters 10 and 11 (on the moral climate for nursing practice), Chapter 18 (on ethics in organizations and policy), and Chapter 19 (on ethical issues in home care). For now, let us return to our consideration of Ethics in Practice 5-1. As a theoretical lens, feminist ethics raises somewhat different considerations than those we have discussed so far in relation to ethics from a cultural view.

Power Relations

For one, feminist ethics reminds us to consider the power relations that might be at play in the situation in Ethics in Practice 5-1. We ought to inquire about the quality of the relationship between the patient, her husband, and the rest of the family. The patient and her husband may be living in situations of unequal balance of power related to decision-making and control of their lives, and we ought to be sensitive to the fact that she (or any other patient) *may* be living in an abusive situation. As would be the case in any patient assessment, it was important for the nurse to ensure that the woman had some time alone with herself or another health care provider and a translator who was not a member of her family. It takes strong clinical and communication skills to make this kind of assessment without jeopardizing the relationships between the health care providers, the patient, and the family. We ought *not* to proceed with the inaccurate (but widely held) stereotype that only women who come from immigrant, Aboriginal, or impoverished families experience violence (Varcoe 2001; 2004; Varcoe and Einboden in press). As we have said earlier, the husband's preference for non-disclosure may well have come from a sincere desire to protect his wife.

Other power relations we ought to consider include how, in Ethics in Practice 5-1, the nurse may have internalized prejudices about people from particular ethnocultural groups, how the staffing and rapid pace in the emergency department made it difficult for her to sit down and listen to the patient, and the pressure she may have experienced from her colleagues and managers to operate "efficiently" and not spend too much time talking with patients and their families (Rodney and Varcoe in press; Varcoe 2001). Feminist theory will also help us to understand why nurses in that emergency department—and in almost every other arena of health care delivery—are so excessively stretched (see also Chapters 9, 10, 11, 12, 18, and 19).

Relational Autonomy

Feminist ethics has also shifted our notion of the ethical principle of autonomy. Conventional views of autonomy hold that an autonomous individual has the capacity to (1) be "sufficiently competent" to make a decision; (2) choose reasonably from the available options; (3) obtain adequate information and demonstrate understanding of the information related to the options available; and (4) not be coerced by others (Sherwin 1998). When we think of this principle in light of a contextual approach to ethics, the application of autonomy as a guide to ethical decision-making becomes far more complex. An important challenge we face is that, in Western societies, the value of respect for autonomy as a principle of ethical practice has tended to be accepted as a universal truth (Burgess et al. 1999). Furthermore, conventional perspectives on autonomy have been challenged by feminist theorists in reaction to notions of Kantian individualism and claims related to invariant developmental sequencing of moral orientations (Gilligan 1982; Sherwin 1998).

Sherwin (1998) draws our attention to what a broader and more contextualized understanding of what autonomy might mean in health care decision-making. She posits an alternative view that she terms *relational autonomy*. Sherwin defines relational autonomy as "a capacity or skill that is developed (and constrained) by social circumstances. It is exercised within relationships and social structures that jointly help to shape the individual while also affecting others' responses to her efforts at autonomy" (36; see also Baylis, Kenny, and Sherwin 2008; Ho 2008; and Mackenzie 2008).

Conventional views of autonomy have also been disputed by post-structural theorists, who suggest that the very idea of autonomy is a sort of illusion of the Enlightenment conception of person (Mackenzie 2000). Whereas feminist theorists tend to support a more relationally composed understanding of autonomy, post-structural theorists insist that understandings of self and identity, and consequently of autonomy, are products of language and power.[18] Post-structuralist and feminist theorists therefore remind us to think about the power dynamics of the sociopolitical contexts we operate in as moral agents. And feminist theorists (especially Sherwin) remind us to consider the complex network of relationships that the persons we serve—and we ourselves—are embedded in. In Ethics in Practice 5-1, for instance, relational autonomy can help us to better appreciate the network of relationships in the patients' family and community, and the network of relationships in the nurse's work location and health region. The models of ethical decision-making we articulate later in this text are designed to help to assess both power and relationships (see Chapter 13 as well as Appendices A and B).

Social Justice

Furthermore, feminist ethics will help us to further explore the ethical principle of *justice* in situations such as Ethics in Practice 5-1. As was identified in Chapter 4, justice is a poorly operationalized principle in health care ethics (Anderson et al., 2009; Bekemeier and Butterfield 2005; Reimer Kirkham and Browne 2006; Yeo, Rodney, and Moorhouse, 2010). At the heart of feminist ethics is the ideal of achieving *social* justice. Feminist ethics therefore brings greater understanding to the concept of justice. One feminist theorist, Young (1990), argues that contemporary theories of justice are dominated by a distributive paradigm and that it is a mistake to reduce social justice to distribution, claiming that the distributive paradigm "tends to ignore the social structures and institutional context that often help determine distributive patterns" (15). She argues that notions of distributive justice cannot illuminate class relations or provide critical analysis of such relations: "The concepts of domination and oppression, rather than the concept of distribution, should be the starting point for a conception of social justice" (16). Domination and oppression are not always overt. They can be manifested in policies and structures that create covert barriers to health care access (Browne et al. 2011; Henry et al. 2000; Pauly 2008b). Further, the social determinants of health—income, education, secure employment, secure housing, and so forth—have a tremendous impact on access to the resources for *health* as well as health care (Baylis, Kenny, and Sherwin 2008; Coburn 2010; Daniels et al. 2004; Macklin 2008; Marmot 2004; Powers and Faden 2006; Sherwin 2003; 2011; Young 2004).[19] And *postcolonial* feminist theorizing reminds us to consider the impact of the history of Western colonization of Aboriginal peoples in Canada and other countries (Browne, Smye, and Varcoe 2005; Racine 2009a; 2009b; Reimer-Kirkham and Anderson 2010). In Chapter 21 Pauly explores what theorizing about social justice means for enacting social justice in nursing practice, and in Chapter 18 Rodney and co-authors explore what this means for enacting social justice in policy.

Reflecting back on Ethics in Practice 5-1 from a social justice lens, we ought to consider questions such as how the patient's lack of fluency in English affected her access to prenatal care, whether she and her family were able to afford transportation to health care services, whether they were able to afford adequate nutrition, what their immigration experiences in relation to Canadian authorities had been, and so forth. As was identified at the beginning of this chapter, the challenge before us in health care ethics is to better understand and address the personal, social, and cultural aspect of health as well as the socio-political climate of health care delivery. We agree with Sherwin's (2011) claim that

> Bioethics is (or ought to be) concerned with ethical questions relating to health and life, and at least some bioethicists ought to be engaged in critically evaluating the institutional and policy ways in which societies seek to promote and protect health. (78)

What our analysis has suggested is that feminist ethics, through new understanding and insights into justice, has much to offer in addressing this challenge.

Process

Feminist theory also contributes to the study and debate of ethical questions by introducing diversity in *how* health care ethics is pursued and by encouraging the exploration of ethics from many different perspectives (DeRenzo and Strauss 1997; Tong 1997; Wolf 1994b). In feminist theory, attention is paid to how people relate in ethics discussions (Warren 1989). Discussions in health care ethics in the past were too often demeaning—focused on someone "winning" rather than on finding meaning or truth (Warren 1989). In other words, feminist ethics now asks us to consider how we treat each other and our patients and their family members as well as the power dynamics in the organizational and societal structures in which we operate. Returning to Ethics in Practice 5-1, then, this would mean that the process by which ethics resources were offered to the patient and her family (and all others in the emergency department) as well as the nurses, other health care professionals, and managers in the department ought to be inclusive, respectful, and responsive. We will say more about how such processes might be achieved in Chapters 10 and 13 in this text.

Enacting an authentic feminist process also requires that we consider the manner in which we conduct ourselves as we practice, study, teach, and/or do research and policy work in health care ethics. All the remaining chapters in this text take this challenge up.

Summary

Feminist ethics draws our attention to important contextual features of peoples' lives and social circumstances. It especially draws our attention to particulars involving gender, power, and justice. Returning to Daniels' (1996) proposal for the use of diverse sources of theory in ethics, we note that his second premise is "Because there are many types of problems and a division of moral labor is reasonable, many people from many different disciplines and training backgrounds can expect to make important contributions in bioethics" (112; see also Fox and Swazey 2008; McCarthy 2006 and Yeo 2010). We suggest that cultural and feminist approaches can help us to engage more effectively in health care ethics. As this chapter has indicated, we need insights from anthropologists, sociologists, Aboriginal scholars, Buddhist and other scholars, and feminist theorists, as well as scholars in nursing and the other health care professions. Their insights can complement the insights from bioethicists and human rights scholars and advocates we reviewed in Chapter 4 and help to move up toward more ethical practice and policy.[20] Susan Sherwin (2011) puts the local to global ethical challenge this way:

> If bioethicists are to respond effectively to the evidence that links ill health with social and economic injustice, militarism, and environmental damage, we need to rethink our conceptual tools. We need to search out different theoretical starting points and different analytical strategies—ones that direct our attention to the population and not only to the individuals who constitute it. Our major challenge in the next twenty-five years of bioethics work is to find new methods and frameworks that will allow us to contribute effectively to badly needed societal conversations about the big picture. (80)

A Wider Terrain: Toward Relational Ethics

In concluding this chapter, we wish to reflect on a wider terrain foreshadowed in contextual approaches to ethics. For instance, in thinking of culture we are reminded to think of the unique meaning systems held by individuals, families, communities, and health care institutions. In thinking of feminism we are reminded to consider relationships and power dynamics in organizations and the wider society. Furthermore, both feminist and cultural analyses point us to societal values and expectations as well as global considerations. This means that the theoretical diversity in health care ethics that Daniels (1996) calls for (and that we support) ought to include more organizational, ecological, human rights, and political contributions, which we will address further in Chapters 11, 18, 19, 20, and 21 in particular. This is necessary if those of us engaged in health care ethics are to better understand and deal with the complex sociopolitical climates in which health care is delivered and in which resources for health are embedded.

Relational ethics is a newly emerging conceptual approach informed by such theoretical lenses as culture, ethics, feminism, phenomenology, pragmatism, and radical hermeneutics that can encompass all of the above. Relational ethics asks us to consider context at every level—from the individual through to the larger society within and between nations, and to constructively address power inequities at every level (Austin, Bergum, and Dossetor 2003; Baylis, Kenny, and Sherwin 2008; Gadow 1999; Hartick Doane and Varcoe 2005; Kunyk and Austin 2011; Olmstead et al. 2010; Sherwin 1998).[21] Relational ethics reminds us to be reflective about our own positionality, and to embrace complexity and diversity on moving toward a moral horizon. Chapter 7 by Bergum and Chapter 8 by Hartrick Doane and Varcoe offer two different and complementary views of this important and growing field of ethical theory.

In the meanwhile, we close this chapter with the words of Cree elder Willie Ermine (2007), who is helping all of us from our various cultural locations to find our way forward relationally through his articulation of the notion of *ethical space*:

> . . . the idea of the ethical space, produced by contrasting perspectives of the world, entertains the notion of a meeting place, or initial thinking about a neutral zone between entities or cultures. The space offers a venue to step out of our allegiances, to detach from the cages of our mental worlds and assume a position where human-to-human dialogue can occur. The ethical space offers itself as the theatre for cross-cultural conversation in pursuit of ethically engaging diversity and disperses claims to the human order. (202)

Ermine further notes that:

> The idea of an ethical space, produced by contrasting perspectives of the world, entertains the notion of 'engagement'. Engagement at the ethical space triggers a dialogue that begins to set the parameters for an agreement to interact modeled on appropriate, ethical and human principles. (202)

We believe that the theoretical and applied reviews we have provided in Chapters 1 through 5 of this text—as well as all the chapters that follow—take up the kind of engagement Ermine calls for. Singly and together the chapters contribute to a rich and growing dialogue in nursing ethics and health care ethics more broadly.

For Reflection

1. In reflecting on your own personal values and beliefs, how do you think they influence your approach to ethical problems in health care? What are the implications for you as a moral agent?

2. Culture is more than ethnicity. Identify cultural characteristics (shared values and beliefs) of a health care specialty you are familiar with. What are some of the consequences of those characteristics?

3. What do you think a feminist analysis of the under-reporting and under-treatment of mental health problems might address?

4. As we noted above, Susan Sherwin (2011) claims that "Our major challenge in the next twenty-five years of bioethics work is to find new methods and frameworks that will allow us to contribute effectively to badly needed societal conversations about the big picture" (80). What do you think such methods and frameworks should look like? Who should be involved in creating them?

Endnotes

1. As it was defined in Chapter 4, the method of wide reflective equilibrium

   seeks coherence among three divisions of moral thought: our considered moral judgments, a set of principles designed to rationalize and order these judgments, and a set of relevant background theories or understandings about subjects such as human nature and psychology, the workings of the law and procedural justice, conditions for social stability and change, and the socio-economic structure of society. (Winkler 1996, 64)

2. Winkler's (1993) definition may be somewhat narrow, since contextualism does not always proceed by comparative case analysis and may, in fact, also use ethical standards additional to specification of institutional and professional norms and virtues. Nonetheless, Winkler's definition is helpful in starting to delineate the field of contextual ethics.

3. Casuistry is an inductive approach to ethics that proceeds through case analyses (Arras 1991; Jonsen 1995). Inductivism is a more general term referring to the use of qualitative and quantitative data to inform ethical theorizing (Hoffmaster 1993; Jameton and Fowler 1989). Narrative bioethics has emerged as a means to use story to inform ethical practice (Brody 2002; Frank 1998; Tschudin 2003; see also Chapter 6). Care-based ethics entails a primary focus on relationships and care (Edwards 2009; Flanagan 1991; Gilligan 1982; van Hooft 2003), while relational ethics entails a primary focus on human meaning, connectedness, and power dynamics (Austin, Bergum, and Dossetor 2003; Baylis, Kenny, and Sherwin 2008; see also Chapters 3, 7, and 8).

4. For a thoughtful analysis of ethical relativism, see Susan Sherwin's (1992) chapter on "Feminism and Moral Relativism" (58–75). For an interesting critique of debates in philosophy and anthropology about cultural relativism, see Clifford Geertz's (2000) chapter on "Anti-Anti Relativism" (42–67).

5. For a comprehensive resource on diverse methodologies see Denzin and Lincoln (2011).

6. Over time, writers both inside and outside of nursing have chronicled their observations of the culture of the nursing profession. See, for example, Ashley 1976; Chambliss 1996; Growe 1991; Picard 2000; Gordon 2005; and Street 1992.

7. There are three Aboriginal (Indigenous) populations of people in Canada: First Nations, Inuit, and Métis. There is a rich diversity of history, traditions, and beliefs among these peoples. All three groups do, however, share an unfortunate history of dominance and colonization by Anglo-European settlers.

8. We would like to thank an anonymous reviewer of the first edition of this chapter for emphasizing the importance of this history.

9. Chapter 22 in this text provides a discussion of globalization and ethics. See also Austin (2003; 2004) and Benatar and Brock (2011) for further discussions of globalization and ethics and Browne (2001) for a discussion of neoliberalism. Chapters 10, 11, 12, 18, 19, 20, and 21 in this text elaborate on the impacts caused by such global ideologies.

10. The Canadian philosopher Charles Taylor has provided insightful critiques of our current era in terms of what he calls the malaise of modernity (1991) as well as its increasing secularization (2007). See also Chapter 18.

11. Vandenberg (2010) provides a useful overview of the history of theorizing about culture in nursing.

12. See Chapter 4 for a discussion of human rights and informed consent.

13. In an actual case review we would, of course, need much more information. We are extrapolating on the basis of our knowledge of the rest of the focus group interview, related research, and our own experiences in ethics consultations and policy work.

14. In Chapter 13 we talk about the use of ethical decision-making models that can assist in the fuller exploration of morally relevant features in ethical situations. Two such models (Michael McDonald's Ethical Decision-Making Framework for Individuals and Janet Storch's Model for Ethical Decision-Making for Policy and Practice) are available in Appendices A and B of this book.

15. Edward Said (1993) was an insightful and highly influential commentator on cultural imperialism, linking culture to narration. He explained:

    The main battle in imperialism is over land, of course; but when it came to who owned the land, who had the right to settle and work on it, who kept it going, who won it back, and who now plans for its future—these issues were reflected, contested, and even for a time decided in narrative. (xii–xiii)

    We believe that a similar claim can be made about health care ethics. That is, we see similar contested questions about who owns the "correct" ethical theory, who has the right to use their theory, and where, and how that theory should evolve. Such questions involve issues of Western dominance over non-Western, traditional, and Aboriginal cultures and are at least in part reflected by how we narrate our approaches to health care ethics (see also deVries 2004; Fox 1990; Fox and Swazey 2008; Kleinman 1995; Weisz 1990).

16. This is not an argument for cultural appropriation of Aboriginal philosophy or ethics. Instead, we are suggesting that an egalitarian and ongoing dialogue between theorists and practitioners in Western, non-Western, traditional, and Aboriginal cultures could help to move theory and theorizing ahead in health care ethics. This is a point that Aboriginal elder Willie Ermine (2007) makes and that we return to at the closing of this chapter.

17. Feminist theory is by no means a homogenous whole. See Jaggar (1991) and Tong (1997) for interesting historical descriptions of some of the various forms of feminist theory. See also Racine (2009a; 2009b) and Reimer-Kirkham and Anderson (2010) for contemporary examinations of feminist theory in nursing.

18. It should be noted that the relationship between post-structuralism and ethics is an uneasy one. Post-structuralism is one of the facets of postmodern theorizing and can be interpreted as being nihilistic (Brown 1994; Crotty 1998; Squires 1993). Nonetheless, post-structuralist inquiry in nursing has generated some useful insights for practice, policy, and theory (see, for example, Cheek and Porter 1997 and Purkis and Bjornsdottir 2006).

19. This is an important area of emerging inquiry in ethics, nursing, and other health-related disciplines. For further study see also Anderson et al. (2009); Canadian Nurses Association (2009); Farmer (2003); Frankish et al. (2005); Peter (2011); Reimer Kirkham and Browne (2006); Rodney (2011); Sen (2009); Varcoe, Pauly, and Laliberté (in press); and the World Health Organization (2008a; 2008b).

20. One of the ways by which such progress is happening—and will continue to happen—is by the thoughtful reciprocity between empirical inquiry and theoretical ethical inquiry. See van der Scheer and Widdershoven (2004), Carnevale (2007), Rodney (2011), and Yeo (1994).

21. The theoretical approach to relational ethics by each of the groups of authors cited here is not homogenous. All the groups of authors share a commitment to looking at relational connections at all levels, but each group deals somewhat differently with assumptions about agency, power dynamics, and other theoretical constructs.

References

Anderson, J.M., Rodney, P., Reimer-Kirkham, S., Browne, A.J., Khan, K.B., and Lynam, M.J. 2009. Inequities in health and healthcare viewed through the ethical lens of critical social justice: Contextual knowledge for the global priorities ahead. *Advances in Nursing Science, 32* (4), 282–294.

Ashley, J.A. 1976. *Hospitals, paternalism, and the role of the nurse.* New York: Teacher's College Press.

Austin, W. 2003. Using the human rights paradigm in health ethics: The problem and the possibilities. In V. Tschudin (Ed.), *Approaches to ethics: Nursing beyond boundaries* (pp. 105–114). Edinburgh: Butterworth Heinmann. (Reprinted from *Nursing Ethics* 2001; *8* (13), 183–195).

Austin, W. 2004. Global health challenges, human rights, and nursing ethics. In J. Storch, P. Rodney and R. Starzomski (Eds.), *Toward a moral horizon: Nursing ethics for leadership and practice* (pp. 339–356). Toronto: Pearson Prentice Hall.

Austin, W.J. 2011. The incommensurability of nursing as a practice and the customer service model: An evolutionary threat to the discipline. *Nursing Philosophy, 12,* 158–166.

Austin, W., Bergum, V., and Dossetor, J. 2003. Relational ethics: An action ethic as a foundation for health care. In V. Tschudin (Ed.), *Approaches to ethics: Nursing beyond boundaries* (pp. 45–52). Edinburgh: Butterworth Heinmann.

Baylis, F., Kenny, N.P., and Sherwin, S. 2008. A relational account of public health ethics. *Public Health Ethics, 1* (3), 196–209.

Bekemeier, B. and Butterfield, P. 2005. Unreconciled inconsistencies: A critical review of the concept of social justice in 3 national nursing documents. *Advances in Nursing Science, 28* (2), 152–162.

Benatar, S. and Brock, G. 2011. *Global health and global health ethics.* Cambridge: Cambridge University Press.

Bhabha, H.K. 1994. *The location of culture.* London: Routledge.

Brody, H. 2002. Narrative ethics and institutional impact. In R. Charon and M. Montello (Eds.), *Stories matter—The role of narrative in medical ethics* (pp. 149–153). New York: Routledge.

Brown, R.H. 1994. Reconstructing social theory after the postmodern critique. In H.W. Simons and M. Billig (Eds.), *After postmodernism: Reconstructing the ideology critique* (pp. 12–37). London, UK: Sage.

Browne, A.J. 2001. The influence of liberal political ideology on nursing science. *Nursing Inquiry, 8*, 118–129.

Browne, A.J., Smye. V.L., and Varcoe, C. 2005. The relevance of post-colonial theoretical perspectives to research in Aboriginal health. *Canadian Journal of Nursing Research, 37* (4), 16–37.

Browne, A.J., Smye, V.L., Rodney, P., Tang, S.Y., Mussell, B., and O'Neill, J. 2011. Access to primary care from the perspective of Aboriginal patients at an urban emergency department. *Qualitative Health Research, 21* (3), 333–348.

Burgess, M. 1999a. Part III: Introduction: Ethical issues in the delivery of health care services. In H. Coward and P. Ratanakul (Eds.), *A cross-cultural dialogue on health care ethics* (pp. 157–159). Waterloo, ON: Wilfrid Laurier University Press.

Burgess, M. 1999b. Part III: Conclusion: Ethical issues in the delivery of health care services. In H. Coward and P. Ratanakul (Eds.), *A cross-cultural dialogue on health care ethics* (pp. 207–209). Waterloo, ON: Wilfrid Laurier University Press.

Burgess, M., Rodney, P., Coward, H., Ratanakul, P., and Suwonnakote, K. 1999a. Pediatric care: Judgments about best interests at the outset of life. In H. Coward and P. Ratanakul (Eds.), *A cross-cultural dialogue on health care ethics* (pp. 160–175). Waterloo, ON: Wilfrid Laurier University Press.

Canadian Nurses Association. 2008. *Code of ethics for registered nurses.* Ottawa, ON: Authors.

Canadian Nurses Association. 2009. *Position statement: Determinants of health.* Ottawa, ON: Authors.

Canales, M.K. 2010. Othering: Difference understood?? A 10-year analysis and critique of the nursing literature. *Advances in Nursing Science, 33* (1), 15–34.

Carnevale, F.A. 2007. [Guest editorial and discourse.] Relating the "is-ought problem" to nursing inquiry. *Canadian Journal of Nursing Research, 39* (4), 11–17.

Chambliss, D.F. 1996. *Beyond caring: Hospitals, nurses, and the social organization of ethics.* Chicago: The University of Chicago Press.

Cheek, J. and Porter, S. 1997. Reviewing Foucault: Possibilities and problems for nursing and health care. *Nursing Inquiry, 4*, 108–119.

Coburn, D. 2010. Health and health care: A political economy perspective. In T. Bryant, D. Raphael, and M. Rioux (Eds.), *Staying alive: Critical perspectives on health, illness, and health care* (2nd ed.; pp. 65–91). Toronto, ON: Canadian Scholars' Press.

Commission on the Future of Health Care in Canada. 2002. *Building on values: The future of health care in Canada.* Ottawa, ON: Authors.

Coward, H. and Ratanakul, P. 1999. Introduction. In H. Coward and P. Ratanakul (Eds.), *A cross-cultural dialogue on health care ethics* (pp. 1–11). Waterloo, ON: Wilfrid Laurier University Press.

Crotty, M. 1998. *The foundations of social research: Meaning and perspective in the research process.* London: Sage.

Daniels, N. 1996. Wide reflective equilibrium in practice. In L.W. Sumner and J. Boyle (Eds.), *Philosophical perspectives on bioethics* (pp. 96–114). Toronto: University of Toronto Press.

Daniels, N., Kennedy, B., and Kawachi, I. 2004. Health and inequality, or, why justice is good for our health. In S. Anand, F. Peter, and A. Sen (Eds.), *Public health, ethics, and equity* (pp. 63–91). Oxford: Oxford University Press.

Denzin, N.K. and Lincoln, Y.S. (Eds.) 2011. *The Sage handbook of qualitative research* (4th ed.). Thousand Oaks, CA: Sage.

DeRenzo, E.G. and Strauss, M. 1997. A feminist model for clinical ethics consultation: Increasing attention to context and narrative. *HEC Forum, 9* (3), 212–227.

De Vries, R. 2004. How can we help? From "sociology in" to "sociology of" bioethics. *Journal of Law, Medicine & Ethics, 32,* 279–292.

Dodds, S. 2005. Gender, ageing, and injustice: Social and political contexts of bioethics. *Journal of Medical Ethics, 31,* 295–298.

Edwards, S.D. 2009. Three versions of an ethics of care. *Nursing Philosophy, 10,* 231–240.

Ellerby, J.H. 2008. Aboriginal bioethics. In P.A. Singer and A.M. Viens (Eds.), *The Cambridge Textbook of bioethics* (pp. 383–390). Cambridge: Cambridge University Press.

Ermine, W. 2007. The ethical space of engagement. *Indigenous Law Journal, 6,* (1), 193–203.

Farmer, P. 2003 *Pathologies of power: Health, human rights, and the new war on the poor.* Berkeley: University of California Press.

Flanagan, O. 1991. *Varieties of moral personality: Ethics and psychological realism.* Cambridge, MA: Harvard University Press.

Fox, R.C. 1990. The evolution of American bioethics: A sociological perspective. In G. Weisz (Ed.), *Social science perspectives on medical ethics* (pp. 201–217). Philadelphia: University of Pennsylvania Press.

Fox, R.C. and Swazey, J.P. 2008. *Observing bioethics.* Oxford: Oxford University Press.

Frank, A.W. 1998. First-person microethics: Deriving principles from below. *Hastings Center Report, (July-August),* 37–42.

Frankish, C.J., Hwang, S.W., and Quantz, D. 2005. Homelessness and health in Canada: Research lessons and priorities. *Canadian Journal of Public Health, 96* (S2), S23–S29.

Frenk, J., Chen, L., Bhutta, Z.A., Cohen, J., Crisp, N., Evans, T., et al. 2010. Health professionals for a new century: Transforming education to strengthen health systems in an interdependent world. *The Lancet, 376,* 1923–1958.

Gadow, S. 1999. Relational narrative: The postmodern turn in nursing ethics. *Scholarly inquiry for Nursing Practice, 13* (1), 57–70.

Geertz, C. 1984. "From the native's point of view": On the nature of anthropological understanding. In R.A. Shweder and R.A. Levine (Eds.), *Culture theory: Essays on mind, self, and emotion* (pp. 123–136). Cambridge: Cambridge University Press.

Geertz, C. 2000. *Available light: Anthropological reflections on philosophical topics.* Princeton: Princeton University Press.

Gilligan, C. 1982. *In a different voice: Psychological theory and women's development.* Cambridge, MA: Harvard University Press.

Gordon, S. 2005. *Nursing against the odds: How health care cost cutting, media stereotypes, and medical hubris undermine nurses and patient care.* New York: Cornell University Press.

Growe, S.J. 1991. *Who cares? The crisis in Canadian nursing.* Toronto: McClelland & Stewart.

Hartrick Doane, G. and Varcoe, C. 2005. *Family nursing as relational inquiry: Developing health promoting practice.* Philadelphia: Lippincott, Williams and Wilkins.

Henry, F., Tator, C., Mattis, W., and Rees, T. 2000. *The colour of democracy: Racism in Canadian society* (2nd ed.). Toronto: Harcourt.

Ho, A. 2008. The individualistic model of autonomy and the challenge of disability. *Bioethical Inquiry, 5,* 193–207.

Hoffmaster, B. 1993. Can ethnography save the life of medical ethics? In E.R. Winkler and J.R. Coombs (Eds.), *Applied ethics: A reader* (pp. 366–389). Oxford: Blackwell.

Hoffmaster, B. 2001. Introduction. In B. Hoffmaster (Ed.), *Bioethics in social context* (1–11). Philadelphia: Temple University Press.

Jaggar, A.M. 1991. Feminist ethics: Projects, problems, prospects. In C. Card (Ed.), *Feminist ethics* (pp. 78–104). Lawrence, Kansas: University of Kansas Press.

Jameton, A. 1990. Culture, morality, and ethics: Twirling the spindle. *Critical Care Nursing Clinics of North America, 2* (3), 443–451.

Jameton, A. and Fowler, M.D.M. 1989. Ethical inquiry and the concept of research. *Advances in Nursing Science, 11* (3), 11–24.

Jonsen, A.R. 1995. Casuistry: An alternative or complement to principles? *Kennedy Institute of Ethics Journal, 5* (3), 237–251.

Keown, D. 2008. Buddhist bioethics. In P.A. Singer and A.M. Viens (Eds), *The Cambridge Textbook of bioethics* (pp. 391–396). Cambridge: Cambridge University Press.

Kleinman, A. 1995. *Writing at the margin: Discourse between anthropology and medicine.* Berkley: University of California Press.

Kunyk, D. and Austin, W. 2011. Nursing under the influence: A relational ethics perspective. *Nursing Ethics,* 1–10. Published online 6 June 2011. DOI: 10.1177/0969733011406767.

Lebacqz, K. 1991. Feminism and bioethics: An overview. *Second opinion: Health, faith and ethics, 17* (2), 10–25.

Liaschenko, J. and Peter, E. 2003. Feminist ethics. In V. Tschudin (Ed.), *Approaches to ethics: Nursing beyond boundaries* (pp. 33–43) Edinburgh: Butterworth Heinmann.

Macklin, R. 2008. Global justice, human rights, and health. In R.M. Green, A. Donovan, and S.A. Jauss (Eds.), *Global bioethics: Issues of conscience for the twenty-first century* (pp. 141–160). Oxford: Clarendon Press.

Marmot, M. 2004 Social causes of social inequalities in health. In S. Anand, F. Peter, and A. Sen (Eds.) *Public health, ethics, and equity* (pp. 37–61). Oxford: Oxford University Press.

McCarthy, J. 2006. A pluralist view of nursing ethics. *Nursing Philosophy, 7* (3), 157–164.

Mckenzie, C. 2008. Relational autonomy, normative authority and perfectionism. *Journal of Social Philosophy, 39* (4,), 512–533.

Myrick, F. 2004. Pedagogical integrity in the knowledge economy. *Nursing Philosophy 5,* 23–29.

Ng, R. 1993. Sexism, racism, Canadian nationalism. In H. Bannerji (Ed.), *Returning the gaze: Essays on racism, feminism, and politics* (pp. 223–241). Toronto: Sister Vision Press.

Olmstead, D.L., Scott, S.D., and Austin, W.J. 2010. Unresolved pain in children: A relational ethics perspective. *Nursing Ethics, 17* (6), 695–704.

Pauly, B. 2008a. Shifting moral values to enhance access to health care: Harm reduction as a context for ethical nursing practice. *International Journal of Drug Policy, 19*, 195–204.

Pauly, B. 2008b. Harm reduction through a social justice lens. *International Journal of Drug Policy, 19,* 4–10.

Peter, E. 2011. Discourse: Fostering social justice: The possibilities of a socially connected model of moral agency. *Canadian Journal of Nursing Research, 43* (2), 11–17.

Peternelj-Taylor, C. 2004. An exploration of othering in forensic psychiatric and correctional nursing. *Canadian Journal of Nursing Research, 36* (4), 131–146.

Picard, A. 2000. *Critical care: Canadian nurses speak for change.* Toronto: HarperCollins.

Powers, M. and Faden, R. 2006. *Social justice: The moral foundations of public health and health policy.* Oxford: Oxford University Press.

Purkis, M.E. and Bjornsdottir, K. 2006. Intelligent nursing: Accounting for knowledge as action in practice. *Nursing Philosophy, 7,* 247–256.

Racine, L. 2009a. Examining the conflation of multiculturalism, sexism, and religious fundamentalism through Taylor and Bahktin: Expanding post-colonial feminist epistemology. *Nursing Philosophy, 10,* 14–25.

Racine, L. 2009b. Applying Antonio Gramsci's philosophy to postcolonial feminist social and political activism in nursing. *Nursing Philosophy, 10,* 180–190.

Ratanakul, P. 1999. Buddhism, health, disease, and Thai culture. In H. Coward and P. Ratanakul (Eds.), *A cross-cultural dialogue on health care ethics* (pp. 17–33). Waterloo, ON: Wilfrid Laurier University Press.

Reimer-Kirkham, S. and Anderson, J.M. 2010. The advocate-analyst dialectic in critical and post-colonial feminist research: Reconciling tensions around scientific integrity. *Advances in Nursing Science 33* (3), 196–205.

Reimer Kirkham, S. and Browne, A.J. 2006. Toward a critical theoretical interpretation of social justice discourses in nursing. *Advances in Nursing Science, 29* (4), 324–339.

Report of the Royal Commission on Aboriginal People. 1996a. *Volume 1, Looking forward, looking back*. Ottawa: Author.

Report of the Royal Commission on Aboriginal People. 1996b. *Volume 3, Gathering strength*. Ottawa: Author.

Report of the Royal Commission on Aboriginal People. 1996c. *Volume 4, Perspectives and realities*. Ottawa: Author.

Rodney, P. 2011. [Guest editorial]. Nursing inquiry to address pressing empirical and ethical questions. *Canadian Journal of Nursing Research, 43* (2), 7–10.

Rodney, P., Doane, G.H., Storch, J., and Varcoe, C. 2006. Workplaces: Toward a safer moral climate. *Canadian Nurse, 102* (8), 24–27.

Rodney, P. and Varcoe, C. in press. Constrained agency: The social structure of nurses' work. In F. Baylis, J. Downie, B. Hoffmaster, and S. Sherwin (Eds.), *Health care ethics in Canada* (3rd ed.). Toronto: Nelson. (Revised version of Varcoe, C. and Rodney, P. 2009. Constrained agency: The social structure of nurses' work. In B. S. Bolaria and H. D. Dickinson (Eds.), *Health, illness, and health care in Canada* (4th ed.; pp. 122–151). Toronto: Nelson Education.)

Rorty, R. 1999. *Philosophy and social hope*. London: Penguin.

Said, E.W. 1993. *Culture and imperialism*. New York: Vintage.

Sanders, K., Pattison, S., and Hurwitz, B. 2011. Tracking shame and humiliation in accident and emergency. *Nursing Philosophy, 12*, 83–93.

Saul, J.R. 2005. *The collapse of globalism and the reinvention of the world*. Toronto, ON: Penguin Canada.

Saul, J.R. 2008. *A fair country: Telling truths about Canada*. Toronto, ON: Viking Canada.

Sen, A. 2009. *The idea of justice*. Cambridge, MA: The Belknap Press.

Sewell, W.H. 1992. A theory of structure: Duality, agency, and transformation. *American Journal of Sociology 98* (1), 1–29.

Sherwin, S. 1992. *No longer patient: Feminist ethics and health care*. Philadelphia: Temple University Press.

Sherwin, S. 1998. A relational approach to autonomy in health care. In S. Sherwin and the Feminist Health Care Ethics Research Network (Eds.), *The politics of women's health* (pp. 19–47). Philadelphia: Temple University Press.

Sherwin, S. 2011. Looking backwards, looking forward: Hopes for bioethics' next twenty-five years. *Bioethics 25* (2), 75–82.

Shestowsky, B. 1993. *Traditional medicine and primary health care among Canadian Aboriginal people: A discussion paper with annotated bibliography*. Ottawa: Aboriginal Nurses Association of Canada.

Shweder, R.A. 1984. Preview: A colloquy of culture theorists. In R.A. Shweder and R.A. Levine (Eds.), *Culture theory: Essays on mind, self, and emotion* (pp. 1–24). Cambridge, UK: Cambridge University Press.

Squires, J. 1993. Introduction. In J. Squires (Ed.), *Principled positions: Postmodernism and the rediscovery of value* (pp. 1–13). London: Lawrence & Wishart.

Stein, J.G. 2001. *The cult of efficiency.* Toronto: Penguin.

Stephenson, P. 1999. Expanding notions of culture for cross-cultural ethics in health and medicine. In H. Coward and P. Ratanakul (Eds.), *A cross-cultural dialogue on health care ethics* (pp. 68–91). Waterloo, ON: Wilfrid Laurier University Press.

Storch, J.L. 2010. Canadian healthcare system. In M. McIntyre and C. McDonald (Eds.), *Realities of Canadian nursing: Professional, practice, and power issues,* (3rd ed.; pp. 34–55). Philadelphia: Wolters Kluwer Health.

Storch, J., Hartrick, G., Rodney, P., Starzomski, R., and Varcoe, C. 2001. *The ethics of practice: Context and curricular implications for nursing.* Research study, University of Victoria School of Nursing.

Street, A.F. 1992. *Inside nursing: A critical ethnography of clinical nursing practice.* Albany, NY: State University of New York Press.

Tait, C. L. 2008. Ethical programming: Towards a community-centred approach to mental health and addiction programming in Aboriginal communities. *Pimatisiwin: A Journal of Aboriginal and Indigenous Community Health, 6* (1), 29–60.

Tarlier, D. S., Browne, A. J., and Johnson, J. L. 2007. The influence of geographical and social distance on nursing practice and continuity of care in a remote First Nations community. *Canadian Journal of Nursing Research, 39* (3), 126–148.

Taylor, C. 1992. *Multiculturalism and "the politics of recognition."* Princeton: Princeton University Press.

Taylor, C. 2001. *The malaise of modernity.* Toronto: House of Anansi Press.

Taylor, C. 2007. *A secular age.* Cambridge, MA: Belknap Press.

Thorne, S., Bultz, B., and Baile, W. 2005. Is there a cost to poor communication in cancer care? A critical review of the literature. *Psycho-Oncology, 14,* 875–884.

Tong, R. 1997. *Feminist approaches to bioethics: Theoretical reflections and practical applications.* Boulder, CO: Westview.

Tschudin, V. 2003. Narrative ethics. In V. Tschudin (Ed.), *Approaches to ethics: Nursing beyond boundaries* (pp. 61–72) Edinburgh: Butterworth Heinmann.

Vandenberg, H.E.R. 2010. Culture theorizing past and present: Trends and challenges. *Nursing Philosophy, 11,* 238–249.

van der Scheer, L. and Widdershoven, G. 2004. Integrated empirical ethics: Loss of normativity? *Medicine, Health Care and Philosophy 7,* 71–79.

van Hooft, S. 2003. Caring and ethics in nursing. In V. Tschudin (Ed.), *Approaches to ethics: Nursing beyond boundaries* (pp. 1–12) Edinburgh: Butterworth Heinmann.

Varcoe, C. 2001. Abuse obscured: An ethnographic account of emergency nursing in relation to violence against women. *Canadian Journal of Nursing Research, 32* (4), 95–115.

Varcoe, C. 2004. Widening the scope of ethical theory, practice, and policy: Violence against women as an illustration. In J. Storch, P. Rodney, and R. Starzomski (Eds.), *Toward a moral horizon: Nursing ethics for leadership and practice* (pp. 414–432). Toronto: Pearson-Prentice Hall.

Varcoe, C. and Einboden, R. in press. Family violence and ethics. In J. Humphreys and J. Campbell (Eds.), *Family violence and nursing practice*. New York: Springer.

Varcoe, C., Pauly, B., and Laliberté, S. in press. Intersectionality, social justice and policy. In O. Hankivsky (Ed.), *Intersectionality-type health research in Canada*. Vancouver BC: UBC Press.

Walker, M.U. 2003. *Moral contexts*. Lantham Mayland: Rowman & Littlefield.

Warren, V.L. 1989. Feminist directions in medical ethics. *Hypatia, 4* (2), 73–87.

Weisz, G. 1990. Introduction. In G. Weisz (Ed.), *Social science perspectives on medical ethics* (pp. 3–15). Philadelphia: University of Pennsylvania Press.

Willms, D.G., Lange, P., Bayfield, D., Beardy, M., Lindsay, E.A., Cole, D.C., and Johnson, N.A. 1992. A lament by women for "The People, The Land" [Nishnawbi-Aski Nation]: An experience of loss. *Canadian Journal of Public Health, 83* (5), 331–334.

Winkler, E.R. 1993. From Kantianism to contextualism: The rise and fall of the paradigm theory in bioethics. In E.R. Winkler and J.R. Coombs (Eds.), *Applied ethics: A reader* (pp. 343–365). Oxford: Blackwell.

Winkler, E. 1996. Moral philosophy and bioethics: Contextualism versus the paradigm theory. In L.W. Sumner and J. Boyle (Eds.), *Philosophical perspectives on bioethics* (pp. 50–78). Toronto: University of Toronto Press.

Wolf, S.M. 1994. Shifting paradigms in bioethics and health law: The rise of a new pragmatism. *American Journal of Law & Medicine, 20* (4), 395–415.

World Health Organization. 2008a. *Closing the gap in a generation: Health equity through action on the social determinants of health.* (Final Report of the Commission on Social Determinants of Health). Geneva: Authors.

World Health Organization. 2008b. *World Health Report 2008: Primary health care: Now more than ever.* Geneva: Authors.

Yeo, M. 1994. Interpretive bioethics. *Health and Canadian Society, 2* (1), 85–108.

Yeo, M. 2010. A primer in ethical theory. In M. Yeo, A. Moorhouse, P. Khan, and P. Rodney (Eds.), Concepts and cases in nursing ethics, (3rd ed.; pp. 37–72). Peterborough, ON: Broadview Press.

Yeo, M., Rodney, P., Moorhouse, A., and Khan, P. 2010. Justice. In M. Yeo, A. Moorhouse, P. Khan, and P. Rodney (Eds.), *Concepts and cases in nursing ethics* (3rd ed.; pp. 293–316). Peterborough, ON: Broadview Press.

Young, I.M. 1990. *Justice and the politics of difference.* Princeton: Princeton University Press

Young, I.M. 2004. The ideal of community and the politics of difference. In C. Farrelly (Ed.), *Contemporary political theory: A reader* (pp. 195–204). London: Sage Publications. (From Young, I.M. 1986 The ideal of community and the politics of difference, *Social Theory and Practice 12* (1), 1–26. Excerpts from pp. 1–2, 14–23. Also from Young, I.M. 2000. *Inclusion and democracy.* Oxford: Oxford University Press. Excerpts from pp. 21–26.)

CHAPTER 6

Narrative Ethics in Health Promotion and Care

Jeffrey Nisker

It is only with the heart that one can see truly, for what is essential is invisible to the eye. (de Saint-Exupéry 1943)

My conversion from a theories-and-principles-based (Beauchamp and Childress 1994) to a narrative-based approach to moral exploration, ethics education, and research occurred with the reading to my children of the above line in *The Little Prince* (de Saint-Exupéry 1943). With epiphanic clarity, this line opened the imperative to ask health professionals and students to hear the hearts of the persons who come to our care and, with our hearts, to strive to promote better health for our patients and our communities. This line also encouraged me in classrooms and conference rooms to explore ethical issues with the hearts of health professionals and students rather than just cognating moral issues or teaching the cognition of moral issues in the same manner health professionals and students cognate symptoms and signs of disease (Nisker 1997a).

Hearing our patients' stories brings us to the inherent beauty of the persons too often confined within a diagnosis (Nisker 2001a; 2010a). Hearing our patients' stories allows us to appreciate the position of the woman or man or child for whom the moral exploration is occurring and see their beauty within (Nisker 2001a; 2010a).

In this chapter, I will begin by suggesting the value of narratives and by supporting John Arras' contention that narrative is "an essential element in any and all ethical analysis [and] constitutes a powerful and necessary corrective to the narrowness and abstractness of some widespread versions of principle- and theory-based ethics" (Arras 1997, 84). I will describe the types of narrative used in health ethics, which will lead me to a discussion of the advantages of "thick" narratives and how "thick" narratives improve traditional presentation of "cases."[1] I will continue by exploring the uses of narratives in health ethics exploration, education, policy development, and research.

THE VALUE OF NARRATIVE

Exploring ethical issues through the narratives of a person at the centre of the issue helps us to better understand the person and the ethical issues involved in that person's care. Next to being a patient, or spending considerable time truly caring for the person who is our patient, hearing narratives is the best way a health professional can experience what the persons in their care feel, how they want to be treated, and what they want to know.

Narratives assist in clinical and moral decision-making because they bring us closer to understanding the uniqueness of the persons we serve.[2]

Story has provided moral footing for thousands of years. We experience moral learning when reading Greek mythologies, epic literary works such as Homer's *Odysseus*, and religious texts such as the Bhagavad Gita, Old Testament, and Quran, as well as Jesus' parables and the Gospels. Unfortunately, many great works, especially those created by women, and those created by women and men from non-Western cultures, have been lost. Those that have survived the filter of time can, in a compelling manner, engage health professionals and students, bringing us insight into the moral problems inherent in humanness. Over the centuries, poets and novelists have continued to surface ethical issues and help their readers explore right action. Telling our own stories[3] allows us to share our unique health care experiences with other caregivers, ethics explorers, policy-makers, and the general public.

Stories remain an engaging and memorable vehicle for moral learning, much more so than didactic, topic-based approaches. Stories may be fictional compilations of insights and feelings, or true stories of an illness experience. Anna Quindlen, former *New York Times* Op Ed columnist and author of the health-related novels *One True Thing* (1995) and *Black and Blue* (1998a), stated when she left journalism for novels that "Facts sometimes need fiction to be told truly" (1998b). Nadine Gordimer, Nobel Laureate, goes further, stating, "There is always more truth in fiction" (1999).

For fictional works to significantly contribute to moral exploration in health care, it is not necessary that they describe medical moments, health care settings, or illness experiences. It *is* necessary, however, that they powerfully surface the feelings of the persons involved and explore humanness in a manner that can be absorbed for later understanding to assist other persons who are (or will be) confined beneath the medical microscope. "The universalizing tendency of the moral imagination is encouraged by the very activity of novel-reading of itself, with its alternations between identification and sympathy" (Nussbaum 1990, 166). This can be challenging to some health professionals and students for, as Philips suggests, to "engage with a narrative requires a leap of faith that suspends disbelief in order that what is told can be heard" (1994, 10). Although I find that this is true for some individuals in all health professional disciplines, it is especially true for medical students and practitioners, culturally hardened to computer-like objectivization of data input.

Nonfiction stories and memoirs are also extremely valuable. In the writings of illness experience by Arthur Frank (1991; 1995; 2004), we have personal stories and personal reflections beautifully juxtaposed. They are at once self-reflective, compelling to the reader, and informative as to what can be learned from the author's personal experience. In scholarly texts such as Howard Brody's *Stories of Sickness* (1987; 2003), the power of story as it relates to the provision of better health care is elegantly described.

Knowing as much as possible of the life stories of the persons for whom we care allows us to understand from where those persons' actions, hopes, and desires come and how we can best help those persons achieve their goals in relation to their illness experience. Let me say more about the various forms the stories may take.

Thick and Thin Narratives

We have had a tendency in health professions to present "cases" that are "thin" on everything except medical data (Murray 1997). These "thin" stories, by revealing only a smattering of family and social information, are rarely adequate to help us understand who the person *qua* patient[4] is or what her desires for the present and future are—that is, the essentials in assisting with her health care. "Thick" stories, whether fictional, true, or fictional based on truth, bring us to the deeper understanding we require as health professionals.

Through "thick" narratives rather than the "thin" narratives in "cases," we are able to develop "empathetic imagining" (Halpern 2001) for each person we are hoping to help. "Thick" narratives do not need to be longer than "thin" narratives. Indeed, a poem, the densest form of narrative through its precision of words and the power of imagery per word, can concisely bring us to a person's condition. Short stories, short plays, and even novellas (and longer forms of each when there is sufficient time) are also very useful tools for imbuing insight in ethics exploration. Further, "thick" narratives can also be expressed in film, in song, and even in media where no words are used (such as paintings, photographs, other visual arts, and instrumental music).[5]

TYPES OF NARRATIVE IN HEALTH ETHICS

Narratives useful in ethics exploration, education, research, and policy development can be divided by their type or by their utility. Types of narrative can be categorized according to the form of presentation, such as a poem, play, short story, or film, or described in terms of content (see Exhibit 6-1).

EXHIBIT 6-1

Types of Narratives in Health Ethics

I. Narratives Described in Terms of Presentation Form

- poem
- short story
- play
- film

II. Narratives Described in Terms of Content

Benner, Tanner, and Chesla (1996)

- *constitutive or sustaining narratives:* "depict situations that constitute the person's understanding of what it is to be a nurse" and "capture the significance of the practice and demonstrate meaning-laden clinical episodes that convey the worth of the work" (237)
- *narratives of learning:* subdivided into "narratives about being open to experience" (241), "narratives of learning the skill of involvement" (242), "narratives of disillusionment" (245), "narratives about facing death and suffering" (248), and "liberation narratives" (249)

Frank (1995)

- *restitution narratives:* dominate the stories of both those who are sick and are focusing on being healthy again, and how "contemporary culture treats health as the normal condition that people ought to have restored" (77)

- *chaos narratives:* "the opposite of the restitution [narrative, their] plot imagines life never getting better" (like a Holocaust story) (97)
- *quest narratives:* "stories meet suffering head on; they accept illness and seek to use it" (115)
- *memoirs:* combines "telling the illness story with telling other events in the writer's life" (119)
- *manifestos:* "the truth that has been learned is prophetic, often carrying demands for social action" (120)
- *automythologies:* like the Phoenix myth, "where the protagonist reinvents herself from the ashes of the fire of [her] own body" (122)

Nelson (2001)

- *counter stories:* stories "that [resist] an oppressive identity and [attempt] to replace it with one that commands respect" (6)
- *master narratives:* "stories found lying about in our culture that serve as summaries of socially shared [understanding which over the years have 'exercised'] a certain authority over our moral imaginations and play a role in informing our moral intuitions" (6)

Smythe and Murray (2000)

- *personal narratives:* biographies, autobiographies, and works of fiction that are "centred on the individuality of a central main character or person . . . told from a consistent, personal perspective and is aimed at revealing the unique, idiosyncratic character and life circumstances of a particular individual" (327)
- *archetypal narratives:* stories "of mythological and religious texts" in which "the focus is not human individuality, as such, but . . . timeless human motifs that reflect fundamental spiritual, existential, and moral concerns" (327)
- *typal narratives:* based on "psychological and social" themes, in which the "principal aim is neither to capture the individuality of persons in detail nor to bring out archetypal human themes, but rather to concretely exemplify the theory-laden categories of contemporary social science" (327)

Presentation Forms

Poetry is the most concise narrative form. Each word, by itself or in phrases, is calculated to convey maximum feeling—imagery created through similes and metaphors profoundly painting feeling through our hearts and minds. Many of my students prefer song to poetry, as it is more accessible and, for the many students with talent in music, easier to present.

Short stories are best presented in a "readers' theatre" format in which each participant takes a turn reading a paragraph or stanza. These literary works might be selected from anthologies, such as *Literature and Aging* (Kohn, Donley, and Wear 1992). By involving the members of the class or conference participants in the narrative presentation, an ownership of the material and capacity to engage in moral exploration is achieved. The acting of plays similarly offers the opportunity to immerse many members of the class or conference in ethics exploration.

Film (video) is also a very valuable surfacing tool for narrative ethics exploration. Whether the central character is a nurse, as in *The English Patient*; a physician, as in *The Doctor*; or a family member, as in *Marvin's Room* and *What's Eating Gilbert Grape?*, film is an engaging vehicle for surfacing ethical issues for the person *qua* caregiver or person *qua* patient relationships (as in the films suggested above).

A specific exploration of an ethical issue may use several narratives. For example, in exploring "end-of-life decision-making," I begin with a readers' theatre format of Earle Birney's poem "David." The poem brings participants to the position of David, not only as he is, lying quadriplegic on a rocky precipice after falling from a mountain, but, through the reflection of the narrator (David's friend), as he was throughout his life and while climbing the mountain. We are also placed in the position of the narrator as an unwilling substitute decision-maker. I also use several films to explore end-of-life issues (see Chapter 17) including *The Sea Inside* (Amenábar 2004), *Barbarian Invasions* (Arcand and Potashnik 2003), and *Wit* (Edson 2001).

Narrative-surfacing vehicles may vary in length from Rilke's three-stanza poem, "The Dwarf's Song," to student-performed plays of varying length, to two-hour films (usually viewed in the week before the ethics exploration). Narratives allow learning through participation in the presentation, as well as in the discussion of the ethical issues surfaced.

USES OF NARRATIVE IN HEALTH ETHICS

Stories, whether true, fictional, or fictional based on truth, can help bring the reader or audience member to the position of the person requiring health care, thus allowing a much deeper appreciation of that person's needs, rights, and desires than is possible in health care and philosophy tomes. By approximating empathy for the person at the centre of the decision-making, we can better contribute to moral resolution of the issue at hand, and provide better care.

Martha Montello tells us that "drawing on readers' own desires, memories, psychological defenses and imaginations enables readers to experience and understand things entirely unfamiliar, offering virtually limitless opportunities to engage their faculties in different ways of perceiving the world" (1997, 189). These different ways of perceiving the world should allow us "readers" to participate in more sensitive, and indeed informed, decision-making regarding the person and the issues affecting that person. Our participation in turn enables more depth in our analysis and more empowerment of future persons *qua* patients to inform future decision-making. Further, these different perceptions could be used to promote clinical discussions and public discussion of an ethical issue, national policy development, or specifically, for ethics education purposes.

EXHIBIT 6-2

Purposes of Narratives in Health Ethics

Arras (1997)

- to supplement principle-driven approaches
- to function as "the very ground of all moral justification" (73) (as described

by MacIntyre and Hauerwas, e.g., MacIntyre 1981; 1988; Burrell and Hauerwas 1977)

- in a "postmodern ethical stance" in which "narrative and the authenticity of the narrator appear to play the role of substitutes for ethical justification" (68)

Montello (1997)

- to "reframe . . . the issues by focusing attention on the context of a patient's and family's life in all its moral complexity" (186)
- to "have long-term effects on the structure of the self by extending a reader's psychic map to include unfamiliar territory, taking in new values and knowledge and knowledge of other ways of seeing the world" (188–190)

Nelson (2001)

- "(1) to teach us our duties; (2) to guide morally good action; (3) to motivate morally good action; (4) to justify action on moral grounds; (5) to cultivate our moral sensibilities; (6) to enhance our moral perception; (7) to make actions or persons morally intelligible; and (8) to reinvent ourselves as better persons" (36)
- for compassionate health care decision-making
- for health ethics education
- for health ethics research
- for health policy development

Narrative for Moral Exploration

Patricia Benner (1994) writes that "Narratives and narrative knowing allow us to examine practical moral reasoning and to get beyond abstractions" (59). Ann Hunsaker Hawkins (1997) describes narratives as a "counter [to] the tendency in philosophy-based ethics to overemphasize moral principles and rules in considering a particular ethical situation" (154).

Narratives can be written specifically for readers to use to begin their moral exploration of a particular issue or as stand-alone explorations in which authors use narratives as their argument. An example of the latter is my narrative exploration of the ethics of using economically disadvantaged women who request *in vitro* fertilization as "oocyte donors" for wealthier women who have delayed childbearing and have run out of eggs (Nisker 1997b). In this narrative exploration, I offered stories from multiple literary genres as analogies for what economically disadvantaged women (offered the opportunity to "share" their eggs in return for "free" IVF) have shared with me and others.

Another way to use narrative in moral exploration is that suggested by Rita Charon (1994; 1997; 2006; 2008) and other scholars (Jones 1998; Montello 1997; Nussbaum 1990) in which the principles of literary critical analysis are used to help health professionals better understand a patient's story and better practise medicine. As Martha Montello writes, "the same literary skills that critical readers use to interpret the meaning of events in a story allow clinicians to see the way ethical issues are embedded in the individual and continent nature of people's beliefs, cultures and biography" (1997, 186).[6]

Compassion Ethics

The utility of a narrative to bring compassion to the exploration of an ethical issue lies in its ability to approximate empathy for the person at the centre of the ethical issue (Nisker 2001a; 2010a). By developing a sensitivity to the position of the other, we are able to provide better care, not only for that person but for all those who come to our care

(Nisker 2001a; 2010a). Indeed, though the purpose of using narrative in health ethics can vary, the shared power of narratives lies in their link to compassion: "we see and hear and feel the same thing the characters do and from their perspective, so that when we close the book to render our own lives, that set of emotions and way of knowing is embedded in us, a part of us" (Montello 1997, 194). Defending the importance of compassion in ethics, David Thomasma argues that "not only rationality, but also emotional compassion, is an important teacher of bioethical decision making . . . our compassion can lead us to truths beyond reason and its analysis" (1994, 124). In the introduction to her book *From Detached Concern to Empathy* (2001), Jodi Halpern argues that by allowing patients to move us, we "gain access to a source of understanding illness and suffering that can make [us] more effective healers" (xi–xiii). The empathizer must be sufficiently affected by the patient "to be able to recognize and appreciate, in some quasi first-person way, how the rain and sun feel" (Halpern 2001, 67–68). Lois LaCivita Nixon, drawing on the work of Jones (1994), suggests that narratives function to "illuminat[e] ethical dilemmas with fictional materials that stretch the 'intuitive and imaginative faculties of mind' . . . [so that we] empathize with others, understand more fully what it means to be human, and develop moral wisdom" (Nixon 1997, 245).

I agree with Arthur Frank (1995) that stories are ends in themselves, but the writing of these stories is also a means to an end for the author—an exploration of self, of a relationship, of an issue. Indeed, the sharing of our stories with colleagues is a means to several ends: surfacing ethical issues for discussion, increasing awareness of an individual person's position (*qua* patient or *qua* health professional), increasing sensitivity and compassion in members of a health professional team, and even bringing the health professional team closer together.

In 1997, I wrote the play *Orchids: Not Necessarily a Gospel* (Nisker 2001b), a two-hour musical, originally with a cast of health professionals and students, to bring audience members to the position of women immersed in the ethical issues of new reproductive-genetic technology. This play was remounted in 2005 with a professional cast for a national citizen deliberation on regulating this technology as described below under "Narrative to Surface Ethical Issues in Health Policy Research." The play explores what is considered "normal" in "genetic technology's magic mirror" and how "disabled" people and "normal" people see their reflections. The play encourages audience members to approximate empathy for the two women having to make decisions regarding genetic testing, for persons living with disabilities, and indeed for all persons. The final line in the closing song of *Orchids*, "Help compassion happen every day" (Nisker 2001b), was spontaneously sung over and over by audience members along with the original cast.

The term "compassion ethics" is frequently used to describe my narrative ethics courses because bringing the ethics explorer to the person's position imbues compassion for the person. Students in the health professions carry a "cargo" (Spiro 1996) of compassion into their chosen disciplines. It is important that the "miles of medical ink" and the "consuming call schedules" consistent with health professional training not be allowed to evaporate any of this cargo (Nisker 1997a, 689).

Obstacles to compassion are both macro and micro in nature. In Canada, health professionals face workplaces where the climate of compassion (and thus the moral climate) is deteriorating due to reduced resources for patient and family care (Nisker 2003a; 2003b;

2007; 2008b; see Chapters 10 and 11). Staff shortages result in excessive workloads, loss of clinical leadership, and other efficiency-driven changes (see Chapter 9; as well as Janice Stein's 2001 *Cult of Efficiency*).

Although most health professionals are aware of their one-on-one obligation to those in their care, "out-of-the-box" moral obligations of health professionals are less appreciated. As we will not be able to provide compassionate health care at the micro level if macro-level policy decisions are void of compassion, understanding our "out-of-the-box" moral imperatives is as important as our imperatives in the professional–patient relationship. In particular, we ought to challenge "efficiency"-based health policy (Nisker 2003c).

Narrative in Health Ethics Education

Ethics education is an integral part of undergraduate and post-graduate health professional curricula and continuing professional development. Thomasma (1994) worries that students in the health professions, many of whom have a science background, are attracted to the principles-and-theories approach to ethics because the thought process is similar to clinical decision-making. This is true, but rather than committing to a principles-and-theories approach, ethics educators should take advantage of another characteristic of health professionals and students. That is, they should take advantage of our most essential characteristic: a desire to care for others that brings us eagerly to stories of illness, of compassion, of others' needs, of caring for others. In a narrative-based ethics curriculum, students eagerly come to class to share in an experience that might not only deepen their insight into ethical issues but also enhance their ability to understand their future patients' position so as to afford them compassionate care.

Scholars such as Charon (1994; 1997; 2006; 2008), Frank (1991; 1995; 2004), Montello (1997), and Lindemann (Nelson 2001) emphasize the importance of narratives to help students in the health professions become better health professionals. Narrative fosters "empathetic imagining" (Halpern 2001, 185–190), whether as part of a narrative ethics or health care humanities curriculum, or indeed, in the form of the first-hand stories of the persons for whom we care (Nisker 2010a). Empathetic imagining also helps us write narratives to help others experience empathy for the persons in our care. Martha Nussbaum (1990) suggests that "[b]y cultivating our ability to see vividly another person's distress, to picture ourselves in another person's place—we make ourselves more likely to respond with the morally illuminating and appropriate sort of response" (39). Narrative can help conserve compassion (Nisker 1997a) or even increase compassion through the years of undergraduate, post-graduate, and health professional education.

Writing "Thick" Narratives for Health Professional Education

Just as health professional education has evolved in the past 20 years from disease-based learning, to problem-based learning (PBL),[7] to patient-centred care (PCC) (Stewart et al. 1995), so too has the type of "case" evolved from cases consisting of diagnosis-driven facts, to relatively "thin cases" that include superficial reference to social circumstances and relationships, to "thick" narratives revealing the story of the person experiencing the health care issue through images that give deep insight into the social circumstances and relationships that surround the clinical condition. "Thick" narratives can assist in the evolution from PBL to PCC, forging a new person-centred learning. By keeping the story of the person for whom we are caring as the centre of our focus, we acknowledge the uniqueness of that person.

It is not hard to convert "thin" stories to "thick" stories or, more accurately, to ensure that a person's story is not sliced down to its medical thread. In the workshops and seminars in which I suggest writing "thick" stories, I am always impressed with how quickly the participants are able to rewrite the "thin" cases I provide into "thick" narratives. Special talent or skill is not required, just a gentle reminder that there is a person inside that patient (Nisker 2001a). However, I also include the following suggestions:

1. Write from your heart, using "empathetic imagining" (Halpern 2001) to intuit what it is like to be in the person's position.

2. When possible, write in a first-person voice to more intimately bring to the reader what the person feels.

3. Use expressive adjectives, as well as similes and metaphors to create strong images.

4. Include tactile, auditory, and visual clues to imbue what the person is feeling, as in "I stopped the *coarseness* of the hospital's washcloth, as the *grating* sound of *yellowing* curtains opened me to the world."

5. Use a setting with which the participants can identify.

6. Make sure you include all necessary clinical information, but immerse it within the person's story.

7. When information from additional characters is necessary, reveal their words in the protagonist's recollection of a conversation that he or she had with them or that they had with others (i.e., an overheard conversation).[8]

Readers' Theatre

I find readers' theatre an extremely effective vehicle through which to bring poems and short stories to health ethics explorers. Members of a class or participants in a conference are able to immerse themselves in the narrative and take mutual ownership in the discussion that follows the presentation. Ethics educators can write short stories specifically to be presented in a readers' theatre format. Dramatic phrasing, tending to purple (almost Shakespearean) prose seems particularly embracing. These short stories can be specifically written for subjects to be discussed in the classroom or conference auditorium. For example, to bring participants to the position of a 12-year-old boy suffering chemotherapy, I wrote the short story "Philip" (Nisker 2003b). (See also Chapter 16.)

Victorian Parlour Game

A useful tool to develop compassion through group poetry writing is the Victorian parlour game I learned at a Centre of Literature in Medicine workshop at Hiram College in August 1994. This game is a useful tool for both imbuing empathy and bringing together groups of students or professionals for moral exploration. Each Victorian guest (or seminar participant) is instructed to write one line in response to, "Imagine if you were in the position of a person in . . . [the ethical dilemma being explored]. How would you feel?" The first participant writes his or her line on the top of the page and folds the paper over the line (to conceal his or her response) and then passes the paper to the next person, who writes his or her line below the one already written and then folds the paper over again and passes it to the next person—and onward in succession until the last person (usually me) is charged to weave the lines into a group poem. In larger audiences, it may be necessary to have the paper passed down each row and (possibly) to construct a group poem for each row, or weave all the lines into one long poem. The poem constructor may change the order of the lines and, when necessary, the participants' words or phrases in order to achieve consistent tensing and rhythm and to avoid repetition, but may not introduce any new thoughts or images. This synthesis usually occurs after the class or on a break at a conference. The final poem is then presented to the group at the next session.

Let me provide an illustration. When exploring ethical issues of persons living with disabilities, I share with session participants the story of the woman confined by illness to moving only her facial muscles (Nisker 2001a; 2010a). I then ask the participants to imagine themselves in this woman's position and to write one line each about how they would feel, after which these collections of lines are shaped into poems. Below are two of the 12 poems created at the 2000 Canadian Association of Critical Care Nurses (CACCN) Meeting in response to this question.[9]

CACCN Poem 1

I feel like an insect
Trapped in a glass jar.
It is warm,
I have air to breath,
But I am not free.
Time crawls incessantly.

CACCN Poem 3

I watch an elastic raindrop
Struggle out of a puddle.
I watch an energetic fly
Struggle through a screen.
The fly is scared,
I am encouraged;
Give me a small opening
And I will soar.

"Yick Factor"

I encourage students to recognize their "gut feelings" as one of the important assessors of moral appropriateness. I have offered my students a "yick factor" (i.e., upsetting) scale (from 0 to 10, but as logarithmic as the Richter seismograph scale) as an impression of the appropriateness of a specific action, request, policy, or procedure. We also use the scale as a measure of the discomfort of participants when imagining themselves in the position of the person *qua* patient or person *qua* caregiver in the narrative. A high "yick factor" rating immediately draws the students to the need for ethics exploration. The use of this scale supports Nixon's view that ethics education has a role in helping students "gain practice in experiencing unsettling ideas and events" (1997, 247). In fourth year my students write a story exploring an ethical dilemma they faced during their clerkship (Kelly and Nisker 2010).

NARRATIVES IN HEALTH ETHICS RESEARCH

In this section, I will reflect on both some of the promise that narrative holds for health research and the problems particular to narrative research.

Narrative to Present Research

Narrative has been used by social scientists to present their research (Denzin 1997; McCall 2000) in scholarly journals (Cox 2003), books directed primarily to scholars (Frank 1991; 1995; 2004; Kuhl 2002), or primarily to the general public in books such as John Howard Griffin's *Black Like Me* (1961) and William H. Whyte's *The Organization Man* (1956). The books of Frank (1991; 1995; 2004) and Kuhl (2002), drawing on personal experience, and patient interviews respectively, are extremely important to health professionals.

Theatre is also a useful way of presenting research (McCall 2000). In collaboration with Vangie Bergum we brought her research on "The experience of becoming mother through birthing, adopting, and placing a child" (Bergum 1997), and my research and concerns regarding the use of economically disadvantaged women as surrogate mothers and as oocyte donors (Nisker 1996; Rodgers and Nisker 1997) was juxtaposed on Bergum's research to explore ethical issues common to both areas of research (Nisker 1997b; Rogers et al. 1997) in the play titled *A Child on Her Mind*.

Similarly, Christina Sinding and Ross Gray have used theatre (Gray and Sinding 2002) to bring their research on women living with breast cancer (Gray, Sinding, and Fitch 2001) to audiences of health professionals, cancer patients, and the general public.

Narrative for Research

As an ethics **research** tool, narrative can not only bring the research of scientists and scholars to the public but also engage the public to provide multiple and diverse thoughts and perspectives as research data. There has been increasing interest in arts-based research (Cahnmann-Taylor and Siegesmund 2007; Knowles and Cole 2008; Leavy 2009; Pierson and Stephanson 2010). Alongside researchers who use photography (Mitchell and Allnutt 2008), installations (Cole and McIntyre 2008), music (Bresler 2008), and other artistic representations in their research, I explore narrative in general, and theatre in particular, as a research strategy (Nisker 2008a). Theatre as a research tool has been used to investigate attributes of specific health problems and areas of inquiry, for example, Alzheimer's disease (Cole, McIntyre, and Burns 2006; Johnson 2010), hereditary breast cancer (Nisker et al. 2006), genetics (Cox, Kazubowski-Houston, and Nisker 2009), and reproductive sciences (Nisker 2010b).

Narrative to Surface Ethical Issues in Health Policy Research

Ethical health policy development requires that a large number of citizens, representing different perspectives, participate in the development of health policies that will affect them personally, members of their community, and citizens in general (Coleman and Gøetze 2001; Garland 1999; Lenaghan 1999; Nisker et al. 2006; Rowe and Frewer 2000; Webler and Renn 1995). In addition, it is important that the citizens participating in health policy development be provided with all the scientific, clinical, and social information required to help them internalize the issues and voice their views to health policy developers (Brunger and Cox 2002).

The idea that narrative may serve as a site of dialogical inquiry for policy has precedent in the seminal work of Augusto Boal (1998), *Legislative Theatre: Using Performance to Make Politics*. In this book, Boal describes theatre as a powerful tool for engaging the public to create a true form of democracy and effect social change. Theatre can surface ethical issues in health policy research (Cox et al. 2009; Nisker et al. 2006; Nisker 2008a). Through the perspectives of persons immersed in health ethics policy issues, theatre can recruit the thoughts of the public, health professionals, and policy-makers toward health policy development (Cox et al. 2009; Nisker et al. 2006). Theatre can engage the public for health policy development (Cox et al. 2009; Nisker et al. 2006; Nisker 2008a), rather than the "expert" engagement that currently forms the basis of health policy development (Brunger and Cox 2002; Buchanan et al. 2000, 305).

In 2001, we began an exploration of the use of a full-length play as a possible public engagement tool for ethical health policy development (Nisker et al. 2006). I based the script for *Sarah's Daughters* on interviews with women who were themselves immersed in issues of adult predictive testing for BRCA gene mutation-related breast cancer, and those making policy decisions in this area (Nisker et al. 2006). The play provides information to audience members about the scientific, social, and clinical issues of adult predictive genetic testing, and attempts to immerse them in the position of the women I interviewed (Nisker et al. 2006). The play was followed by audience members sharing their comments with the researchers and other audience members (Nisker et al. 2006), knowing that their comments were being taped and transcribed for qualitative analysis (Strauss and Corbin 1994), and would be published (Nisker et al. 2006).

More than 1000 Canadians were engaged through the research tour of *Sarah's Daughters* (Nisker et al. 2006). The qualitative analysis of audience members' comments (Strauss and Corgin 1994) indicated that they were engaged both cognitively and emotionally, both in the position of the central character and in health policy issues (Nisker et al. 2006).

In 2005, Canada's first theatre-based citizen deliberation to develop health policy was funded by the Canadian Institutes for Health Research (CIHR) and Health Canada

(Cox et al. 2009) to develop a national policy on preimplantation genetic diagnosis (Handyside et al. 1989; Nisker and Gore-Langton 1995), using an updated iteration of my late 1990s play *Orchids*. Susan Cox, a sociologist, ethicist, and qualitative researcher at the University of British Columbia, joined me as co-principal investigator on this research. Important for democratic health policy development, all 16 research performances of *Orchids* were free, and occurred in level-access theatres that were easily reachable through public transportation. The results of this theatre-based citizen deliberation were submitted to Health Canada in a formal report (Nisker, Cox, and Kazubowski-Houston 2006; Cox et al. 2009). We believe senior citizens, disabled persons, and citizens from rural and remote locations were underrepresented in this citizen deliberation and have suggested strategies to overcome this shortcoming (Cox et al. 2009).

Ethics of Using Narrative for Research and Policy Development

When using narrative as a research tool, "traditional **ethical principles governing research** with human participants offer insufficient guidance in dealing with our [qualitative research] unique dilemmas" (Smythe and Murray 2000, 312). Smythe and Murray draw our attention to the fact that "potential risks invoked by narrative research have to do with subtle and often unforeseen consequences of writing about other people's lives" (321) and that "extensive precautions often are necessary to protect the integrity of participants' reputations and their ongoing relationships with the others who figure in their stories" (321). This is an important warning as to how to go about achieving permission to tell a patient's story, or whether we should attempt to do so in a research or education or even moral exploration aegis.

Under what circumstances is it appropriate to present the narrative of a person we know, including persons who are (or have been) in our care or in the care of our colleagues (Nisker and Daar 2006)? I am concerned not only when these stories are used for research or policy development purposes, but also when these narratives are used in classrooms, at rounds, at conferences, or other educational venues. In the clinician–patient relationship (Baylis 1990; Kenny 1994; Sherwin 1994), but also in other relationships such as in families, **power differentials** inexorably exist and exceed standard differentials in the researcher–research subject relationship (Nisker and Daar 2006; see also Chapter 14). I have become increasingly concerned that stories in which the medical condition has a genetic basis—especially if the inheritance pattern is autosomal dominant or x-linked recessive, rather than an autosomal recessive or polygenic inheritance pattern that is less likely to identify family members—are quite different from other stories (Nisker and Daar 2006). This is because such stories may inadvertently violate not only the privacy of the person whose story is being told, but also family members'; and that sacrifice of privacy may threaten the person's ability to access life insurance and employment opportunities (Nisker and Daar 2006). Striving for maximum camouflage of the persons kind (and brave) enough to allow us to tell their story not only requires changing names but also geographic locations and even at times factual material.

I believe it important in order to promote informed choice of the research participants *qua* audience members, to include as much information as possible about the play and the research in the invitations to participate (playbills, advertisements, posters, brochures, e-mail, etc.) and in the theatre lobby. This information should include the subject material of the play, that an audience discussion will follow the performance, that the theatre experience is part of a research project, and that audience members choosing to share their perspectives will have their comments audiotaped and transcribed for research purposes (Cox et al. 2009; Cox and Nisker 2010). Further, when the audience is seated, prior to each play's performance, it is important a reading of a formal (research ethics approved) invitation letter to participate in the research occur, in order to clearly explain the nature of the research in which they are invited to participate, the content of the play, and that they have a choice whether to participate or not. I recommend the contents of the letter be reiterated prior to the audience discussion (Cox et al. 2009; Cox and Nisker 2010). I also recommend including a caution that it may not be possible to show the results of the research to the participants for their approval prior to publication, as the participants were advised to remain anonymous and, indeed only if they were comfortable, indicate from where their perspective was offered (health professional, patient, member of the general public, or policy maker) (Cox et al. 2009; Cox and Nisker 2010).

Another ethical concern is that audience members *qua* research participants may experience emotional harm by viewing the play that is part of the research (Nisker et al. 2006). Emotional harm was suggested in the analysis of audience members' comments following performances of *Sarah's Daughters*, in which audience members learned for the first time information about their personal and family members' genetic risk (Nisker et al. 2006). Cautions posted and read from the stage that this might occur are important, as audience members *qua* research participants may come to see the play because of their personal connection to the subject matter (Nisker et al. 2006). It has also been my practice to have a person capable of counselling in regard to the health issue being explored seated at the back of the theatre, with pamphlets regarding follow-up care should someone leave in distress.

Summary

For almost 20 years the wise fox's words in *The Little Prince*, "It is only with the heart that one can see rightly" (de Saint-Exupéry 1943) has informed not only the way I engage in health ethics education, research, and policy development, but also the way I live my life. I hope you will consider using story to delve deeper into the ethical issues in which we are immersed than a theories-and-principles-based approach allows. I hope you will use narratives to approximate empathy for the persons at the centre of the ethical issue, their families, and their health professionals. I hope you will use narratives to bring the beauty of persons, too often confined within a clinical diagnosis, to classrooms, conference auditoria, and policy tables. For narratives can "help compassion happen."

For Reflection

1. How might "telling stories" of ethics problems assist practitioners working in direct care areas to improve their work environment?

2. How might educators better evaluate ethics learning involving narrative?

3. Think of ways in which you might use various forms of narrative to influence health policy development. Provide specific examples.

4. What measures can be taken to preserve the confidentiality of persons when their stories are presented?

Endnotes

1. The use of the term "thick" narrative parallels Geertz's (1973) concept of "thick description."

2. Benner points out an interesting link to clinical reasoning here. Benner draws attention to Rubin's (1996) observation that "[p]ublic storytelling among practitioners allows for noticing distinctions and clinical learning. The forming of the story, where it begins, how it develops, what concerns shape the story, and how the story ends as well as the dialogue and perceptions of the storyteller present meaningful accounts of practical engaged reasoning" (Rubin's article cited as "in press" in Benner 1994, 58).

3. For the purposes of this chapter I am using the terms "story" and "narrative" interchangeably.

4. I believe the term "person" or "person qua patient" affords more dignity and respect than "case" or "patient" to the person at the centre of the ethical issue or moral exploration.

5. Note that some of these are not precisely qualified under the rubric of narrative.

6. See also Charon and Montello (2002).

7. Credit for the development of problem-based learning goes in large part to the work done at McMaster University, Hamilton, Canada.

8. For a scholarly discussion on writing "thick" case-based narratives, I recommend Chambers (1997).

9. Used with permission of the conference organizer.

References

Amenábar, A. 2004. *The sea inside.* New Line Cinema.

Arcand, D. and Potashnik, J. 2003. *The barbarian invasions.* Miramax.

Arras, J.D. 1997. Nice story, but so what? Narrative and justification in ethics. In H.L. Nelson (Ed.), *Stories and their limits: Narrative approaches to bioethics* (pp. 65–88). New York: Routledge.

Baylis, F. 1990. The ethics of ex utero research on spare "non-viable" IVF human embryos. *Bioethics, 4,* 311–329.

Beauchamp, T. and Childress, J.F. 1994. *Principles of bioethics.* New York: Oxford University Press.

Benner, P.A. 1994. Caring as a way of knowing and not knowing. In S. Philips and P.A. Benner (Eds.), *The crisis of care: Affirming and restoring caring practices in the helping professions* (pp. 42–62). Washington, DC: Georgetown University Press.

Benner, P.A., Tanner, C.A., and Chesla, C.A. 1996. *Expertise in nursing practice: Caring, clinical judgment and ethics.* New York: Springer.

Bergum, V. 1997. *A child on her mind.* Westport, CT: Bergin & Garvey.

Boal, A. 1998. *Legislative theatre: Using performance to make politics.* London: Routledge.

Bresler, L. 2008. The music lesson. In In J.G. Knowles and A.L Cole (Eds.), *Handbook of the arts in qualitative research: Perspectives, methodologies, examples, and issues* (pp. 225–237). Thousand Oaks, CA: Sage.

Brody, H. 1987. *Stories of sickness.* New Haven, CT: Yale University Press.

Brody, H. 2003. *Stories of sickness* (2nd ed.). Oxford: Oxford University Press.

Brunger, F. and Cox, S.M. 2002. Ethics and genetics: The need for transparency. Available online at www.cwhn.ca/groups/biotech/availdocs/4-brun-cox.pdf.

Buchanan, A., Brock, D.W., Daniels, N., and Wikler, D. 2000. *From chance to choice: Genetics and justice.* Cambridge, UK: Cambridge University Press.

Burrell, D. and Hauerwas, S. 1977. From system to story: An alternative pattern for rationality in ethics. In H.T. Engelhardt, Jr. and D. Callahan (Eds.), *Knowledge, value and belief* (pp. 111–152). Hastings-on-Hudson, NY: The Hastings Centre.

Cahnmann-Taylor, M. and Siegesmund, R. 2007. *Arts-based research in education: Foundations for practice.* New York: Routledge.

Chambers, T. 1997. What to expect from an ethics case (and what it expects from you). In H.L. Nelson (Ed.), *Stories and their limits: Narrative approaches to bioethics* (pp. 171–184). New York: Routledge.

Charon, R. 1994. Narrative contributions to medical ethics: Recognition, formulation, interpretation, and validation in the practice of the ethicist. In E.R. Dubose, R.P. Hamel, and L.J. O'Connell (Eds.), *A matter of principles? Ferment in U.S. bioethics* (pp. 260–283). Valley Forge, PA: Trinity Press.

Charon, R. 1997. The ethical dimensions of literature: Henry James's *The Wings of the Dove.* In H.L. Nelson (Ed.), *Stories and their limits: Narrative approaches to bioethics* (pp. 91–112). New York: Routledge.

Charon, R. 2006. *Narrative medicine: Honoring the stories of illness.* New York: Oxford University Press.

Charon, R. 2008. Where does narrative medicine come from? Drives, diseases, attention, and the body. In P.L. Rudnytsky and R. Charon (Eds.), *Psychoanalysis and narrative medicine* (pp. 23–36). Albany, NY: State University of New York.

Charon, R. and Montello, M. (Eds.). 2002. *Stories matter: The role of narrative in medical ethics.* New York: Routledge.

Cole, A.L. and McIntyre, M. 2008. Installation art-as-research. In J.G. Knowles and A.L Cole (Eds.), *Handbook of the arts in qualitative research: Perspectives, methodologies, examples, and issues* (pp. 287–297). Thousand Oaks, CA: Sage.

Cole, A., McIntyre, M., and Burns, L. 2006. *The Alzheimer's project: Living and dying with dignity*. Halifax, NS: Backalong Books.

Coleman, S. and Gøetze, J. 2001. *Bowling together: Online public engagement in policy deliberation*. London: Hansard Society.

Cox, S.M. 2003. Stories in decisions: How at-risk individuals decide to request predictive testing for Huntington Disease. *Qualitative Sociology, 26* (2), 257–280.

Cox, S.M, Kazubowski-Houston, M., and Nisker, J.A. 2009. Genetics on stage: Public engagement in health policy development on preimplantation genetic diagnosis. *Social Science & Medicine, 68* (8), 1472–1480.

Cox, S.M. and Nisker, J.A. 2010. Public understandings of a "healthy" embryo: A citizen deliberation on preimplantation genetic diagnosis. In J. Nisker, F. Baylis, I. Karpin, C. McLeod, and R. Mykitiuk (Eds.), *The "healthy" embryo: Social, biomedical, legal and philosophical perspectives* (pp. 151–169). Cambridge, UK: Cambridge University Press.

de Saint-Exupéry, A. 1943/1993. *The little prince*. San Diego: Harcourt Brace Jovanovich.

Denzin, N.K. 1997. *Interpretive ethnography: Ethnographic practices for the 21st century*. Thousand Oaks, CA: Sage.

Edson, M. 2001. *Wit*. New York: Faber and Faber.

Frank, A. 1991. *At the will of the body*. Boston: Houghton Mifflin.

Frank, A. 1995. *The wounded storyteller: Body, illness, and ethics*. Chicago: University of Chicago Press.

Frank, A. 2004. *The renewal of generosity: Illness, medicine, and how to live*. Chicago: University of Chicago Press.

Garland, M. 1999. Experts and the public: A needed partnership for genetic policy. *Public Understanding of Science, 8*, 241–245.

Geertz, C. 1973. *The interpretation of cultures*. New York: Basic.

Gordimer, N. 1999. Interview on CBC Radio.

Gray, R.E. and Sinding, C. 2002. *Standing ovation: Performing social science research about cancer*. Lanham, MD: AltaMira Press.

Gray, R.E., Sinding, C., and Fitch M. 2001. Navigating the social context of metastatic breast cancer: Reflections on a project linking research to drama. *Health, 5* (2), 233–248.

Griffin, J.H. 1961. *Black like me*. Boston: Houghton Mifflin.

Halpern, J. 2001. *From detached concern to empathy: Harmonizing medical practice*. New York: Oxford University Press.

Handyside, A.H., Pattinson, J.K., Penketh, R.J., Delhanty, J.D., Winston, R.M., and Tuddenham, E.G. 1989. Biopsy of human preimplantation embryos and sexing by DNA amplification. *Lancet, 1* (8634), 347–349.

Hawkins, A.H. 1997. Medical ethics and the epiphanic dimension of narrative. In H.L. Nelson (Ed.), *Stories and their limits: Narrative approaches to bioethics* (pp. 153–170). New York: Routledge.

Johnson, K. 2010. Grafting *Orchids* and *Ugly*: Theatre, disability and arts-based health research. *Journal of Medical Humanities, 31* (4), 279–294.

Jones A.H. 1994. Literature as mirror or lamp? Commentary on literature, medical ethics, and "epiphanic knowledge." *Journal of Clinical Ethics, 5* (4), 340–341.

Jones, A.H. 1998. Narrative in medical ethics. In T. Greenhalgh and B. Hurwitz (Eds.), *Narrative-based medicine*. London, UK: BMJ Books.

Kelly E. and Nisker J.A. 2010. Medical students' first clinical experiences of death. *Medical Education, 44* (4), 421–428.

Kenny, N.P. 1994. The ethics of care and the patient–physician relationship. *Annual of the Royal College of Physicians and Surgeons, 17* (6), 356–258.

Knowles, J.G. and Cole, A.L. (Eds.). 2008. *Handbook of the arts in qualitative research: Perspectives, methodologies, examples, and issues*. Thousand Oaks, CA: Sage.

Kohn, M., Donley, C., and Wear, D. 1992. *Literature and aging: An anthology*. Kent, OH: Kent State University Press.

Kuhl, D. 2002. *What dying people want: Lessons for living from people who are dying*. New York: Public Affairs.

Leavy, P. 2009. *Method meets art: Arts-based research practice*. New York: The Guilford Press.

Lenaghan, J. 1999. Involving the public in rationing decisions. The experience of citizens' juries. *Health Policy, 49* (1–2), 45–61.

MacIntyre, A.C. 1981. *After virtue: A study in moral theory*. Notre Dame, IN: Notre Dame University Press.

MacIntyre, A.C. 1988. *Whose justice? Which rationality?* Notre Dame, IN: Notre Dame University Press.

McCall, M.M. 2000. Performance ethnography: A brief history and some advice. In N.K. Denzin and Y. Lincoln (Eds.), *Handbook of Qualitative Research* (2nd ed.). Thousand Oaks, CA: Sage.

Mitchell, C. and Allnutt, S. 2008. Photographs and/as social documentary. In J.G. Knowles and A.L. Cole (Eds.), *Handbook of the arts in qualitative research: Perspectives, methodologies, examples, and issues* (pp. 251–263). Thousand Oaks, CA: Sage.

Montello, M. 1997. Narrative competence. In H.L. Nelson (Ed.), *Stories and their limits: Narrative approaches to bioethics* (pp. 185–197). New York: Routledge.

Murray, T.H. 1997. What do we mean by "narrative ethics?" In H.L. Nelson (Ed.), *Stories and their limits: Narrative approaches to bioethics* (pp. 3–17). New York: Routledge.

Nelson, H.L. 2001. *Damaged identities: Narrative repair*. New York: Cornell University Press.

Nisker, J.A. 1995. A user-friendly framework for exploration of ethical issues in reproductive medicine. *Assisted Reproduction Reviews, 5* (4), 272–279.

Nisker JA. 1996. Rachel's ladders or how societal situation determines reproductive therapy. *Human Reproduction, 11* (6), 1162–7.

Nisker, J.A. 1997a. The yellow brick road of medical education. *Canadian Medical Association Journal, 156* (5), 689–691.

Nisker, J.A. 1997b. In quest of the perfect analogy for using in vitro fertilization patients as oocyte donors. *Womens Health Issues, 7* (4), 241–247.

Nisker, J.A. 2001a. Chalcedonies. *Canadian Medical Association Journal, 164* (1), 74–75.

Nisker, J.A. 2001b. Orchids: Not necessarily a gospel. In *Mappa mundi: Mapping culture/mapping the world* (pp. 61–109).Windsor, ON: University of Windsor Press.

Nisker, J.A. 2003a. Medical students mirror and hold mirrors. *Journal of Obstetrics and Gynaecology Canada, 25* (12), 995–996.

Nisker, J.A. 2003b. Philip. *Canadian Medical Association Journal, 168*, 746–747.

Nisker, J.A. 2003c. Rebuilding compassionate Canadian healthcare policy. *Journal of Obstetrics and Gynaecology Canada, 25* (1), 7–12.

Nisker J.A. 2007. In their hands. In L.E. Clarke and J.A. Nisker (Eds.), *In our hands: On becoming a doctor* (pp. 19–23). Halifax, NS: Pottersfield Press.

Nisker, J.A. 2008a. Health-policy research and the possibilities of theater. In J.G. Knowles and A.L. Cole (Eds.), *Handbook of the arts in qualitative research: Perspectives, methodologies, examples, and issues* (pp. 613–624). Thousand Oaks, CA: Sage.

Nisker J.A. 2008b. Preface. In J. Nisker (Ed.), *From the other side of the fence: Stories from health care professionals* (pp. 11–15). Halifax, NS: Pottersfield Press.

Nisker, J.A. 2010a. Calcedonies: Critical reflections on writing plays to engage citizens in health and social policy development. *Reflective Practice, 11* (4), 417–432.

Nisker, J.A. 2010b. Theatre and research in the reproductive sciences. *Journal of Medical Humanities, 31* (1), 81–90.

Nisker, J.A., Cox, S.M., and Kazubowski-Houston, M. 2006. *Citizen deliberation on preimplantation genetic diagnosis*. Ottawa: Health Canada.

Nisker, J.A. and Daar, A.S. 2006. Moral presentation of genetics-based narratives for public understanding of genetic science and its implications. *Public Understanding of Science, 15*, 113–123.

Nisker, J.A. and Gore-Langton, R.E. 1995. Pre-implantation genetic diagnosis: A model of progress and concern. *Journal of Obstetrics and Gynaecology Canada, 17* (3), 247–262.

Nisker, J.A., Martin, D.K., Bluhm, R., and Daar, A.S. 2006. Theatre as a public engagement tool for health-policy development. *Health Policy, 78*, 258–271.

Nixon, L.L. 1997. Medical humanities: Pyramids and rhomboids in the rationalist world of medicine. In H.L. Nelson (Ed.), *Stories and their limits* (pp. 238–272). New York: Routledge.

Nussbaum, M.C. 1990. *Love's knowledge: Essays on philosophy and literature.* New York: Oxford University Press.

Phillips, S.S. 1994. Introduction. In S.S. Phillips and P. Benner (Eds.), *The crisis of care: Affirming and restoring caring practices in the helping professions*. Washington, DC: Georgetown University Press.

Pierson, R. and Stephanson, R. (Eds.). 2010. Imagining reproduction in science and history [Special issue]. *Journal of Medical Humanities, 31* (1), 1–9.

Quindlen, A. 1995. *One true thing.* New York: Dell.

Quindlen, A. 1998a. *Black and blue.* New York: Dell.

Quindlen, A. 1998b. Interview on *The Charlie Rose Show.*

Rogers S., Baylis F., Lippman, A., MacMillan J., Parish, B., and Nisker J. Policy statement: Preconception arrangements. *Journal of Obstetrics and Gynaecology Canada, 19* (4), 393–99.

Rowe, G. and Frewer, L.J. 2000. Public participation methods: A framework for evaluation. *Science, Technology and Human Values, 25* (1), 3–29.

Rubin, J. 1996. Impediments to the development of clinical knowledge and ethical judgment in critical care nursing. In P.A Benner, C.A. Tanner, and C.A. Chesla (Eds.), *Expertise in nursing practice: Caring, clinical judgment, and ethics* (pp. 170–192). New York: Springer.

Sherwin, S. 1994. Feminism, ethics, and cancer. *Humane Medicine, 10* (4), 282–290.

Smythe, W.E. and Murray, M.J. 2000. Owning the story: Ethical considerations in narrative research. *Ethics and Behavior, 10* (4), 311–336.

Spiro, H. 1996. *Empathy and the practice of medicine: Beyond pills and the scalpel.* New Haven, CT: Yale University Press.

Stein, J.G. 2001. *The cult of efficiency.* Toronto: House of Anansi Press.

Stewart, M.A., Weston, W.W., Brown, J.B., McWhinney, I.E., McWilliam C., and Freeman T.R. 1995. *Patient-centered medicine.* Thousand Oaks, CA: Sage.

Strauss, A. and Corbin, J. 1994. Grounded theory methodology: An overview. In N.K. Denzin and Y.S. Lincoln (Eds.), *Handbook of qualitative research.* Thousand Oaks, CA: Sage.

Thomasma, D.C. 1994. Beyond the ethics of rightness: The role of compassion in moral responsibility. In S.S. Philips and P.A. Benner (Eds.), *The crisis of care: Affirming and restoring caring practices in the helping professions* (pp. 123–143). Washington, DC: Georgetown University Press.

Webler, T. and Renn, O. 1995. A brief primer on participation: Philosophy and practice. In O. Renn, T. Webler, and P. Wiedemann (Eds.), *Fairness and competence in citizen participation: Evaluating models for environmental discourse* (pp. 17–33). Dordrecht, Germany: Kluwer Academic Publishers.

Weijer, C. 1997. Film and narrative in bioethics: Akira Kurosawa's *Ikuru.* In H.L. Nelson (Ed.), *Stories and their limits: Narrative approaches to bioethics* (pp. 113–122). New York: Routledge.

Whyte, W.H. 1956. *The organization man.* New York: Simon and Schuster.

CHAPTER 7

Relational Ethics for Health Care

Vangie Bergum

If relational space is the location of enacting morality, ethical considerations occur in every situation, every encounter, and with every patient. If all relationships are the focus of understanding and examining moral life, then it is important to attend to the quality of relationships in all professional practices, whether with patients and their families, with other health care professionals, or with administrators and politicians.

The focus of attention in this chapter is on relationship itself, the space where health care professionals and patients make connection. Relational ethics is built on the premise that all relationships as experienced are moral. In each connection one enacts the question of what is the "right thing to do" both for oneself and with and for others. Along with the use of a clinical example, presented as a series of Ethics in Practice scenarios, this chapter highlights four themes useful to increase understanding of a relational ethic: environment, embodiment, mutual respect, and engagement.[1] Breath is used as an example to show the necessary integration of mind and body within a relational ethic.

The clinical example, a story in six parts, begins with "Once upon a time." Story engages the reader with the complexity of a particular situation that sheds light on other particular situations. The example, taken from personal experience with permission of the patient and her family, has distinguishing details changed to protect privacy. One could think that this story is fiction, and in one sense it is, as any recounting captures only part of any person's experience. If the woman, the patient herself, or one of the nurses or doctors had written the story, it would have a different emphasis and language. Use of story invites readers to engage with it from their own perspective, to be touched and challenged with what resonates with their personal experience. In conjunction with the clinical story, "breath" is explored as an example that bridges physiological realities with personal, psychological, and social concerns. The breath, and the ability to breathe, also bridges individual, community, and ecological issues. The chapter concludes with a discussion of dialogue, the place where relational ethics is vividly enacted.

RELATIONAL ETHICS

Relational ethics is an action ethic. A relational ethic is, as Peacock (1999) suggests, "an evolving thing, expanding in scope and effectiveness as our collectively shared experience grows—and is always a bit tentative, even when it must guide us in life-and-death situations" (703). There is no clear high mountain vantage point from which to view a situation with complete objectivity. Nor is there clear certainty found in the valley of subjective experience. In a relational ethic, one is "inescapably, dialogically, in the midst," and it is this relational space that gives moral meaning to our actions (Gaita 1991, 142).

Ethical action from the perspective of relationship is a move away from direct attention to epistemology, virtues, or problems. Rather, attention is given to the moral space created by one's relation to oneself and to the other (Austin 2007; Bergum in press; Bergum and Dossetor 2005; Ermine 2007). Relational space, as a moral space, is where one enacts responsiveness and responsibility not just for oneself *or* for the other, but within the space of being for and with both oneself *and* the other (Jopling 2000).

In relationships, where intersubjectivity is a goal, there is no assumption that the other person is like ourselves, but rather, through dialogue we may come to see the other as radically different. The opportunity of intersubjectivity is to encounter another as "absolutely foreign" without making the other an object or meshing oneself with another (Jopling 2000, 153). Through dialogue something new is made possible because of the uniqueness of each partner. Within the "logic of dialogue" we listen and attend to another human being, "a dimension that encompasses and supports all of our reason and thought" (Gadamer 1996, 167). Dialogue builds on the presupposition "that the other may not just have *a* right but may actually *be* right, may understand something better than we do" (Gadamer 1996, 82, italics added). Even the definition of just who is "other" alters relationships. Disparities of health and illness, wealth and poverty are not experienced only as problems to be solved, but as questions to be asked: "Women, students, the mad, the ill, the poor, blacks, the suffering, the marginalized of every sort" (Caputo 1989, 61) lead to ethical questions precisely because it is often marginalized people who challenge the meaning of relational commitments. A relational ethic must genuinely embrace, cherish, and celebrate difference (Olthuis 2000).

With relational space as the location of enacting morality, we consider ethics in every situation, every encounter, and with every patient. If relationships are the focus of understanding and examining moral life, it is important to attend to the *quality* of relationships in all practice, whether with patients and their families, with other health care professionals, or with administrators and politicians. The practice of relational ethics affects all levels of health care. In a world where people are increasingly isolated from each other and communities are divided against each other, it is not surprising that a relational approach to ethics has been gaining interest and credibility (Ermine 2007). With governments' and organizations' focus on dollars and cents, it would be easy for relationships to be seen as a nice "add on" to the primary economic concerns. The harsh reality of the need to attend to rising costs of health care can overshadow the equally harsh reality of human suffering. Both realities need research and development. Relational ethics demands attention in order to improve the human condition.

Attention to relationship does not take away from the need to distinguish between different ethical foci: practical ethics, professional ethics, nursing and medical ethics, bioethics, or health ethics. Nor does it erase the need to learn about ethical principles such as respect for autonomy, beneficence, preventing harm, truth-telling, or distributive justice. Placing the focus of ethics at different levels of the health system—micro, meso, or macro (see Chapter 4)—is also helpful in providing the language for ethics of the health care system. Yet attention to relationship has a way of dismantling these distinctions and categories for what happens at the bedside is not cut off from the broader issues. Ethics at the bedside and ethics in the system are part and parcel of the same lived universe. The moral community includes each of us as responsible for our actions in relation to the people we care for, educate, supervise, or work with in partnership. In each interaction a relational ethic can flourish.

RELATIONAL THEMES

The four themes of **environment**, **embodiment**, **mutual respect**, and **engagement** explored here are useful in giving language to a relational ethic. The themes come alive in the disorderly realities of practice rather than in the orderly requirements of theory. In practice, too, it is difficult to confine discussion of one theme to one particular section, as in real life the themes show themselves and disappear throughout the whole of experience. Many professionals in health care already practise a relational approach to ethics, yet there remains a need for a well-developed perspective that gives voice to the significance of ethical relationships and how to improve them.

ENVIRONMENT

Within the relational approach, environment is not only "out there" to be manipulated and managed. Instead, environment is "in here," in each of us as a living system that changes through daily action. We are the health care system; we are the environment. Perhaps one reason that studies of the health care system seem to produce little lasting change is that we have been looking in the wrong place. Instead of exploring "out there" we need to look "in here." The clinical example presented in Ethics in Practice 7-1 demonstrates the theme of environment in which all of us are intimately engaged and therefore constantly changing.

ETHICS IN PRACTICE 7-1

The Breath—Connecting the Individual and the Environment

Once upon a time, not so long ago and not so far away, on a quiet spring day on one of Canada's major highways, two vehicles crashed into each other. The drivers of the two vehicles were similar in some ways—driving alone, being of similar age with busy, active lives. Both were severely injured as their smashed vehicles crushed bones and organs. Both individuals were released from their vehicles with the "jaws of life" and rushed off in screaming ambulances to the nearest emergency department (ER), which had recently experienced reduction in staff and resources due to provincial cuts to health care. Each person, now a patient, needed specialized care, and when each was stabilized with open airways and blood, was sent off to a larger regional hospital. Here, they were separated. One patient, a woman, was taken by air ambulance to the next major hospital. Even here the specialists could not attend to the severity of her injuries so she was transferred to a large university centre where the intensive clinical expertise of nurses and doctors saved her life—reduced brain pressures, closed contusions, straightened bones and muscles, added bone transplant materials to reconstruct heels and ankles, and, all the while, monitored all life processes. Each practitioner who touched the injured people enacted the whole of the health care system.

Imagine the scene where nurses rush to assist and start with the process of maintaining the breath of the patient—and perhaps even catching their own breath. As the breath is stabilized, the nurses, along with the doctor and others, work to stop the bleeding, call out the name of the patient, start the intravenous (IV) to administer blood and drugs, align broken bones, and contact the family. The person who witnessed the accident, the ambulance attendant, the nurse, the doctor, and other members of the team are the health care system that attends to each person's needs. As the patient is moved through the various locations to find the best possible care, the system responds through individual action and each action affects the system itself. While there is a need to question whether cutbacks in health care resources affected the care of these patients, there is also a need to question how each patient and each professional acted from a place of being "inescapably in the midst" of the environment that they affect and are affected by.

With this kind of attention to environment, while the persons in the accident become the primary focus, all those who care for them are involved and personally affected as well. The system is enacted through each individual connection to save the patient's life: the nurses and doctors who rush to give attention, which takes attention away from others less in danger of dying; the families of the patients who are stopped in their tracks when they hear the news; or the neighbours who take on the responsibility to tell the children so that the police are not the first to break the news. Even the citizen who decides that health care will be available to all its country's people, and hospitals and professionals that provide expertise, are affected and involved. The undulating vibrations of the ambulance siren are felt far beyond the ears of anyone who hears it, or indeed the life of any one particular person. Looking at environment in this relational way brings us back to individual acts.

In considering the environment and the health care system as an interdependent and complex entity, ethics cannot be understood as just personal, social, or political, but needs also to be ecological (Peacock 1999). Such ecological consciousness is a hopeful sign, says Gadamer (1996), as it includes not only the ability to manage by oneself (autonomy) but also the ability to manage along with other people (community). Such "housekeeping" (Gadamer 1996) encompasses not only individual caretaking but also includes the caretaking of the "house" that is held in common, the health care system, and even the planet as a whole. In such a living relation one begins to see the fluidity between breath of the individual and breath of the universe, between stabilizing each patient's breathing and making sure that the air is pure and toxin free. The breath is in continuous communion, in both its micro and macro circumstances, which in its pure form would be "breathing in tune with the breathing of the entire living universe" (Irigaray 2002, 36).

The breath is the origin of autonomous existence of the living human being as an individual and citizen of the culture. The breath maintains a person's life, yet to breathe for survival is not enough. The ultimate goal for the woman in Ethics in Practice 7-1 is to again breathe on her own, to take her own breath as a particular person who has a name, a history, a family, and a community. As the woman is secured in the reality of having breath maintained by artificial means of intubations and ventilators, the health care team begins the process of moving toward assisting her to become autonomous and take charge of her own breath and her own life. We often speak of the elementary need to eat or drink, but we do not often consider the need to breathe, which, says Irigaray (2002), is our first and most radical need: "Breathing in a conscious and free manner is equivalent to taking charge of one's life, to accepting solitude through cutting the umbilical cord, to respecting and cultivating life, for oneself and for others" (74). The patient, in order to come back to her individual and communal life, will begin to transform the vital breath in the service of survival to the more subtle breath in the service of the heart, of thought, and of speech. Even with this discussion, it is necessary to consider how autonomy can be fostered with those who will never be able to breathe without mechanical support.

During the first moments after the accident the woman's breath is breathed by and with others, through oxygen machines, yet like the umbilical cord that once tied her to her mother, breath is always given. The first ethical task with respect to autonomy is to share the breath and to breathe together. With the breath we begin to see how the individual is autonomous and also how individuals are connected to each other, how they respect and share life. "Community is then composed of autonomous individuals in conscious relation to one another" (Irigaray 2002, 102). Irigaray further reminds us that it is impossible to appropriate breath or air: one can only cultivate it, for oneself and for others (79).

Consider how Gadamer's notion of housekeeping speaks to the relation between the need to live well for oneself and to also live well together (1996). These needs are the same; we can only live well autonomously if we live well together. If we do not attend to our shared home, we will have no home at all. Think about the extensive resources used in the woman's care: the IV and feeding tubes, the sheets and blankets, the detergents, the plastics, and the landfills that take both the benign and toxic waste. The environment (here indicating the health care system) is part of the ecological system. Relational ethics highlights the connection between care of the woman and care of the earth. (See also, Chapter 11).

Nurses have a great deal of power and responsibility in making waste disposal choices, and nurses are taking the lead in creating less hazardous waste (Gonzales 2002). Think of the boxes and boxes of latex gloves that are used each day in our major hospitals as staff don them whenever they touch a patient, to give oral medications, turn the patient, lift blankets to observe wounds and dressings, or to hand the patient a glass of water. The gloves are used to prevent transfer of infection, a practice of vital importance, yet it is possible that the practice can become thoughtless if gloves are overused and discarded with ease. A minor issue, one could say, but when one thinks of the self in the midst of the environment the interconnection between the use of gloves and landfills is no longer minor.

The second theme of relationship that will be highlighted through discussion of the scenario is embodiment. Embodiment shows the patient's lived life, where she is more than an object that needs emergent attention as she is navigated through the various hospitals and the care of many different professionals.

EMBODIMENT

Each person, when brought into hospital by ambulance, is immediately treated, according to Gadow, as "pure object, without interiority . . . [with] no inherent authority over her body [which now] logically . . . belongs to the expert" (1994, 298). Yet, at the same time, even during such critical episodes, patients are still tied to their own lives and worlds. Though the woman is not able to go about her regular activities—drive her car, or call to her children—she is bound to a world in which she was usually forgetful of her body. As the caregivers focus on the woman as an object (as a body), they also know that in actual life there is "absolute inseparability of the living body and life itself" (Gadamer 1996, 71).

Embodiment calls for healing the split between mind and body so that scientific knowledge and human compassion are given equal weight: emotion and feeling are understood to be as important to human life as physical signs and symptoms. It is the family, in the particular instance of our clinical example, which assists the professionals, in their world of objectivity, to be mindful of the embodied reality of the woman. If the woman did not have a family who could readily be present, the professionals would be more actively cognizant of the need to attend to the woman's lived life.

ETHICS IN PRACTICE 7-2

The Breath—Connecting Mind and Body

It so happened that a woman, from her garden, heard the quaver of the sirens and stood to watch two racing ambulances flash by. Little did this mother, grandmother, and great-grandmother realize that from that moment her life would irreversibly change from the quiet enjoyment of planting her garden to the fear of losing her adult child and only daughter. Soon she had a call from the hospital. Now this mother felt the fear. After locating her grandchildren and ensuring their protection and safety, she and the woman's father went to see their daughter, now at the second hospital. There was little recognition of the daughter they loved, with her face and head swollen beyond belief, legs and pelvis mangled, breathing through a ventilator, surrounded by tubes and bags with little evidence of life. Nurses and doctors did what was needed. The parents were told that their daughter would be moved by air to another larger hospital and they made the necessary calls: to the woman's husband working in the North, to her brother on a business trip, to nieces and nephews, and to friends. Life changed for each person. Each experienced a moment of terror that a precious life could be lost.

The focus of attention for professionals in this crisis is on the woman's body—the breath, the blood, the pressure on the brain, and the broken bones—that is now treated as if it were a machine laid out by medical definition. Yet, the focus of attention of the woman's parents is on the lived body, of the daughter and her life with them. Professionals support the reconnection of the "body as object" to the "body as lived" because they recognize that the lived body is as ethically important as the body as an object. While the woman is unconscious the practitioners do for her what throughout her life she has, without thinking, done for herself. They work within the reality of the inseparability of the lived body and the body as object.

The woman needs multiple surgeries carried out by different professional teams. What treatment does she want? She does not even know she has been in an accident. She will not completely grasp this fact for days, indeed months. She cannot make decisions for herself. It is up to those close to her, in particular her husband, to give consent for the various treatments. Her autonomy—her self-knowledge and responsibility—is fostered by her connections to others, to those who know her best. The lived reality of autonomy is achieved through human connections. Our relationships define who we are. The lived body is more important to the principle of autonomy than the object body as there is no autonomy for human beings in isolation from each other. Being alone and independent is primarily experienced because there are others to miss.

Commitment to others is felt in the body. The mother remembers the physical connection to the daughter as she looks to find the face that she loves. The nurse too must become bodily connected to the woman in order to remember the lived body of the woman at the same time as she or he tends to the patient's body as an object (Gadow 1980). Caregivers, too, need to remember their own lived lives and to take time to breathe for themselves. There must be deep ethical commitment to *who* the woman is and not just *how* she breathes. The sharing of the breath reminds nurses and other caregivers that the woman is both embodied and autonomous yet connected to others through the embodiment of the caregiver (Gadow 1989). They acknowledge their own vulnerability as they resonate with the other's pain: the women could be my daughter, my mother, or me. In such situations caregivers remain vigilant to the reality that it is the woman's pain and not their own. A fine balance allows for sensitivity to another's pain as the embodied reality of the other person, while being aware of the reality of one's own embodiment as separate and distinct. This self-knowledge and self-respect is as important as respect for the patient, which is the next relational theme to be discussed.

MUTUAL RESPECT

Mutual respect arises from the reality that people are fundamentally connected to one another. Our experience of the world and of ourselves is shaped by the attitude of others toward us and by our attitude toward others. The challenge of health care, politics, culture, and gender relations is to respect those with differences of opinions, beliefs, values, and activities. Mutual respect includes respect for ourselves as well as others (Dillon 1992).

ETHICS IN PRACTICE 7-3

The Breath—Connecting Self and Other

Time passed. Life unfolded. Nurses, neurologists, orthopedic specialists, physiotherapists, occupational therapists, rehabilitation psychologists, rehabilitation physicians, transfer teams, and laboratory technicians enacted their special knowledge in the care of the woman. Each team member, working alone with the woman but in concert and collaboration with other team members, was directed toward the goal of restoring the woman to a full functioning life. The woman's family, too, worked as a team to connect the woman to the life she had lived prior to the road accident. Her brother rushed to her bedside; her husband arrived after hours in flight. Over the weeks, her mother, children, in-laws, and friends were able to stay at the woman's bedside as she gradually came back to her own world.

Each family member and each friend offered unique qualities and abilities no less important than the professionals, just remarkably different. Each contact was necessary: the technical "wizard" nurses and expert doctor "carpenters" as well as the brother who stood by her bedside, singing and speaking healing words into her ear.

Mutual respect is a central theme of a relational ethic. It sounds so easy: "Of course, everyone deserves respect." Yet with the different teams that looked after this woman, the question of respect needs foreground consideration. Different disciplines and genders, different access to and use of power, and different kinds of knowledge are present in all health care relations and are embodied on any interdisciplinary team, including patients and their families. Right from the beginning there were different teams of specialists taking charge of the woman's care: nurses in the ER and intensive care unit (ICU), on the trauma general ward, on the rehabilitation (rehab) ward, and on various shifts; surgeons for her pelvis, for her left leg, for her right foot, for the facial bone; neurologists for the pressure on her brain and the fracture of her spine; rehab specialists and psychologists to assist with recovering abilities and learning new activities. Each had expertise that was unique yet overlapped with others.

Respect for difference—for example, power, knowledge, beliefs and values, experience, and attitudes—does not come easily. Professionals grounded in their own perspective sometimes find it hard to realize that others also have valuable perspectives, and may, in fact, be right. The word *mutual* directs attention to the interactive and reciprocal nature of respect. To reduce the other person to an object of study, or to see them as no different than oneself, avoids the problem of meeting someone who is different and makes it easier to miss the experience of "letting ourselves be moved, questioned, modified and enriched by the other" (Irigaray 2002, 125). With the theme of mutual respect, we are asked to look for ways to achieve cohabitation or coexistence between people who are different but of equal worth and significance. There is a need to learn ways to engage the other, the *you*, without reducing *you* to the same as *me*, or *me* to the same as *you*.

If mutual respect is the central challenge of relational ethics, then teamwork is the prime opportunity for relational action, with the patient and family taking on important roles. Often the nurse is the coordinator of the team—a tough and sometimes thorny job. Of course, the effort to work in a collaborative way, rather than within hierarchical pockets, is a shared responsibility. The relational theme of engagement focuses attention on being true to oneself while still attending to the other (Austin 2006).

ENGAGEMENT

Ethical action needs to start with an attempt to understand the other's situation, perspective, and vulnerability. This understanding requires a true movement toward the other as a person and to genuine engagement. When engagement does not occur, the lack of involvement of person-to-person needs to be recognized as the ethical issue it is. If we believe that the quality of relationship needs ethical attention, then lack of engagement could be understood as an ethical concern (Austin 2007).

ETHICS IN PRACTICE 7-4

The Breath—Breathing Together

Again, time passed. The woman was now in the hospital where she began her journey. Now she breathed on her own, using her breathing to both ease the pain and ease the anxiety. A feeding tube was inserted in an attempt to give the necessary nutrition to heal the various fractures. Her neck brace was off, leaving her cheekbone as smooth and lovely as before the accident, the external pelvic brace was gone, and her scarred legs began to move through her own effort rather than only with the aide of the continuous rotating machine. Family and professional teams surrounded her, but she was still losing weight, had a rash, felt discouraged, and said she was "so, so sick." Now she demanded drugs to kill the pain, shouted at nurses and doctors and husband. Everyone was worried.

Then came one nurse who heard that the woman's son was a basketball star.

Would she like to go see a game? The social worker arranged the van, the doctors agreed, the nurses helped her dress, and family members came to escort her to the gym under the nurse's guidance and vigilance (done on her own time). As the van carried the woman through her own town, which she had not seen for months, she wept. This event moved the woman to gain new vigour for life. It changed the course of her healing. Realistic and wise, the nurse reminded the woman that ups and downs are part of health and healing, preparing her for the "downs" that were sure to come again. Yet, the nurse also reminded the woman that she or someone else would assist her through difficult times whenever she needed.

The feeding tube and the urinary catheter were soon removed, and the woman wheeled her own chair.

In Ethics in Practice 7-4, the woman begins to be demanding. The word *demand* means to ask urgently and firmly, leaving no chance for refusal. Its root is from the Latin *demandãre*, meaning to entrust (Morris 1978, 350), to give into someone's hand (1527). The woman seems to be asking for more now. She seems to realize that as a person she must now move to take charge of her own life, to more radically take "her own breath" willed by oneself and not by the demands of physiology (Irigaray 2002). However, she still cannot do this alone, so she again entrusts herself to others and gives herself into others' hands *by her own request*. By her demands she asks for engagement. Because she cannot be fully vigilant in all parts of her life she trusts others to assist her to bring herself into harmony with her changed life.

Relational engagement is located in the shared moment when people have found a way to look at something together. They "compose a mutually satisfactory interpretation of their situation . . . freely accepting or declining the interpretation that each other offers, until they reach a meaning that both affirm" (Gadow and Schroeder 1996, 131). This meaning is found in those moments when the nurse comes to understand what the patient really needs, for example, to connect her to her son and to her community. The tears felt by the woman as she was driven through her town acknowledge the reality of mortality and what she had lost, such as walking freely or looking after her children, and what she had gained in reconnecting to her world of love for husband and family and increased awareness of community support. There is power in the experience of people with different perspectives, such as a nurse and patient, coming to understand something together.

How can professionals engage with patients and with one another? There is concern about over-involvement and standing too close, leading to abusive situations. Yet there is a need to be equally concerned about under-involvement and the disengagement that some say has led to a humanitarian crisis in which there is little connection between people, that harms patients and professionals alike. Perhaps engagement is not something that can be required by any professional body, rather, engagement is something that each professional has to consider individually (Frank 2004). In this scenario it was just one nurse, one person, whose action changed the course of care. This is not the only example that could be found, but it is a significant one.

The health care encounter brings into focus a particular kind of relation that connects strangers together in meaningful and even intimate ways. *This* practitioner comes with specific competencies and a commitment to exploring what needs to be done for *this* person who comes for care by respecting autonomy, values, confidentiality, and so forth. When a relationship is engaged, the patient comes with willingness to discuss health care needs in an environment where trust (entrusting) is an essential ingredient. According to Taylor (1985), it is the self-interested focus of modern life and the primacy of techno-logical or instrumental reasoning with its search for control and domination of life and death that fragments community life and leads to general malaise or indifference to the needs of others.

In a technical relationship, one nurse is interchangeable with another nurse and patients are interchangeable as well, identified according to disease or problem. As nurses find that they are expected to do more with insufficient time, and while they want to do good, they find that they cannot do so in the manner they believe is best for their patients (Rodney and Varcoe 2001; Varcoe and Rodney 2009). This reality can lead to a bigger problem, for when patients are treated as objects (diseases or problems) because of too many expectations, professionals become objects as well. They become faceless practi-tioners who mechanically carry out their duties.

Is it possible that when we distance ourselves from others we all lose? Perhaps this is when staff experience "burnout," that feeling of exhaustion and overload that occurs when we take on, either by demand or choice, more than we can handle. Reasons for burnout include the unrecognized separation of body and mind that leads to lack of embodiment; when we are not able to be fully present in the moment; when there is no time for care for the self; and when we become focused only on outcomes and the need to accomplish more. Engagement, attention to *this* moment, *this practitioner*, *this* patient, *this* place offers one way for professionals to renew attention to the meaning found in their work. Engagement offers a way for each to make meaning out of tragic experiences that can only be found by each person in his or her own way. Through the experience of responsiveness to the needs of both oneself and the other, the professional discovers and responds to the moral commitment of relationship.

Bauman (1993) suggests that the moral impulse arises because one person elicits a response from another. Engagement with others allows one to discover abilities that one did not previously know one had: "The Other enables me to do more than I can do" (Lippitz 1990, 59). Such engaged relationships make it possible, not just necessary, to be moral: we gain ourselves, so to speak, and find out what we are capable of. From this point of view, engagement does not ask for *selflessness* on the part of the practitioner as both are recognized as *whole beings*, both self-interested and other-focused, in what Dillon (1992) calls person-directed attention.

The notion of reciprocity, or mutuality, is sometimes hard to grasp for health care professionals because a major impetus for becoming a professional is the desire to do good for others. Yet the moment we step out of mutuality, moral angst and depletion become a danger and we feel we give more than we receive. With engagement, practitioners receive as well as give. Could increased attention to mutuality and engagement with each other lead to a new creativity in professional practice, decreased stress, and increased self-confidence and satisfaction?

A new creativity would require the "imaginative grasp of the relevant webs of inter-dependency" in which "concepts like sufficiency, wholeness, health, participation, diversity, possibility, creativity become the keywords, instead of privation, rationing, authority, centralization, rationalization, downsizing, inevitability, and management" (Peacock 1999, 705, 710). Here we begin to see the rippling effects of a relational ethic; the ethical space that begins between professional and patient needs to extend to organizational spaces as well; an ethic for living life together in a finite and interdependent world.

One difficulty that is frequently raised about engagement is the matter of time. There is just not enough time in the health care environment for engagement. Even with the benefits of technology there is not enough time; or perhaps it is *because* of technology, and its technological attitude, that there is not enough time. Yet the image of patients lined up in emergency rooms gives reality to the fact that time and resources are limited. While it is true that there is need for more time and resources available for staff, resources cannot be the *only* consideration. Would engagement with patients and colleagues in more meaningful ways be helpful, or would it only make matters worse?

With attention to time, it might be useful to think that the measure of an engaged relationship is inner rather than outer. Consider the notion of lived time in which we are fully present to the other person and the needs of the moment. Niebuhr (1963) describes being present to another person as a *time-full* encounter. The time-full self is a "self that is always in the present to be sure, always in the moment, so that the very notion of the present is probably unthinkable apart from some explicit reference to a self, I and now belong together" (93). To be present in *this* moment, the practitioner will need to hold past activities and future responsibilities at bay to be able to be in the moment with the patient. Or, as Niebuhr (1963) states, when one is in the present moment, past, present, and future "are dimensions of the active self's time-fullness" (99). Past and future are part of the present. Being truly present to another through engagement makes it possible to expand the feeling of having enough time, at least for a particular moment.

Tarzian (1998) distinguishes between the Greek notion of non-linear time (*kairos*) and chronological time (*kronos*). With non-linear time, we remain fully present in the moment, to the point of losing track of time or finding that time loses its demands. Tarzian says that when nurses say they *spend time* with patients, they may be focusing on the chronological sense of time. When nurses say that they are *being with* patients, there is a sense of time stopping so that it is time that cannot be "spent." "*Spending* refers to attaching monetary value to an experience and exchanging units of equal value. *Waiting upon* [being with], as a gift, cannot be spent or bought" (Tarzian 1998, 180, italics in original). Nurses often realize that being with patients (*kairos*) at crucial moments will save chronological time (*kronos*) in the end. Being with patients can be actualized by dialogue.

RELATIONAL ETHICS THROUGH DIALOGUE

Genuine dialogue is the place where relational ethics is most easily realized. It is the place where the themes of relational environment, embodiment, mutuality, and engagement are enacted. Dialogue is not a one-sided interview for the purpose of diagnosis so that treatment can begin. Dialogue is the beginning of treatment itself. Dialogue is a conversation that must be sustained throughout the whole process of recovery (Gadamer 1996). Austin (2008) discusses the importance of dialogue amongst caregivers themselves. Using the example of pandemics, such as SARS or flu scares, caregivers talk about the quandary they feel regarding carrying out their responsibilities for patients while at the same time managing their concerns and fears about their own health and the health and safety of their families. Open dialogue, suggests Austin, is important in order to acknowledge fears, raise questions, and explore solutions together.

In Ethics in Practice 7-5, we see that as the woman recovers her breath she becomes more demanding. She begins to speak, to demand. She wants dialogue.

ETHICS IN PRACTICE 7-5

The Breath—Breathing and Speaking Together

And so the days, weeks, and months passed, and the woman was moved to a rehab ward. Her arms were getting stronger, her legs still too fragile, it seemed, to imagine walking or even standing on them. Yet the woman did imagine. She wanted to have a picture taken when she was able to stand on her own. It was the picture she wanted to send to the specialists who had reconstructed her shattered bones. She wanted them to know how grateful she was that she had their unique ability to care for her. And one specialist, too, must have imagined the possibilities of her standing and walking again as she called her family, as well as her current physician, to find out about the patient's recovery. The specialist was concerned that the woman not stand too soon, that she lay on her stomach to avoid contractions of her hips from long periods in the wheelchair. The professionals wanted to know that the work of the team was a success for this woman. The talk continued between husband and family, doctors, nurses, social workers, and rehab therapists. The conversation grew to include brothers and sisters, nieces and nephews, friends, and neighbours. While in hospital, the woman's contact with nurses offered the consistent daily opportunity for conversation.

If dialogue is part of treatment rather than a preparation for treatment or for evaluating treatment, the ethical responsibility to promote, maintain, or revive dialogue is clear. In Ethics in Practice 7-5, dialogue is not merely a mode of communicating instructions or evaluating effectiveness, but is necessary for practitioner and patient to understand together.

We come back to breath. Proper attention to the breath, re-learning to breathe, is, as Irigaray (2002) points out, necessary for us to take charge of our own life, and with this attention we begin to see the relationship between the breath and speech. McPherson (2000), paralyzed due to childhood polio, uses glossopharyngeal breathing in which he activates the muscles of the glossa and the pharynx. This "frog breathing" (McPherson 2000, 30), is a mastered skill that allows him to be free of the respirator while he is awake. With this skill he is able to speak, which makes the connection between breath and speech obvious. According to Irigaray (2002), patriarchal philosophies and religious traditions have immobilized the breath by giving emphasis to words and speech, that is, "have substituted words for life without carrying out the necessary links between the two" (51). One way to recover the links between words and life is to recover the breath, which allows "reciprocally conserving, regenerating, and enriching life and speech" (51). There is a need to take time to breathe, to help practitioners feel grounded in their own bodies so that activities and speech are strong and appropriate to the moment. Jopling (2000) identifies six characteristics of a dialogic encounter that are useful for this discussion:

1. Dialogue is open-textured, not goal oriented. One does not know what will come of it, how each partner will be changed, how self-understandings will be expanded. Nothing is predetermined as there may be unexpected outcomes.

2. In dialogue there is mutual respect in order to encounter the other as other. In mutual respect one regards the other as a responsible partner within established norms of trustworthiness.

3. In dialogue one is forthright. One is present to the other's company. "Language would be a rootless and impersonal system of signs if it were not anchored in the face-to-face confrontation" (156).

4. When dialogue is embodied, feelings such as compassion, anger, sympathy, shame, desire constitute the response. Feelings give body to words and bring back words to the body.

5. Dialogue signals mutual recognition by addressing the other as *you*, which calls forth the personal in *me* as well.

6. Dialogue is found in the ethical moment, when one is present *with* and *for* someone, not merely thinking about them. One is "called into conversation" with an actual other person (152–157).

Through dialogue, which is in the actual words, in the silences, or in touch, patients and practitioners find their own way to connect.

RELATIONAL ETHICS: KNOWING OURSELVES AS WE ENGAGE WITH OTHERS

We began with the proposition that all relationships, as experienced in daily life, are moral. Within such a perspective, it is an ethical responsibility for health care professionals to consider the quality of their relationship with patients and colleagues. The quality of relationship needs to be given as much attention as the quality of science and the quality of clinical competence. Throughout the chapter we used a clinical example to highlight relational themes: environment, embodiment, mutual respect, and engagement. The breath, the most important physical aspect of life, was used to evocatively provide another avenue to connect to the relational themes: environment (the importance of the breath/air for survival of the individual and the world); embodiment (the breath as connecting the body as object, to the body as lived); mutual respect (the need to breathe for oneself and to support the breath of others); and engagement (the need for breath to speak). In the final section of the chapter, we looked more closely at dialogue, a foundational action that explores the ethical space between people. As Ethics in Practice 7-6 illustrates, the bridge between the individual and community brings both together, to the enrichment of both.

ETHICS IN PRACTICE 7-6

The Breath—Bridging Autonomy and Community

Not long after the woman settled in the fourth hospital, she received, at her home address in Canada, a bill from the third hospital, an American hospital, where she spent less than two hours. The bill was for services rendered at a cost of more than U.S. $14 000. Because the woman was Canadian this bill was paid by the Canadian health care system. Neither the woman nor her family could have managed to pay this huge cost of just one short episode in her care. Mentioning the financial support needed for all patients demonstrates the connection between the life of the individual and the life of the community. The woman, through the concrete financial support of the health care system and the competent physical, emotional, and social support of professional staff and family, moved from bed to wheelchair, to crutches, and to canes in her desire to walk again. Unlike a fairy tale, this story does not end with a statement that the woman lived happily ever after. Nor does it tell the story of the other person in the accident whom the woman met again as they both worked at recovering their own lives. Rather this story shows the need for individual and community to support each other on the road to health. Health and healing cannot happen alone.

Readers will recognize that relational ethics is not a panacea for easy ethical care; rather the focus on relationship may make ethical considerations even more complex. Yet individual professionals, who number in the hundreds in the months and years of this woman's care, each had opportunity to practise relational ethics. Each had the opportunity to enact the health care environment, embodiment, mutual respect, and engagement through the daily care of the person who experiences illnesses, traumas, and even death. For the woman in our six-part clinical example, professionals, and the community, were integral to her healing and growth, and perhaps the relationship of professionals with this woman may have also assisted them to come to know themselves better. "Not only does dialogue open the self to itself by opening it to the other person; it is by means of reflective dialogue that persons are 'talked into' knowing who they are" (Jopling 2000, 157). Relational ethics reminds caregivers to consider how important it is to continue to know more about one's self. In that self-knowledge and openness, we can care for and know others.

For Reflection

1. Consider how relational ethics is already part of health care practice using the relational themes of environment, embodiment, mutual respect, and engagement.

2. How, specifically, can professionals support a relational approach to ethics in working with other members of the health care team, including patients?

3. While ethical principles and virtues are already a part of ethical teaching, how might a focus of relational ethics be learned?

4. How can relational values be fostered in health care organizations so that professionals are better supported in enacting a relational ethic?

Endnote

1. The themes discussed here are an outcome of a relational ethics research project that spanned a number of years and a number of projects at the University of Alberta (for more specific details of the project and the identified themes, see Bergum and Dossetor (2005).

References

Austin, W. 2006. Engagement in contemporary practice: A relational ethics perspective. *Texto Contexto Enferm, Florianópolis 15* (Esp), 135–141.

Austin, W. 2007. The ethics of everyday practice. Healthcare environments as moral communities. *Advances in Nursing Science, 30*, (1), 81–88.

Austin, W. 2008. Ethics in a time of contagion: A relational perspective. *Canadian Journal of Nursing Research, 40*, (4), 10–24.

Bauman, Z. 1993. *Postmodern ethics.* Oxford: Blackwell.

Bergum, V. in press. Quickening practice: The ethical space of action. In M. Riemslagh, M. Burggraeve, R. Corveleyn, and A. Liegeois (Eds.), *After you.* Leuven-Dudley Peeters.

Bergum, V. and Dossetor, J. 2005. *Relational ethics. The full meaning of respect.* Hagerstown, MD: University Publishing Group.

Caputo, J.D. 1989. Disseminating originary ethics and the ethics of dissemination. In A.B. Dallery and C.E. Scott (Eds.), *The question of the other: Essays in contemporary continental philosophy* (pp. 55–62). Albany, NY: State University of New York Press.

Dillon, R.S. 1992. Respect and care: Toward moral integration. *Canadian Journal of Philosophy, 22* (1), 105–132.

Ermine, W. 2007. The ethical space of engagement. *Indigenous Law Journal, 6* (1), 193–203.

Frank, A. F. 2004. Ethics in medicine. Ethics as process and practice. *Internal Medicine Journal, 34*, 355–357.

Gadamer, H-G. 1996. *The enigma of health.* Stanford, CA: Stanford University Press.

Gadow, S. 1980. Existential advocacy: Philosophical foundation of nursing. In S. Spicker and S. Gadow (Eds.), *Nursing: Images and ideals: Opening dialogue with the humanities* (pp. 79–101). New York: Springer.

Gadow, S. 1989. Clinical subjectivity: Advocacy with silent patients. *Nursing Clinics of North America, 24* (2), 535–541.

Gadow, S. 1994. Whose body? Whose story? The question about narrative in women's health care. *Soundings: An International Journal, 77* (3–4), 295–307.

Gadow, S. and Schroeder, C. 1996. An advocacy approach to ethics and community health. In E.T. Anderson and J. McFarlane (Eds.), *Community as partner: Theory and practice in nursing*, (2nd ed.; pp. 123–137). Philadelphia: J.B. Lippincott.

Gaita, R. 1991. *Good and evil: An absolute conception.* London: Macmillan.

Gonzales, A. 2002. Hospitals adopting new methods of handling waste. *Sacramento Business Journal.* Available online at www.bizjournals.com/sacramento/stories/2000/03/06/focus2.html.

Irigaray, L. 2002. *Between east and west. From singularity to community.* S. Pluhácek (Trans.). New York: Columbia University Press.

Jopling, D.A. 2000. *Self-knowledge and the self.* New York: Routledge.

Lippitz, W. 1990. Ethics as limits of pedagogical reflection. *Phenomenology and Pedagogy, 8*, 49–60.

McPherson, G. 2000. *With every breath I take. One person's extraordinary journey to a healthy life and how you can share it.* Edmonton: Author.

Morris, W. (Ed.). 1978. *The American heritage dictionary of the ethics language.* Boston: Houghton Mifflin.

Niebuhr, H.R. 1963. *The responsible self: An essay in Christian moral philosophy.* New York: Harper and Row.

Olthuis, J.H. (Ed.). 2000. *Towards an ethic of community: Negotiations of difference in a pluralist society.* Waterloo, ON: Wilfrid Laurier University Press.

Peacock, K.A. 1999. Symbiosis and the ecological role of philosophy. *Dialogue, 38*, 699–717.

Rodney, P. and Varcoe, C. 2001. Towards ethical inquiry in the economic evaluations of nursing practice. *Canadian Journal of Nursing Research, 33* (1), 35–37.

Tarzian, A. 1998. *Breathing lessons: An exploration of caregiver experiences with dying patients who have air hunger.* Unpublished doctoral dissertation. University of Maryland, Baltimore, MD.

Taylor, C. 1985. *Philosophy and the human sciences.* Volume 2 of *Philosophical Papers.* New York: Cambridge University Press.

Varcoe, C. and Rodney, P. 2009. Constrained agency: The social structure of nurses' work. In B.S. Bolaria and H.D. Dickinson (Eds.), *Health, illness, and health care in Canada* (4th ed.; pp. 122–151). Toronto: Nelson Education Inc.

CHAPTER 8

Relational Practice and Nursing Obligations[1]

Gweneth Hartrick Doane and Colleen Varcoe

By the close of the twentieth century, the image of the "lady with the lamp" administering tender loving care to a wounded soul had faded. More contemporary images depict nurses rushing between too many patients, grappling with technology, paperwork, and limited resources. These changing images reflect not only a shift in the nature of nursing practice but the changing contexts of health care—contexts that are reflected throughout the chapters of this book, but particularly Chapters 2, 10, 11, 12, and 18 through 21. Moreover, the changing images highlight the need for broader understandings of contemporary nursing relationships, including the integral connection between "therapeutic" relationships and "ethical" relationships.

Relationships in nursing typically have been understood in congruence with liberal individualism and its companion, paternalism. That is, the relationship between the individual nurse and individual patient is seen as the relationship of importance, the nurse is considered an autonomous agent with free will who is able to make choices, there is an assumption of therapeutic intent on the part of the nurse, and responsibility for achieving health outcomes through "good" relationships is vested in the nurse. As Browne and her colleagues argue, such ideologies underpin much of nursing theory and practice (Anderson et al. 2010; Browne 2001; 2005).

Understanding relationships in this way ascribes responsibility to the nurse to foster therapeutic relationships and thus to provide better care and achieve better outcomes. Supporting this understanding is a wealth of literature focused on concepts and behaviours that have the potential to enhance relational engagement. For example, concepts such as respect, presencing, trust, mutuality, and so forth are frequent topics in the relationship literature in nursing. Less common in that literature are discussions of the multitude of factors that shape and at times determine the connection between any individual patient and nurse. Yet, these other personal and contextual factors frequently make trusting, respectful, therapeutic relationships challenging. For example, workload, patient acuity, staffing ratios, and supportive (or unsupportive) collegial relationships can shape whether a nurse even views "presencing" with a particular patient as an option. Further, a nurse's personal identity and social location shapes his or her interpretations, willingness, and capacity to be in-relation with particular patients in particular situations.

In this chapter we argue that although nurses are handed the responsibility and obligation for therapeutic nurse–patient relationships, and are given descriptive indicators of "good" relationship behaviours, often missing is an examination of how nurses might meet this nursing obligation within highly complex, multi-faceted, and contextually dependent moments. Specifically we wish to consider nurse–patient relationships using a relational lens that takes multiple contexts and relationships into account. Moreover we highlight the way in which familiar relationship concepts such as trust, empathy, and respect work in concert with ethical concepts such as obligation, responsibility, and "good" action. We critically examine the concept of obligation, and using a relational understanding, suggest three obligations underlying nursing relationships. It is our contention that responsive, compassionate, therapeutic relationships and ethical and competent nursing practice are integrally connected and that relational inquiry can support the enactment of both. Our intent is to examine the way in which a relational lens of inquiry can enhance nurses' capacity and ability to navigate through the challenges and competing obligations of contemporary relationships in health care.

CONNECTING RELATIONSHIPS, ETHICS, AND NURSING EFFECTIVENESS

Gastmans (2002) contends that relationship is "a foundational condition of nursing practice" (495). Tschudin (1999) describes relationships as "salutogenic" in the sense that they contribute to health more essentially than we often are aware (35). Similarly, Tarlier (2004) contends that responsive relationships are one way nurses "make a difference" and influence clinical outcomes.

Tarlier (2004) outlines that within the nursing literature "good" relationships are conceptualized as being founded on three essential elements: respect, trust, and mutuality. *Respect* includes five characteristics: (1) treating others as inherently worthy and equal, (2) acceptance of others, (3) willingness to listen to others, (4) genuine attempts to understand another and the other's situation, and (5) sincerity (Browne 1995). *Trust* is developed through the processes inherent in respect. At the same time trust rests on the patient's belief that the nurse will assist him or her in achieving a good outcome (Tarlier 2004). Baier (1986) defines trust as "reliance on others' competence and willingness to look after, rather than harm, things one cares about which are entrusted to their care" (25). Further, Baier describes trust as involving a "reliance on another's good will not just dependable habits" (234). *Mutuality*, according to Tarlier, refers to a relationship as a negotiated, collaborative process where both people participate, choose, and act.

Armstrong (2006) contends that nurse–patient relationships typically have been viewed in terms of human interactions, communication skills, and collaborative action. However, describing the significance of relationships to ethical nursing practice in Chapter 7 of this text, Bergum purports that in essence, relationships are a moral space where one enacts not only responsiveness but also responsibility. Similarly Nortvedt (2001) argues that nurse–patient relationships are the site where moral responsibilities and professional duties are generated (see also Nortvedt 2004). As Gilligan (1982) described, "the most basic questions about human living—how to live and what to do—are fundamentally questions about human relations, because people's lives are deeply connected, psychologically, economically, and politically" (14). Everyday interactions between patients and nurses, between nurses and other health practitioners, and between nurses and their practice contexts involve complicated networks of mutual dependencies. Bergum contends that "with relational space as the location of enacting morality, we need to consider ethics in every situation, every encounter, and with every patient" (Chapter 7 in this text, p. 128).

A review of the literature reveals that overall nurses in "good" relationships are considered not only more responsive to others in the sense of being more respectful and trustworthy, but also results in more ethical and effective care. *It is this integral connection of relationships, ethics, and effective nursing practice that we wish to highlight and explore further.* Within both the relationship literature and the ethics literature it is argued that nursing practice requires a deep sensitivity to what is significant to patients in particular situations. Until recently there has been little integration of these different bodies of literature. Subsequently there has been very little discussion about what is required to develop and enact that sensitivity and/or the knowledge, capacities, and skills required for ethical and responsive nursing relationships within the complexities of current health care milieus. For example, as social inequities deepen and neo-liberal ideologies hold individuals responsible for their own health and well-being—regardless of how poverty, disability, remote geographical locations, or other inequities determine health—notions of obligation, responsibility, accountability, and efficiency are as vital to nursing relationships as are notions of compassion, responsiveness, trust, and respect. Thus, nurses require a broader understanding of relationships and their significance to ethical nursing practice. The story in Ethics in Practice 8-1 will help us to illustrate what we mean.

ETHICS IN PRACTICE 8-1

Interaction in the Emergency Department

During a long wait in the emergency waiting room to have a laceration sutured, I watched an elderly woman and her mature adult daughter get increasingly impatient "to be seen" and have the mother's injured leg attended to. At one point the daughter went to the reception window to declare in an exasperated voice that they had been waiting for close to three hours, she was not sure how much longer her mother could tolerate sitting in the chair and that if they were not seen soon they would just leave. The nurse behind the window replied in an assertive voice that the emergency policy was to see patients in order of medical priority, not waiting time, and they would be seen as soon as was possible. Shortly afterward I was called into the stretcher area. A few minutes later as I lay on the stretcher after having my laceration sutured, another nurse popped her head into my cubicle saying that she would be with me in a minute to apply a dressing, she was just going to assist a patient onto a stretcher. From behind the curtain I could hear that the other patient was the elderly woman. As the nurse assisted her onto the stretcher the nurse exclaimed, "That's quite a gash on your leg." In response, the elderly woman began to tell the story of falling at home. The nurse quickly interjected, cutting the story off by stating, "Well, at least it isn't too serious and we will be able to suture that up fine." In response, the woman ignored the nurse's words and once again began to tell the story of her fall. Once again the nurse interjected to keep the focus of the discussion on the leg wound. At this point the daughter spoke up saying, "She fell two days ago and just called me this afternoon—imagine she was home by herself with this and she didn't even call me." As I lay in the next cubicle I could "hear" the nurse in that moment making an important relational decision. There were a few seconds of silence (where I believe she was weighing her promise to return to me with the more compelling obligation to listen and respond to the elderly woman and her daughter) and then she replied, "You live alone do you?" Through those few words the nurse entered into relationship in a meaningful way, simultaneously letting the woman know that she was "seen" and acknowledging the significance of her injury within the larger contextual/personal underpinnings of her life. Although the "easily fixed wound" was the physical evidence of her trauma, there were much more meaningful elements that needed attention relationally for healing to occur. As the elderly woman accepted the nurse's invitation and began to reveal the "whole" of her experience through her story, she communicated her shock in falling, her fear and vulnerability as an elderly woman living on her own, and the fierce independence, strength, and capacity she had. By creating the relational space for the woman to tell her story the nurse provided an opportunity for the elderly woman to weave the various elements of her experience together and narrate herself and her situation into a manageable form. By the end of the story (which took a matter of approximately two or three minutes) the woman concluded much as the nurse had initially concluded—that the wound was easily fixed and she would be fine to return home on her own.

This story exemplifies the significance of a nurse–patient relationship and the profound difference it can make in promoting health and healing. At the same time, the story highlights the competing and at times conflicting obligations through which nurses find themselves navigating. Although the woman had come to the emergency department to have her leg sutured, what was most meaningful and what she needed to sort through, was what the fall and injury meant within the context of her life. That is, as an elderly woman living alone the fall underscored her vulnerability and called her independence into question. Thus for the relationship to be therapeutic and nursing practice to be effective in addressing the woman's health and healing needs, the relational space for this contextual understanding needed to be created. However the story also highlights how personal and contextual elements (e.g., a nurse's sense of responsibility, feeling obligated to another waiting patient, the normative values of health care culture) shape what happens in any nursing moment and how the pressures of competing demands and values can lead to certain things being privileged over others (e.g., privileging treatment and procedures over the promotion of health and healing). The story also draws attention to the competing obligations that nurses may face as they try to "do good" within competing values, demands, and expectations. The nurse in the story was obligated to both patients—yet attending to one meant not immediately fulfilling her promise to the other. At the same time, emergency department norms pressured her to function in certain ways.

As nurses we are obligated to ensure that our nursing actions promote health and healing, and are ethical and safe. However, determining what actually constitutes "ethical," "safe" and "health/healing promoting" practice in particular situations can be challenging since the specific behaviours and responses are arrived at in the particularities of the relational moment—as we engage with and respond to specific patients in particular situations. For example, promoting the health and healing of the elderly woman in the above story required that the nurse create the relational space for the woman to reach the "outcome" that she was able to continue to function independently in her life. In contrast, as a patient in the next cubicle, the nurse's pleasant demeanour and dressing application were sufficient to address my health and healing needs.

RELATIONSHIPS, ETHICS, AND NURSING OBLIGATIONS

Nursing obligations are the site where the integral connection between responsive relationships and ethical practice comes to the foreground. Peter and Liaschenko (2004) highlight that proximity to others is one way that nurses understand what their obligations are. "Proximity beckons moral agents to act, and therefore has an impact on moral responsiveness" (219; see also Peter 2011).

Armstrong (2006) writes that the concept of obligation "runs deep in contemporary western society" (115) and has dominated much of existing ethical theory and practice. Subsequently, obligation-based ethics (e.g., principle approaches grounded in consequentialism and/or deontology) have been popular within nursing and remain so (see Bergum in Chapter 7 of this text). Within the philosophical and ethical literature, obligations have been conceptualized as external to the person (Armstrong 2006) and most often are articulated in the form of codes or principles such as the obligations of beneficence, nonmaleficence, autonomy, and justice (see also Chapters 4 and 5). As externally derived and sanctioned entities, obligations in the form of codes are expected to reinforce professional and societal values and give coherence to professional behaviour by disclosing the profession's values and duties (Thompson 2002). The norms included in codes are determined by the nursing philosophy of a particular country, and at the same time are influenced by the moral problems nurses face in their everyday work (Dobrowolska et al. 2007).

One of the main criticisms of existing conceptualizations of obligation-based ethics and the principles/codes that arise from them is that they usually present overly simplistic understandings of ethical practice. For example, obligation-based ethics focus on right and wrong action (Armstrong 2006) and theoretically assume that there is a definitive "right" response to a situation (Thompson 2002). At the same time as implying that a right answer and/or response can be determined, most existing codes that express nursing obligations do not elaborate enough on how nurses might actually enact their ethical obligations in their everyday practice (Armstrong 2006; Thompson 2002; Pattison 2001; MacDonald 2007). Codes are usually confined to idealistic prescriptions that only partially explain how the concepts relate to actual practice and provide limited guidance for particular nurses in particular relational moments (Dobrowlska 2007). Further, within extant liberal orientations, codes of ethics tend to promote the values of individualism. In the U.S. and Canadian contexts respectively, Bekemeier and Butterfield (2005) and Kirkham and Browne (2006) argue that codes of ethics encourage us to presume Western societies are essentially egalitarian, and while we are directed to be aware of broader social issues, we are not committed by our professional values to action. Peter raises similar concerns in 2008 in response to the latest revision of the Canadian Nurses Association (2008) *Code of Ethics for Registered Nurses* and in a recent research discourse (2011).

OBLIGATIONS AS EXTERNAL ENTITIES

At the same time that existing conceptualizations of nursing obligations have been criticized for not offering practical direction, the conceptualization of obligation as an external and universal entity has been criticized for failing to address important features that shape ethical practice including context, historical changes, culture, character, and relationship (Thompson 2002). In not addressing these features, obligation-based ethics cover over certain types of questions that are integral to everyday nursing practice and may also disguise the lack of agreement about values that dominate nursing situations (Thompson 2002). For example, Provis and Stack (2004) describe how caring work is ripe with conflicting obligations and how the interface of personal and organizational obligations can cause uncertainty about what is the "right thing to do" when those obligations run counter to each other. They offer the example of a caregiver who, interpreting her use of bath towels through the values and norms of the organization, worried that she was being "extravagant." "You're always told how much it costs for linen and that sort of thing . . . I like to put an extra towel over their shoulders to keep them warm while I dry them with the other towel, so that may not be cost conscious" (6). Even in the smallest moments, various obligations pull us in different directions. Yet obligation-based ethics do not address what happens when nurses are obligated in conflicting ways, when, for example, their obligations to different patients are in tension and/or when their obligation to their organization is at odds with the obligations they feel to patients.

Interestingly, Pattison (2001) highlights that although obligation-based ethics and ethical codes in particular rest on the assumption of the "thoughtful, autonomous, 'ethical' practitioner who possesses independent critical judgment, practical wisdom and the capacity to act responsibly and with regard to the hinterland of wider human values and principles" (7), codes of obligation may actually militate against the emergence and survival of such practitioners. For example, following a review of "the inherent ethical defects of a number of codes" Pattison concluded that codes may "do little to develop or support the active independent critical judgement and discernment . . . (and) may, in fact, be in danger of engendering confusion, passivity, apathy and even immorality" (8). Indeed, in our teaching of ethics, despite our attempts to support enactment of all values simultaneously, nursing students (both new to nursing and experienced nurses) using codes often revert to a "pick one value" mentality, wherein they use one value (e.g., one related to autonomy) to override other values, and support their chosen direction rather than guide their choices. Similarly, research has highlighted how viewing ethics and obligation as something that is rationally determined outside of one's own practice can lead to confusion and inaction (Doane 2004; Varcoe et al. 2004).

Nurses have not been alone in articulating the limitations of existing conceptualizations of obligation. Within the broader field of philosophy writers offer criticisms and alternative conceptualizations. In particular John Caputo (1987; 1993) addresses the need for an understanding of obligation that raises questions rather than prescribes answers, opens space for the complexity and difficulty of ethical decision-making, and offers direction for how ethics and "good" relationships might be lived within the challenges of everyday life. Caputo's reframing of obligation has informed our view of obligations and relationships in nursing.

REFRAMING OBLIGATION

Bauman (1993) describes that within philosophy, ethics has been dominated by a modernist approach to the search for truth that has focused on looking for absolutes and universals of morality (see also Chapters 4 and 5). According to Bauman, modern thinkers believed that rather than being a natural trait of human life, morality was something that needed to be created and injected into human conduct. Obligation, conceptualized through this universal perspective, resulted in a decontextual, depersonalized understanding of obligation. It also resulted in ethical challenges being responded to through normative regulation (Bauman 1993). In contrast, Caputo's (1987) discussion locates obligation and ethics *in the relational moment*— for example, in the moment when a nurse finds him or herself in the midst of people, contexts, and multiple, competing demands. Drawing on deconstructive hermeneutics, Caputo calls for a way of understanding and responding to obligations that entails both interpretation and deconstruction.

In contrast to the understanding of obligations as something external to the person Caputo (1987) contends that obligations are local events—they are matters of flesh and blood. According to Caputo (1987), obligation is the feeling that comes over us in very binding ways when others need our help or support and we feel bound to respond. "When I feel obliged something demands my response. It is not a matter of working through a set of principles to conclude whether one is obliged" (22). Caputo (1987) asks "Does one really 'conclude' that one is obliged, or does one not just find oneself obliged, without so much as having been consulted or asked for one's consent?" (22). Caputo's description echoes the experience of the emergency room (ER) nurse in the above story. Although the nurse initially attempted to extricate herself from the situation she ultimately felt bound to listen and create the relational space for the elderly woman to "do her healing."

While one may find one's self obliged, one's personal values and contextual constraints may mute the sensing of those obligations. For example, initially the ER nurse in the above example seemed more "bound" by her obligation to the organizational norms. Similarly, how the nurse values elderly persons will shape her sense of her obligations in this case. What if the elderly woman had been, for example, intoxicated? Would the nurse's sense of obligation and her actions change? Should they change? This example highlights how determining our obligation to particular patients in particular moments of relationship involves looking carefully at our own responses, "thinking hard" (Armstrong 2006, 115) about the nursing values and obligations to which we are committed, and inquiring into the particularities of the moment and the various elements that are shaping that moment to ensure that our relational goals and behaviours are aligned with the nursing values and obligations we espouse. "Thinking hard" includes thinking about our own biases and to whom we are obligated. It is our contention that nurses are obligated to all persons, most immediately on an individual basis to all those within their care, but also collectively to those who require their care. Thus, a relational conception of obligation applied to nursing relationships suggests that new conceptualizations of nursing obligations and relationships are required.

BRINGING A RELATIONAL INQUIRY LENS TO RELATIONSHIPS

Although existing conceptualizations of relationships that emphasize concepts such as respect, trust, and mutuality offer a good starting point for therapeutic relationships, a relational inquiry lens expands the understanding and thereby the potential of relationships. This inquiry lens highlights that enhancing nurse–patient relationships requires more than individual nurses taking up caring attitudes or presencing behaviours. In contrast to a de-contextual view of relationships that considers the nurse to be an autonomous agent who exercises free and intentional choice, *relational inquiry foregrounds the way in which personal and contextual forces shape both nurses' and patients' capacities for relational connection and thereby health and healing*. Relational inquiry involves a reflexive process where one is always assuming and looking for the ways in which people, situations, contexts, environments, and processes are integrally connecting and shaping each other. This inquiry process rests on the assumption that people are contextual beings who exist in relation with others and with social, cultural, political, and historical processes. Within this contextual existence, each person has a unique personal, sociohistorical location that affects and shapes that person's identity, experience, interpretations, and way of being in the world. It is assumed that the values, knowledge, attitudes, practices, and structures that dominate the socio-cultural world within which each person lives are passed on through relational interactions. Subsequently, peoples' experiences, interpretations, and actions are products of a multitude of relational interactions and processes. In this way people are both shaped by and shape other people's responses, situations, experiences, and contexts. Not only nurses, but patients, their families, other health care providers, and actors beyond the immediate health care context (such as policy makers and the media) continuously negotiate and shape one another. Nursing practice as a process of inquiry focuses on the question "How might I most responsively and effectively be in-relation to promote health and healing?" (Hartrick Doane & Varcoe 2005).

Using this inquiry lens, relationships between people are viewed as sites, opportunities, and/or vehicles for meaningful experience and response. It is possible to be in a relationship with another person without practicing responsively in the sense we are discussing. For example, one can enter into a relationship in ways that distance or objectify people ("The GI bleed in room 8"; "At risk youth") as is the case in many health care relationships. Thus there is an important distinction between relationships that are determined and regulated primarily by the adoption of dominant social customs and practices, and relationships that are purposefully shaped through a relational inquiry where one consciously chooses within the apparent possibilities for action, or even works to create new possibilities. Overall, relational inquiry directs a more in-depth look at the values, experiences, goals, and concerns shaping action within particular moments of practice and a conscious consideration of possibilities and intentional, responsive action.

The Significance of Context

Relational inquiry requires that we move beyond the surface(s) of people, situations, and relationships—beyond the "iceberg" pattern of interaction where a substantial portion of the elements shaping the interaction are unseen and/or ignored. For example, the iceberg pattern of relationship may include a nurse engaging with a smiling, friendly demeanour while going about the tasks of morning care, yet never really connecting with the patient in a meaningful way to inquire into what the patient is experiencing. Although a friendly, cheerful demeanour can certainly be responsive, it may also serve as a veneer that at best covers over and at worst does not allow space for people to be themselves, express their experience, and/or reveal what is particularly salient. A cheerful smile and a friendly demeanour can be used to effectively dismiss a patient's request for care that a nurse does not feel he or she has time to provide.

Particular contexts contribute to this iceberg pattern of relationship because the normative patterning within those contexts cue certain behaviours and responses. For example, health care contexts contain strong messages about what is and is not of importance. The business-driven, economic, cost-efficient values combined with the devaluing of nurses for being "too emotional" or "too involved" offers strong pressure to pattern one's actions in ways that enable the organization to work (Armstrong 2006; Austin 2011; Rodney and Varcoe in press). Similarly, the intricate combination of conflicting values, goals, and desires that the particular nurse brings to the relationship can serve to contribute to the iceberg pattern of interaction. For example, if a patient is in pain, the situation is ambiguous and/or there is no clear cut best way to respond, nurses may pull back as a result of their own vulnerability and uncertainty (Soderburg, Gilje, and Norberg 1999). Being unable to "make it better" or "stop the tears," nurses might focus their attention on other more controllable and concrete tasks. Or, as a result of the combination of practising within a service model "fix-it" culture and their own compassionate desire to alleviate suffering, nurses may take up the treatment-cure values and goals and shape their relationships with patients accordingly. A nurse may focus on a laceration rather than the lacerated person. Feeling a sense of responsibility and a desire to "help" they may attempt to use relationships as a means to an end—to "do to," treat, and fix the patient or to meet the needs of the organization (Gastmans 2002; Bergum, Chapter 7 in this text). Within these dynamics, nurses may be inclined to distance themselves from situations that they see as "unfixable"—such as people who under liberal ideology are seen as creating their own suffering, people with addictions, people in poverty, women in abusive relationships, and so on. Relational inquiry requires us to look beyond the tip of the iceberg when engaging with patients because, whether nurses are aware of the influence of contextual and personal elements or not and whether nurses attend to them or not, those elements shape the health and healing experience (Hartrick 2002; Hartrick Doane and Varcoe 2005; Soderburg, Gilje, and Norberg 1999).

RELATIONAL INQUIRY AND NURSING OBLIGATIONS

Such an inquiry process is underpinned by three nursing obligations, all of which are predicated on the overarching obligation to all persons, regardless of their circumstances or characteristics. *These include the obligation (a) to be reflexive and intentional, (b) to open the relational space for difficulty, and (c) to act at all levels to effect the potential for health and healing.* Although for the purpose of discussion we separate these three obligations, it is important to emphasize that not only do these obligations overlap and complement each other, but also they form a synergistic whole. For example, being reflexive and intentional provides the access to and a way of being in difficulty. Similarly, acting at all levels effects the contextual and personal factors that impede reflexive and intentional practice and so forth.

The Obligation to Be Reflexive and Intentional

Nortvedt (2001) contends that *"relationship itself* is a source of special responsibilities and professional qualities" (116), and that through relationships nurses see patients' needs and interests as particular reasons to act. However, seeing patients' needs and interests as particular reasons to act requires conscious and intentional participation and, as we have argued, involves looking beyond the surface of people and situations. For example, in the story above, the nurse did not initially respond to the elderly lady's need to tell the story of her fall. Furthermore, looking beyond the surface requires looking critically through the veil created by biases (such as ageism), structures (such as how health care is organized), and ideologies (such as individual responsibility).

Similar to Walker's (2003) description of moral oblivion where there is a lack of awareness of the moral demands that are being made, when nurses are oblivious to the relational elements (e.g., the personal and contextual elements) shaping their decisions and actions, they are more likely to be at the mercy of those influences, and thereby less likely to exercise their clinical judgment effectively. That is, they are more likely to be practising *in relational oblivion*. Practising without relational awareness impacts nursing care in a very practical way and ultimately makes meeting nursing obligations all but impossible.

As Provis and Stack (2004) report, sensitivity and compassion are often at odds with organizational directives. Nurses increasingly find themselves rationing their care in ways that marginalize meaningful relational engagement (Austin 2011; Nortvedt 2001; Rodney and Varcoe in press). Nortvedt (2001) contends that what is often central to nursing practice is not how to give the best care for one's patients but how to minimize harm to patients created by socio-contextual circumstances. For the emergency department nurse, apparently it was her felt sense of obligation that overrode the competing demands of a patient in the next cubicle and the organizational press to treat the physical injuries of patients quickly and efficiently. And, this obligation sparked the nurse to reflexively consider her options and intentionally decide to create the relational space for the woman to tell her story. As Bauman (1993) has described, "when competing moral demands arise in the moment it is the moral self which feels, moves and acts within the context of that ambiguity" (34).

In essence Caputo's (1987) deconstructive hermeneutic approach to obligation requires nurses to be humanly involved and interpreting, yet simultaneously critically analyzing, and at times deconstructing the values, structures, and processes that are constraining ethical nursing responsiveness. This reflexive process requires acknowledgement of the ambiguity of relationships, ethics, and nursing care. Moving beyond both prescriptive regulation and personal interpretation, it involves the nurse "activating herself as a knowledgeable practitioner" (Purkis and Björnsdóttir 2006, 255) to critically examine the values, goals, and intents shaping the nursing moment and ultimately relationships. It involves not only using knowledge and information but also practical judgment, and approximates what Aristotle termed *phronesis* (Caputo 1993; Flaming 2006).

Simply put, reflexivity enlists the moral self and simultaneously enlists nursing knowledge, experience, and judgment. In so doing reflexive inquiry moves nurses to look at both what they are doing and how they are doing it. It creates the space for a self-conscious consideration of the relational means and ends and consideration of how nurses are conserving, renewing, inventing, and/or changing those means and ends. For example, a nurse might more consciously weigh conserving towels in relation to conserving warmth and comfort of her patients and in relation to the consequences of providing (or not) such comfort. As such, relationships are enhanced through a reflexive process of intention, attention, interpretation, critical scrutiny, and reconstruction. That is, relational practice involves a conscious intent to act toward the espoused values and goals of nursing, attention to the particularities of people and situations, a critical consideration of one's own and others' interpretations, and very often a reconstruction of decisions, actions, and norms that may be at odds with the values and goals of nursing.

The Obligation to Open Relational Space for Difficulty

As nurses respond to their obligation to be reflexive and intentional they simultaneously find themselves obligated to "be in difficulty." As they look beyond the surface of relational encounters and begin to see people and situations through a relational lens they find themselves in close proximity to and/or experiencing the inherent difficulties of health and healing situations. For example, they may come into closer proximity with suffering, uncertainty, and/or conflict. Similarly, they may find themselves experiencing intense emotional responses—both their own and of others. Caputo describes the challenge of being in the abyss of difficulty—and the suffering that is part of that experience. He describes this difficulty and suffering as something that "humbles us, brings us up short, stops us in our tracks . . . something which both strikes us down and draws us near" (1987, 275). At the same time Caputo (1993) contends that within the abyss of difficulty

> There is suffering and there is suffering. Short-term suffering may easily belong to long-term flourishing, to a larger economy of pain and suffering which is understood by anyone who understands the economy of life itself. To spare others pain and hard work and suffering may easily mean to spare them everything that gives their life worth and a greater long-term felicity. (29)

It is for this reason that Caputo argues for the importance of being in difficulty as it presents itself and of entering the abyss of difficulty and suffering not to succumb or surrender but to be "instructed by the abyss, to let the abyss be, to let it play itself out" (1987, 278). It is only by opening the relational space to be in the difficulty that one is able to move beyond breaking down or detaching (Doane 2003).

Along a similar vein, Mitchell and Bunkers (2003) argue that the danger to nurses is not in witnessing difficulty and suffering but rather in turning away when suffering appears. In contrast to others who have earlier argued that experiencing suffering and difficulty over time may lead to what is discussed in nursing literature variously as "burn out," "care giver fatigue" (Bakker et al. 2000; Demerouti et al. 2000; Taylor and Barling

2004) or in the case of violence, vicarious trauma (Collins and Long 2003; Crothers 1995; Rosenberg et al. 2000), these authors support Caputo's contention that if one enters into nursing situations without the need to fix or make the difficulty/suffering better but rather to open, be in, witness, and be instructed by it, the difficulty/suffering can be a pathway toward meeting the relational obligations to both our patients and ourselves.[2]

Nursing has long focused on suffering, both at an individual and a social level. Yet within the neo-liberal dominance of Western thinking, where individualism is central and biomedicine powerful, suffering that arises from physical pathology has received greater attention. Our obligation to be in the difficulty also extends to examining and acting on suffering as it arises through relational dynamics. To return again to the situation of the elderly woman with the laceration, the example illustrates how understanding the way institutional power operates to limit the nurse's time to attend to the woman's needs allows the nurse to work against these dynamics to alleviate, rather than be complicit with or further suffering. Furthermore, the nurse can inquire as to how other social forces—such as ageism or poverty or gender—might be operating in this woman's life to foster suffering and might be operating to shape the nurse's own sense of her obligations and her actions.

Difficulty and/or our experience of suffering is not separate from who we are—from our own interpretive frames and the interpretive frames that dominate the larger social world in which we live and practise (Doane 2003). How we understand any situation and how we define it and attend to it are subject to our individual and collective understandings and interpretations, and the systems that shape those understandings/interpretations. There is a tendency to think of difficulty and suffering as something negative and as something to be avoided. However, *difficulty is at the heart of ethically responsive nursing care.* Framing difficulty as an inherent feature of nursing relationships paves the way, not only for more ethical but also for more effective and efficient nursing relationships. For example, the emergency department nurse in the story above reflexively and intentionally created the relational space for the difficulty within the situation to "play itself out" (e.g., she opened the space for the woman's fear, vulnerability, and the nurse's own competing obligations to come into relation) and in a matter of two or three minutes she not only supported the woman's health and healing but also responded to her own feelings and needs by making a nursing decision to provide the care she felt was required. Thus, she was able to conclude the encounter with her identity as an ethical "good" nurse intact (Bergum, Chapter 7 in this text).

Understanding "difficulty and suffering" as windows into meaningful relationships and as the base for ethical decision-making and responsive nursing care creates the relational space for nurses to better understand multiple and competing obligations, goals, and perspectives; to raise questions and inquire into the particularities of each situation; and ultimately develop the clarity and courage to act in health-promoting ways.

The Obligation to Act at All Levels to Effect Health and Healing

Bergum (Chapter 7 in this text) contends that attention to relationship as an ethical endeavour has a way of dismantling the distinctions of different levels of care. " . . . [W]hat happens at the bedside is not cut off from the broader issues," (p. 128). Because each nursing moment is shaped by our own actions, by the actions and responses of others, and by the contexts within which we work, relational practice involves the nursing obligation to act at all levels including the intrapersonal, interpersonal, and contextual. *Developing relational nursing practice requires that we continually think through not only what it is we are doing, but also what it is that is shaping and influencing what we are doing.* At the same time it requires that we closely examine how we are responding in particular situations and intentionally act toward nursing values, goals, and obligations.

The emergency department story highlights how relational action is required at all levels. Although the nurse was able to act both intrapersonally (reflexively questioned herself and her options) and interpersonally (responded to the woman's need to tell her story) to affect the situation and possibly prevent similar situations in the future, action at the organizational level is required. For example, the policy that people are seen according to medical priority may not adequately address the needs of elderly patients. To assume that it is equitable to treat a 20-year-old in good health and an 80-year-old in frail health the same in terms of waiting time is not health promoting (see also Sellman 2009).

The nursing obligation to act at all levels requires accepting that we cannot control all conditions of practice and at the same time not abandoning the attempt to exert influence. Margaret Urban Walker (2003) argues that "our thinking about responsibility must encompass the reality that our impact on the world and each other *characteristically* exceeds our control and foresight" (15). As Walker notes, our "potent but blinkered agency" requires considerable effort and skill to achieve the understanding required to fulfill our obligations adequately. Neither fatalistic acceptance of the wider conditions of practice nor naïve underappreciation of the power of those conditions will be an adequate basis for meaningful action.

Overall the nursing obligation to act at all levels rests on the understanding that relational concepts such as respect, trust, mutuality, and presencing require and in many ways can only be enacted through action at all levels. For example, to enact trust—to be trustworthy—requires action at all levels. Potter (2002) describes a trustworthy person as someone who can be counted on to take care of those things that others entrust to that person. An interesting distinction that Sellman (2006) makes when examining the concept of trust is the distinction between trusting nurses as individual people, and trusting them as representatives of nursing and of an institution. From a relational practice perspective this distinction is an important one. Provis and Stack (2004) point out that given the nature of health care situations, patients, in their vulnerability and need, are left with little choice when it comes to having to put their trust in nurses. For example, when they present at an emergency department with a deep laceration that needs suturing, patients have no choice but to stay and wait to get stitched up and to put their trust in the nurses and other members of the health care team. Yet, as the emergency department story depicts, in many cases there may be a conflict between what a patient ultimately needs and what the institutional policies direct. It is at this disjuncture between individual and institutional levels of action where "the difficulty" of enacting trust and of being trustworthy also arises for nurses and where it becomes evident that the enactment of trust necessitates action at all levels. For example, if the way in which patient care is organized does not allow for nursing practice that is adequate to address the health care needs of patients, as was the case for the elderly woman with the laceration, how do nurses meet the nursing obligation to be trustworthy without addressing the organizational constraints? If health care institutions are truly about promoting health and healing, nurses' obligations/trustworthiness as individuals and as representatives of nursing and a particular institution need to be aligned. Thus, the nursing obligations to be trustworthy and "take care" of those things with which patients are entrusting nurses ultimately means that nurses are obliged to attend to issues of workload, acuity, organizational guidelines, availability of resources, and so on. These are policy challenges taken up in many of the chapters in this text, particularly Chapters 10, 11, 13, and 18.

As Walker (2003) describes, at the larger contextual level it is imperative to create active, accessible moral-reflective spaces so that ongoing inquiry and deliberation takes place. Close "relational" inspection of the contexts of practice may reveal how "good practice" is constrained. In a study we conducted with nurses in different practice settings (Rodney et al. 2006), the fact that unmanageable workloads and high patient acuity made good practice very difficult took most of the nurses' attention, and overshadowed ideas about possible actions the nurses might take. In one setting, the nurses initially focused almost exclusively upon how their manager made "good practice" more difficult—how, for example, making decisions without consulting the nursing staff led to less effective care. Changing a certain kind of IV tubing, a seemingly small decision, led to lengthy delays for patients and increased the nurses' workload unnecessarily. The level of frustration and anger with the manager initially overshadowed examination of other influences on practice—for example, how relationships among the nurses themselves might have contributed to an unsupportive work environment and ironically to confrontational relationships within which the manager was increasingly reluctant to consult with staff. Thus, looking critically at the context of practice not only *involves looking at wider influences, but also how we ourselves practise in relation to those influences.*

Summary

Nortvedt (2001) explains that several philosophers have elucidated how relational proximity and the face-to-face encounter generate particular kinds of moral responsibilities. Encounters with vulnerability, pain, and suffering compel a response. "To encounter a patient's pain or the worries of a relative is to be addressed morally" (Nortvedt 2001, 117; see also Nortvedt 2004). Although the close proximity of nurse–patient relationships may serve to "address us morally" and heighten the feeling of obligation, Bauman (1993) argues that proximity to others can also lead to a mixture of ambiguous responses. On the one hand, proximity is what calls us to action, what compels us to help. At the same time, such proximity can overwhelm and spark the flight response. Nursing relationships and the enactment of nursing values and goals in contemporary health care contexts is incredibly challenging. Thus, an understanding of relationships that turns attention to the connection between attitudes, intentions, judgment, and action—one that connects responsibilities, roles, and identities to relationships—is required (Bjorklan 2006). Such an understanding highlights not only our obligations, but also the ways we might better meet those obligations. By looking beyond the surface of one-to-one encounters and by considering what shapes those encounters—nurses and patients, colleagues and contexts—we can act more intentionally and direct our actions in ways that foster trust, respect, compassion, and mutuality in contexts as well as in ourselves and with others.

Endnotes

1. This chapter is a revised version of Hartrick Doane, G. and Varcoe, C. 2007. Relational practice and nursing obligations. *Advances in Nursing Science 30* (3), 192–205. It is used with copyright permission of Wolters Kluwer Health.

2. See Chapter 9 for a discussion of how to support nurses as moral agents as they engage in such difficulty, and Chapter 10 for a discussion of how to improve the overall moral climate for relational practice. See also Chapter 13 for an exploration of ethical practice from a relational lens and Chapter 18 for an exploration of organizational and policy action from a relational lens.

References

Anderson, J.M., Browne, A.J., Reimer-Kirkham, S., Lynam, M.J., Rodney, P., Varcoe, C., Wong, S., Tan, E., Smye, V., McDonald, H., Baumbusch, J., Khan, K.B., Reimer, J., Peltonen, A., and Brar, A. 2010. Uptake of critical knowledge in nursing practice: Lessons learned from a knowledge translation study. *Canadian Journal of Nursing Research, 42* (3), 106–122.

Armstrong, A.E. 2006. Towards a strong virtue ethics for nursing practice. *Nursing Philosophy, 7,* 110–124.

Austin, W.J. 2011. The incommensurability of nursing as a practice and the customer service model: An evolutionary threat to the discipline. *Nursing Philosophy, 12,* 158–166.

Baier, A. 1986. Trust and antitrust. *Ethics, 96,* 231–60.

Bakker, A.B., Killmer, C.H., Siegrist, J., Schaufeli, W.B. 2000. Effort-reward imbalance and burnout among nurses. *Journal of Advanced Nursing, 31* (4), 884–891.

Bauman, Z. 1993. *Postmodern ethics.* Oxford, UK: Blackwell.

Bekemeier, B. and Butterfield, P. 2005. Unreconciled inconsistencies: A critical review of the concept of social justice in 3 national nursing documents. *Advances in Nursing Science, 28* (2), 152–162.

Bjorklund, P. 2006. Taking responsibility: Toward an understanding of morality in practice. A critical review of the empirical and selected philosophical literature on the social organization of responsibility. *Advances in Nursing Science, 29* (2), E56–E73.

Browne, A. 1995. The meaning of respect: A First Nation's perspective. *Canadian Journal of Nursing Research 27,* 95–109.

Browne, A.J. 2001. The influence of liberal political ideology on nursing practice. *Nursing Inquiry 8* (2), 118–129.

Browne, A.J. 2005. Discourses influencing nurses' perceptions of First Nations patients. *Canadian Journal of Nursing Research, 37* (4), 62–87.

Canadian Nurses Association. 2008. *Code of ethics for registered nurses.* Ottawa: Authors.

Caputo, J. 1987. *Radical hermeneutics: Repetition, deconstruction and the hermeneutic project.* Bloomington, Indiana: Indiana University Press.

Caputo, J. 1993. *Against ethics.* Bloomington, Indiana: Indiana University Press.

Collins, S., Long, A. 2003. Working with the psychological effects of trauma: Consequences for mental health-care workers—A literature review. *Journal of Psychiatric and Mental Health Nursing, 10* (4), 417–424.

Crothers, D. 1995. Vicarious traumatization in the work with survivors of childhood trauma. *Journal of Psychosocial Nursing and Mental Health Services, 33* (4), 9–13, 44–45.

Demerouti, E., Bakker, A.B., Nachreiner, F., Schaufeli, W.B. 2000. A model of burnout and life satisfaction amongst nurses. *Journal of Advanced Nursing, 32* (2), 454–464.

Doane, G. 2003. Reflexivity as presence: A journey of self-inquiry. In L. Finlay and B. Gough (Eds.), *Reflexivity: A practical guide for researchers in health and social sciences* (pp. 93–102). Oxford: Blackwell Publishing.

Doane, G. 2004. Being an ethical practitioner: The embodiment of mind, emotion and action. In J. Storch, P. Rodney, and R. Starzomski (Eds.), *Toward a moral horizon: Nursing ethics for leadership and practice* (pp. 433–446). Toronto, ON: Pearson-Prentice Hall.

Dobrowolska B., Wronska I., Fidecki W., and Wysijubski, M. 2007. Moral obligations of nurses based on the ICN, UK, Irish and Polish codes of ethics for nurses. *Nursing Ethics, 14* (2), 171–180.

Flaming, D. 2006. Using phronesis instead of "research-based practice" as the guiding light for nursing practice. *Nursing Philosophy, 2*, 251–258.

Gastmans, C. 2002. A fundamental ethical approach to nursing: Some proposals for ethics education. *Nursing Ethics, 9* (5), 494–507.

Gilligan, C. 1982. *In a different voice.* Cambridge, MA: Harvard University Press.

Hartrick, G.A. 2002. Beyond interpersonal communication: The significance of relationship in health promoting practice. In L. Young and V. Hayes (Eds.), *Transforming health promotion practice. Concepts, issues and applications* (pp. 49–58). Philadelphia: F.A. Davis.

Hartrick Doane, G. & Varcoe, C. 2005. *Family nursing as relational inquiry: Developing health promoting practice.* Philadelphia: Lippincott, Williams and Wilkins.

Kirkham, S.R. & Browne, A.J. 2006. Toward a critical theoretical interpretation of social justice discourses in nursing. *Advances in Nursing Science, 29* (4), 324–339.

MacDonald, H. 2007. Relational ethics and advocacy in nursing: Literature review. *Journal of Advanced Nursing, 57* (2), 119–126.

Mitchell, G.J. and Bunkers, S.S. (2003). Engaging the abyss: A miss-take of opportunity. *Nursing Science Quarterly, 16* (2), 121.

Nortvedt. P. 2001. Needs, closeness and responsibilities: An inquiry into some rival moral considerations in nursing care. *Nursing Ethics, 2*, 112–121.

Nortvedt, P. 2004. Emotions and ethics. In J. Storch, P. Rodney, and R. Starzomski (Eds.), *Toward a moral horizon: Nursing ethics for leadership and practice* (pp. 447–464). Toronto: Pearson-Prentice Hall.

Pattison, S. 2001. Are nursing codes of practice ethical? *Nursing Ethics, 8* (1): 5–18.

Peter, E. 2008. Seeing our way through the responsibility vs. endeavour conundrum: The code of ethics as both product and process. *Canadian Journal of Nursing Leadership, 21* (2), 28–31.

Peter, E. 2011. Discourse: Fostering social justice: The possibilities of a socially connected model of moral agency. *Canadian Journal of Nursing Research, 43* (2), 11–17.

Peter, E. and Liaschenko, J. 2004. Perils of proximity: A spatiotemporal analysis of moral distress and moral ambiguity. *Nursing Inquiry, 11* (4), 218–225.

Potter, N.N. 2002. *How can I be trusted? A virtue theory of trustworthiness*. Lanham, MD: Rowan and Littlefield.

Provis, C. and Stack, S. 2004 Caring work, personal obligation and collective responsibility. *Nursing Ethics, 11* (1), 5–14.

Purkis, M.E. and Björnsdóttir K. 2006. Intelligent nursing: Accounting for knowledge as action in practice. *Nursing Philosophy, 7*, 247–256.

Rodney, P., Doane, G.H., Storch, J. and Varcoe, C. 2006. Workplaces: Toward a safer moral climate. *Canadian Nurse, 102* (8), 24–27.

Rodney, P. and Varcoe, C. in press. Constrained agency: The social structure of nurses' work. In F. Baylis, J. Downie, B. Hoffmaster, and S. Sherwin (Eds.), *Health care ethics in Canada* (3rd ed.). Toronto, ON: Thompson/Nelson. (Revision of Varcoe, C. and Rodney, P. 2009 Constrained agency: The social structure of nurses' work. In B.S. Bolaria, H.D. Dickinson (Eds.), *Health, illness, and health care in Canada* (4th ed.; pp. 122–151). Toronto: Nelson Education.)

Rosenberg, H.J., Rosenberg, S.D., Wolford, G.L., Manganiello, P.D., Brunette, M.F., and Boynton, R.A. 2000. The relationship between trauma, PTSD, and medical utilization in three high risk medical populations. *International Journal of Psychiatry and Medicine, 30* (3), 247–59.

Sellman, D. 2006. The importance of being trustworthy. *Nursing Ethics, 13* (2), 105–115.

Sellman, D. 2009. [Editorial] Ethical care for older persons in acute care settings. *Nursing Philosophy, 10*, 69–70.

Soderberg, A., Gilje, F., and Norberg, A. 1999. Transforming desolation into consolation: The meaning of being in situations of ethical difficulty in intensive care. *Nursing Ethics, 6* (5), 357–373.

Tarlier, D. 2004. Beyond caring: The moral and ethical bases of responsive nurse-patient relationships. *Nursing Philosophy, 5*, 230–241.

Taylor, B. and Barling, J. 2004. Identifying sources and effects of carer fatigue and burnout for mental health nurses: A qualitative approach. *International Journal of Mental Health Nursing, 13* (2), 117–125.

Thompson, F. 2002. Moving from codes of ethics to ethical relationships for midwifery practice. *Nursing Ethics, 9* (5), 522–536.

Tschudin, V. 1999. *Nurses matter*. London: Macmillan.

Varcoe, C., Doane, G., Pauly, B., et al. 2004. Ethical practice in nursing—Working the in-betweens. *Journal of Advanced Nursing, 45* (3), 316–325.

Walker, M.U. 2003. *Moral contexts*. Lanham, MD: Rowman & Littlefield.

CHAPTER 9

Moral Agency: Relational Connections and Support

Patricia Rodney, Susan Kadyschuk, Joan Liaschenko, Helen Brown, Lynn Musto, and Nickie Snyder

The dominant rationalist view . . . has given us a model of ourselves as disengaged thinkers. (Taylor 1995, 63)

The dominant rationalist view with its focus on disengaged thinkers, which Canadian philosopher Charles Taylor critiqued in the quote above, has not served nursing well. It tends to reduce moral problems to binary solutions,[1] thereby diminishing the interface of moral problems with the human experiences of nurses, their clients, and their colleagues in other professions. Moreover, it provides a limited conceptual vantage point from which to understand the interface of nurses with the complex—and increasingly problematic—sociopolitical health care environments in which they practice.[2] This has rendered nurses' moral agency largely invisible (Rodney and Varcoe in press). In this chapter we will argue that understanding the intersection between nursing knowledge and nursing work helps us to better appreciate the moral situation of nurses. We will further argue that nurses' enactment of their moral agency is influenced by gender and context, and is profoundly dialogical and relational. Lastly, we will argue that authentic presence and trust are important elements of the network of relationships within which nurses enact their moral agency. We close by reflecting on the implications of our arguments for supporting nurses as moral agents and for collaborative practice. Throughout the chapter, it is our premise that unless nurses are able to enact their moral agency, they will have difficulty fulfilling their professional responsibilities. Such difficulty is to the detriment of patient, family, and community care, and to the detriment of nurses and other health care providers.[3]

Nurses are not disengaged thinkers, and neither are the rest of the persons they encounter in their practice. It is encouraging to note that current scholarship from nursing, ethics, and other disciplines is increasingly reflecting this realization about professionals as moral agents. Here we wish to contribute to the growing dialogue by providing our own analyses of nurses as moral agents. In subsequent chapters of this text—particularly Chapters 10, 11, and 18—we will say more about how nurses' moral agency is constrained by the moral climate of their workplaces, with suggestions as to how we might improve that climate and hence improve nursing practice, interprofessional practice, and patient, family, and community care.

We start this chapter with an account of practice from nurses in direct care. We then visit the everyday nature of nursing knowledge, linking this knowledge to nurses' work. This leads us to a more detailed explication of nurses' moral agency, including the influence of gender, context, and relationships. We subsequently look at nurses' relational connections, including moral agency in a collaborative context and the impact of moral distress and moral residue. In so doing, we draw on research focused on nursing ethics to show how nurses work in an interconnected web (matrix) of relationships with their colleagues in nursing and other disciplines. Using a second account from a new graduate, we explicate how we might better support new as well as experienced nurses in the enactment of their moral agency. We conclude by emphasizing the importance of trust in sustaining relationships with colleagues. Overall, this chapter identifies theoretical themes that are picked up in different ways through the remaining chapters of the book. In the subsequent chapters, these themes are enriched by the diverse theoretical and practice backgrounds of the various authors.

CONCEPTUALIZING MORAL AGENCY

Before we proceed, we will make more explicit what we mean by moral agency. Within the overall field of ethics, the traditional view of an agent is that of a person who is capable of deliberate action and/or who is in the process of deliberate action (Angeles 1981, 6). An agent may engage in deliberate action with or without moral overtones. It is the former variety that we are interested in, which we will term "moral agency." Characteristics that have been used by philosophers to define moral agency include rationality, autonomy, and (limited) self-interest (Sherwin 1992, 41). Thus, traditional perspectives on moral agency reflect a notion of individuals engaging in self-determining or self-expressive choice (Taylor 1992, 57). Those perspectives have been greatly influenced by Immanuel Kant, who placed human dignity and rationality at the centre of his moral view (Taylor 1989, 364).[4]

Over the past two decades or so, critiques within philosophy and health care ethics have raised concerns about theories of moral agency. Feminist and other contextual theorists have come to understand agency as enacted through relationships in particular contexts. For instance, Sherwin (1998, 2011) and Walker (2003) critique traditional perspectives on ethics and moral agency that arise in the form of ethical theory dominating contemporary Anglo-American philosophy (see also McGee 2003). *One problem with traditional perspectives on moral agency is that they presuppose a "level playing field" in which moral agents are seen to be independent and similarly situated* (Rodney 1997). This misses the multiple kinds of relationships that exist within society in which there is an asymmetry of power between agents (Baier 1994; Peter 2011; Sherwin 1992); for instance, it misses adult–child relationships and nurse–patient relationships.[5] Such asymmetries are not unusual in health care and have diverse causes. Moral agents in health care (patients, families, and professionals/providers) are not as "equal" and autonomous as the traditional perspectives might assume.

Secondly, the traditional focus on rationality and self-interest neglects the relational, contextual nature of moral agency (Peter 2011; Rodney 1997; see also Chapter 16). This abstract neutrality is particularly objectionable from the perspective of feminist ethics, which demands an explicit focus on the social and political contexts of individuals in its moral deliberations (Sherwin 1992, 40). Women "are assumed to fall under the general rubric of 'the agent,' but the moral concerns that are examined are always those most salient from the male perspective" (Sherwin 1992, 44).

In fact, feminists are especially interested in constraints on women's agency. While there are various forms of feminist theory that pursue questions about agency in different ways, in this chapter (and in this book overall) we are particularly interested in *relational* approaches (see also Chapters 5, 7 and 8). Such approaches "focus attention on the need for a more fine-grained and richer account of the autonomous *agent*" (Mackenzie and Stoljar 2000b, 21, italics in original). While the work we have cited above focuses on women, it is our premise throughout this chapter and this book that relational understandings of moral agency apply to men as well as women, and to people from diverse contexts in terms of sexual orientations, ethnicity, age, ability, and so forth. Mackenzie and Stoljar (2002b) further explain,

> . . . [A]n analysis of the characteristics and capacities of the self cannot be adequately undertaken without attention to the rich and complex social and historical contexts in which agents are embedded; they point to the need to think of autonomy as a characteristic of agents who are emotional, embodied, desiring, creative and feeling, as well as rational, creatures; and they highlight the ways in which agents are both psychically internally differentiated and socially differentiated from others. (21)

Agents are seen as relational "because their identities or self-conceptions are constituted by elements of the social context in which they are embedded" and "because their natures are produced by certain historical and social conditions" (Mackenzie and Stoljar 2000b, 22). Another way of putting this is to say that we ought to attend to the interrelationships between *structure* and agency, where structures are "mutually sustaining cultural schemas and sets of resources that empower and constrain social action" and agents are empowered (or disempowered) by structures because of the access to resources those structures facilitate or constrain (Sewell 1992, 27).

As can be seen from the above, there is an important reciprocity between structure and agency. There is also an important reciprocity between agency and autonomy. Sherwin (1998) explains that "[t]o exercise agency, one need only exercise reasonable choices" (32), while to be autonomous means, minimally, "to resist oppression" (Sherwin 1998, 33). When autonomy is threatened, we see moral agency as being constrained.

Further, the exercise of agency is *embodied*. As Taylor (1995) explains,

> Our body is not just the executant of the goals we frame, nor just the locus of causal factors shaping our representations. Our understanding itself is embodied. That is, our bodily know-how, and the way we act and move, can encode components of our understanding of self and world. (170)

This requires us to consider not only the kinds of choices that agents make, but also the circumstances, feelings, and relationships that are affecting their ability to make those choices (see also Chapters 7 and 8).

Recent work by nurse scholar Elizabeth Peter has continued to enrich our understanding of nurses' moral agency. Together with Liaschenko, she has defined moral agency as "the capacity to recognize, deliberate/reflect on, and act on moral responsibilities" (Peter and Liaschenko 2004, 221). And in a recent academic discourse, Peter uses feminist political theorist Iris Marion Young's (2011) writing about socially connected moral responsibility to offer this interpretation of a relational understanding of moral agency:

> With a feminist approach . . . (which conceptualizes persons as connected and interdependent), it is possible to think of moral agency as more than a characteristic possessed by an aggregate

of individuals. It is possible to think of agency as a relational or socially connected characteristic of individuals in such a way that we can, at least to some extent, recognize, reflect on and act on moral responsibilities as a collective. (Peter 2011, 12)

For the purposes of this chapter, then, our conceptualization of moral agency includes *rational and self-expressive choice, embodiment, identity, social and historical relational influences, and autonomous action within wider societal structures. That action requires recognition of and reflection on moral challenges, and is expressed at collective as well as individual levels.*

NURSES' VOICES

In an early ethnographic study of nurses practising on two acute medical units conducted by Rodney, nurses spoke of the importance of the relationships they had with their colleagues in nursing and other disciplines, as well as with patients and their family members. Consistent with what Peter (2011) articulated in the quotation above, a sense of *connectedness* and *trust* in these relationships enabled them to feel more ready to deal with ethical problems in their practice (Rodney 1997). Two nurses from the study talked in separate interviews about the ethics of their practice (see Ethics in Practice 9-1). While they did not explicitly use the language of ethics, they said a great deal about how they operate as moral agents—that is, how they act to promote what they see as "the good" of patients and patients' families.[6] The first nurse participant, a relatively inexperienced nurse, talked of how much she relied on her experienced nurse colleagues to help her with patient crises. The second participant, who had years of nursing experience on an acute medical unit, talked of how she continued to rely on her colleagues to help her "see a pattern."

ETHICS IN PRACTICE 9-1

Working Together

First Nurse Participant: You know, the thing is that you often get ways of working around [dealing with a patient crisis]. . . . [O]ther nurses have lots of experience and so you work together to figure out what to do. There's some things written in the policy and procedure, but yet, that's not really [enough]. I mean, it works out fine in the end but if you come up with a situation that you've never seen before or nobody has seen before then you can run into a problem.

Second Nurse Participant: I think, you know, [with] really critically ill people and really anxious scenarios we, we have to take our leads from what is being said . . . by the family and that and go from there till we can

see a pattern, and the pattern may not show up for a week or two sort of thing, . . . especially where we have so many of our own personnel involved because we're all [working eight-hour shifts] and so there's a lot of turnover and everybody works and sees things through different eyes. . . . Well, what we also do . . . is ask for feedback among ourselves like, "What do you think . . . ?" or "How do you see this?" . . . [S]ometimes you wonder if it's your own perception or maybe it's . . . a pattern that's coming up in [the perception of] . . . other staff members as well and that's . . . why we have conferences too sometimes or . . . why we leave notes for one another . . . just so that we don't get misled. (Rodney 1997, 142)

Both nurses in Ethics in Practice 9-1—and every other nurse in that study as well as all others Rodney has conducted since—emphasized the importance of their relationships with their colleagues. We will say more about this as we proceed in this chapter, and revisit these nurses' words periodically throughout our analysis. At this point we turn to examine the relationships between nursing knowledge and nurses' work as essential for understanding nurses' enactment of moral agency and ethical nursing practice.

NURSES' KNOWLEDGE AND NURSES' WORK

Knowledge is a critical aspect of moral action (Audi 1997; Flanagan 1991). We act in accordance with what we know or believe to be the case about the material and social world. Responsibility for our actions can be influenced by the knowledge we have about the situation and moral agents involved. A moral agent can be released from responsibility for their actions, or held less responsible for them, if they lacked knowledge that would have led them to judge and act differently. On the other hand, we can be held responsible for knowledge we should have had in specific situations. This sounds straightforward and uncomplicated enough. However, as the two nurse participants in Ethics in Practice 9-1 indicated, acquiring knowledge is a process fraught with uncertainty ("if you come up with a situation that you've never seen before or nobody has seen before" and "everybody works and sees things through different eyes"). Acquiring knowledge is complicated and involves appreciation of cultural norms, experience, the particular circumstances, consequences, and other features. And, when moral agents are set in highly complex social organizations with multiple moral agents in multiple relational networks, the relations between knowledge and morality are even more complex (Liaschenko 1997a; Liaschenko and Fisher 1999).

When many people are involved in working to produce an outcome, the knowledge is typically distributed along a continuum that depends not only on formal divisions specified by educational requirements and licensing but also on other features. These other features include, for example, experience and location. *Experience* is necessary for the transformation of a novice to an expert (Benner 1984; 1991; Benner, Tanner, and Chesla 1996). *Location* of the work is relevant because locations bind knowledge in particular ways (Stein-Parbury and Liaschenko 2007). Indeed, the nurses in Ethics in Practice 9-1 emphasized the importance of experience ("other nurses have lots of experience and so you work together to figure out what to do"), and they were speaking from their specialized location of an acute medical unit. Understanding how knowledge is distributed therefore helps us to understand some of the social and historical contexts in which nurses as moral agents are embedded, and it helps us to understand some of their differentiation from moral agents in other professions.

In direct patient care the key moral agents involved are those closest to the patient and the patient's family: nurses, physicians, and their colleagues in other professions. Knowledge essential to patient care includes (but is not limited to) knowledge of anatomy and physiology, the pathophysiology of disease, therapeutics, and human responses to illness (*case knowledge*). It also requires knowledge of how the disease is manifest in this particular patient, any unique features of anatomy and physiology in this patient, and how this patient responds to the treatments of choice (*patient knowledge*). It may or may not require knowledge of the patient's unique biography and how he or she understands the meaning of the disease and its treatment in his or her life (*person knowledge*) (Liaschenko and Fisher 1999). None of this knowledge is exclusive to any particular discipline among health care providers. If it were, the work could not be done. However, there are clearly levels of emphasis, focus, and legal parameters in how the knowledge is distributed. Patient care also typically requires knowledge about how to get things done within an institutional setting—or a relational network that may involve many institutions or settings, such as in-patient practices, programs, and community care networks (Liaschenko 1998).

Critical to the implementation of case, patient, and person knowledge is *social knowledge*. By social knowledge we mean knowledge of human beings in situations in which the individual is a subject (i.e., a moral actor) and not an object. In other words, it includes knowledge about social relations. The difference is particularly relevant to patient knowledge because patient knowledge can be knowledge of the patient primarily as an object or primarily as a subject. For example, certain kinds of measures of a patient's response to treatment, such as blood oxygenation or hematocrit, are knowledge of the *patient as an object*. However, knowledge of the *patient as a subject* would be, for example, knowing that the patient does not take medication in the way prescribed because the patient is resisting the establishment of a routine that disrupts his or her previously known life. Even case knowledge is social, in the important sense that human beings work together to produce case knowledge. *Who* the people are is critical. In nursing, for instance, knowing the individual physician is an important piece of knowledge that nurses use in caring for surgical intensive care unit patients (Liaschenko and Fisher 1999). In other words, knowledge of the "who" influences how nurses build/shape their arguments and "make the case" for a particular intervention or approach to a plan of care, and knowing the physician is similarly "used" by nurses in caring for a patient.[7]

For nurses, all forms of knowledge are central to their location within a complex system. This knowledge both informs and arises from moral action and makes it possible. For instance, nurses have and require knowledge of other moral agents, the routines that make up the everyday flow of activities that are health care work, and how to get things done (Liaschenko 1998). What this means is that *if we are to understand the nature of nurses' moral work, we must better understand the nature of knowledge used by nurses in their practice* (Liaschenko and Fisher 1999; see also Canam 2008; Manias and Street 2001). The work of nursing can best be captured in an integration of the language of the everyday work of caring for patients *and* the language of science (Liaschenko and Fisher 1999). Similarly, the nature of knowledge is inseparable from nursing work—reflective of the historical invisibility and silencing of what counts as nursing knowledge (Liaschenko 1997a; see also Rodney and Varcoe in press).

NURSES' ENACTMENT OF THEIR MORAL AGENCY

The previous description of the intersection between nursing knowledge and nursing work helps us to understand the moral situation of nurses, since both nursing knowledge and nursing work are socially mediated processes embedded within the contextual realities of nursing practice. Here we would like to further explore the notion of nurses' enactment of their moral agency. Health care professionals such as nurses are considered to have a particular kind of moral agency because of the unique knowledge and skills—and hence power—they hold (Rodney 1997). Yet our knowledge of the ethics of professional practice in nursing and other fields is incomplete. As an anonymous reviewer of the first edition of this chapter noted, we need to understand more about what "enactment" entails. This remains true eight years later, though, as Peter's (2011) discourse demonstrates, there has been some thoughtful theorizing and empirical work in nursing over those years. *In this chapter we argue that relational knowledge and trust are important, as well as virtues, professional values, experience, and other qualities.* Answering questions about enactment more fully requires the kind of composite approach to ethical theory argued for in Chapters 5, 13 and 18 of this text—a composite approach that we implicitly draw on throughout this chapter.

Nurses' actions arise from a primary commitment to patients (Brown 2008). This commitment is therefore an important site for inquiry about moral agency and ethical practice. Nursing has as its foremost mandate a professional and ethical commitment to promoting the health and well-being of patients. Since nurses' primary ethical and professional commitment is to patients, the nurse–patient relationship is often viewed as the moral foundation of nursing practice (Peter and Morgan 2001) and, therefore, represents a central site of nursing work (Brown 2008; Gadow 1980). This commitment means that nursing by its very nature is a moral endeavour (Bishop and Scudder 1990; Liaschenko 1995; Smith and Godfrey 2002). A commitment to patients, coupled with the fact that nurses are the largest group of health care providers consistently with patients, help to delineate the importance of nurses' status as moral agents (Oberle and Raffin Bouchal 2009; Yarling and McElmurry 1986; Yeo et al. 2010; see also Hartrick Doane and Brown 2011). Yet that status remains contested.

Contested Agency

Gender and Context

The nature of nursing work is mediated by the social location of nursing as a predominately women's profession. As will be highlighted in different ways in several chapters in this text, this social location has a profound impact on nurses' enactment of their moral agency. *Questions about the social status of women and nursing mark the landscape of what nursing is about, both historically and for the future* (Liaschenko 2008). Many of the contemporary assumptions regarding nursing work have their roots in the cultural tradition of the 19th century—a tradition in which women and men had unequal status, and which emphasized hierarchical social organization and authoritarian lines of command (Kuhse 1997; see also Chapter 2). Nursing has been described as a metaphor for subordinated femininity, and most often described as a "natural" extension of a woman's role such that the status afforded to women and nurses has been and continues to be compared (David 2000). Women's historic invisibility and the language that sustains such invisibility are long-standing problems for nursing as a female-dominated profession. Since nursing has a history of subordination in health care settings, and of being composed primarily of women, we believe that any analysis of the socialization and practice of nursing work must thoughtfully attend to historically constructed experiences. At the same time we ought to also attend to the too often marginalized positions of men in nursing, of those who are people of colour, and of those with non-heterosexual orientations. Paying attention to the diverse experiences of women and men in nursing can expose how language and power intersect, which can facilitate a language of constructive social change in nursing (David 2000; Latimer 2000).

Caring Theory

Social discourses shaping nursing work that are particularly relevant in an exploration of nurses' moral agency are the textual and social conversations arising from locating caring as *the* moral foundation for nursing (Brown 2008). Caring language, as it is taken up in nursing, both legitimizes and marginalizes different subject positions (David 2000; see also Edwards 2009). The texts of caring in nursing have frequently constructed caring as evolving from a nurse's character and individual motivation for caring while ignoring both the material conditions and power relations in the particular contexts (the structure) where nurses work (MacPherson 1991). As the feminist theorists whom we cited at the outset of this chapter have claimed, the material conditions and power relations matter. For example, the nurses in Ethics in Practice 9-1 were attempting to provide (even basic) nursing care for elderly and critically ill patients on the acute medical unit where they worked, yet the nursing staffing was such that their work was characterized by a race against the clock (Rodney 1997; see also Rodney and Varcoe in press). The nurses themselves had almost no say in administrative decisions about their conditions of work. Care, with its gendered connotation in Western culture, is all too easily, in our view, reduced to feminine character and virtue and evaluation of what it means to be a "good nurse." Attention is neither paid to the sociopolitical context of that work nor to the apparent unreasonableness of being overworked (Austin 2011; see also Chapters 10, 11, and 18). For these reasons, care and the related social practices it entails become problematic as *the* moral foundation for nursing when issues of power, social justice, and domination remain obscured and unaccounted for (Bowden 2000; Edwards 2009; Liaschenko and Peter 2003).[8]

It is clear that since nursing is a profession predominantly (although not exclusively) pursued by women, a disciplinary, social, cultural, political, *and* gender-based analysis of nursing is necessary when examining the moral work of nursing and nurses' moral agency. *In other words we will not be able to understand—and hence support—nurses' enactment of their moral agency if we think of nurses as isolated, rational individuals who are discharging their ethical obligations.*

Nurses are constrained by the structures in which they operate, yet we also need to recognize nurses' own roles in (paradoxically) perpetuating some of the very structures that constrain them as moral agents. We will explore what we mean here by first looking at an interview segment from a nurse who participated in a study of ethical practice in emergency department nursing (Ethics in Practice 9-2).[9]

ETHICS IN PRACTICE 9-2

Pulled Like a Piece of Toffee

Sometimes you get pulled like a piece of toffee. You know. People calling you names, the phones are ringing, you're having to put out a fire or you're having to start a fire under somebody, keep things moving, dealing with the administration, and that's the biggest problem is trying to get something going throughout the day so you can get your day done (staff nurse interview, *Ethics in Action*, 2005; reported in Rodney and Varcoe in press. See also Endnote 9).

As can be seen in the transcript above, the emergency nurses we interviewed and observed were struggling daily with significant contextual constraints to their agency.[10] The department was overwhelmed with seriously ill and chronically ill patients who had to be held in the department for too long; angry backlogs of patients and their families in the waiting rooms; chronic short-staffing; and persistent conflict with management about how best to provide care. The nurses from the department who joined us in our action research helped us to understand, though, that at times it was their own feelings and behaviours that made the constraints for themselves and their colleagues worse— for example, by criticizing their more junior colleagues for not being efficient (see also Varcoe 2001). Over time, and in conversation with these nurses, we came to understand that nurses were to some extent internalizing the emergency department's constraints to their agency. *In other words, nurses (and other moral agents) certainly experience external constraints in the enactment of their moral agency, but they also experience internal constraints when their own moral compasses start to shift*—processes that are not yet well enough understood, but may include errors in judgment or a "weakness or crimp in one's character such as a pattern of 'systemic avoidance'" (Webster and Baylis 2000, 218). Corley and Goren (1998) have termed this nursing's "dark side" (see also Rodney and Varcoe in press).

Moral Sequelae

Moral Distress and Moral Residue

We have argued that nurses' socio-political position influences what they are able to accomplish as moral agents, and that there is some reciprocity between what they experience as external constraints and what they internalize, though we do not yet fully understand that reciprocity. While nurses have great capacity and resilience— and are quite skilful in navigating the complexities of the practice world—they are too often limited in their autonomy as moral agents. There are significant moral sequelae for such problems with autonomy. And there is an expanding theoretical and empirical literature in nursing tracking sequelae such as moral distress and moral residue. Further, this literature is now being taken up and applied by our colleagues in other professions.

Moral distress is a concept that started to gain prominence in the nursing literature as a result of the work of the American ethicist Andrew Jameton (1984). Essentially, Jameton's early definition focused on what nurses (or any moral agents) experience when they are constrained from moving from moral choice to moral action—an experience associated with feelings of anger, frustration, guilt, and powerlessness. It is important to note that more recent conceptualizations have focused less on external constraints alone and more on the complex interplay of structure and agency. Moral distress has become characterized as the result of an incoherence between values and action and possibly also outcome (Webster and Baylis 2000), and (as we have indicated above) also as a result of nurses internalizing external constraints such that their own moral identities may shift, sometimes leading to coercive and/or harmful nursing practice (Pauly et al. 2009; Pauly et al. 2010; Rodney and Varcoe in press; Varcoe, Rodney, and McCormick 2003). In other words, it is not just external constraints such as excessive workloads that get in the way of moral action. It is also how interconnected individuals act in relation to each other to facilitate or constrain moral action, which is closely linked to nurses' moral integrity (Yeo et al. 2010).

It is our contention that internal and external constraints to nurses' autonomy as moral agents, and their resultant moral distress, threaten the well-being of nurses and the well-being (and likely also the safety) of patients and families. We need to understand more about nurses' integrity challenges as well as nurses' strengths so as to promote more ethical practice. Not surprisingly, then, in recent years there has been growing interest in the theoretical development of moral distress as a concept and empirical measurement of that concept in nursing and other professions.

Research over the past two and a half decades has shown that the experience of moral distress in nursing is pervasive, especially in end-of-life decision making (Austin 2007; Corley 2002; Epstein and Hamric 2009; Hamric 2000; 2007; Hefferman and Heldig 1999; Fry et al. 2002; Rushton 2006), and more recent research has shown that this distress is also shared by physicians and other members of the health care team in various arenas of practice (Austin et al. 2005; Brazil et al. 2010; Corley et al. 2005; Hamric and Blackhall 2007; Pauly et al. 2009; Pavlish et al. 2011; Ulrich, Hamric and Grady 2010).

There is also work being done implementing and evaluating a moral distress scale so as to measure moral distress and evaluate practice and policy challenges (Corley et al. 2001; Hamric et al. 2007; Pauly et al. 2009). Moral distress is of concern not just because of the human impact on health care providers but also because moral distress is now being shown to be associated with staff conflict, staff attrition, and likely patient safety (Beagan and Ells 2007; Rodney et al. 2006; Storch 2005; see also Sanders, Pattison, and Hurwitz 2011).

Notwithstanding the conceptual and empirical progress we have noted above, it is important to point out that most of the research on moral distress had been conducted with acute care nurses working in specialty areas such as critical care, oncology, and medical/surgical units (Austin et al. 2005; Corley et al. 2001; Corley et al. 2005; Raines 2000), with little attention given to the areas of mental health, community, long-term care and so forth. Notable exceptions are studies by Austin et al. (2005), Deady and McCarthy (2010), and Lützén and Schreiber (1998), whose research has focused on nurses' experience of moral distress in mental health. Exhibit 9-1 provides a mental health illustration from the masters thesis of one of this chapter's authors (Musto).

EXHIBIT 9-1

Research Illustration: "Doing the Best I Can Do"

In her recent nursing master's thesis Musto (2010) explored the process used by mental health nurses working with adolescents to ameliorate the nurses' experience of moral distress. Using grounded theory methodology, Musto found that the basic social process that nurses used when experiencing moral distress (often after a patient safety event) was "doing the best I can do," whereby participants described enacting their day-to-day practice against the backdrop of the elements nurses bring to the nurse–patient relationship. These elements included the concepts of keeping the adolescent safe, providing individualized care, practising from a theory base, practising according to the professional standards, and emotional engagement. *Engaging in dialogue* was the primary means nurses used to work through the experience of moral distress—an ongoing process whereby nurses sought out dialogue with a variety of people as they tried to make sense of their experience. If participants expressed having a more positive experience of dialogue, they experienced a *shifting perspective* from viewing the safety incident as a result of their own personal practice, to seeing the incident within the broader context of health care delivery and the factors that contributed to that safety event. *Resolution* for these participants meant they were able to answer the question, "Is this the best I can do?" and continue working with adolescents with a renewed focus on the therapeutic relationship. If participants had a negative experience of dialogue, they were not able to view the incident from a broader perspective of the context of health care delivery and the factors that contributed to the safety incident and could *not* answer the question "Is this the best I can do?" For these participants, resolution meant they either left the unit or agency, or they talked about leaving.

The results from Musto's thesis work as portrayed in Exhibit 9-1, as well as the account from the emergency nurse in Ethics in Practice 9-2, underscore the seriousness of moral distress. Yet, as our discussion of moral agency in general has implied, we still have a great deal to learn about moral distress and the phenomena associated with it. For one, it is probably not a linear process of cause (constraints) and effect (moral distress), and nurses' own identities and integrity are likely implicated in how they respond to and possibly confound morally conflicting situations. *Regardless of the particular conceptualization of moral distress, though, the cumulative effects of moral distress are being recognized as a serious concern.* The fact that the nurses described in Exhibit 9-1 who had unresolved moral distress left the unit or agency or talked about leaving, reinforces this concern. Two Canadian ethicists, Webster and Baylis (2000), have claimed that unresolved moral distress can lead to moral compromise and subsequently *moral residue*—moral residue being what we carry with us when we knew how we should act but were unwilling and/or unable to do so (see also Epstein and Hamric 2009; Mitchell 2001; Rodney and Varcoe in press). Webster and Baylis acknowledge that the experience of moral residue can encourage the moral agent to reflect on and improve his or her practice, but they also warn that the moral agent may move toward denial, trivialization, or unreflective acceptance of the incoherence between beliefs and action (224–226).

There are certainly areas we need more focused inquiry in. For example, as we note in Chapter 18, the moral positions of managers in our current health care system are fraught with challenges. The few studies we have related to them indicate that managers experience significant moral distress related to their "in between" position relative to direct care staff and senior administration (see, for example, Gaudine and Beaton 2002; Mitton et al. 2011). It is also the case that we should be careful not to overextend the concept of moral distress. McCarthy and Deady (2008) offer the following caution:

> Although we are confident that the language of moral distress can offer new ways of engaging with and understanding the moral realm of nurses and health professionals generally, we are also concerned that the nursing discourse on moral distress may sometimes be confusing and counterproductive. We are worried that some of the research on moral distress to date: (1) lacks conceptual clarity; and (2) perpetuates the dominant or meta-narratives about the professional identity of nursing that, we think, ought to be challenged. (258)

In other words, we will not be able to support nurses such as the ones we have learned from in Ethics in Practice 9-1 and 9-2 and Exhibit 9-1 if we overextend the notion of moral distress, or encourage nurses to play moral distress like a "trump card" in all situations of conflict. Moral distress is important because it points to significant values-based conflicts. It has been our observation that our colleagues in medicine, psychology, pharmacy, and a number of other fields are looking to follow nursing's lead to better understand the phenomenon. We have a good beginning at a theoretical and empirical base from which we ought to proceed with caution.

Moral Disengagement

Our warnings above about nurses' possible internalization of moral constraints leads us to reflect on a concept that has emerged from cognitive theory and has only recently been applied to nursing (Kadyschuk 2007; see also Pask 2005). The concept of moral disengagement has its roots in Albert Bandura's social cognitive theory (1986), a significant aspect of which is self-regulation. *Moral disengagement may help explain what we have alluded to above in terms of some nurses' shifting moral identities.* According to Bandura (2002), through the process of socialization, people adopt moral standards that serve as both deterrents and guides for conduct. If they act against accepted moral standards, they employ mechanisms of moral disengagement to avoid the self-condemnation that normally accompanies behaving in ways they think are wrong.

Bandura (1986) argues that through cognitive restructuring of behaviour, distorting the relationship between behaviour and causal effects, and devaluing the recipients of amoral behaviour, individuals are able to avoid the self-condemnation that usually accompanies abdication of moral agency. If people choose to act in accordance with their moral standards, they remain morally engaged; conversely, they morally disengage if they choose to act in opposition to these same standards. How are people able to do this and what are the ramifications for health care and nursing today? The concept of moral disengagement sheds light on this from a psychological perspective. Similar to concepts such as ethical drift (Kleinman 2006) and moral erosion (Glover 1999), moral disengagement is a progressive process, with gradual weakening of self-sanctions that may initially go unnoticed until, eventually, few barriers remain to dissuade individuals from behaviour once thought of as amoral, and at which point little distress is experienced when carrying out such behaviour (Bandura 1990). *We believe that moral disengagement may be behind erosions of nurses' integrity and "normalization" of inadequate resources to provide safe, competent, compassionate, and ethical care* (see also Bandura 2006 and Chapters 10, 11, and 18).

Bandura (1986; 1990; 2002) argues that the processes by which moral disengagement operate include a combination of moral justification, euphemistic language, and advantageous comparison. Assigning moral qualities to a decision or behaviour the agent knows to be immoral in order to justify it is *moral justification*. Moral justification poses a significant threat to health care, nursing, and patient care because the more an unethical act is justified as ethical or moral, the more the perception of the act changes until what once was considered unethical is now considered ethical, and reservations about engaging in such practice are eroded. For example, the inappropriate use of restraints on the elderly is often justified as way to keep patients safe without looking at better staffing and other interventions that would prevent the need for restraints. *Euphemistic language* camouflages the actual meaning of an unethical behaviour to make it appear ethical. Like moral justification, euphemistic language threatens health care by distorting the moral implication of an action through cloudy or deceptive language. For example, early discharge of vulnerable patients from hospitals without adequate home support is justified as being "efficient" patient care (see also Anderson et al. 2010; Austin 2011 as well as Chapter 18 and Chapter 19). *Advantageous comparison* exploits the contrast principle whereby an unethical behaviour is made to seem more palatable by comparing it to something even worse. For example, in acute care advantageous comparison is illustrated by claims that a "hallway bed" is better than no bed at all.

Bandura states that a second set of mechanisms used by people to disengage morally from their conduct allows people to obscure responsibility for their behaviour by *diffusing or displacing responsibility* for their actions, thereby obscuring the relationship between their actions and their causal effects (1986; 1990; 2002). Displacement of responsibility allows people to blame their behaviour on the dictates of others; in other words, surrendering responsibility for their own actions. Diffusion of responsibility often operates in organizations, where actions or change stemming from decisions made at higher levels are diffused throughout the organization. Individuals may "own" responsibility for single components of a change or behaviour, but are able to claim ignorance about the sum of the components; thereby excusing themselves of any injurious effects. In the example above, for instance, the early discharge of patients is seen to be a decision made from "higher up." Conversely, according to Bandura, moral control operates most strongly when people acknowledge that their actions will harm others.

The third set of disengagement mechanisms—*minimizing or disregarding injurious consequences*—works on the principle that if people are able to minimize or disregard the harm their behaviour causes, they are able to avoid the self-censure that normally accompanies behaviour known to be injurious to others (Bandura 1986; 1990; 2002). Key to this mechanism is distance from recipients of injurious behaviour: it is easier to deny the potential harm of an action if the person conducting it does not witness any injurious effects. An administrator who creates a bed utilization policy, for example, may not witness the experiences of patients and family members who are sent home from hospital before they are ready. Finally, people disengage morally from their actions by *dehumanizing or blaming the victims of their actions*. Bandura (1999) suggests that dehumanization is cultivated in a modern society by factors such as increased bureaucratization. At the level of patient care, dehumanization is illustrated by patients being identified in terms of diagnoses and/or potential for discharge or transfer, rather than as human beings. Worse yet, patients who require frequent acute care because of chronic physical or mental illness, age, and so forth may be labelled as "bed blockers." People are also able to disengage morally from their actions by blaming the recipients of their actions for the actions themselves. This can also be illustrated at the level of patient care, where patients such as IV substance users may be accused of "bringing it upon themselves," thereby justifying provision of poor care by health care professionals (see also Browne et al. 2011).

Moral disengagement is a gradual process that may go unnoticed (Bandura 1986; 1990; 2002) by individuals and organizations, and hence strategies of moral disengagement become normalized in health care. Clearly, we need more theoretical and empirical research on how constructs such as moral agency, nursing knowledge, moral distress, moral residue, moral disengagement, and normalization of poor practice might be related. Given our premise that moral disengagement may be behind erosions of nurses' integrity and the "normalization" of inadequate resources, it is crucial that we learn how to better support nurses as moral agents and that we learn how to foster ethical practice in organizations as well as ethical policy development. We address the latter two in Chapter 18.

Interestingly—and possibly as a counterpoint to the prevalence of moral distress, moral residue, and moral disengagement—a concept that is getting more attention in nursing and ethics literature now is that of *moral courage*. Moral courage can be understood as "the pinnacle of ethical behavior; it requires a steadfast commitment to fundamental ethical principles despite potential risks" (Murray 2010, 2; see also Day 2007). While we ought not to require that nurses or other health care providers become heroic in order to uphold ethical standards, moral courage is a concept worth more exploration. And in the meanwhile, we certainly need to be proactive in supporting *all* nurses as moral agents.

SUPPORTING NURSES AS MORAL AGENTS

Nurses' Relational Connections

Nurses' moral work is profoundly embedded in the interconnectedness and relationships of the structure of everyday health care encounters—sometimes to the detriment of the autonomy and integrity of nurses as moral agents, as we have discussed above. We see embodied, empathic relations as an essential site in which moral agency is enacted and nursing knowledge is deployed—embodied relations with their support for the moral relevance of personal involvement, values, emotions, intersubjectivity, moral sensitivity, and experience (Benner 2000; Hartrick Doane and Brown 2011; Nortvedt 2001; 2004; see also Chapters 7 and 8). A relational focus in nursing ethics means that the notion of nurses as moral agents can be articulated within the dialectic of nurses' normative and particular commitment to doing good in nursing practice (see also Gadow 1999). For instance, nurses' work is about both being with and doing for/with patients at times when they are made vulnerable by illness, suffering, and treatment, and requires the kind of knowledge work we explored earlier in this chapter. Yet the emotional work of nursing has been rendered invisible and has been systematically devalued while the more technical work becomes visible and valued (Henderson 2001; Rodney and Varcoe in press). *The important paradox here is that the emotional work of nursing and the technical work both affect one another.* In other words, expertise in nursing practice is about being both humanly involved in relationships and responsive and capable to respond to the emotional, physiologic, and treatment needs of another.

Let us illustrate by saying more about the ethnographic study of nurses practising on an acute medical unit that we introduced at the outset of this chapter (Ethics in Practice 9-1). In this study, Rodney (1997) came to understand that moral agency was not just enacted by individual nurses per se, but was enacted by a matrix of individual nurses working in interdependent relationships (see also Varcoe, Rodney, and McCormick 2003). For instance, as one of the nurses in Ethics in Practice 9-1 said, "What we also do . . . is ask for feedback among ourselves." Rodney used the concept of *relational matrix* to illustrate the connectedness and interdependence of individuals working in relationship with each other in an organizational context. The connectedness was not linear. Further, it was embedded in the particularities of the patient care context, and, when working well, lent support to the work of individuals. For example, one of the nurse participants on the acute medical unit told the story of a distraught family trying to decide whether or not to continue treatment with their mother, whose condition was irreversible (Rodney 1997). The nurse was on an evening shift, and was not able to reach the attending physician, and so reached the physician on call, whom she had never met. The physician came to see the nurse and the family immediately. Over the course of the evening, the family, nurse, and on-call physician worked together in (what the nurse described as) an egalitarian manner to try to make sense of the best interests of the dying woman. While the experience was emotionally draining, the nurse reported that the family, she, and the physician felt that they had arrived at the best possible decision for the patient. In this situation, the individuals involved (including the family) were connected and interdependent in a manner that was based only in part on their roles. They came together on the basis of a shared concern and were able to work around formal and informal hierarchies (for instance, on the unit being studied, norms about on-call physicians being less involved in family support and team decision-making, and the common trend for physicians not to consult with nurses).

Rodney (1997) found that the relational matrix may or may not be supportive of nurses' efforts to effect their moral intentions, and it seemed that the nature of the relationships between individuals in the matrix made a significant difference. Disrupted and/or conflicted relationships between even a couple of individuals were problematic. Moreover, *who* was part of the matrix was not a given. Individuals from a variety of professions were involved, depending on the particular practice context—in the example above, the family, the on-call physician, and the evening nurse. Counter to this example, though, despite their shared responsibility in patient care, physicians were often not perceived to be part of the relational matrix. In particular, they were often not accessible to help nurses deal with ethical problems in their practice, and/or their absence created ethical problems for the nurses.

However, as our earlier discussion of moral distress and moral disengagement has foreshadowed, the problems nurses experienced in the relational matrix were also caused by fellow nurses (Rodney 1997), which was apparent in the more recent study in the emergency department that we cited earlier in this chapter. And when physicians *were* available and *were* perceived to be supportive and respectful, nurses described the positive impact that this had on the care of patients and families (as in the evening nurse's story). Knowing each other was beneficial, though not required, as the on-call physician illustrates and as we discussed earlier in this chapter. There were also accounts where individuals were well known but seemed to have a profoundly negative impact on the relational matrix—for instance, a physician who "yelled at" nursing staff regularly and a group of nurses who were difficult to approach for help. It seemed that being *authentically present* for each other made a tremendous difference for the quality of relationships within the matrix. Authentic presence meant being respectful and listening as well as being willing to be available to help (whether in person or over the telephone or through other means). The research studies cited in Ethics in Practice 9-1 and Exhibit 9-1, where nurses emphasized the importance of dialogue with their colleagues, point to something similar.

What Rodney's (1997) study also illustrated was that who was in the relational matrix changed over even short periods of time. In other words, the boundaries of the relational matrix were not fixed, but were fluid. Significantly, Rodney (1997) found that the relationships in the relational matrix worked best when they were founded on trust. Furthermore, it appeared that authentic presence helped trust to flourish. The nurses in Ethics in Practice 9-1, for instance, clearly identified that in order for them to draw on their colleagues' expertise, they had to trust that those colleagues were both knowledgeable and approachable. For the nurses in Ethics in Practice 9-2, trust in each other and in emergency room physicians was a major point of emphasis—as was distrust in administration.

Trust

The feminist philosopher Annette Baier (1994) defines trust as "reliance on others' competence and willingness to look after, rather than harm, things one cares about which are entrusted to their care" (128).[11] Rodney (1997) came to think of trust as the "glue" that holds the relational matrix together, and authentic presence as a major constituent of that glue. She saw the relational matrix in terms of the connectedness and interdependence of individuals working in relationship with each other in an organizational context. The connectedness was not linear, but was, rather, embedded in particular contexts, and lent support to the work of individuals.

In continuing to reflect on the relational matrix, we do not wish to say that when there is trust between most individuals the relational matrix will support every health care professional's/provider's or patient's/family member's enactment of their moral agency. Nor is it to deny that there could be some trusting matrices where individuals are authentically present for each other, but where the resultant standards of care are unethical. Having large groups of individuals who have unresolved moral residue and who are morally disengaged could certainly be a problem. And, of course, not all individuals uphold the knowledge, skill, or other attributes they are being trusted to embody.[12] *What we have underscored here is the importance of trust for its influence on nurses' abilities to enact their moral agency* (see also Peter 2011 and Peter and Morgan 2001). The strategies we suggest as we close this chapter, as well as those in Chapters 10, 13, and 18 will, we hope, strengthen trust within and between nurses and other health care providers, as well as the individuals, families, and communities they serve.

In summary, we started this chapter with a conceptualization of moral agency as inclusive of rational and self-expressive choice, embodiment, identity, social and historical relational influences, and autonomous action within wider societal structures. We claimed that the action above requires recognition of and reflection on moral challenges, and is expressed at collective as well as individual levels. We have contributed some details to adapt this conceptualization for nursing, first by locating our analysis within the nature of nurses' knowledge and nurses' work. We identified nurses as engaged actors who draw on their various sources of knowledge as they live their nursing work. Following this, we commented on constraints to nurses' autonomous agency and emphasized the seriousness (and complexity) of moral distress, moral residue, and moral disengagement. We then posited that nurses and other individuals operate within a relational matrix as moral agents, and that this matrix flourishes with authentic presence and trust. In other words, to work together as moral agents requires more than just sharing information and using a decision-making process to arrive at solutions (Rodney 1997). It requires that we come closer to what is meaningful in each other's experiences, and that such proximity become the basis for enacting moral agency in nursing practice. This is true for nursing and other health care providers.

Toward Collaborative Practice

How does focusing on authentic presence and trust as essential for enactment of nurses' moral agency point toward particular implications for practice? Nurse ethicist Carol Taylor (1997) claims that a commitment to responding to the unique needs of patients requires that nurses collaborate with each other and with multiprofessional teams. We fully agree.

Within nursing, one of the most important sites for collaboration is with/for our students and new graduates. In Exhibit 9-2 below we recount the experiences that one of us (Snyder) encountered as a new graduate so as to explore what supporting new graduates as moral agents should entail.

EXHIBIT 9-2

Narrative: A New Graduate's Journey

When I first started working as an RN, I quickly realized that I needed a way to separate my work life from my private life. Perhaps it was because I was so new, but I cared so much about my patients and would sometimes find myself fretting about them on my days off. The shower became my solution. Everyday when I finished my shift, I would come home and shower off all the germs of the hospital, but also shower off my patients. Once I got out of the shower, I could no longer think about my patients. My routine worked well and I was quite proud of myself!

About six months into my practice, my five minute showers started becoming longer. We had a patient on our unit who was deemed medically futile, but the family refused to consider a terminal wean from treatment. In fact, it seemed like they tried to blame the physicians for everything that was going wrong, rather than accepting that their father was dying. Due to the skill mix on our unit, I ended up caring for this patient often. With all my new graduate optimism, I would try to gently speak to the family about their father. I tried to explain that he was no longer responsive, and only alive because of the machines. I felt like I never got anywhere. At home, I would replay these conversations over and over in my mind as I stood under the hot water of my shower. My five-minute showers were becoming 15 minutes. . . . Soon they were 30 minutes.

One day in particular I sat down with the patient's daughter and explained to her how all of his systems were failing. I told her that his skin was in very poor condition due to all the vasopressors that we had to give him in order to maintain his blood pressure. She sat there nodding and listening. I thought that I was finally getting through to her! But in the next moment she burst my bubble by asking why had a dermatologist not seen him. I had failed. She did not understand. That day my shower was 45 minutes.

It took me a while to see the correlation between my lengthening showers and my patient assignment at work. Finally, after a month of increasingly long showers, it dawned on me—this was moral distress. I had learned about it in school, and had been able to define it and apply it to an essay question on an exam, but applying it to my life had been a bit harder. As I analyzed the situation I realized that I could not enact my moral agency, and this was causing distress. The other nurses and I all felt that a terminal wean [taking the patient off the ventilator so that he could die] was the most humane option. We felt our job was to provide comfort and care, not needlessly prolong suffering. However due to the family's anger we believed that we could not enact this. So I was left to provide care that I morally disagreed with.

Being able to define my experience as moral distress did provide some comfort. I felt less alone, and more normal when I realized that I was not the only one who experienced this. Despite this, I still did not discuss my feelings at work because I was afraid of being seen as the "weak" new graduate.

After two months, the patient finally deteriorated to a point where he died. I was his nurse that day. Even as he was dying, with his daughters by his side, they wanted to know if we were still "forcing the air in." They still wanted everything done. Once he had died, I excused myself, went to the bathroom, and burst into tears. I can only guess now at what his daughters were going through . . .

In the narrative above there are clearly complex issues around the need for appropriate treatment at the end of life, palliative care, support of families, and support of health care providers, all of which are explored throughout this text, particularly in Chapters 13 and 17. In the meanwhile, though, we would like to emphasize that as a new nurse the narrator was left feeling alone and angry with the family. Her moral distress was, by her own account, significant. And without the kind of thoughtful reflection she undertook after the event she would have been in danger of morally disengaging from families in future situations of conflict.

What do new graduates need to support the enactment of their moral agency? This is an important question and one that we believe has not been addressed enough in nursing or ethics research and literature. Snyder found people who listened to and supported her, and later became active in mentoring other new graduates through a new graduate support program. Musto's research in Exhibit 9-1 emphasizes that the need for supportive dialogue with colleagues is prevalent in a variety of practice contexts, which is also clear through every study Rodney has ever been engaged in. *So we would argue that the first step is to* name *the importance of supporting new graduates, starting with when they are students.* We do not do enough to support undergraduate students to learn to care for themselves (Anthony and Yastik 2011; Barbarosa 2009), as Snyder's account indicates (the showers were necessary but not sufficient). This is true for the entire profession. We need to acknowledge our vulnerabilities as individuals and as a profession overall (see also Chapter 10 as well as Kunyk and Austin 2011). We need to foster safe places for regular dialogues—for instance, through regular, pre-structured debriefing sessions (Serrano, Martin, and Rodney 2011; Storch et al. 2009a; 2009b). And there is likely a role for mind-body-spirit disciplines such as mindfulness meditation, yoga, and karate to help nurses deal with the challenges they face as embodied moral agents (Hanlon 2011).

In terms of *multiprofessional teams* it is, of course, important to start by acknowledging that collaboration with physicians, social workers, dieticians, physiotherapists, and many others is a significant prerequisite to nurses' enactment of their moral agency. To illustrate, the nurses in Ethics in Practice 9-1 identified that for them to draw on their colleagues' expertise, they had to trust that those colleagues were knowledgeable as well as approachable. The nurses in the relational matrix needed case knowledge as well as the situated or particular knowledge of the patient, person, and social context (Liaschenko and Fisher 1999). All these forms of knowledge were tied to context and, therefore, reflected differences in time and space, or geography. And all required interdisciplinary collaboration. For instance, nurses needed case knowledge (e.g., the resistance of a particular strain of pneumococcus to antibiotics), patient knowledge (e.g., the progression of this patient's pneumonia and response to the antibiotic), person knowledge (e.g., the meaning that the patient and family attached to the pneumonia and subsequent hospitalization), and social knowledge (e.g., how to get physician assistance quickly if the patient's oxygenation dropped). From this illustration we can say that for nurses to be able to acquire and work with all these forms of knowledge as moral agents, they need to have a supportive relational matrix of colleagues for collaboration within and outside of nursing. *Yet the theoretical and practical barriers to collaboration are pervasive.* Physicians and nurses operate from quite different forms of knowledge and quite different interpretations of what ethical practice is (Manias and Street 2001). Moreover, under conditions of uncertainty—when the uncertainty entails diagnostic and management work that is split between disciplines—collaboration can break down (Stein-Parbury and Liaschenko 2007). This leaves us with a number of challenges if we are to foster nurses' enactment of their moral agency within the context of interdisciplinary teams, especially in today's cost-constrained health care environment. As we said earlier in this chapter, the socio-political context matters. And, as Chapters 10, 11, 12 and 18 will illustrate, that socio-political context is currently fraught with problems, such as short-staffing, loss of clinical leadership, and inadequate services for patients and families, to name a few (Austin 2011).

Since the first edition of this text in 2004, there is now more research about *how* to reduce moral distress and foster collaborative practice (e.g., Centre for American Nurses 2008; Day 2007; Pauly, Storch, and Varcoe 2010; Rushton 2006; Serrano, Martin, and

Rodney 2011; Storch et al. 2009a; 2009b; Wiskow, Albreht, and de Pietro 2010; see also Chapter 10). Fostering collaborative practice ought to be a focus of continued investigation, action, and evaluation now and in the future. Helping moral agents to navigate the complex structural—and internal—barriers they face in health care delivery is going to be a long-term endeavour, and will need to be supported through the ethics resources we address in the chapters throughout this text, including Chapter 13 (see also Bell and Breslin 2008). In the meanwhile, we will close this chapter by positing a number of conclusions and subsequent recommendations.

Individuals, we have said, must be present to be effective moral agents—present in the sense that they are involved in the here-and-now of the actual patient care situation, and present in the sense that they are trying to understand what their colleagues and/or patients and family members are experiencing, as was evident in the new graduate's narrative in Exhibit 9-2. Individuals need to be authentically present for each other so that their relationships can be built on a foundation of trust. In order for this to happen—or be sustained in places where it is already occurring—it is our belief that at least the following changes are required:[13]

1. Workload and staffing patterns in all areas of practice must provide *time* for nurses, physicians, and other health care providers to meet regularly, share perspectives, and engage in planning for treatment and care. Time also needs to be built in for patients/clients and their family members to engage in regular dialogue with members of the health care team. While electronic and other media can supplement such meetings, they should not replace face-to-face contact if at all possible (see also Chapters 10 and 13).

2. Time is necessary but it is not sufficient in itself. Nurses, physicians, and other health care providers also need help to *critically reflect on the quality of their interactions* within and between disciplines, and with patients/clients and their family members. In order to enhance their ways of being with each other they ought to be cognizant of the implicit and explicit power relationships that are always at play in health care encounters, with the aim of being more authentically present for each other. Skills in communication techniques can be helpful, but must arise from a philosophical stance of mutual respect. There must be awareness of the vulnerability that arises in relationships of unequal power (see also Chapters 7 and 8).

3. Health care providers should be *more proactive in engaging patients/clients and their family members* in discussions about the *meaning* of their treatment and care, related concerns, expectations and aspirations, and so forth. It is difficult to build or retrieve trust with patients/clients and their family members if such discussions are fragmented, late, or non-existent (see also Chapters 13, 16 and 17).

4. *Leadership in clinical practice* is required to ensure the successful implementation of these first three changes. Most health care providers require some mentoring in how to be more present for their colleagues, patients/clients, and their family members. Clinical leadership is also required to ensure that the structure of the work environment makes it possible for individuals to be able to connect with each other and find ways to collaborate in taking moral action. Further, if clinical leaders are to be effective, they

must also be *authentically present* for providers, patients/clients, and their family members. This means that their management portfolios ought not to be so huge that they are inaccessible (see also Chapters 12 and 18).

5. *Education about collaboration, authentic presence, and trust* ought to be built into preparatory and continuing education programs for all health care providers (see also Chapters 6 and 15).

Summary

Although it is not difficult to articulate the recommendations above on paper, it is, of course, much more difficult to implement and/or sustain such action in practice. Many of the chapters in this book will offer insights into the current socio-political climate within which nurses enact their moral agency, including ideas about how to improve that climate. It is important that we believe in our capacity as moral agents individually and collectively. Indeed, "our potential to act is likely underestimated " (Peter 2011, 14).

For Reflection

1. Think of an area of clinical practice you are familiar with, and identify examples of the case, patient, person, and social knowledge used.

2. We have argued that embodiment is an important part of moral agency. Identify some examples of how that plays out in clinical practice.

3. What actions can nurses take as individuals to strengthen their autonomy as moral agents? As members of organizations? In professional groups?

4. What strategies can support nurses who have recently graduated to strengthen their enactment of their moral agency?

5. Remember (or imagine) a policy initiative that was meant to improve collaborative practice. What are the most important characteristics of the initiative? What helped it to work or not work?

Endnotes

1. By binary solutions we mean, for instance, yes/no or treat/do not treat. See also Chapter 13.

2. See also Chapter 5 and Chapter 18.

3. This is a premise that is provided with empirical support in Chapter 10.

4. As Taylor explains, Kant's moral view was that

   Rational beings have a unique dignity. They stand out against the background of nature, just in that they are free and self-determining. (Taylor 1989, 364)

   See also Chapter 4 and Chapter 5.

5. See also Chapter 16 as well as Brown 2008; McPherson 2007; and Varcoe and Einboden 2010.

6. Our use of the term "the good" is congruent with an Aristotelian notion of ethics, where ethics is seen as integral with character, action, and practice (Aristotle c.320 BC/1985; Benner, Tanner, and Chesla 1996; Sher 1987). As Benner and her colleagues have claimed,

even in clinical situations, where the ends are not in question, there is an underlying moral dimension: the fundamental disposition of the nurse toward what is good and right and action toward what the nurse recognizes or believes to be the best good in a particular situation. (Benner, Tanner, and Chesla 1996, 6)

Nurses' notions of the good therefore provide a value-based direction for their practice.

7. We would like to thank an anonymous reviewer of the second edition of this chapter for this paraphrase.

8. These are not the only reasons. Locating caring as the main (or only) theory for nursing ethics would have the potential to overlook the importance of caring in other professions and in other societal roles. The relationship of care to justice is also significant and problematic (Bowden 2000). While we do not want to argue that conceptualizations of care do not have a role, we believe that nursing ethics needs more than just care theory, and that the care theory we do employ ought to come from feminist theorists. Se also Chapter 5 for an argument supporting a composite approach to ethical theory.

9. In order to learn more about how to address the ethical problems we had identified in earlier studies we embarked on a participatory action research (PAR) study of nursing practice ("Ethics in Action") conducted in an emergency unit and a medical oncology unit (2003–2006). This study (funded by the Social Science and Humanities Research Council and the University of Victoria) involved three years of participant observation, interviews, focus groups, meetings, workshops, and informal work within the two practice settings (Hartrick Doane, Storch, and Pauly 2009; Rodney et al. 2006). At each site, the research team included staff nurses and academic investigators working in partnership. Along with qualitative data collection through focus groups and interviews, regular meetings with staff were conducted at each site to discuss, debrief, and to plan for change. The research process was geared to supporting staff to initiate changes in their workplaces toward ethical practice (the summary above is cited in Rodney and Varcoe in press). Rodney was a principal investigator in this study and Brown was a research assistant.

10. For a powerful account of emergency department constraints in a recently reported United Kingdom–based narrative analysis see Sanders, Pattison, and Hurwitz 2011.

11. Baier (1994) builds her conceptualization of trust on David Hume's theory of moral sentiment and Carol Gilligan's theory of care.

12. These are questions that Baier (1994) takes up in her writing about trust.

13. These recommendations are based on the analysis provided in this chapter as well as on the authors' study and experiences in practice, education, research, and ethics consultation.

References

Anderson, J.M., Browne, A.J., Reimer-Kirkham, S., Lynam, M.J., Rodney, P., Varcoe, C., et al. 2010. Uptake of critical knowledge in nursing practice: lessons learned from a knowledge translation study. *Canadian Journal of Nursing Research, 42* (3), 106–122.

Angeles, P.A. 1981. *Dictionary of philosophy*. New York: Barnes & Noble.

Anthony, M. and Yastik, J. 2011. Nursing students' experiences with incivility in clinical education. *Journal of Nursing Education 50* (3), 140–144.

Aristotle. 1985. *Nicomachean ethics* (T. Irwin, Trans.). Indianapolis, IL: Hackett. (Original work published c. 320 B.C.).

Audi, R. 1997. *Moral knowledge and ethical character*. New York: Oxford University Press.

Austin, W. 2007. The ethics of everyday practice: Healthcare environments as moral communities. *Advances in Nursing Science, 30* (1), 81–88.

Austin, W.J. 2011. The incommensurability of nursing as a practice and the customer service model: An evolutionary threat to the discipline. *Nursing Philosophy, 12*, 158–166.

Austin, W., Lemermeyer, G., Goldberg, L., Bergum, V., and Johnson, M.S. 2005. Moral distress in healthcare practice: The situation of nurses. *HealthCare Ethics Committee Forum, 17* (1), 33–48.

Baier, A.C. 1994. *Moral prejudices: Essays on ethics.* Cambridge, MA: Harvard University Press.

Bandura, A. 1986. *Social foundations of thought and action: A social cognitive theory.* Englewood Cliffs, NJ: Prentice Hall.

Bandura, A. 1990. Selective activation and disengagement of moral control. *Journal of Social Issues, 46* (1), 27–46.

Bandura, A. 1999. Moral disengagement in the perpetration of inhumanities. *Personality and Social Psychology Review, 3*(3), 193–209.

Bandura, A. 2002. Selective moral disengagement in the exercise of moral agency. *Journal of Moral Education, 31* (2), 101–119.

Bandura, A. 2006. Toward a psychology of human agency. *Perspectives on Psychological Science, 1* (2), 164–180.

Barbarosa, V. 2009. *Exploring sustainability: Supporting the mental health of student nurses.* Unpublished undergraduate directed studies paper, University of British Columbia School of Nursing, Vancouver, BC.

Beagan, B. and Ells, C. 2007. Values that matter, barriers that interfere: The struggle of Canadian nurses to enact their values. *Canadian Journal of Nursing Research, 39* (4), 37–57.

Bell, J. and Breslin, J.M. 2008. Healthcare provider moral distress as a leadership challenge. *JONA'S Healthcare Law, Ethics, and Regulation, 10* (4), 94–97.

Benner, P. 1984. *From novice to expert: Excellence and power in clinical nursing practice.* Menlo Park, CA: Addison-Wesley.

Benner, P. 1991. The role of experience, narrative, and community in skilled ethical comportment. *Advances in Nursing Science, 14* (2), 1–21.

Benner, P. 2000. The roles of embodiment, emotion and lifeworld for rationality and moral agency in nursing practice. *Nursing Philosophy, 1*, 1–14.

Benner, P.A., Tanner, C.A., and Chesla, C.A. (with contributions by H.L. Dreyfus, S.E. Dreyfus, and J. Rubin). 1996. *Expertise in nursing practice: Caring, clinical judgment, and ethics.* New York: Springer.

Bishop, A.H. and Scudder, J.R. 1990. *The practical, moral and personal sense of nursing: A phenomenological philosophy of practice.* Albany: State University of New York Press.

Bowden, P. 2000. An "ethic of care" in clinical settings: Encompassing "feminine" and "feminist" perspectives. *Nursing Philosophy, 1* (1), 36–49.

Brown, H. 2008. *The face to face is not so innocent: Into interpersonal spaces of maternal-infant care.* Unpublished doctoral dissertation, University of Victoria School of Nursing, Victoria BC.

Brazil, K., Kassalainen, S., Ploeg, J., and Marshall, D. 2010. Moral distress experienced by health care professionals who provide home-based palliative care. *Social Science & Medicine, 71,* 1687–1691.

Browne, A.J., Smye, V.L., Rodney, P., Tang, S.Y., Mussell, B., and O'Neill, J. 2011. Access to primary care from the perspective of Aboriginal patients at an urban emergency department. *Qualitative Health Research 21* (3), 333–348.

Canam, C.J. 2008. The link between nursing discourses and nurses' silence: Implications for a knowledge-based discourse for nursing practice. *Advances in Nursing Science, 31* (4), 296–307.

Center for American Nurses. 2008. *Lateral violence and bullying in the workplace.* Silver Spring, MD: Authors.

Corley, M.C. 2002. Nurse moral distress: A proposed theory and research agenda. *Nursing Ethics, 9* (6), 636–650.

Corley, M.C., Elswick, R.K., Gorman, M., and Clor, T. 2001. Development and evaluation of a moral distress scale. *Journal of Advanced Nursing, 33* (2), 250–256.

Corley, M.C. and Goren, S. 1998. The dark side of nursing: Impact of stigmatizing responses on patients. *Scholarly Inquiry for Nursing Practice, 12* (2), 99–118.

Corley, M.C., Minick, P., Elswick, R.K., and Jacobs, M. 2005. Nurse moral distress and ethical work environment. *Nursing Ethics, 12* (4), 381–390.

David, B.A. 2000. Nursing's gender politics: Reformulating the footnotes. *Advances in Nursing Science, 23* (1), 83–93.

Day, L. 2007. Courage as a virtue necessary to good nursing practice. *American Journal of Critical Care, 16 (6)*: 613–616.

Edwards, S.D. 2009. Three versions of an ethics of care. *Nursing Philosophy: An International Journal for Healthcare Professionals, 10,* 231–240.

Epstein, E.G., and Hamric, A.B. 2009. Moral distress, moral residue, and the crescendo effect. *Journal of Clinical Ethics, 20*(4), 330–342.

Flanagan, O. 1991. *Varieties of moral personality: Ethics and psychological realism.* Cambridge, MA: Harvard University Press.

Fry, S.T., Harvey, R.M., Hurley, A.C., and Foley, B.J. 2002. Development of a model of moral distress in military nursing. *Nursing Ethics, 9* (4), 373–387.

Gadow, S. 1980. Existential advocacy: Philosophical foundation of nursing. In S.F. Spiker and S. Gadow (Eds.), *Nursing: Ideals and images, opening dialogue with the humanities* (pp. 79–101). New York: Springer-Verlag.

Gadow, S. 1999. Relational narrative: The postmodern turn in nursing ethics. *Scholarly Inquiry for Nursing Practice, 13* (1), 57–69.

Gaudine, A.P. and Beaton, M.R. 2002. Employed to go against one's values: Nurse managers' accounts of ethical conflict within their organizations. *Canadian Journal of Nursing Research, 34* (2), 17–34.

Glover, J. 1999. *Humanity: A moral history of the twentieth century.* New Haven, CT: Yale University Press

Hamric, A.B. 2000. Moral distress in everyday ethics. *Nursing Outlook, 48,* 199–201.

Hamric, A.B. and Blackhall, L.J. 2007. Nurse-physician perspectives on the care of dying patients in intensive care units: Collaboration, moral distress, and ethical climate. *Critical Care Medicine, 35*, (2).

Hanlon, E.S.M. 2011. *Notice, balance and respond: How mind-body-spirit disciplines can help nurses stay in nursing, unharmed*. Unpublished master of science in nursing major essay, University of British Columbia School of Nursing, Vancouver, BC.

Hartrick Doane, G. and Brown, H. 2011. Recontextualizing learning in nursing education: Taking an ontological turn. *Journal of Nursing Education, 50* (1), 21–26.

Hartrick Doane, G., Storch, J., and Pauly, B. 2009. Ethical nursing practice: Inquiry-in-action. *Nursing Inquiry, 16* (3), 1–9.

Hefferman, P. and Heldig, S. 1999. Giving "moral distress" a voice: Ethical concerns among neonatal intensive care unit personnel. *Cambridge Quarterly of Healthcare Ethics, 8*, 173–178.

Henderson, A. 2001. Emotional labor and nursing: An under-appreciated aspect of caring work. *Nursing Inquiry, 8* (2), 130–138.

Jameton, A. 1984. *Nursing practice: The ethical issues*. New Jersey: Prentice Hall.

Kadyschuk, S.K. 2007. *Moral disengagement in healthcare*. Unpublished master of science in nursing major essay, University of British Columbia School of Nursing, Vancouver, BC.

Kleinman, C.S. 2006. Ethical drift: When good people do bad things. *Journal of Nursing Administration's Healthcare Law, Ethics, and Regulation, 8* (3), 72–76.

Kuhse, H. 1997. *Caring: Nurses, women, and ethics*. Oxford: Blackwell.

Kunyk, D. and Austin, W. 2011. Nursing under the influence: A relational ethics perspective. *Nursing Ethics*, 1–10. Published online 6 June 2011. DOI: 10.1177/0969733011406767

Latimer, J. 2000. *The conduct of care: Understanding nursing practice*. Cornwall, UK: Blackwell Science.

Liaschenko, J. 1995. Ethics in the work of acting for patients. *Advances in Nursing Science, 18* (2), 1–12.

Liaschenko, J. 1997a. Knowing the patient? In S.E. Thorne and V.E. Hayes (Eds.), *Nursing praxis: Knowledge and action* (pp. 23–38). Thousand Oaks, CA: Sage.

Liaschenko, J. 1997b. Ethics and the geography of the nurse-patient relationship: Spatial vulnerabilities and gendered space. *Scholarly Inquiry for Nursing Practice: An International Journal, 11* (1), 45–59.

Liaschenko, J. 1998. The shift from the closed to the open body—ramifications for nursing testimony. In S.D. Edwards (Ed.), *Philosophical issues in nursing* (pp. 1–16). London: Macmillan.

Liaschenko, J. 2008. ". . . to take one's place . . . and the right to have one's part matter." In W. Pinch and A. Haddad (Eds.), *Nursing and health care ethics: A legacy and a vision* (pp. 195–202). Washington, DC: American Nurses Association Press.

Liaschenko, J. and Fisher, A. 1999. Theorizing the knowledge that nurses use in the conduct of their work. *Scholarly Inquiry for Nursing Practice: An International Journal, 13* (1), 29–41.

Liaschenko, J. and Peter, E. 2003. Feminist ethics. In V. Tschudin (Ed.), *Ethics in nursing: Issues in advanced practice*. Oxford: Butterworth Heinemann.

Lützén, K., and Schreiber, R. 1998. Moral survival in a non-therapeutic environment. *Issues in Mental Health Nursing, 19* (4), 303–315.

Mackenzie, C. and Stoljar. N. (Eds.), 2000a. *Relational autonomy: Feminist perspectives on autonomy, agency and the social self.* New York: Oxford University Press.

Mackenzie, C. and Stoljar. N. 2000b. Autonomy refigured. In C. Mackenzie and N. Stoljar. (Eds.), *Relational autonomy: Feminist perspectives on autonomy, agency and the social self* (pp. 3–31). New York: Oxford University Press.

MacPherson, K.I. 1991. Looking at caring and nursing through a feminist lens. In R.M. Neil and R. Watts (Eds.), *Caring and nursing: Explorations in feminist perspectives* (pp. 25–42). New York: National League for Nursing.

Manias, E. and Street, A. 2001. The interplay of knowledge and decision making between nurses and doctors in critical care. *International Journal of Nursing Studies, 38,* 129–140.

McCarthy, J. and Deady, R. 2008. Moral distress reconsidered. *Nursing Ethics, 15* (2), 254–262.

McGee, G. 2003. Preface to the second edition. In G. McGee (Ed.), *Pragmatic bioethics* (pp. xi–xvi). Cambridge: MIT Press.

MacPherson, K.I. 1991. Looking at caring and nursing through a feminist lens. In R.M. Neil and R. Watts (Eds.), *Caring and nursing: Explorations in feminist perspectives* (pp. 25–42). New York: National League for Nursing.

McPherson, G. 2007. *Children's participation in chronic illness decision-making: An interpretive description.* Unpublished doctoral dissertation, University of British Columbia School of Nursing, Vancouver, BC. (UMI No. 304706376)

Mitchell, G.J. 2001. Policy, procedure and routine: Matters of moral influence. *Nursing Science Quarterly, 14* (2), 109–114.

Mitton, C., Peacock, S., Storch, J., Smith, N., and Cornelissen, E. 2011. Moral distress among health system managers: Exploratory research in two British Columbia health authorities. *Health Care Analysis, 19,* 107–121.

Murray, J.S. 2010. Moral courage in healthcare: Acting ethically even in the presence of risk. *Online Journal of Issues in Nursing* 15(3): 1 DOI:10.3912/OJIN.Vol15No03Man02

Musto, L.C. 2010. *Doing the best I can do: Moral distress in adolescent mental health nursing.* Unpublished masters thesis, University of Victoria School of Nursing, Faculty of Human and Social Development. Victoria, BC.

Nortvedt, P. 2001. Clinical sensitivity: The inseparability of ethical perceptiveness and clinical knowledge. *Scholarly Inquiry of Nursing Practice, 15* (3), 1–19.

Nortvedt, P. 2004. Emotions and ethics. In J. Storch, P. Rodney, and R. Starzomski (Eds.), *Toward a moral horizon: Nursing ethics for leadership and practice* (pp. 447–464). Toronto: Pearson-Prentice Hall.

Oberle, K. and Raffin Bouchal, S. 2009. *Ethics in Canadian nursing practice: Navigating the journey.* Toronto: Pearson-Prentice Hall.

Pauly, B.M., Storch, J.L., and Varcoe, C. 2010. *Final report: Moral distress in health care symposium.* (Unpublished report to the Canadian Institutes of Health Research, University of Victoria, and University of British Columbia). Victoria, BC: Authors.

Pauly, B., Varcoe, C., Storch, J.L., and Newton, L. 2009. Registered nurses' perceptions of moral distress and ethical climate. *Nursing Ethics, 16* (5), 561–573.

Pask, E.J. 2005. Self-sacrifice, self-transcendence and nurses' professional self. *Nursing Philosophy, 6,* 247–254.

Pavlish, C., Brown-Saltzman, K., Hersh, M., Shirk, M., and Nudelman, O. 2011. Early indicators and risk factors for ethical issues in clinical practice. *Journal of Nursing Scholarship, 43* (1), 13–21.

Peter, E. 2011. Discourse: Fostering social justice: The possibility of a socially connected model of moral agency. *Canadian Journal of Nursing Research, 43* (2), 11–17.

Peter, E. and Liaschenko, J. 2004. Perils of proximity: A spatio-temporal analysis of moral distress and moral ambiguity. *Nursing Inquiry, 11* (4), 218–225.

Peter, E. and Morgan, K.P. 2001. Exploration of a trust approach for nursing ethics. *Nursing Inquiry, 8* (3), 3–10.

Raines, M.L. 2000. Ethical decision making in nurses: Relationships among moral reasoning, coping style, and ethics stress. *JONA's Healthcare Law, Ethics, and Regulation, 2* (1), 29–41.

Rodney, P.A. 1997. *Towards connectedness and trust: Nurses' enactment of their moral agency within an organizational context.* Unpublished doctoral dissertation. University of British Columbia, Vancouver, BC.

Rodney, P., Doane, G.H., Storch, J., and Varcoe, C. 2006. Workplaces: Toward a safer moral climate. *Canadian Nurse, 102* (8), 24–27.

Rodney, P. and Varcoe, C. (in press). Constrained agency: The social structure of nurses' work. In F. Baylis, J. Downie, B. Hoffmaster, and S. Sherwin (Eds.), *Health care ethics in Canada* (3rd ed.). Toronto: Nelson. (Revised version of Varcoe C. and Rodney P. 2009. Constrained agency: the social structure of nurses' work. In Bolaria, B.S., Dickinson, H.D., [Eds.], *Health, illness, and health care in Canada* [4th ed.; pp. 122–151]. Toronto: Nelson Education.)

Rushton, C. 2006. Defining and addressing moral distress: Tools for critical care nursing leaders. *AACN Advanced Critical Care, 17* (2), 161–168.

Sanders, K., Pattison, S., and Hurwitz, B. 2011. Tracking shame and humiliation in accident and emergency. *Nursing Philosophy, 12,* 83–93.

Serrano, E., Martin, L.A., and Rodney, P. 2011. *Final report: Building a moral community for collaborative practice in ambulatory oncology care: Toward improved patient/family and team outcomes.* (Unpublished report to the Canadian Nurses Foundation and the British Columbia Cancer Agency). Vancouver, BC: Authors.

Sewell, W.H. 1992. A theory of structure: Duality, agency, and transformation. *American Journal of Sociology 98* (1), 1–29.

Sher, G. 1987. The nature of moral virtue: Aristotle. In G. Sher (Ed.), *Moral philosophy: Selected readings* (p. 67). San Diego: Harcourt Brace.

Sherwin, S. 1992. Feminist and medical ethics: Two different approaches to contextual ethics. In H.B. Holmes and L.M. Purdy (Eds.), *Feminist perspectives in medical ethics* (pp. 17–31). Bloomington, IN: Indiana University Press.

Sherwin, S. 1998. A relational approach to autonomy in health care. In S. Sherwin and the Feminist Health Care Ethics Research Network (Eds.), *The politics of women's health* (pp. 19–47). Philadelphia: Temple University Press.

Sherwin, S. 2011. Looking backwards, looking forward: Hopes for bioethics' next twenty-five years. *Bioethics, 25* (2), 75–82.

Smith, K.V. and Godfrey, N.S. 2002. Being a good nurse and doing the right thing: A qualitative study. *Nursing Ethics, 9* (3), 301–312.

Stein-Parbury, J. and Liaschenko, J. 2007. Understanding collaboration between nurses and physicians as knowledge at work. *American Journal of Critical Care, 16* (5), 470–77.

Storch, J.L. 2005. Patient safety: Is it just another bandwagon? *Canadian Journal of Nursing Leadership, 18* (2), 39–55.

Storch, J., Rodney, P., Pauly, B., Fulton, T., Stevenson, L., Newton, L., and Makaroff, K.S. (2009a). Enhancing ethical climates in nursing work environments. *Canadian Nurse, 105* (3), 20–25.

Storch, J., Rodney, P., Varcoe, C., Pauly, B., Starzomski, R., Stevenson, L. et al. 2009b. Leadership for ethical policy and practice (LEPP): Participatory action project. *Canadian Journal of Nursing Leadership, 22* (3), 68–80.

Taylor, C. 1989. *The sources of the self: The making of the modern identity.* Cambridge, MA: Harvard University Press.

Taylor, C. (with A. Gutmann, S.C. Rockefeller, M. Walzer, and S. Wolf) 1992. *Multiculturalism and "The politics of recognition."* Princeton: Princeton University Press.

Taylor, C. 1995. *Philosophical arguments.* Cambridge, MA: Harvard University Press.

Taylor, C.R. 1997. Everyday nursing concerns: Unique? Trivial? Or essential to health care ethics? *HealthCare Ethics Committee Forum, 9* (1), 68–84.

Ulrich, C.M., Hamric, A.B., and Grady, C. 2010. Moral distress: A growing problem in the health professions? *Hastings Center Report, 40*(1), 20–22.

Varcoe, C. 2001. Abuse obscured: An ethnographic account of emergency unit nursing practice in relation to violence against women. *Canadian Journal of Nursing Research, 32* (4), 95–115.

Varcoe, C. and Einboden, R. 2010. Family violence and ethics. In J. Humphreys and J.C. Campbell (Eds.), *Family Violence and Nursing Practice* (2nd ed.; pp. 381–410). New York: Springer.

Varcoe, C., Rodney, P., and McCormick, J. 2003. Health care relationships in context: An analysis of three ethnographies. *Qualitative Health Research, 13* (7), 957–973.

Walker, M. U. 2003. *Moral contexts.* Lantham, MD: Rowman & Littlefield.

Webster, G.C. and Baylis, F.E. 2000. Moral residue. In S.B. Rubin and L. Zoloth, (Eds.), *Margin of error: The ethics of mistakes in the practice of medicine* (pp. 217–230). Hagerstown, MD: University Publishing Group.

Wiskow, C., Albreht, T., and de Pietro, C. 2010. *Policy brief 15: How to create an attractive and supportive environment for health professionals.* Copenhagen, DK: World Health Organization.

Yarling, R. and McElmurray, B. 1986. The moral foundation of nursing. *Advances in Nursing Science, 8* (2), 63–73.

Yeo, M., Rodney, P., Khan, P., and Moorhouse, A. 2010. Integrity. In M. Yeo, A. Moorhouse, P. Khan, and P. Rodney (Eds.), *Concepts and cases in nursing ethics* (3rd ed.; pp.349–367). Peterborough, ON: Broadview Press.

Young, I.M. 2011. *Responsibility for justice.* New York: Oxford University Press.

CHAPTER 10

The Moral Climate of Nursing Practice: Inquiry and Action

Patricia Rodney, Barbara Buckley, Annette Street, Elena Serrano, and Lee Ann Martin

Over time, nursing research has consistently raised concerns about the quality of nurses' workplaces, and those concerns are escalating as this chapter goes to press. Researcher Marie Campbell offered a warning in 1987 about nurse staffing that is even truer today:

Recommended as a rational method of improving nurse productivity, I argue that objective needs assessment and staffing procedures result in decisions that are neither as rational as they seem nor more trustworthy than those made on nurses' judgement alone. The objective decisions do, however, mean that nursing-care time can be limited and nurses' work intensified. Such outcomes add stress to nurses' working conditions that, combined with reductions in the scope and level of services able to be offered under new time constraints, threaten the quality of care for hospital patients. (Campbell 1987, 463)

The economic, political, and social contexts of Western health care delivery have undergone rapid and often devastating changes in the more than two decades that have elapsed since Campbell's warning. In Canada and other Western countries, this has led to an era in which there is a widely held assumption that actions to save money in health care and other social services are inherently justifiable. Efficiency considerations have come to trump considerations of quality of care in the implementation of a great deal of health and health care policy (Stein 2001).[1] Thus, patients, families, and communities are experiencing increasing difficulty accessing services appropriate for their needs, and the impact on health care providers—especially nurses—has been close to catastrophic.[2] While our focus in this chapter is on Canada and other Western countries, we would like to note that concerns about the quality of health care workplaces are also a global concern.[3]

MORAL CLIMATE CHANGE

What we take the above to mean is that the phenomenon of climate change has not been limited to global weather patterns—it is also present within the Canadian health care system as a *moral climate change*.[4] Moral climate can be defined as, "the implicit and explicit values that drive health-care delivery and shape the workplaces in which care is delivered" (Rodney et al. 2006, 24; see also Canadian Nurses Association 2008).[5] As we argue in Chapters 9 and 11 of this book, the current health care climate in Canada has presented significant impediments to nurses' abilities to enact their moral agency. The moral climate change over the past two decades and more within health care has negatively impacted nurses, patients, families, and communities because of deteriorations of care within the health care setting. Health care restructuring[6] has resulted in routinized efficiency-driven patient care, deskilling, casualization of nurses, and patient care goals being subordinate to institutional goals. This has created significant—and escalating—moral angst in the nursing profession (Beagan and Ells 2007; Daiski 2004; Pauly et al. 2009; Sanders, Pattison, and Hurwitz 2011; Rodney and Varcoe in press). Nursing is certainly not the only health care profession experiencing such moral angst, which is a point we will return to in addressing solutions. Nor is nursing always an innocent bystander—we have at times also contributed to an over-emphasis on efficiency by remaining silent or actively pursuing efficiency goals at the expense of the well-being of our patients, their families and communities, and our colleagues in nursing and other health care provider groups (Rodney and Varcoe, in press).

Restructuring is an instrument of *corporatism*. The broad philosophical concept of corporatism can be considered as, "an alternative model for civilization" (Saul 1995, xi). According to Saul, corporatism "encourages a society of form over content; management over leadership; of self-interest being rewarded while ethics are marginalized, and decisions being made as part of a narrow linear process, as against broader, more inclusive, even lateral, ways of thinking and acting" (xii). Corporatism is a manifestation of the malaise of modernity (which we explore in Chapter 18 of this book). It has created an environment destructive to morale, it is blamed for nurse shortages, and it has been linked to the creation of moral distress and moral residue in the research literature.[7]

Our Premises

In this chapter it is our intent to discuss some of the implications of contemporary policy shifts for nursing, particularly in terms of the moral climate of nursing practice. It is also our intent to point toward directions nursing can take—and is beginning to take—to improve that moral climate. Let us start by laying out some of our premises.[8] *First, we assume that changes in health care policy per se are not necessarily problematic.* Indeed, the changes are usually driven by positive goals such as making health care delivery more patient-centred, reducing over-treatment, and having more input from regions and communities about what they need. A number of policy initiatives have been beneficial, including, for example, health prevention initiatives such as smoking cessation programs and improved primary, secondary, and tertiary care through initiatives such as chronic disease management programs. However, as we explain in this chapter, our primary concern is that the *processes* by which changes are planned, the processes by which changes are implemented, and the lack of systematic evaluation of the effects of the changes are problematic. A corporate ethos has infused health care policy processes, with resultant power inequities that have generated a number of unintended negative consequences.[9] Second*, we assume that power inequities in contemporary health care policy processes are interfering with nurses' abilities to provide good quality patient/family/community care.* As we indicated in Chapter 9, we see these power inequities as constraints to nurses' enactment of their moral agency—constraints that nurses themselves sometimes internalize and inadvertently perpetuate. Third*, we assume that nurses' difficulties providing good quality care constitute a serious ethical problem.* Providing quality care to patients, families, and communities is an important ethical good—important because it underpins the entire health care enterprise. Therefore, facilitating nurses' abilities to provide care in a manner that is respectful to the nurses themselves and to the values of the nursing profession is also an important ethical good—instrumentally important because it also supports the ethical practice of other health care providers and ultimately helps to promote the health and well-being of the public. In this chapter we will therefore profile some research data warning what happens to the health and well-being of the public when nurses are unable to provide quality care. Fourth, *it is our premise that in addressing our own moral climate in nursing we ought to join and share leadership with our colleagues in other health care professions.*

In expanding on our premises we commence with illustrations of relevant nursing research examples from Canada and other countries. This will lead us to a reflection on the impact of Western economic, political, and social changes on health care delivery, and particularly on nursing practice. Following this we will link power inequities in health care policy processes to the moral climate of nursing practice. In concluding, we will posit a number of strategies that can help to improve that climate, including what we have learned from our own programs of participatory action research. We will also point to areas for future nursing inquiry.

Inquiry into the Moral Climate of Nursing Practice

Early nursing ethics research tended to focus on naming ethical issues and on understanding nurses' patterns of moral reasoning (Rodney 1997). Thus, as Chapter 9 on nurses' moral agency pointed out, our understanding of the complex socio-political contexts in which nurses and other health care providers enact their moral agency is relatively recent. Our profession now has a burgeoning body of research on the serious challenges to nurses' workplaces arising from the socio-political contexts in which we practice—including some of nursing's strengths in negotiating these contexts. We will highlight some relevant nursing research here and then reflect on the implications for the moral climate of nursing practice.

Starting with a Metaphor: Moral Winter

A growing body of Canadian and other Western research tells us that restructuring, a lack of human and structural resources, altered work environments, increased patient acuity with offloading of care to families, and the uncritical adoption of a rigid corporate business ethos in the Canadian health care system have created a significant level of moral chaos in the nursing profession (Austin 2007; Austin 2011; Rodney and Varcoe in press; Rudge 2011; Walston, Lazes, and Garcia Sullivan 2004; Zboril-Benson 2007). The prevalence of this moral chaos within the practice of nursing has, we believe, led to a *moral winter* (Buckley 2007) for the profession. According to our co-author Buckley (2007), the metaphor of moral winter speaks to a moral landscape of nursing practice that has become frozen, lying dormant and buried beneath layers of contextual constraints. When nurses see themselves as unable to stop moral wrongdoing they themselves have become frozen, and when substandard practice becomes normalized such that deteriorations in practice standards are not overtly challenged, a moral winter has arrived.[10] As we show later in this chapter, current nursing practice environments continue to show signs of moral climate change from ongoing restructuring and health care reform initiatives. Overtly unethical behaviours that result have been chronicled as including misuse of power by coercion or force; withholding care; failure to document medication errors or falsifying documentation to cover errors; and performing inappropriate procedures (Garon 2006). However, we also believe that a moral winter holds the promise of spring (Buckley 2007), which we will say more about later in this chapter when we talk about our action research.

To further illustrate, in a study that one of us (Rodney) was engaged in, a research team undertook a qualitative study of the meaning of ethics for nurses providing direct care, for nurses in advanced practice positions in nursing, and for students in nursing (Rodney et al. 2002; Storch et al. 2002; Varcoe et al. 2004).[11] Our research team was also interested in how these three groups of nurses/student nurses described their enactment of ethical practice. Our findings included insights about how the organizational context influenced nurses' abilities to uphold the ethics of their practice—that is, their ability to work toward a moral horizon (Rodney et al. 2002).[12] Throughout our study, nurses in every practice context identified their practice as frequently constrained—and, fortunately, also assisted—by influences outside of their immediate control. In subsequent research in a medical oncology unit and a busy emergency department we witnessed similar issues (Rodney et al. 2006; Rodney and Varcoe in press) that are reflective of a moral winter. Ethics in Practice 10-1 provides a sample of a focus group interview with nurses practising on an acute medical unit, which is representative of our findings in our overall program of research. The nurses are discussing end-of-life care.

ETHICS IN PRACTICE 10-1

On the Medical Unit

First Medical Unit Nurse: . . . [I]n the last few cases . . . I said [to the doctor], "Well, they've got a hospital bed now, they're not going to get a hospice bed, that's the way the system works." . . . And in a very rare case, the squeaky wheel does get greased and they get a hospice bed, but it's a very rare case. Those two [patients waiting for a hospice bed] that we had both died on the ward, waiting and wanting to go to hospice. I'm not saying that we didn't make them comfortable. Because we do a lot of hospice care on our floor, just like they do in [the hospice]. But you know, they [the patients] really, in their mind, they'd gone through the hospice program, they got the [information], they wanted to die in hospice, they had the tour, that's where they wanted to spend their last days and they couldn't do that because somewhere in the communication, they ended up getting sent to the hospital.

Second Medical Unit Nurse: I think everyone's so busy, that everyone's running around. And that's why it's too bad there's not one person on the unit looking over all of it. I think that would be wonderful. I don't know, I think things would run so much smoother . . . because from casual nurse to part-time to full-time . . . you're not as familiar as you would like to be. But if there was one designated person on the unit that could oversee that . . .

Third Medical Unit Nurse: There used to be the head nurse to do all the discharge planning. . . .

First Medical Unit Nurse: There's nothing more frustrating, and we've all done it, it's going in to see a patient in the morning and they say, "Okay, I'm supposed to see L," or whoever [the] social worker happens to be that day, "at 2:15 today and meet with so-and-so." And you have no clue. Let alone why. . . . And so then they [the patient] think, "Oh, this one's stupid."

Second Medical Unit Nurse: Yeah, I often sometimes feel very stupid. Like in the last two days that it's been so busy on the unit. I don't know their names and I don't know their diagnosis.

First Medical Unit Nurse: All of a sudden they become a bed: "[Bed 4] and he wants . . . " I know . . . I think a lot of that has to do with the fact that there's so much going on. And we try, I mean we make these new forms . . . and here's a new discharge planning form and a new form for this and that's fine, it might put everything together, but unless we use them and have the time to use them, they're useless (Storch et al. 2001).

In Ethics in Practice 10-1, the medical unit nurses were trying to navigate to a place where they could offer their patients meaningful choices in end-of-life care and help to coordinate activities with other colleagues (such as social workers)—the kind of ethical practice that we advocate in Chapter 13 and Chapter 17 and other chapters of this book (see also Stajduhar 2011). However, the corporate ethos meant that nurses' time to communicate or plan was not valued, and they were required to care for as many patients as they could as quickly as possible. Thus, the corporate emphasis on efficiency trumped considerations of patient/family well-being, interdisciplinary team cohesion, or nurse satisfaction. Time for quality nursing care became a prized and contested commodity (Rodney et al. 2002; Rodney and Varcoe in press). In the transcript above, for instance, the paperwork required to implement a new discharge planning process was felt to be too time-consuming to implement, especially in the absence of unit-based nursing leadership. The consequences of not being able to move toward a moral horizon were more than just dissatisfaction. The nurses felt exhausted and demoralized ("stupid"), which they spoke of more as the focus group interview progressed. We have heard similar kinds of concerns echoed in every focus group with nurses (and more recently other health care providers) involved in direct care that our team has done over several years of research.[13]

Fortunately, in Ethics in Practice 10-1 there were also situations in which the prevailing currents facilitated nurses' attempts to navigate toward a moral horizon (Rodney et al. 2002). Supportive colleagues in nursing and other disciplines were a major positive influence, as were professional guidelines and standards and access to ethics education. While our initial focus in this chapter is primarily the problems that nurses encounter, understanding such assets is also important.

The impact of the constrained organizational context on patients, families, and communities is significant, and the evidence we do have indicates that it is profound. For example, in an ethnographic study with 60 patients and 56 health care professionals in a large teaching hospital in a major Canadian city, nurses found "difficulties in ensuring patients' basic care needs were met," particularly "when care needs of patients changed unexpectedly, when new care needs arose, when patients did not follow the 'usual' progression of recovery or when they had needs that had not been considered" (Lynam et al. 2003, 123). Furthermore, researchers noticed that while patients generally expressed satisfaction with the care they received in hospital, rapid discharge from hospital left many of them vulnerable when they returned home. Patients and families were not prepared, there were often inadequate resources in the home, and the families were not sure whom to call if they ran into difficulty. Families who did not speak English and who were not well off economically were especially vulnerable (Lynam et al. 2003; see also Anderson et al. 2010). Another researcher (Stajduhar 2003) raised similar concerns about the impact on patients and families in an ethnographic study of home-based palliative caregiving (with 12 dying patients, 13 family members, and 47 caregivers as well as 28 health care providers and 10 administrators). She warned that "restructuring of home support resulted in some caregivers losing familiar home support workers they trusted" and that "policy changes to accommodate provincial standards for home support resulted in reduced numbers of subsidized home support hours for families" (31). Stajduhar shed light on a chilling picture in the following interview segment from a retired woman on a small pension:

> I was told that if he wasn't dead before November 1st that I wouldn't have any more support hours left . . . If he's not dead before November 1st, I don't know what I'll do. (Stajduhar 2003, 31)

Such challenges in the quality of care that patients receive and erosions in the conditions of nurses' work are continuing (Rodney and Varcoe in press). As we will expand on later in this chapter, *poor work climates are linked in the nursing literature to nurse illness and attrition, burnout, poor patient care practices, and growing patient safety challenges* (Canadian Nurses Association and Registered Nurses Association of Ontario 2010; Laschinger and Leiter 2006; Mallidou, Cummings, Estabrooks and Giovanetti 2011; Wynne 2003). Further, inequities in access to care for patients, families, and communities are continuing to widen, especially for groups that have been marginalized in our society (Anderson et al. 2009; Health Council of Canada 2008). For instance, in their study of the experiences of access to primary care services from the perspective of Aboriginal people seeking care at an emergency department in a large Canadian city, Browne et al. (2011) collected data over 20 months of participant observation and in-depth interviews with 44 patients who were triaged as stable and non-urgent. Their research findings indicated that in addition to having difficulty with providers' stereotyped assumptions about them, patients frequently had chronic pain that was poorly treated. The patients' difficulties in accessing adequate health care was confounded by poverty, racialization, and other forms of disadvantage.

What policy processes have led to the kinds of problems for nurses, patients, and families we have illustrated above?[14] The nurses in Ethics in Practice 10-1 also spoke of the absence of nursing leadership on their unit, which is a common occurrence in today's health care environments (Canadian Nursing Association 2010; MacPhee et al. 2010). Gaudine and Beaton (2002) focused on ethical practice and leadership in their qualitative study of 15 nurse managers in an eastern Canadian province. Their findings add a disturbing overlay to the concerns expressed in the other studies we have cited so far.[15] The authors articulated four themes of ethical conflict arising between nurse managers and their organizations, including voicelessness, where to spend the money, rights of individuals versus needs of the organization, and unjust practices on the part of senior administration and/or the organization (Gaudine and Beaton 2002). Significantly, the theme of voicelessness was identified in every interview. It reflected a widespread sense of powerlessness on the part of the nurse managers. Ethics in Practice 10-2 provides a transcript quotation from one of the nurse managers.

ETHICS IN PRACTICE 10-2

The Manager

There doesn't seem to be knowledge [by senior administration] with regards to why we need nursing, why we need to have a good float pool, why we need to have permanent staff versus casual staff . . . The bottom line is always the dollar and the cents and I keep going back saying, "Well, you know, this is a business, but it's a health care business, and when you forget that you have forgotten why we're here." And of course everybody looks at me like I'm from another planet . . . I really don't think that they want to get it (Gaudine and Beaton 2002, 23).

Given that supportive nursing leadership is prerequisite to a safe and competent workplace (Canadian Nurses Association and Registered Nurses Association of Ontario 2010; Health Canada Office of Nursing Policy 2001; Health Canada 2002; Storch 2010), the absence and/or demoralization of nurse leaders portrayed in Ethics in Practice 10-1 and Ethics in Practice 10-2 (and also portrayed or implied in most of the other studies we have cited thus far) is a major concern (see also McCutcheon et al. 2009). In fact, Gaudine and Beaton's (2002) entire study is a graphic portrayal of the power inequities inherent in the corporate ethos that has come to dominate health care delivery. Nurses' voices are apparently not heard in the planning, implementation, or evaluation of health care policy—and this has been a problem for some time now across Canada.

Ethics in Practice 10-2 is a bleak contrast to the finding almost 30 years ago from research with "magnet hospitals" in the United States, where:

> Nursing . . . has a voice at the top decision-making level of the hospital, and there is a perception that others at that same level fully understand and value the contribution that the profession makes not only to patient care but also to the institution's reputation in the community. (McClure et al. 1983, 85)

What happened? Our colleagues in the United States have certainly been experiencing similar erosion and demoralization of nursing leadership (and attendant problems for nurses, patients, and families) that we have in Canada in the almost three decades since McClure et al. published their findings. Understanding the values shifts that have created such problems requires stepping back to do a broader analysis of Western health care. In other words, the policy and power shifts that have hit Canadian nurses are shared across national borders.

Revisiting International Research on Nurses' Workplaces

Thus far, the research we have cited from Canada portrays significant constraints and power inequities in the organizational contexts within which nurses work, and raises worrisome questions about the negative impacts on patients, families, and communities. Over the past two decades nurses in Australia, the United Kingdom, the United States and other countries have provided research evidence of similar problems (e.g., Auditor General Victoria 2002; Heath 2002; Rudge 2011; Sanders et al. 2011; Weiss et al. 2002).

There is an important body of international research that added other relevant insights. This international research looked at the quality of nurses' work environments and the impact of those environments on nurses and the patients they serve. Although not conceptualized in moral or ethical terms, the research had a great deal to say about the moral climate of nurses' work.

In 1998, an international team of investigators led by Dr. Linda Aiken from the United States launched a program of research to better understand the impact of health care restructuring on the nursing workforce and patient outcomes. There were seven sites in the research program, including Pennsylvania in the United States; British Columbia, Alberta, and Ontario in Canada; Scotland and England in the United Kingdom; and Germany in the European Union (Clarke at al. 2001, 51). The conceptual framework of Aiken et al.'s research was based on the earlier research with magnet hospitals that we mentioned above. The findings were consistent and alarming. They revealed that the cost constraint measures that swept through Western health care in the late 1980s and early 1990s—which include rapid restructuring with limited nursing input, increased registered nurse/patient ratios, casualization of the nursing workforce, loss of nurse leaders, and limited continuing education opportunities—harmed patients as well as nurses. *More specifically, the results showed increased morbidity and mortality of patients (including "failure to rescue" or failure to stop a preventable complication), reduced patient satisfaction, reduced nurse satisfaction, skyrocketing nurse illness and injury, and widespread nurse attrition* (Aiken, Clarke, and Sloane 2000; Aiken et al. 2002; Clarke et al. 2001; Dunleavy, Shamian, and Thomson 2003; Estabrooks et al. 2005; Shamian et al. 2002).

There was a period of positive progress following the research program led by Aiken and her colleagues—for instance, through the creation of new nurse leadership positions and through better support programs for new nursing graduates. Unfortunately, as this revised chapter goes to press we are in another wave of escalating cost constraints in Canada that have followed the 2008 and apparently ongoing recession (Canadian Nurses Association 2009; Canadian Nurses Association and Registered Nurses Association of Ontario 2010; Pringle 2009; Rodney and Varcoe in press). One of the major impacts is "substituting practical nurses and non-regulated workers for RNs" in "'new care models'" (Pringle 2009, 14). In British Columbia, according to the British Columbia Nurses Union (BCNU) health care cuts in B.C. have resulted in the widespread replacement of registered nurses (RNs) with licensed practical nurses (LPNs) for case manager positions, public health immunization clinics, detoxification services, and senior care facilities (BCNU 2011).

Perhaps one of the most significant insights from the program of research done by Aiken and her colleagues was their observation that *so little* research had been done in the planning or evaluation of the reforms that swept through health care in the 1990s. Aiken and her colleagues warned:

> What we know about changes in organization and structure and the potential for those changes to affect patient outcomes pales by comparison to what we do not know. However, this is itself an important finding: we are subjecting hundreds of thousands of very sick patients to the unknown consequences of organizational reforms that have not been sufficiently evaluated before their widespread adoption. (Aiken, Clarke, and Sloane 2000, 463).

This remains true today. In fact, in our current Canadian context, *Canadian Journal of Nursing Leadership* editor-in-chief Dr. Dorothy Pringle (2009) warns that:

> In the mid-1990s we had little research on the effects on patient outcomes of varying proportions of RNs versus practical nurses and unregulated health workers. We have much more now, and hospitals ignore it at their peril. (14)

Pringle goes on to say that to "ignore the evidence of the effect of high ratios of RN staffing on patient care is administrative malpractice and should be acknowledged as such" (15). *Yet we are currently practicing in a health care system where there is alarmingly little evaluative follow up of the impact of past and current cost constraint measures for patients, families, communities, nurses, other health care providers, and the health care system as a whole.*

Implications for the Moral Climate of Nursing Practice

While the international research by Aiken and her colleagues on nurses' workplaces and Pringle's current warning did not include an explicit moral or ethical analysis, they do inform value-based inquiry. That is, they tell us about problems in the moral climate for nursing practice that make it difficult for nurses to enact their moral agency. As we indicated at the outset of this chapter, by "moral climate," we mean the implicit and explicit values inherent in nurses' workplaces. Those values operate at individual, organizational, and societal levels, and affect the structural and interpersonal resources available for nursing practice.

It is important to note that the constraints nurses experience in accessing structural and interpersonal resources are not just external features of the environment, but are also part of the culture of the organizational context in which they practice. As is identified in Chapters 5 and 13, culture is more than just ethnicity. It permeates health care delivery and influences implicit and explicit values. The longstanding disempowerment of nurses as a cultural group within health care is remarkable, given the extent of our professional responsibilities and the importance of nursing care for patient well-being (Chambliss 1996; Jameton 1990; Liaschenko 1993; Picard 2000; Street 1992; Storch 2010). For instance, in Ethics in Practice 10-1, it was taken for granted that the nurses would work largely without the benefit of access to other members of the health care team (e.g., social workers) because of the lack of mechanisms such as regular interdisciplinary rounds. Such rounds were not a part of the culture of the unit they worked on, whereas dying patients in the culture of a palliative care unit would have had access to an interdisciplinary team that met regularly (see also Stajduhar 2011). The reason for the difference was not patient needs—the patient needs were often equivalent in both places. The resultant sense of powerlessness of the nurses on the so-called non-specialty (medical) unit is not new. But coupled with erosions in staffing, loss of nursing leadership, and high turnover, it has certainly become more problematic. *In other words, longstanding cultural problems in health care delivery have been exacerbated by the current corporate ethos with its own set of power inequities.*

Our illustrations of ethical research from Canada and workplace studies from international research indicate that problems with the moral climate for nursing practice have become endemic in Western health care, and that we are only beginning to grasp their consequences. While our illustrations are drawn from a limited number of studies, they are by no means idiosyncratic. As we have shown, similar findings of situational constraints interfering with nurses' ability to practice according to the ethical standards of their practice are increasingly evident in the research literature throughout Western health care. This is not to say that the *only* constraints nurses face enacting their moral agency are external and out of their control. As we have indicated earlier in this chapter and in Chapter 9, nurses are sometimes complicit in reinforcing situational constraints (e.g., by undermining their colleagues' attempts to provide emotional support to patients), and they sometimes engage in unjust rationing of their care (e.g., because of judgments that a patient is not worthy) (see also Chapters 8, 9, and 21). But it is to say that the moral climate to support nursing practice has—notwithstanding some periods of positive progress—deteriorated significantly over the past two decades and more. Unfortunately, as we write this revised chapter in 2011, Pringle's (2009) warning above tells us (and we have witnessed) that after a period of some warming the moral winter in Canada has been getting colder.

Nurses experience moral distress when they find themselves in situations where they know what the right thing to do is but where institutional constraints and their own internal and interpersonal conflicts make it difficult to follow through (Austin 2007; Corley et al. 2005; Hamric and Blackhall 2007; Jameton 1984; Pauly et al. 2009). Moral distress is a pervasive problem that can cause unwanted moral residue for nurses and impact the quality of care they provide (Webster and Baylis 2000; see also Chapter 9).

Nursing's historical position as a (primarily) women's occupation in a gender-biased culture has rendered it vulnerable to the economic forces sweeping through health care. And our history of difficulties with nurse–physician collaboration has not helped.[16] Because nurses are the most numerous professionals and are the professionals who are most consistently present with the recipients of health care, their ability to practice ethically has a profound effect on the health and well-being of patients/ clients, families, and communities. And their ability to practice ethically has a profound effect on the functioning of the entire health care team. Clearly, any deterioration in the quality of nursing and health care received by the recipients of health care is of concern. What is also of concern is the impact on nurses as professionals and as human beings.

Thus, nurses, as well as other health care providers, administrators, and policy-makers need to strive for a more ethical work environment. The ideology that health care is a commodity, in which nurses are discussed in terms of scarcity and supply, must be challenged (Austin 2011; Rodney and Varcoe in press; Rudge 2011). Right now a significant proportion of nurses are trying to provide ethical care to patients in an under-resourced, severely strained, and poorly managed health care system. Moreover, nurses are trying to maintain their moral integrity in environments that are becoming increasingly characterized by conflict and disagreement (Centre for American Nurses 2008; Johnstone 2002).

We turn now to some ideas about how a more positive moral climate can be fostered—and defended where it currently exists. This is relatively new and important territory for nursing inquiry. While we now have extensive documentation of problems in the moral climate of nursing practice, we do not yet have a great deal of research about *how* to deal with those problems.

TAKING ACTION TO IMPROVE THE MORAL CLIMATE OF NURSING PRACTICE

Fostering Moral Communities

Perhaps the first step to improve the moral climate for nursing practice (and, hence, for health care delivery overall) is to *name* it as a goal. That is, "we want, as participants in institutional culture, to be able to notice our moral problems and to cope with them with sensitivity and integrity and to keep our health care institutions responsive to their moral goals" (Jameton 1990, 450). Thinking of ourselves as members of a moral community is a way of linking the goal to action. As one nurse ethicist has explained:

> Nurses and others who contribute to delivery of nursing care should identify themselves as citizens of a moral community, a specialized community of individual moral agents with shared values and goals within the broader community of health care. (Aroskar 1995, 134)

A moral community is a place where ethical values are made explicit and shared, where ethical values direct action, and where individuals feel safe to be heard (Aroskar 1995; Canadian Nurses Association 2008; Corley and Goren 1998; Jameton 1990; Rodney et al. 2002; Storch 2010; Webster and Baylis 2000; see also Chapter 18).[17] Fostering a moral community involves organizational, political, and research-based action.

Organizational Action

It is clear that the moral climate for nursing practice has suffered from economically driven reductions in staffing and leadership and rapid, repeated changes with little nursing input. The program of research from Aiken and her colleagues tells us that "the most important hospital characteristics predictive of nurses' emotional exhaustion and [dis]satisfaction with their jobs are nurses not having control over their work environment, including not having sufficient resources, and not having effective nursing leadership" (Clarke et al. 2001, 54). They add that good nurse–physician collaboration and sufficient length of nursing experience on the hospital unit are also significant (54). *A minimal requirement for improving the moral climate for nursing practice and fostering the development of nursing as a moral community is to turn the negative characteristics around and strengthen the positive characteristics.* Thus, nurses' workplaces require better resources, including adequate staffing, regular work schedules, job security, positive interdisciplinary relationships, educational support, and available nurse leaders (Canadian Nurses Association and Registered Nurses Association of Ontario

2010; Clarke et al. 2001; Health Canada 2002; Laschinger et al. 2000; Storch 2010; Storch et al. 2002; see Exhibit 10-1 below).

EXHIBIT 10-1

Quality Workplace Attributes for Nurses

(Adapted from the Canadian Nurses Association and Canadian Federation of Nurses Unions 2006)

- Good communication and collaboration
- Consistent responsibility and accountability
- Realistic workloads

- Strong, accessible leadership
- Support for information acquisition and knowledge development
- Ongoing professional development opportunities
- Positive workplace culture

Resources will certainly help, but part of the challenge is also to tackle the taken-for-granted values that have helped to disenfranchise nurses as well as other health care providers, patients, families, and even communities. For example, the nurse managers in Ethics in Practice 10-2 also felt devalued—sometimes even by the nurses they were supposed to represent. Weiss et al. (2002) note that "besides the physical dimensions, the . . . moral dimensions of institutions can increase or decrease the likelihood that a community of practitioners, organized around common goals, will adopt the standards and visions of good practice" (115). In other words, structural organizational changes are necessary but not sufficient. *We also need to have positive values-based change if nursing is to move forward as a moral community.*

How to promote values-based change is by no means entirely clear. A starting point is to help nurses to find their moral voices (Liaschenko 1993; Rodney et al. 2002; Storch et al. 2002). Helping nurses to find their moral voices means assisting them to use the language of ethics in a way that supports the values in their practice. Ethics education for nurses (Bell and Breslin 2008; Hartrick Doane et al. 2004; Myrick 2004; Storch et al. 2009; Varcoe et al. 2004)[18] and, indeed, for *all* heath care providers (Frenk et al. 2010) is essential for this to happen. While much of this education is beginning to flourish in preparatory and graduate nursing programs, a great deal can also be done in the workplace (see Exhibit 10-2).

EXHIBIT 10-2

Educational Strategies to Promote Nurses' Moral Voices in the Workplace

Strategies from Raines (2000, 40):

1. Start a nursing ethics library and/or a nursing ethics journal club;
2. Sponsor a nursing ethics committee and/or a nursing research committee;

3. Support a nursing ethics grand round and plan for interdisciplinary participation;
4. Provide an annual ethics educational program for all staff;
5. Circulate a nursing ethics article of the month and foster related discussion;

6. Do a biannual survey of staff to assess the ethical issues they are facing;

7. Send representatives of nursing staff to other agencies to learn about their strategies; and

8. Ensure that there are nurse representatives on the agency's ethics committee and research review board (see also Chapter 13).

To this list we (the authors) would add:

9. Encourage networking between community, hospital, long-term care, and other health care agencies to share nursing ethics resources;

10. Promote discussion of nursing ethics at regional, national, and international nursing association meetings; and

11. Work to ensure that nursing has a strong presence on regional, national, and international interdisciplinary ethics bodies such as the Canadian Bioethics Society.

Political Action

Organizational resources will not be liberated, and positive value shifts will not happen, however, without political action. What do we mean by political action? Clearly, we are not just talking about lobbying local and national governments, essential though such activities are. We are talking about a notion of politics that includes individual as well as group action. "Political theory tells us what can happen when people act in concert in certain ways" (McGowan 1998, 178). Acting in concert takes place, for instance, every day at the bedside, in a client's home, in a primary school office, in a hospital administrative meeting, at a regional health board meeting, and at a nursing association conference as well as in a national government house (see also Chapter 18).

Political action should foster respect for all individuals so that they can have meaningful participation in decisions that will affect the community that they live and/or work in (Mann 1994; McGowan 1998). This means promoting a constructive dialogue that embraces diverse viewpoints—processes that equalize power and are at the heart of democracy (Chinn 2008; Mouffe 1993; see also Chapter 18). What we have presented about the moral context of nurses' practice indicates that democratic processes are not functioning all that well in health care policy construction and health care delivery throughout Western health care. The nurse manager quoted in Ethics in Practice 10-2, for example, found that rather than having her expertise valued and her perspective incorporated in senior administrative meetings, she felt as if "everybody was looking at her like she was from another planet."[19]

How can nurses engage in concerted political action? Every one of us in the profession has a role to play, and many have embarked upon significant political work throughout nursing's history. It is important to note that our codes of ethics can be political as well as ethical tools—they are based on the assumption that quality practice environments are foundational for ethical practice (Canadian Nurses Association 2008). Waving a copy of the Canadian Nurses Association's Code of Ethics at administrative meetings might not help the nurse manager in Ethics in Practice 10-2, but the knowledge that she has a professional ethical obligation to advocate for safe, competent, ethical, and compassionate care can help her to feel more confident about the validity of her moral stance. This confidence may also help her to seek support from peers, professional nursing associations, academic colleagues, and other sources.

Political action takes place at all levels of health care (see also Chapter 18). At the *macro* level of societal influence, as nurses we ought to be more proactive in challenging socio-political ideologies that disenfranchise nurses and those for whom they provide care—for instance, by hosting national and international conferences on health reform and cultivating strong media support. The current corporate ideology, with its prevalent marketplace metaphors, needs to be challenged (Rodney and Varcoe in press). As Pringle (2009) reminds us in her recent alert, our "weapon to resist a return to the 1990s is knowledge" (15), and so continuing to strengthen our academic and research strength is crucial. Fortunately, these are both areas that our profession has made significant progress in over the past two decades—our graduate programs in nursing are flourishing, and as a profession we have numerous accomplished researchers in the fields of health and health care.

At the *meso* level of organizational/regional influence, we especially need to improve the moral foundations of health policy (Giacomini, Kenny, and DeJean 2009; see also Chapter 18). Such policy work takes nursing expertise and nursing leadership (Johnstone 2002; Malone 1999; Mitchell 2001; Rodney et al. 2002; Storch 2010). The need for expertise was evident, for instance, in the nurses' concerns about patient and family choices at the end of life in Ethics in Practice 10-1. Further, we need to follow expert professional recommendations to improve the quality of nurses' workplaces (see Exhibit 10-1).

At the *micro* level of individual and interpersonal influence, *we should learn to listen to diverse viewpoints and treat all others with respect—whether they are managers, other health care providers, patients, family members, or nursing colleagues.* Interpersonal conflict, especially if it is demeaning or bullying, has an important interactive effect on the moral climate. Such conflict is worsened by problems with resources and power inequities, but in turn exacerbates these problems (Center for American Nurses 2008; Corley and Goren 1998; Rodney et al. 2002; Rodney and Varcoe in press). In Ethics in Practice 10-2, for example, the managers in Gaudine and Beaton's (2002) study claimed that feeling unsupported by staff nurses made it much harder for them to do their job.

Research Action

We can use the growing expertise in philosophical inquiry and research methodologies in nursing (and in other disciplines such as philosophy and sociology) to support nursing's evolution as a moral community. This can take place in at least three ways. *First,* we can use philosophical inquiry[20] as well as empirical inquiry to continue to articulate the nature (and importance) of nursing. At the heart of nursing's disempowerment in current health care policy processes lie implicit assumptions about the nature of nursing—that it can be reduced, parcelled out, and directed by non-nurses. To rebut these assumptions we need to better articulate the unique nature of nursing; that is, we need to better articulate what we do and why it matters (Mitchell 2001; Nagle 1999; Thorne 2011; see also Chapter 3). *Second,* we can do some conceptual work to further our research about nurses' work environments and the moral climate of nursing practice. In their work with a measurement tool for the international nursing outcomes research project, Estabrooks et al. (2002) have noted that such clarification is needed in future. They argue that:

> A longer-range and more ambitious goal involves the systematic examination of the concepts of organizational culture, organizational climate, and practice environment from both conceptual and measurement perspectives. (267)

We agree, and we would add that the concepts of moral agency, moral climate, and moral community ought to be considered at the same time—as is apparent throughout this chapter, the problems in nurses' workplaces have significant moral dimensions. *Third*, we can promote action research to help to improve the moral climate of nursing practice.

Action Research to Improve the Moral Climate of Nursing Practice

Four of the authors of this chapter (Martin, Rodney, Serrano and Street) have been part of different research teams involved in a number of action initiatives through which we have learned a great deal about how to improve the moral climate of nursing and interprofessional practice (including the complexity of such action work). Action research is an umbrella term for a range of research methodologies that share (1) a common commitment to political and strategic action that values human flourishing; (2) a focus on the relationship between knowledge and action; (3) inclusion of the participation of all relevant stakeholders in the conduct and decision-making of the research; and (4) the goal of addressing practical problems to improve a situation (Ladkin 2004; Reason and Bradbury 2001; Street 2002). Drawing on the work of Habermas (1971), Park (2001) argues that the "full realisation of human life in society requires the mobilization of rationality that includes knowledge of moral values relevant in everyday living" (86). Action research is a process that is increasingly being adopted by nurses interested in identifying shared values and working together to improve a health care situation, particularly one characterized by injustice (Kelly and Simpson 2001). *It offers significant promise in helping to redress some of the power dynamics that have led to our current moral climate challenges.*

The research process begins with a preliminary investigation with individuals in direct care and other roles to explore the literature and the politics of the health care context (Street 1995). Strategic action is planned, implemented, and monitored. Analysis of the findings is followed by collaborative critical reflection on the success of the plan or the need to modify it and begin another cycle of planning, implementation, data collection, analysis, and reflection. Participants continue to work though this cyclical process until the situation has improved (Street 1999). The outcomes of action research in health care are context-specific (Dickson 2000; Tobin 2000) and may be focused on improving a clinical situation (Rose et al. 1999), addressing policies (Roy and Cain 2001), or informing changes in the health care culture (Kelly and Simpson 2001; Wadsworth 2001).

The knowledge gained through these processes provides practical moral criteria for comprehending the complexity of health care situations and discerning appropriate, acceptable, and feasible plans to implement change (Park 2001). In consequence, co-researchers (involved stakeholders) reflect on their own values and on the consistency between these values and the action they have implemented through a process of critical reflection (Goodson 1997). In turn, this group deliberation leads to opportunities to uncover the exercise of power relations and its consequences for the nurses and those for whom they provide care.

Rodney, Storch, Varcoe, Pauly, Doane and other colleagues—including Martin and Serrano—have been involved in a program of participatory action research in B.C. over the past eight years. In order to learn more about *how* to address the ethical problems we had identified in earlier studies, we embarked on a participatory action research (PAR) study of nursing practice ("Ethics in Action") conducted in an emergency unit and a medical oncology unit (2003–2006). This study (funded by the Social Science and Humanities Research Council and the University of Victoria) involved three years of participant observation, interviews, focus groups, meetings, workshops, and informal work within the two practice settings (Hartrick Doane, Storch, and Pauly 2009; Rodney et al. 2006; Rodney and Varcoe in press). At each site, the research team included direct care nurses and academic investigators working in partnership. Along with qualitative data collection through focus groups and interviews, regular meetings with staff were conducted at each site to discuss, debrief, and to plan for change. The research process was geared to supporting staff to initiate changes in their workplaces toward ethical practice.

Our PAR work has been continuing as the result of a British Columbia province-wide project to generate action initiatives (Storch et al. 2009a; 2009b). One such initiative, *Building a Moral Community for Collaborative Practice in Ambulatory Oncology Care,* was a participatory action study recently completed by an interdisciplinary team in an outpatient oncology clinic (2007–2010), and was funded by the British Columbia Cancer Agency and the Canadian Nurses Foundation. In this study Rodney, Serrano, and Martin and their interdisciplinary colleagues at the B.C. Cancer Agency used qualitative and quantitative methods to assess health care providers' moral climate, work with them to generate strategies for positive change, and evaluate the effectiveness of those changes (Serrano, Martin, and Rodney 2011; see also Rodney and Varcoe in press). Research participants included all the categories of direct care providers at a busy outpatient oncology unit in B.C.[21] The research team learned how changes in cancer care delivery across Canada have resulted in increasing pressures on all health care providers to deliver complex treatments in rapid-paced outpatient settings with little time to appreciate each other's roles and little time to keep up with the knowledge explosion in their specialty. Providers experienced moral distress related to their concerns about the significant needs of patients and their family members who were going to have to manage their own care at home, and about how providers delivering services have little input into the restructuring of cancer care systems.

The cancer care providers we worked with during our research helped us to generate a number of strategies to improve the moral climate of their practice, and we were supported by administration in the funding, design, and conduct of the research. The strategies we tested included interactive and supportive interdisciplinary rounds, interdisciplinary workshops on symptom management, and communicating the need for better transparency in decision making to senior administration (see Exhibit 10-3). Our evaluation of the effectiveness of the action strategies has shown significant promise, and as this chapter goes to press we are currently working on planning follow-up knowledge translation to assist with sustainability and transferability of what we have learned thus far.

EXHIBIT 10-3

Interdisciplinary Action Strategies

(Adapted from Serrano, Martin, and Rodney 2011)

- Regular, pre-structured debriefing sessions with safe facilitators
- Built-in rounds to learn "from, with and about"[22] each other
- Transparent, reciprocal feedback between all levels of staff and administration

- Ethics support and related policy initiatives for complex end-of-life situations
- Advocacy work through professional associations to improve resources for cancer *care* as well as treatment in all settings (outpatient, hospital, and home).

Overall, action research provides the opportunity to learn more about *how* to foster the development of moral communities for nursing and interdisciplinary practice, and hence move out of the moral winter we find ourselves in. Such research generates organizational as well as political action. While we still have a lot to learn, the voices of nurses and other health care providers in our action research show us that there is hope. Interestingly, the participants in our action research studies have consistently told us that being listened to and respected through the research is itself a source of hope.

Summary

Trace the word **professional** *back to its origins and you will find that it refers to someone who makes a "profession of faith" in the midst of a disheartening world (Palmer 2007, 212).*

To move forward does, as educational theorist Parker Palmer indicates in the quote above, take faith. In this chapter we have argued that power inequities in contemporary health care policy processes have interfered with nurses' abilities to provide good quality patient/family/community care. We have claimed that those power inequities have worsened the moral climate of nursing practice, and have been harmful to nurses as well as patients/families/communities. We have further claimed that fostering a stronger sense of moral community—in which ethical values are made explicit and shared, direct action is valued, and individuals feel safe to be heard—can help us to improve the moral climate of nursing practice. And we have posited some organizational, political, and research-based strategies that can help us to move toward a healthier moral community—strategies that build on hope and faith.[23] Indeed, *all* the chapters in this book provide analyses and strategies that can move us in this direction.

While not exhaustive, the strategies we have articulated in this chapter nonetheless point to an important turning point for nursing inquiry. A growing number of nurse researchers, nurse leaders, and colleagues in other disciplines are beginning to focus more on *how* to improve nurses' workplaces. Our profession, all other health care professions, and most especially our patients and their families and communities, need much more of this kind of work. We ought to continue to imagine and work toward a moral community that values nursing expertise for patient/family/community well-being, has a strong nursing leadership presence, is supportive of continuing education, and has a commitment to adequate staffing as well as good retention and recruitment programs. And we ought to continue to imagine and work toward equitable access to resources for patients/families/ communities, regardless of attributes such as age, gender, sexual orientation, ability, ethnicity, and language fluency. Let us close with the words of our American nursing colleagues Phillips and Benner:

> We believe it is essential to recover the vision of what is possible in actual practices today in order to discover the mandates for reshaping our institutional structures, environments, and economics to serve attentive, sustaining, and healing relationships. (1994, vii)

Their words are as true today as they were in 1994. And the vision they call for is essential if we are to move from the moral winter we find ourselves in toward the promise of spring.

For Reflection

1. What is it about "non-specialty" contexts (such as acute medical wards) that make them especially vulnerable to contemporary cost constraints?

2. Think back to the quotation from the nurse manager (from Gaudine and Beaton's [2002] study) in Ethics in Practice 10-2. How could the staff on the units for which the manager was responsible support the manager in her attempts to advocate for improving their conditions of work?

3. How do you think that nurses ought to use evidence about bad outcomes for patients/ clients and nurses to make a political argument for improved resources? Include some ideas at the micro, meso, and macro levels of health care policy.

4. Participatory action research is built on democratic processes of participation. How might the insights we gain about such processes help nurses and other health care professionals to become more involved in health policy work?

Endnotes

1. Stein (2001) also critiques the impact of efficiency in education. Palmer (2007), whom we have drawn on for a closing quote for this chapter, raises similar concerns in his quest for educational reform.

2. References supporting this claim include: Anderson et al. (2009); Austin (2011); Beagan and Ells (2007); Corley et al. (2005); Canadian Nurses Association and Registered Nurses Association of Ontario (2010); Coburn (2010); Dodds (2005); Health Council of Canada (2008); Marmot (2004); Mitchell (2001); and Rodney and Varcoe (in press). See Storch (2010) for an insightful overview of the history of economic, political, and social changes in Canada and their impact on health care delivery, as well as Moorhouse and Rodney (2010) for a sketch of the contemporary challenges these changes have created for nurses. In this text, Chapters 9, 11, 12, 18, 19, 20, and 21 (in particular) also address constraints in the resources for health and health care and the resultant impact on individuals, families, and communities as well as health care providers.

3. See Frenk et al. (2010); Macklin (2008); Oulton (2007); Sherwin (2011); Wiskow, Albreht, and de Pietro (2010); and World Health Organization (2008a; 2008b). See also Austin (2003; 2004) and Benatar and Brock (2011) for discussions of global health.

4. An anonymous reviewer for the second edition of this chapter has (quite rightly) cautioned us that there are those who deny climate change. This comment has caused us to wonder if similar processes might lie behind an implicit denial of moral climate changes in health care such that cost constraints are continuing despite rising concerns about equity—and even safety—in health and health care.

5. Other terms found in the literature to describe moral climate include *ethical climate*, *ethical culture*, and *ethical environment*. The terms *moral* and *ethical* tend to be used interchangeably, as do *culture* and *environment*.

6. We use the term *restructuring* to include all forms of structural adjustment such as cutbacks, cost reductions, downsizing, cost containment, reorganization, fiscal restraint, offloading, and reallocation.

7. By *corporate ethos* (or ideology) we mean the taken-for-granted acceptance that a market approach to health care is best. The values of the marketplace come to dominate, such that hierarchy, efficiency, and "the bottom line" implicitly replace values related to human well-being, personal integrity, and social justice (see also Annas 1995; Austin 2011; Commission on the Future of Health Care in Canada 2002; Hiraki 1998; Myrick 2004; Rodney and Varcoe in press; and Sellman 2011). This is not to say that corporations are without positive human values—indeed, there is a thriving literature on, and a growing practice in, business ethics. Rather, it is to say that the taken-for-granted acceptance of a limited (and misapplied) set of marketplace values for health care policy processes is highly problematic.

8. The authors wish to thank an anonymous reviewer of the first edition of this chapter for an initial draft of these premises.

9. As we argue in Chapter 9, this corporate ethics can also create significant moral angst for managers and administrators. We address this later in this chapter.

10. See also Chapter 9 on moral disengagement. In Chapter 9 we examine the repercussions for nurses' sense of agency and well-being.

11. This research (and other studies Rodney, Storch, Varcoe, and Doane have conducted since) did not employ one particular conceptual framework. Rather, the researchers used a composite approach to ethical theory that is consistent with Daniels' (1996) notion of wide reflective equilibrium (see also Chapters 4, 5, 13, and 18). Ethical practice was defined in terms of Benner, Tanner, and Chesla's (1996) Aristotelian notion of the "good" in practice. In exploring the meaning of ethics with nurses we therefore asked them to tell us about what helped or hindered them in "doing good" in their practice. (See also Rodney et al. 2002). More recently we have been conducting our research from an explicit ethics lens of *relational ethics* (see also Chapters 5, 7, and 8).

12. In the research that generated Ethics in Practice 12-1 we were explicitly using a metaphor of navigating toward a horizon. Our adoption of the metaphor of winter in this chapter is based on more recent contributions by Buckley (2007). In relation to Buckley's metaphor of winter, we would like to thank an anonymous reviewer for the second edition of this chapter, who told us that "I often have nurses come forward in conferences with cases that have been haunting them, sometimes for years . . . they were frozen then and remain frozen, not knowing how they should have intervened, or could have intervened." See also Chapter 9 regarding moral residue.

13. Hartrick Doane, Storch, and Pauly (2009); Rodney (1997); Rodney et al. (2006); Rodney and Varcoe in press; Rodney et al. (2002); Serrano, Martin, and Rodney (2011); Storch et al. (2009a); Storch et al. (2009b); Varcoe et al. (2004).

14. See Chapter 18 for an exploration of ethics and policy work.

15. See also Mitton et al. 2011.

16. For insightful analyses of the gender-based history of nursing, including conflicts with physicians, see Ashley (1976); Corley and Mauksch (1988); David (2000); Street (1992); and Thompson, Allen, and Rodrigues-Fisher (1992).

17. Terms used in the literature to discuss moral community sometimes include *moral or ethical climate* and *moral or ethical environment*.

18. See De Wolf Bosek and Savage (2007) for an example of a comprehensive ethics resource for nursing education as well as Grace (2009) for comprehensive ethics resources for advanced practice nurses.

19. Whether that was actually the perspective of the nurse manager's administrative colleagues is an empirical question. Nonetheless, the other studies we have cited also consistently portray the disempowerment of nurses in organizational decision making.

20. Chapter 3 provides an overview of philosophy in nursing, including philosophical inquiry. See also Chapter 2 on the evolution of nursing ethics.

21. The total number of participants was approximately 40. Care provider groups included care aides, dietitians, nurses working in radiation therapy, nurses working in systemic therapy, oncologists, patient/family counsellors, pharmacists, and radiation therapists. Most participants were direct care providers but a number were also middle managers.

22. This three-part phrasing has been adapted from the University of British Columbia's Interprofessional Studies program.

23. An interesting concept worth more exploration as applied to improving the moral climate of nursing practice is that of *moral repair*. See Walker (2006).

References

Aiken, L.H., Clarke, S.P., and Sloane, D.M. 2000. Hospital restructuring: Does it adversely affect care and outcomes? *Journal of Nursing Administration, 30* (10), 457–465.

Aiken, L.H., Clarke, S.P., Sloane, D.M., Sochalski, J., and Silber, J.H. 2002. Hospital nurse staffing and patient mortality, nurse burnout, and job dissatisfaction. *Journal of the American Medical Association, 288* (916), 23–30.

Anderson, J.M., Browne, A.J., Reimer-Kirkham, S., Lynam, M.J., Rodney, P., Varcoe, C., Wong, S., Tan, E., Smye, V., McDonald, H., Baumbusch, J., Khan, K.B., Reimer, J., Peltonen, A., and Brar, A. 2010. Uptake of critical knowledge in nursing practice: Lessons learned from a knowledge translation study. *Canadian Journal of Nursing Research, 42* (3), 106–122.

Anderson, J.M., Rodney, P., Reimer-Kirkham, S., Browne, A.J., Khan, K.B., and Lynam, M.J. 2009. Inequities in health and healthcare viewed through the ethical lens of critical social justice: Contextual knowledge for the global priorities ahead. *Advances in Nursing Science, 32* (4), 282–294.

Annas, G.J. 1995. Reframing the debate on health care reform by replacing our metaphors. *New England Journal of Medicine, 332* (11), 744–747.

Aroskar, M.A. 1995. Envisioning nursing as a moral community. *Nursing Outlook, 43* (3), 134–138.

Ashley, J.A. 1976. *Hospitals, paternalism, and the role of the nurse.* New York: Teacher's College Press.

Auditor General Victoria. 2002. *Nurse workforce planning.* Melbourne, AU: State of Victoria.

Austin, W. 2003. Using the human rights paradigm in health ethics: The problem and the possibilities. In V. Tschudin (Ed.), *Approaches to ethics: Nursing beyond boundaries* (pp. 105–114). Edinburgh: Butterworth Heinmann. (Reprinted from *Nursing Ethics* 2001; *8* (13), 183–195.)

Austin, W. 2004. Global health challenges, human rights, and nursing ethics. In J. Storch, P. Rodney, and R. Starzomski (Eds.), *Toward a moral horizon: Nursing ethics for leadership and practice* (pp. 339–356). Toronto: Pearson Prentice Hall.

Austin, W. 2007. The ethics of everyday practice: Healthcare environments as moral communities. *Advances in Nursing Science, 30* (1), 81–88.

Austin, W.J. 2011. The incommensurability of nursing as a practice and the customer service model: An evolutionary threat to the discipline. *Nursing Philosophy, 12*, 158–166.

Beagan, B. and Ells, C. 2007. Values that matter, barriers that interfere: The struggle of Canadian nurses to enact their values. *Canadian Journal of Nursing Research, 39* (4), 37–57.

Bell, J. and Breslin, J.M. 2008. Healthcare provider moral distress as a leadership challenge. *JONA'S Healthcare Law, Ethics, and Regulation, 10* (4), 94–97.

Benatar, S. and Brock, G. 2011. *Global health and global health ethics.* Cambridge: Cambridge University Press.

Benner, P.A., Tanner, C.A., and Chesla, C.A. (with contributions by H.L. Dreyfus, S.E. Dreyfus, and J. Rubin). 1996. *Expertise in nursing practice: Caring, clinical judgment, and ethics.* New York: Springer.

British Columbia Nurses Union. 2011. *BCNU position statement on provision of nursing care.* Burnaby, BC: Author.

Browne, A.J., Smye, V.L., Rodney, P., Tang, S.Y., Mussell, B., and O'Neill, J. 2011. Access to primary care from the perspective of Aboriginal patients at an urban emergency department. *Qualitative Health Research 21* (3), 333–348.

Buckley, B.J. 2007. *Moral winter.* Unpublished major paper, University of British Columbia School of Nursing, Vancouver, BC, Canada.

Campbell, M.L. 1987. Productivity in Canadian nursing: Administering cuts. In D. Coburn, C. D'Arcy, G.M. Torrance, and P. New (Eds.), *Health and Canadian society: Sociological perspectives* (2nd ed.; pp. 463–475). Markham, ON: Fitzhenry & Whiteside.

Canadian Nurses Association. 2008. *Code of ethics for registered nurses.* Ottawa, ON: Authors.

Canadian Nurses Association. 2009. *Tested solutions for eliminating Canada's registered nurse shortage.* Ottawa, ON: Author.

Canadian Nurses Association and Canadian Federation of Nurses Unions. 2006. *Joint position statement: Practice environment: Maximizing client, nurse and system outcomes.* Ottawa, ON: Author.

Canadian Nurses Association and Registered Nurses Association of Ontario. 2010. *Nurse fatigue and patient safety: Research report.* Ottawa, ON: Canadian Nurses Association.

Centre for American Nurses. 2008. *Lateral violence and bullying in the workplace.* Silver Spring, MD: Authors.

Chambliss, D.F. 1996. *Beyond caring: Hospitals, nurses, and the social organization of ethics.* Chicago: The University of Chicago Press.

Chinn, P.L. 2008. *Peace and power: Creative Leadership for building community* (7th ed.). Boston: Jones and Bartlett.

Clarke, H.F., Laschinger, H.S., Giovannetti, P., Shamian, J., Thomson, D., and Tourangeau, A. 2001. Nursing shortages: Workplace environments are essential to the solution. *Hospital Quarterly* (Summer), 50–57.

Coburn, D. 2010. Health and health care: A political economy perspective. In T. Bryant, D. Raphael, and M. Rioux (Eds.), *Staying alive: Critical perspectives on health, illness, and health care* (2nd ed.; pp. 65–91). Toronto, ON: Canadian Scholars' Press.

Commission on the Future of Health Care in Canada. 2002. *Building on values: The future of health care in Canada.* Ottawa, ON: Authors.

Corley, M.C. and Goren, S. 1998. The dark side of nursing: Impact of stigmatizing responses on patients. *Scholarly Inquiry for Nursing Practice, 12* (2), 99–118.

Corley, M.C. and Mauksch, H.O. 1988. Registered nurses, gender, and commitment. In A. Statham, E.M. Miller, and H.O. Mauksch (Eds.), *The worth of women's work: A qualitative synthesis* (pp. 135–149). Albany, NY: State University of New York Press.

Corley, M.C., Minick, P., Elswick, R.K., and Jacobs, M. 2005. Nurse moral distress and ethical work environment. *Nursing Ethics, 12* (4), 381–390.

Daiski, I. 2004. Changing nurses' disempowering relationship patterns. *Journal of Advanced Nursing, 48* (1), 43–50.

Daniels, N. 1996. Wide reflective equilibrium in practice. In L.W. Sumner and J. Boyle (Eds.), *Philosophical perspectives on bioethics* (pp. 96–114). Toronto: University of Toronto Press.

David, B.A. 2000. Nursing's gender politics: Reformulating the footnotes. *Advances in Nursing Science, 23* (1), 83–93.

De Wolf Bosek, M.S. and Savage, T.A. (Eds.). 2007. *The ethical component of nursing education: Integrating ethics into clinical experience.* Philadelphia: Lippincott, Williams and Wilkins.

Dickson, G. 2000. Aboriginal grandmothers' experience with health promotion and participatory action research. *Qualitative Health Research, 10* (2), 188–213.

Dodds, S. 2005. Gender, ageing, and injustice: Social and political contexts of bioethics. *Journal of Medical Ethics, 31*, 295–298.

Dunleavy, J., Shamian, J., and Thomson, D. 2003. Workplace pressures: Handcuffed by cutbacks. *Canadian Nurse, 99* (3), 23–26.

Estabrooks, C., Mididzi, W., Cummings, G., Ricker, K., and Giovanetti, P. 2005. The impact of hospital nursing characteristics on 30-day mortality. *Nursing Research, 54* (2), 74–84.

Estabrooks, C.A., Tourangeau, A.E., Humphrey, C.K., Hesketh, K.L., Giovannetti, P., Thomson, D., Wong, J., Acorn, S., Clarke, H., and Shamian, J. 2002. Measuring the hospital practice environment: A Canadian context. *Research in Nursing and Health, 25*, 256–268.

Frenk, J., Chen, L., Bhutta, Z.A., Cohen, J., Crisp, N., Evans, T., et al. 2010. Health professionals for a new century: Transforming education to strengthen health systems in an interdependent world. *The Lancet, 376*, 1923–1958.

Garon, M. 2006. The positive face of resistance: Nurses relate their stories. *Journal of Nursing Administration, 36* (5), 249–258.

Gaudine, A.P. and Beaton, M.R. 2002. Employed to go against one's values: Nurse managers' accounts of ethical conflict within their organizations. *Canadian Journal of Nursing Research, 34* (2), 17–34.

Giacomini, M., Kenny, N., and DeJean, D. 2009. Ethics frameworks in Canadian health policies: Foundation, scaffolding, or window dressing? *Health Policy, 89*, 58–71.

Goodson, I. 1997. Action research and "The Reflexive Project of Selves." In S. Hollingsworth (Ed.), *International action research: A casebook for educational reform* (pp. 204–218). London: The Falmer Press.

Gordon, S. 2005. *Nursing against the odds: How health care cost cutting, media stereotypes, and medical hubris undermine nurses and patient care.* New York: Cornell University Press.

Grace, P.J. (Ed.). 2009. *Nursing ethics and professional responsibility in advanced practice.* Sudbury MA: Jones and Bartlett.

Habermas, J. 1971. *Knowledge and human interests.* Boston: Beacon Press.

Hamric, A.B. and Blackhall, L.J. 2007. Nurse-physician perspectives on the care of dying patients in intensive care units: Collaboration, moral distress, and ethical climate. *Critical Care Medicine, 35,* (2), 422–429.

Hartrick Doane, G., Pauly, B., Brown, H., and McPherson, G. 2004. Exploring the heart of ethical nursing practice: Implications for ethics education. *Nursing Ethics 11*(3), 240–253.

Hartrick Doane, G., Storch, J., and Pauly, B. 2009. Ethical nursing practice: Inquiry-in-action. *Nursing Inquiry, 16* (3), 1–9.

Health Canada. 2002. *Final report of the Canadian Nursing Advisory Committee.* Ottawa: Author.

Health Canada Office of Nursing Policy. 2001. *Healthy nurses, healthy workplaces.* Ottawa: Author.

Health Council of Canada. 2008. *Rekindling reform: Health care renewal 2003–2008.* Toronto: Author.

Heath, P.C. 2002. *National Review of Nursing Education 2002: Our Duty of Care.* Melbourne, AU: Commonwealth Department of Education, Science and Training, Commonwealth of Australia.

Hiraki, A. 1998. Corporate language and nursing practice. *Nursing Outlook, 46*, 115–9.

Jameton, A. 1984. *Nursing practice: The ethical issues.* New Jersey: Prentice Hall.

Jameton, A. 1990. Culture, morality, and ethics: Twirling the spindle. *Critical Care Nursing Clinics of North America, 2* (3), 443–451.

Johnstone, M.-J. 2002. Poor working conditions and the capacity of nurses to provide moral care. *Contemporary Nurse, 12* (1), 7–15.

Kelly, D. and Simpson, S. 2001. Action research in action: Reflections on a project to introduce clinical practice facilitators to an acute hospital setting. *Journal of Advanced Nursing March, 33* (5), 652–659.

Ladkin, D. 2004. Action research. In C. Seale, G. Gobo, J.F. Gubrium, and D. Silverman (Eds.), *Qualitative research practice* (pp. 536–548). London: Sage Publications.

Laschinger, H.K.S. and Leiter, M. 2006. The impact of nursing work environments on patient safety outcomes: The mediating role of burnout engagement. *Journal of Nursing Administration, 36* (3), 259–267.

Laschinger, H.K.S., Finegan, J., Shamian, J., and Casier, S. 2000. Organizational trust and empowerment in restructured healthcare settings: Effects on staff nurse commitment. *Journal of Nursing Administration, 30* (9), 413–425.

Liaschenko, J. 1993. Feminist ethics and cultural ethos: Revisiting a nursing debate. *Advances in Nursing Science, 15* (4), 71–81.

Lynam, M.J., Henderson, A., Browne, A., Smye, V., Semeniuk, P., Blue, C., Singh, S., and Anderson, J. 2003. Healthcare restructuring with a view to equity and efficiency: Reflections on unintended consequences. *Canadian Journal of Nursing Leadership, 16* (1), 112–140.

Macklin, R. 2008. Global justice, human rights, and health. In R.M. Green, A. Donovan, and S.A. Jauss (Eds.), *Global bioethics: Issues of conscience for the twenty-first century* (pp. 141–160). Oxford: Clarendon Press.

Mallidou, A.A., Cummings, G.C., Estabrooks, C.A. and Giovanetti, P.B. 2011. Nurse specialty subcultures and patient outcomes in acute care hospitals: A multiple-group structural equation modeling. *International Journal of Nursing Studies, 48*, 81–93.

Malone, R.E. 1999. Policy as product: Morality and metaphor in health policy discourse. *Hastings Centre Report,* (May–June), 16–22.

Mann, P.S. 1994. *Micro-politics: Agency in a postfeminist era.* Minneapolis: University of Minnesota Press.

Marmot, M. 2004. Social causes of social inequalities in health. In S. Anand, F. Peter, and A. Sen (Eds.), *Public health, ethics, and equity* (pp. 37–61). Oxford: Oxford University Press.

MacPhee, M., Jewell, K., Wardrop, A., Ahmed, A., and Mildon, B. 2010. British Columbia's provincial workload project: Evidence to empowerment. *Canadian Journal of Nursing Leadership, 23* (1), 54–63.

McClure, M.L., Poulin, M.A., Sovie, M.D., and Wandelt, M.A. 1983. *Magnet hospitals: Attraction and retention of professional nurses.* Kansas City, MO: American Academy of Nursing.

McCutcheon, A.S., Doran, D., Evans, M., McGillis Hall, L., and Pringle, D. 2009. Effects of leadership and span of control on nurses' job satisfaction and patient satisfaction. *Canadian Journal of Nursing Leadership, 22* (3), 48–67.

McGowan, J. 1998. *Hannah Arendt: An introduction.* Minneapolis: University of Minnesota Press.

Mitchell, G.J. 2001. Policy, procedure and routine: Matters of moral influence. *Nursing Science Quarterly, 14* (2), 109–114.

Mitton, C., Peacock, S., Storch, J., Smith, N., and Cornelissen, E. 2011. Moral distress among health system managers: Exploratory research in two British Columbia health authorities. *Health Care Anal, 19*, 107–121.

Moorhouse, A. and Rodney, P. 2010. Contemporary Canadian challenges in nursing ethics. In M. Yeo, A. Moorhouse, P. Khan, and P. Rodney (Eds.), *Concepts and cases in nursing ethics*, (3rd ed.; pp. 73–101). Peterborough, ON: Broadview Press.

Mouffe, C. 1993. *The return of the political.* London: Verso.

Myrick, F. 2004. Pedagogical integrity in the knowledge economy. *Nursing Philosophy, 5*, 23–29.

Nagle, L.M. 1999. A matter of extinction or distinction. *Western Journal of Nursing Research, 21* (1), 71–82.

Oulton, J. 2007. Nursing in the international community: A broader view of nursing issues. In D.J. Mason, J.K. Leavitt, and M.W. Chaffee (Eds.), *Policy & politics in nursing and health care* (5th ed.; pp. 966–981). St. Louis, MO: Saunders Elsevier.

Palmer, P.J. 2007. *The courage to teach: Exploring the inner landscape of a teacher's life* (10th Anniversary ed.). San Francisco, CA: John Wiley & Sons.

Park, P. 2001. Knowledge and participatory research. In P. Reason and H. Bradbury (Eds.), *Handbook of action research: Participative inquiry and practice* (pp. 81–90). London: Sage.

Pauly, B., Varcoe, C., Storch, J.L., and Newton, L. 2009. Registered nurses' perceptions of moral distress and ethical climate. *Nursing Ethics, 16* (5), 561–573.

Phillips, S.S. and Benner, P. 1994. Preface. In S.S. Phillips and P. Benner (Eds.), *The crisis of care: Affirming and restoring caring practices in the helping professions* (pp. vii–xi). Washington, DC: Georgetown University Press.

Picard, A. 2000. *Critical care: Canadian nurses speak for change.* Toronto, ON: HarperCollins.

Pringle, D. 2009. Alert—Return of 1990s healthcare reform. *Canadian Journal of Nursing Leadership, 22* (3), 14–15.

Raines, M.L. 2000. Ethical decision making in nurses: Relationships among moral reasoning, coping style, and ethics stress. *Journal of Nursing Administration's Healthcare Law, Ethics, and Regulation, 2* (1), 29–41.

Reason, P. and Bradbury, H. 2001. Introduction: Inquiry and participation in search of a world worthy of human aspiration. In P. Reason and H. Bradbury (Eds.), *Handbook of action research: Participatory inquiry and practices* (pp. 1–14). London: Sage.

Rodney, P.A. 1997. *Towards connectedness and trust: Nurses' enactment of their moral agency within an organizational context.* Unpublished doctoral dissertation, University of British Columbia, Vancouver, BC.

Rodney, P., Varcoe, C., Storch, J.L., McPherson, G., Mahoney, K., Brown, H., Pauly, B., Hartrick Doane, G., and Starzomski, R. 2002. Navigating toward a moral horizon: A multi-site qualitative study of nurses' enactment of ethical practice. *Canadian Journal of Nursing Research 34* (3), 75–102.

Rodney, P., Doane, G.H., Storch, J., and Varcoe, C. 2006. Workplaces: Toward a safer moral climate. *Canadian Nurse, 102* (8), 24–27.

Rodney, P. and Varcoe, C. in press. Constrained agency: The social structure of nurses' work. In F. Baylis, J. Downie, B. Hoffmaster, and S. Sherwin (Eds.), *Health care ethics in Canada* (3rd ed.). Toronto: Nelson. (Revision of Varcoe, C. and Rodney, P. 2009 Constrained agency: The social structure of nurses' work. In B.S. Bolaria and H.D. Dickinson (Eds.), *Health, illness, and health care in Canada* (4th ed.; pp. 122–151). Toronto: Nelson Education.)

Rose, K., Waterman, H., McLeod, D., and Tullo, A. 1999. Planning and managing research into day-surgery for cataract. *Journal of Advanced Nursing June, 29* (6), 1514–1519.

Roy, C.M. and Cain, R. 2001. The involvement of people living with HIV/AIDS in community-based organizations: Contributions and constraints. *AIDS Care, 13* (4), 421–432.

Rudge, T. 2011. The "well-run" system and its antimonies. *Nursing Philosophy, 12*, 167–176.

Sanders, K., Pattison, S., and Hurwitz, B. 2011. Tracking shame and humiliation in accident and emergency. *Nursing Philosophy, 12*, 83–93.

Saul, J.R. 2005. *The collapse of globalism and the reinvention of the world.* Toronto: Penguin Canada.

Sellman, D. 2011. Professional values and nursing. *Medical Health Care and Philosophy, 14*, 203–208.

Serrano, E., Martin, L.A., and Rodney, P. 2011. *Final report: Building a moral community for collaborative practice in ambulatory oncology care: Toward improved patient/family and team outcomes.* Unpublished research report to the Canadian Nurses Foundation and the British Columbia Cancer Agency. Vancouver, BC: Authors.

Shamian, J., Kerr, M.S., Laschinger, H.K.S., and Thomson, D. 2002. A hospital-level analysis of the work environments and workforce health indicators for registered nurses in Ontario's acute-care hospitals. *Canadian Journal of Nursing Research, 33* (4), 35–50.

Sherwin, S. 2011. Looking backwards, looking forward: Hopes for bioethics' next twenty-five years. *Bioethics, 25* (2), 75–82.

Stajduhar, K.I. 2003. Examining the perspectives of family members involved in the delivery of palliative care at home. *Journal of Palliative Care, 19* (1), 27–35.

Stajduhar, K.I. 2011. Discourse: Chronic illness, palliative care, and the problematic nature of dying. *Canadian Journal of Nursing Research, 43* (3), 7–15.

Stein, J.G. 2001. *The cult of efficiency.* Toronto: Penguin.

Storch, J.L. 2010. Canadian healthcare system. In M. McIntyre and C. McDonald (Eds.), *Realities of Canadian nursing: Professional, practice, and power issues* (3rd ed.; pp. 34–55). Wolters Kluwer Health: Philadelphia.

Storch, J., Hartrick, G., Rodney, P., Starzomski, R., and Varcoe, C. 2001. *The ethics of practice: Context and curricular implications for nursing.* Unpublished research report to the Associated Medical Services Inc. and the University of Victoria School of Nursing. Victoria BC: Authors.

Storch, J., Rodney, P., Pauly, B., Brown, H., and Starzomski, R. 2002. Listening to nurses' moral voices: Building a quality health care environment. *Canadian Journal of Nursing Leadership, 15* (4), 7–16.

Storch, J., Rodney, P., Pauly, B., Fulton, T., Stevenson, L., Newton, L., and Makaroff, K.S. (2009a). Enhancing ethical climates in nursing work environments. *Canadian Nurse, 105* (3), 20–25.

Storch, J., Rodney, P., Varcoe, C., Pauly, B., Starzomski, R., Stevenson, L., Best, L., Mass, H., Fulton, T.R., Mildon, B., Bees, F., Chisholm, A., MacDonald-Rencz, S., McCutcheon, A.S., Shamian, J., Thompson, C., Makaroff, K.S., and Newton, L. 2009b. Leadership for ethical policy and practice (LEPP): Participatory action project. *Canadian Journal of Nursing Leadership, 22* (3), 68–80.

Street, A.F. 1992. *Inside nursing: A critical ethnography of clinical nursing practice.* Albany, NY: State University of New Your Press.

Street, A.F. 1995. *Nursing replay: Researching nursing culture together.* Melbourne, AU: Churchill Livingstone.

Street, A.F. 1999. Bedtimes in nursing homes: Exploring an action research approach for gerontic nursing. In R. Nay and S. Garrett (Eds.), *Nursing older people: Issues and innovations* (pp. 353–368). Sydney, AU: MacLennan and Petty.

Street, A.F. 1992. *Inside nursing: A critical ethnography of nursing practice*. Albany, NY: State University of New York Press.

Thompson, J.L, Allen, D.G., and Rodrigues-Fisher, L. (Eds.). 1992. *Critique, resistance, and action: Working papers in the politics of nursing*. New York: National League for Nursing Press.

Thorne, S. 2011. Theoretical issues in nursing. In J. C. Ross-Kerr and M.J. Wood (Eds.), *Canadian nursing: Issues and perspectives* (5th ed.; 85–104). Toronto: Elsevier.

Tobin, M. 2000. Developing mental health rehabilitation services in a culturally appropriate context: An action research project involving Arabic-speaking clients. *Australian Health Review, 23* (2), 177–184.

Varcoe, C., Doane, G., Pauly, B., Rodney, P., Storch, J.L., Mahoney, K., McPherson, G., Brown, H., and Starzomski, R. 2004. Ethical practice in nursing: Working the in-betweens. *Journal of Advanced Nursing, 45* (3), 316–325.

Walker, M.U. 2006. *Moral repair: Reconstructing moral relations after wrongdoing*. Cambridge: Cambridge University Press.

Walston, S.L., Lazes, P., and Sullivan, P.G. 2004. Improving hospital restructuring: Lessons learned. *Health Care Management Review, 29* (4), 309–319.

Webster, G.C. and Baylis, F.E. 2000. Moral residue. In S.B. Rubin and L. Zoloth (Eds.), *Margin of error: The ethics of mistakes in the practice of medicine* (pp. 217–230). Hagerstown, MD: University Publishing Group.

Weiss, S.M., Malone, R.E., Merighi, J.R., and Benner, P. 2002. Economism, efficiency, and the moral ecology of good nursing practice. *Canadian Journal of Nursing Research, 34* (2), 95–119.

Wiskow, C., Albreht, T., and de Pietro, C. 2010. *Policy brief 15: How to create an attractive and supportive environment for health professionals*. Copenhagen, DK: World Health Organization.

Wadsworth, Y. 2001. The mirror, the magnifying glass, the compass and the map: Facilitating participatory action research. In P. Reason and H. Bradbury (Eds.), *Handbook of action research: Participatory inquiry and practice* (pp. 420–432). London: Sage.

World Health Organization. 2008a. *Closing the gap in a generation: Health equity through action on the social determinants of health*. (Final Report of the Commission on Social Determinants of Health). Geneva: Authors.

World Health Organization. 2008b. *World Health Report 2008: Primary health care: Now more than ever*. Geneva: Authors.

Wynne, R. 2003. Clinical nurses' response to an environment of health care reform and organizational restructuring. *Journal of Nursing Management, 11,* 98–106.

Zboril-Benson, L.R. 2002. Why nurses are calling in sick: The impact of health-care restructuring. *Canadian Journal of Nursing Research, 33* (4), 89–107.

CHAPTER 11

Building Moral Community: Fostering Place Ethics in Twenty-First Century Health Care Systems for a Healthier World

Patricia Marck

I had my boss come and see what's going on in the unit. . . . We don't have any storage for anything. We have commodes that are being used that no one wipes down, that no one knows whether they are fresh, clean, dirty . . . there is nobody doing that job; that's a missing piece. Or you have four beds in every room, well on top of that you don't have four beds, you've got wheelchairs, you've got four walkers, you've got four IV poles, so the rooms are so cluttered there is no ability to move people around freely. So nurses are hurting themselves, patients are falling, tripping over things, so that is a safety issue. (Social Sciences and Humanities Research Council [SSHRC] Workshop Participant 2006, Table B, Discussion 2, 10)[1]

INTRODUCTION

As this text goes to press, there is widening global consensus that environmental issues will constitute the top health concerns of the twenty-first century (Canadian Nurses Association 2009; United Nations Educational, Scientific and Cultural Organization 2009; World Medical Association 2009). A variety of professional associations have also recognized the need to reduce wasteful practices in health care and society that negatively impact environmental and human health (Association of Canadian Academic Healthcare Organizations et al. 2009; World Medical Association 2010). These long needed global developments within health care and the health professions are encouraging, as they speak to the requirement to reverse societal patterns of consumption and waste that progressively degrade the health of ecosystems, and therefore, human health (Dauvergne 2008). *However, the central thesis of this chapter is that from an ethical perspective, these movements are vital, but not sufficient.* In particular, they fail to address equally consumptive and wasteful approaches to resource allocation and service delivery within complex health systems that severely dilute our collective capacity to effectively respond to the linked concerns of ecological and human health.

The consumptive patterns of resource allocation and service delivery critiqued are evident across the continuum of care. For example, over 90 percent of Canadian health system funding is allocated to the acute care sector (Edwards and Riley 2006) where millions are lavished on a few spacious centres of excellence at the same time as three patients are squeezed into two-bed hospital rooms to accommodate chronic emergency department over-capacity.[2] In the community settings, governments continue to fund expensive, inefficient patterns of solo medical practice instead of establishing optimum numbers of primary health care teams across the continuum of care. Throughout society, the gap between rich and poor widens, and most Canadians living with challenges such as disabilities, poverty, family violence, homelessness, mental illness, or addictions are persistently marginalized (see also Chapter 18 through 21). For these citizens, there is little or no access to preventative outreach. Further, early intervention programs in homes, schools, and communities cost a fraction of what recurring emergency visits, incarcerations, and other reactive services require.

All of these paradoxes fuel deepening patterns of inequity, inefficiency, and preventable harm within Canada's "advanced" health systems, along with inevitable and considerable moral distress, as is discussed in Chapter 9. Furthermore, the shortsighted, unsustainable thinking and practices that characterize health systems are equally evident in a blinkered approach to the connections between ecological and human health. In Alberta, for example, world-class scientific research now demonstrates that problematic rates of pollution from Alberta's tar sands to surrounding air, snow pack, and water have not been adequately detected by government monitoring programs (Kelly et al. 2010). Across this land, many Aboriginal communities still await the reliable provision of such basic health determinants as safe drinking water (Westra 2008). Almost a decade after the world's first brush with Severe Acute Respiratory Syndrome (SARS) in 2002–2003, under-regulated factory farming practices in North America—as well as in many impoverished countries that are linked to the genesis of mutant microbes like the SARS coronavirus—continue unabated (Liebler et al. 2009; PEW Commission 2008; Waldvogel 2004). Clear evidence of the links between poverty, over-industrialization, and environmental devastation is ignored, as we witness human suffering across the globe that arises from related famines, wars, and forced migrations (Benatar et al. 2003; Sachs 2007; Westra 2009). *Common to all these scenarios of human and ecological loss is a repeated failure to connect the dots between how we mismanage human health and how we mismanage the health of our world.*

Perhaps it should be no surprise that ethical comportment within health systems significantly mirrors the way we comport ourselves in the wider world in several worrisome ways. Yet, if we continue to ignore our maladaptive management of health systems, it is surely naive at best to expect a markedly better approach in how we manage ecosystem health, and thus ultimately the health of all life on earth. With this twenty-first century version of a persistent "ecomedical disconnection syndrome" in view (as Whitehouse first called it in 1999) what should galvanize us is that these linked human endeavours are both in urgent need of reform. *The central message of this chapter is therefore a call to reconnect our efforts in health care and health care ethics with a more ecologically literate understanding of and respect for our place within nature* (Orr 1992), with the aim of rehabilitating the complex, reciprocal relationship between human and ecological health (Butler and Oluoch-Kosura 2006; Hansen-Ketchum et al. 2009; 2011; McMichael et al. 2008). To accomplish this reconciliation project, I argue that we need to develop an ethic of place within today's health care systems that motivates us to care for the connections between our health and the health of our world.

In calling for the adoption of *place ethics* in health care, I seek the active, democratic engagement of moral communities that share an ethical commitment to treat each other and the places they share with greater ecological wisdom (Buell 2001; Engel 1998; Higgs 2003; Marck 2004a; Marck et al. 2006a; 2008). By *ecological wisdom*, I mean the ability to "think like a system" (Gunderson et al. 2002, 19) in order to wisely conserve and use our collective resources to strengthen and sustain ecological and therefore human health. A robust place ethic is therefore both *local* and attentive to our immediate surroundings, and *global* in its attention to the ecological implications of our local actions for the wider world. It is equally global in its recognition of how under-regulated markets, proliferating production of bio-technology for profit, industrial farming, and other cross-border system phenomena can impact how health care is patterned and practised in local contexts. I contend that this form of system wisdom is largely gained through the intentional development of *ecological sensibilities* that strengthen our capacity to appreciate and nurture the reciprocal relationship between ecological and human health (Brown and Bell 2007; Hansen-Ketchum et al. 2009; Pooley and O'Connor 2000). The expansion of such sensibilities, I maintain, is essential to generating the individual and collective moral imagination we need to create more ethical ways of caring for each other and for nature, which remains our only viable home. The balance of this chapter is devoted to exploring how we might reach these ethical goals.

GENERATING PLACE ETHICS IN TWENTY-FIRST CENTURY HEALTH SYSTEMS

> Our behaviour toward the land is an eloquent and detailed expression of our character, and the land is not incapable of reflecting these statements back. We are perfectly bespoken by our surroundings . . . nobody consciously sets out to wreck a piece of land, but that is a common result of our accustomed habits of land use. (Mills 1995, 3–4)

In health systems, as in other environments, fostering a place ethic requires attention to several principles that help us to think and act in ways that are more ethically, scientifically, practically, and therefore ecologically sound (Marck 2000; 2004a; in review; Marck et al. 2008). These principles are not only adapted primarily from work in ecological restoration, nursing, and interdisciplinary health systems research, but also draw on thinking in philosophy of technology, environmental ethics, health care ethics, environmental writing, geography, and ecosystems management. The field of ecological restoration is concerned with the study, repair, and sustainability of ecosystems that have been degraded, damaged, or destroyed (Society for Ecological Restoration International 2004). Restorative endeavours incorporate knowledge from philosophy, ethics, history, anthropology, economics, the biological and ecological sciences, and other fields in order to effect lasting repairs (Higgs 1999). To assess the ecological integrity or overall health of a given ecosystem, restorationists gather information about a number of considerations, including, but not limited to:

- the diversity of life forms;
- the processes and structures for birth, growth, death, and renewal;

- the regional and historical context for socio-economic development; and
- the cultural practices that sustain or erode ethical relations within communities and with the land (Society for Ecological Restoration International 2004).

As thinkers in restoration, environmental writing, and other fields have noted, our ongoing tendency to neglect the links between ecological and human health is fuelled by a collective failure of imagination, a failure to envision the myriad ways that cultural integrity and ecological integrity are critically intertwined (Buell 2001; Higgs 2005; 2003; 1999; Marck et al. 2006b; 2008; Marck 2000; 2004b; Mills 1995). *Restoration efforts are therefore directed at strengthening local and regional relations, practices, and structures that enable living systems and their inhabitants to thrive* (Gunderson, Holling, and Light 1995; Higgs 2003; 1999a). When Mills (1995) wrote about the need to recognize how our own character shapes the character of the places we inhabit, she was drawing on decades-old counsel from conservationist Aldo Leopold, who urged his fellow American citizens in 1949 to "think like the mountain" instead of "thinking like a clear cut logging operation". Essentially, Leopold argued that when we "think like" instead of "look at" the over-harvested mountain, we regain a sense of the vulnerable state we have created with our excessive exploitation and consumption, and begin to re-experience the mountain landscape as a home place that we need to re-inhabit in ways that are more ethically and scientifically sound. We notice the deepening damage of excessive logging, including lost topsoil, declining species, proliferating pulp mills, and polluted rivers, and we recognize complex connections between our own health and the health of the land. Principles of good restoration therefore stimulate us to ask: *What relations and practices foster the integrity and sustainability of the communities and places we share?*

If we want to tap in to the wisdom of restoration to strengthen the integrity and sustainability of health care environments, distinguishing between technically proficient as opposed to good restorations is critical. Specifically, Higgs (1999) notes that in technically efficient restoration projects such as cosmetic repairs to an industrial park, practitioners tend to "green" the landscape of a damaged ecosystem without actually arresting underlying pollution, waste, and other environmental decay. In contrast, he asserts, practitioners who seek good, lasting restorations must work to address fundamental ethical issues of excessive industrialization and pollution, over-extraction of natural resources, and consumptive human habits. However, Higgs (1999) proposes that several technological tendencies within contemporary society favour the execution of transient technical repairs over the completion of restorations that are more ethically and scientifically sound. These tendencies include

- a pervasive "cult of efficiency" that automatically favours the achievement of short-term efficiencies over more sustainable levels of production and benefit (eco-efficiency) for the longer term;
- a relentless "speed-up" of activity characterized by an excessive pace, volume, and fragmentation of human work; and
- an insidious form of "reverse adaptation" (Winner 1977) to the pressures of efficiency, speed-up, and fragmentation where people focus more on the rapid performance of

disjointed tasks than on the fundamental goals that the work was originally intended to achieve (Marck 2000; 2004a; 2004b).

As one senior manager articulates in a study we conducted that was funded by the Social Sciences and Humanities Research Council (SSHRC), the technological tendencies that threaten good restorations are equally evident in the acute care environment that she navigates every day:

> . . . [T]he re-engineering language of the 1990s was full of things like just-in-time staffing, okay, and maximum output, and we are oppressed in the acute care with the maximum throughput, which means maximum volume possible of elective patients in and out as fast as possible. So even the language conveys that same expectation of not optimum or sustainable, but maximum; we are always trying to operate at the maximum. (SSHRC Participant, 2006, Table D, Discussion 1, 7)

Higgs (1999) notes that, at root, achieving good restoration is fundamentally an ethical endeavour that "requires at the outset a clarity about goals: What are we after?" (19). Urging us to resist the toxic effects of technological tendencies on restoration practice, Higgs (1999) calls for an "ethical counterpoise" that includes more communal management of the land, a much more sustainable pace of resource consumption, and the re-development of cultural practices that nurture each other and the places we call home. These principles require us to *respect and seek the wisdom* of indigenous community members who carry local knowledge about the history and nature of a particular place; *engage* in individual and communal practices that nourish and sustain our surroundings; and *actively resist* factory farming, non-biodegradable packaging, drive-only neighbourhoods, and other consumptive tendencies within our technological societies that threaten our ecological and human health. In other words, sustaining ecological integrity (and therefore, ecosystem and human health) requires us to act with individual and communal integrity that can serve as an ethical counterpoise to a consumptive technological world (see also Exhibit 11-1).

EXHIBIT 11.1

Matters of Integrity in Place Ethics

- From a restoration perspective, matters of **integrity** refer to both **cultural integrity** (individual–personal, individual–professional, collective–professional, communal, organizational, system, and societal) and **ecological integrity** (of local surroundings, larger ecosystems, and the earth). In all of these scenarios, critical concerns of integrity include those discussed by philosophers, such as sustaining wholeness and soundness, and preserving fundamental characteristics in an uncorrupted, unimpaired condition

(Cox, La Caze and Levine 2008). Integrity in this sense is necessary for health and healing throughout interwoven cycles of human–ecological life (Marck 2004a).

- For better and for worse, **cultural integrity** and **ecological integrity** reciprocally shape each other within the places we co-inhabit, and within the larger world (Higgs 2005). The degree to which we perpetuate ecologically harmful patterns of consumption and waste within our communities is reflected in the social, economic, and health inequities that we tolerate within our societies and around the globe. The degree to which we live in more ecologically literate and therefore more equitable ways with each other is reflected in corresponding improvements to the conditions of the communities and ecosystems that are the source of health for us and our world.

• The **healing capacities** of people and their environments refer to the potential for adaptive responses to a variety of threats in order to recover conditions that are more whole (Marck 2004a). Healing does not disrupt or prevent progression through cycles of life, for ecosystems or for people. As indigenous peoples have always understood (Battiste 1996; Tuhiwai Smith 1999) and the ecological sciences have demonstrated (Gunderson and Holling 2002; Gunderson, Holling, and Light 1995), the way of nature is birth, growth, death, and renewal. Ecologically speaking, then, achieving health for all relies on developing accountable patterns of consumption that equitably reflect our respective human place within larger cycles of ecosystem life.

When we contemplate the growing gaps between elite, gated "communities" and neglected inner city neighbourhoods, or between a select few centres of excellence and the rest of our care environments, the parallel technological tendencies that characterize the corporate greening of degraded ecosystems and the corporate redesigns of today's health systems become apparent. Across recurring waves of technically driven health systems re-engineering, resource allocations to environmental health, public health, community outreach, mental health, home care, continuing care, and assisted living remain heavily outweighed by the funding pocket for acute care (Edwards and Riley 2006). Stressful work environments, nursing workforce attrition, and related shortages of health care professionals also remain prevalent (Canadian Health Services Research Foundation 2006; Rodney et al. 2009; see also Chapters 9 and 10). As we struggle with the short-lived material efficiencies of episodic workforce cuts and the accelerating ecological deficiencies of our turbulent health systems, we can use Higgs' (1999) observations about restoration work to ask: What are we after in health care? Can we use the development of deeper ecological sensibilities and more ecologically literate moral imaginations to create and sustain places within health systems and within ecosystems that heal? These, and related questions (see Exhibit 11-2), ask us to critique our current ethically deficient patterns of health system re-engineering in order to find a path forward to more equitable and sustainable health system reform.

EXHIBIT 11-2

Place Ethics for System Healing: Guiding Questions for Reflection

1. **What are equitable goals of health and healing** for people, families, communities, populations, and the places we share?
2. **What forms of integrity are at risk** (personal, professional, ethical, scientific, ecological, systemic) in the way we currently manage health systems, and in what ways are they at risk?
3. **How do we activate each other's moral imaginations** to collectively envision

feasible paths toward better ecological (which includes human) health?

4. **What moral violations must be prevented or addressed** to safeguard the integrity of people and the places they share?

5. **What strengthens our capacities** to maintain individual and systemic integrity, recognize and resolve inequities, prevent or redress moral violations, and further the goals of healing care?

CREATING HEALING PLACES: A RESTORATIVE TASK

. . . [I]t was a different place to come to in January . . . it seemed to progress over the year; it just turned around, with these orientations. To me, it appeared that they started to see that their voice mattered and they were so welcoming to the students. And they were so willing to teach them and it just was really nice to see the turnaround from September to April. [When] we ended off [in April], it was a completely different unit than September. (Participant F802)[3]

Recently, one of our Alberta research teams completed a project to create a joint faculty–hospital clinical learning unit (CLU) in a busy, inner-city ward that serves a high population of complex, vulnerable medical patients (Marck et al. 2010). Drawing on socio-ecological thinking from restoration and other sources, we used a participatory research approach with senior administration, funding partners, unit personnel, faculty, and students to collaboratively create a place where everyone could practise and learn together as one engaged patient care team. Among other goals, we sought to enhance student and staff learning opportunities, strengthen clinical leadership, reduce staff and faculty turnover, conserve scarce faculty and staff resources, and provide quality care. In sum, we wanted to create a safe place to learn about, give, and receive care (see also Chapter 10).

Even though our CLU unit underwent a precipitous, turbulent health system de-regionalization along with the rest of the province just as we proceeded with implementation (Lewis 2011), we achieved all of our aims. With diverse voices, participants have indicated that the unit is a different place than before it became a CLU. Practitioners, students, and faculty are all willing to teach and learn from each other, and all report that they feel like valued members of one team. Patients and families express satisfaction with their care. There are cost savings in that there is less staff turnover and lower absenteeism than on any other medical unit. Others want to join the CLU, or create a CLU of their own. Everyone from senior leaders to faculty, staff, and students articulates that they have stronger relationships with each other across the organizations than they experienced before the CLU, and everyone wants to see the CLU concept spread to other care environments (Marck et al. 2010). Another offshoot of the project was the attainment of subsequent provincial funding to create three inter-professional CLUs for a rehabilitation hospital, an acute hospital stroke unit, and a continuing care setting that are now also in operation.[4]

As we evaluate the project approach and outcomes in order to support the future spread of CLUs across the continuum of care, it is clear that we heightened our ecological sensibilities toward our pilot unit by attending to several principles of good restoration. In particular:

1. *We acknowledged the value of striving for eco-efficiency in every aspect of our work.* We are all too familiar with the "doing more with less" ethos that permeates the short-lived

efficiencies of so many health care re-engineering initiatives. In contrast, good restorations aim for true eco-efficiency, which is characterized by investing sufficient social, economic, and other forms of capital at the right times to achieve longer-term, sustainable goals. For instance, time that organizations might otherwise expend on separate endeavours to improve staff or student practice was instead deliberately spent on building intra-organizational relationships oriented toward the common goal of improving the practice environment for students and staff. Similarly, both organizations collaborated on grant writing to gain funds to purchase computers for student and staff learning. The longer-term efficiencies that were realized included savings in human, intellectual, and economic capital as staff turnover decreased, several team members sought further education related to their clinical roles, and students and faculty enhanced their ability to contribute to the provision of care.

2. *We understood the need to cross boundaries.* Building on previous experiences of intra-organizational collaboration to make eco-efficient use of our shared resources to provide student research experiences (Marck et al. 2007), provide ethics education (Marck 2006), and conduct collaborative research (Marck et al. 2006b; 2008; 2010;), we recognized that creating a different clinical environment for faculty, students, staff, leaders, and patients was a shared enterprise. Our shared enterprise required us to design, fund, and conduct the research as one team. This principle of cross-fertilization between communities, organizations, people, and cultures to support the repair and renewal of habitats is well recognized in the fields of ecosystems management (Gunderson and Holling 2000; Gunderson, Holling, and Light 1995) and restoration (Higgs 2005). As all parties invested their intellectual and social capital into the work, our strengthened relationships built new bridges between our organizations (Hofmeyer and Marck 2008) that continue to thrive.

3. *We valued the centrality of indigenous knowledge.* Community members' local knowledge of the places they share provides essential wisdom that we need to take care of each other and our world. Places, and the people who inhabit them together, carry rich stories that illuminate important historical, contextualized understanding of what was, what is, and what could be. Respecting and nurturing this narrative, continuity of places and their inhabitants is key to building sufficient moral community to preserve what matters in the face of inevitable threats and ongoing systems change (Higgs 2003). Indigenous knowledge provides a critical counter-balance to global technological knowledge by forcing us to contextualize general evidence and policy to specific places. As such, *indigenous knowledge is de-colonizing knowledge* that does not privilege generalizable scientific knowledge over particularized knowledge, but rather uses a community's place sense to thoughtfully determine how and when other forms of knowledge may be ethically applied in order to progress (Cypher and Higgs 1997; Marck in review). To honour the narrative continuity of a hospital CLU whose past included a diploma school of nursing that closed in the 1990s, we discussed with unit staff how we could best respect the past of their unit, learning from that history to strengthen future clinical experiences for everyone concerned. As Higgs notes,

good restorations always seeks and attends to the story of a place over time, because "the depth of our engagement with a place depends on our connections both forward and backward in time" (2003, p. 285). This valuing and remembering of the unit's history allowed us to plan as a community how we could incorporate the close clinical mentoring, teamwork, and pride of identity that were viewed as significant parts of their past hospital-based nursing program into our future CLU.

4. *We expected that cultural integrity and ecological integrity would co-evolve.* As we tackled the task of creating a shared culture by inviting patients, staff, students, and faculty to tell us their vision of a good unit and then using those findings to collectively design and implement the CLU with joint faculty and staff orientations, we watched a better place come into being. We were proceeding on the premise that as people develop a heightened awareness and understanding of the character of a place, they more deeply appreciate what matters for that place, and why (Buell 1995; Higgs 1999; 2003; Worster 1984). As that appreciation grows, so does their shared attachment to that place and to each other. From such simple steps as students and staff sitting beside each other at nursing report to more challenging activities such as conducting collaborative Ethics in Practice sessions (see Ethics in Practice 11-1), we were intentionally building the kinds of equitable and sustainable relationships that we need in health care *and* in our world.

ETHICS IN PRACTICE 11-1

"Please Let Me Go"

I am a third-year nursing student on this medical unit. I am asked by my instructor to search for the agency policy regarding restraints, as my patient for the week has a restraints order. Mr. F. is an 88-year-old male, with an admitting diagnosis of delirium not yet diagnosed. He also has a history of aphasia (stroke), cardiac arrhythmias, hypertension, COPD, and renal failure. He is not violent or aggressive and poses no immediate threat to himself and or others. During report the previous week, we are told that when he is not restrained, Mr. F. pulls off his condom catheter and urinates on the floor. I check the site policy, but it is somewhat vague regarding the criteria, procedure, assessment, and discontinuing the use of restraints. The other document I find is a mental health services policy that specifically states the patient is to be assessed frequently and restraints re-ordered

every 24 hours. I then check the professional association's position statement, which indicates that all other options should be exhausted before the initiation of restraints (College and Association of Registered Nurses of Alberta 2009). The next day while I care for Mr. F., my instructor supports my decision to leave Mr. F. unrestrained except when he is left alone for long periods of time. However, when I leave at the end of my shift, I still have many concerns and questions:

- Why is the local information regarding the criteria for, assessment of, and discontinuation for the use of restraints so vague and inexact, and why does it conflict with current professional association policy?
- Is this a case of choosing convenience over appropriate patient care? Are we

worried about patient safety, or about having to clean up urine?
- Have we really explored all other avenues for providing safe care to Mr. F. other than restraints?

- *What could happen if Mr. F. is left unattended for long periods of time and is unable to reach a call bell, or gets tangled up, or soils himself, or needs a drink?*

Using place ethics to explore the ethical dilemmas illustrated in Ethics in Practice 11-1 with students, faculty, staff nurses, clinical educators, and managers allows us to uncover many other salient details about the conditions that give rise to questionable restraint practices in acute care settings. Specifically, when we explore our goals for care, we recognize that along with fundamental goals of ensuring safety and preventing harm, we seek to ensure that Mr. F. experiences respect, maintains his dignity, and is able to trust in the relationships that he has with the health care team. If we then ask what kinds of integrity are at stake (Exhibit 11-1) in considering the use of restraints, we realize that Mr. F.'s personal integrity, our professional integrity, and the integrity of the organization and the system within which we work are all at risk should our decisions to restrain Mr. F. be less than thoroughly ethically justifiable. It becomes clear in our discussion that the use of restraints can violate a client's dignity, trust, and safety, motivating us to activate each other's moral imaginations to ask things like: What funds (if any) are available for hospitals to provide desirable environmental modifications and appropriate equipment (e.g., comfortable, safe, geriatric chairs) that current research recommends for a growing population of older hospitalized patients (Parke and Friesen 2010)? What can we do as a unit to ensure that we obtain the necessary resources, education, and policy to deliver safe care to older patients? When will health systems fund sufficient access to alternate levels of care so that elderly people who do not benefit from acute care treatment can be transferred to home or continuing care settings with adequate supports? Furthermore, in the absence of the optimum resources and environments for acute care of the elderly, what is the most ethical way to treat those who are in our care? *Pursuing potential responses to such questions allows us to explore various theoretical concepts that are critical to place ethics, such as building community, developing place sense, and using ethical problems to create adaptive learning and growth.*

The thinking, relations, and practices we adopted in the CLU project and related research all share one common critical feature. Specifically, by adopting common goals that are more ecologically literate, we become one moral community across organizational, educational, funding, and other borders, using our collective moral imagination to resourcefully take better care of each other and the places we share. As we widen our imagination, we expand our moral horizon (Rodney et al. 2002) in terms of what we can envision for health and health care. This kind of citizen science (Marck 2006; Marck et al. 2008) is a post-colonial form of health systems research (Gregory 2005)—one that aims to abide by similar principles as those articulated by Tuhiwai Smith (1999), Battiste (1996), and Browne and colleagues (2005) for research with First Nations peoples. The principles are ones of valuing partnerships and the voice of the community, conducting praxis-oriented inquiry, respecting how history shapes our present and potential futures, and recognizing and guarding against "the colonizing potential of research" that does not adequately honour the knowledge and culture of those whom science is intended to serve (Browne et al. 2005, 16). *In other words, just as we need to decolonize our thinking about and work with Aboriginal peoples in oppressive societies, we need to decolonize our thinking about and work with practice communities in oppressive technological systems, if we hope to move forward together into healthier places and better health care.*

EXPANDING MORAL HORIZONS: FOSTERING ECOLOGICALLY LITERATE MORAL IMAGINATIONS TO STRENGTHEN SYSTEMS OF CARE

The first commandment for living successfully in nature—living for the long term at the highest possible level of moral development—is to understand how the round river and its watershed work together and to adapt our behaviour accordingly. Taking a narrow economic attitude toward water, on the other hand, is the surest way to fail in that understanding. (Worster 1984, 57)

When Stan Worster wrote his critique of industrialized farming practices in 1984, he was imploring readers to recognize that when we fail to adequately imagine the moral consequences of our habits of production and consumption, both the river and those who draw on it for sustenance will pay. Restoration scholars Jennifer Cypher and Eric Higgs argue that consumer societies are characterized by a technological "colonization of the imagination" (1997, 107) that encourages us to content ourselves with, if not actively favour, artificial facsimiles of, rather than actual experiences of, real wilderness (Borgmann 1984; Cypher and Higgs 1997; Higgs 1999; 2003). They further assert that these repressed ways of thinking accelerate the degree of disconnect between man and nature that I and others critique (Borgmann 1984; Hansen-Ketchum et al. 2009; Higgs 1999; 2003; Potter 1999; Whitehouse 1999). Re-establishing connections between the moral and the ecological helps us to see again how the world actually works, and therefore, to re-imagine how we could and should endeavour to work with it, as opposed to simply satisfying ourselves with "making it work" for the achievement of short-sighted, unsustainable, inequitable ends.

To inhabit the earth with an ethically robust sense of nature and our place within it is to use our moral imaginations to exercise good *ecological citizenship*, working with human and natural systems in participatory, place-aware, equitable ways that promote the attainment of ecological sustainability and hence, health for all. To continue to occupy the world in our current state of nature deficit disorder (Louv 2008) is to preside over the decline of our earth while taking no adequate steps toward fundamental reform. In discussing Thoreau's study of the economy of Walden Pond, Buell (1995) notes that before the term *ecology* was coined in 1866, the word *economy* was its closest pre-scientific synonym. Can we really afford to incur more false economies like the massive layoffs of the 90s in the absence of fundamental primary health care reform—the same short-sighted and even shorter-lived "efficiencies" that now fuel escalating overtime, illness, injury, and attrition in the health care workforce and growing issues with access to appropriate, timely care? Is it not past time to consider how a more eco-efficient health care system might operate, and to set about a course for making it so? To continue with Worster's observations about the care of water sources for sustainable farming:

> In a strictly economic appraisal, water becomes merely the commodity H_2O, bulked here as capital to invest some day, spent freely when the market is high. It comes to be seen as a "cash flow," no longer as the lifeblood of the land. Then we begin to do foolish things with our streams and rivers, such as diverting creeks and altering flows with no understanding of the long-term consequences. . . . The elementary need in learning how to farm water effectively, Leopold would have said, is to stop thinking about the problem exclusively as economists and engineers and to begin learning the logic of the river. (1996, 58)

Carl Elliott asserts that the profits at stake in the health care marketplace mean that too many who work in bioethics are subject to increasingly problematic influences on their work, and cautions against practising bioethics as a bureaucratic exercise in service of the "new machine" of modern technological health care (2005, 379). Arguing that it is easier to respond to questions on a corporate health care agenda about how technologies should be used than to carry out the intellectual work of raising important ethical questions about *who is served* by the current system, he urges ethicists to ask themselves what their work should be about at its core, and for whom. If our work in health care ethics is about *equity* rather than about the commodification of health, surely our most urgent task is to attend to the wisdom of First Nations elders who have warned us repeatedly that our health, and our efficient use of resources to support health, will improve in direct relation to the extent that we are willing to take care of the health of our world (Matthew 2000).

However, we cannot achieve what we cannot envision. To liberate our imaginations from the bureaucratic confines of technologically colonized health care systems, we may first need to focus on actively re-engaging with nature (Hansen-Ketchum et al. 2009) if we hope to become capable of recovering a deeper, decolonized understanding of the most pressing ethical questions in an over-industrialized, ecologically neglected world. Fortunately, as a vital form of engaging with nature, participating in ecological restoration is one of the best ways to nourish one's own moral imagination as well as the health of the land. As Higgs observes: "By restoring ecosystems we regenerate old ways or create new ones that bring us closer to natural processes and to one another. This is the power and promise of ecological restoration" (2003, 2). Whether it is clearing debris from a city park, creating community gardens from abandoned urban spaces, or other nourishing acts of ecological citizenship, perhaps we need to take part in restorations to open the necessary space in our hearts, our minds, and our health systems for place ethics to take root and thrive.

LOCATING PLACE ETHICS IN THE HEALTH CARE ETHICS LANDSCAPE

Significant overlap and synergy is evident between various tenets of place ethics and one or more other theoretical "places" within the landscape of nursing and health care ethics. Yet there are some important distinctions. In many ways, place ethics (along with several other ethical schools of thinking) can, when considered in concert, enrich the way that we think ethically about nursing and health care. If, as Sherwin (1999) suggests, we benefit from applying a range of theoretical lenses to any given ethical scenario, a discussion of theoretical linkages and gaps is warranted here (see also Chapters 4 and 5 for a review of ethical theory per se).

Beginning with the more obvious differences, in comparison with other ethical theories that are more focused either on the consequences of individual actions (consequentialism), the intentions of individual actions (deontology), or the moral character of individual agents (virtue ethics), *place ethics* is much more concerned with our collective commitment and actions as fellow citizens with responsibilities to the places we share. Some scholars have used virtue ethics as a way to approach environmental ethics, arguing that first and foremost, how we treat the environment is a reflection of how moral we are as people (Sandler 2007), an argument that place ethics would not dispute (see also Chapter 18 for a discussion of virtue ethics as applied to organizations). *Where place ethics and environmental virtue ethics may diverge is on the locus for change to advance their shared aim of improving ecosystem health.* Specifically, while the arguments in environmental virtue ethics may largely focus on the nature of and reason for embracing the virtue of taking better care of the earth (Sandler 2007), the focus in place ethics is more directed toward outlining what we can do as citizens and communities to achieve that goal.

Moving onto other areas of meaningful theoretical convergence, there is substantive overlap between *place ethics* and *narrative ethics* as ways to understand what is ethically at stake. For place ethics as for narrative ethics, story matters because of what is told, how it is told, and why (Charon and Montello 2002; Jones 1999; see also Chapter 6 in this book). However, whereas narrative ethics largely concentrates on narratives of individual experience, place ethics draws on the stories that individuals tell about a place that matters to them as members of that same community. The focus in the latter form of narrative is on what this place means to us, and in what ways, and why—and therefore, what we owe to each other and to it as citizens of this place. In seeking out those stories of place, we also glean a great deal about individual experiences, but the focus is on developing narrative continuity or understanding over time about a whole community as opposed to a particular person. In both forms of inquiry, though, some picture of the culture that shapes the storytellers emerges, as does some sense of the relationships that may be important.

Questions of culture and relationships bring us to other ethical perspectives that share important links with place ethics, including *communitarian* ethics and *relational* ethics. In the case of communitarian ethics, the salient commonality is the recognition of the importance of culture and shared values in shaping both individual and communal actions (Bellah 1985; Etzioni 1998). The distinction between place ethics and communitarianism, however, is that the emphasis in the latter perspective is on achieving human well-being through communal values and action, whereas the emphasis in place ethics is on understanding and acting upon the reciprocal nature of human–ecological well-being. In the case of relational ethics, the most critical intersection is the recognition that how we treat each other fundamentally creates the environment within which we live out our ethical commitments (Bergum and Dossetor 2005; see also Chapters 7 and 8). Another key area of agreement between relational and place ethics is that an adequate ethics in health care must be an ecological one (Bergum 2004). Perhaps the greatest distinction between these closely linked schools of thinking is that relational ethics devotes most of its theorizing to how we can engage with one another to live out our ethical commitments to each other and to the environment, whereas *place ethics tends to devote the bulk of its theorizing to how we can collectively engage with nature in order to concurrently live out our ethical obligations to each other and to the places we share.*

A strong degree of overlap for place ethics with other schools of ethical thinking is also found in ethical theories focused on *equity* and *social justice*. Strong critiques of neoliberal approaches to the economic governance of public goods are common to both equity and ecological ethical lenses (Abassi 1999; Damian and Graz 2001; Higgs 2003; Marck 2000; Ostrum et al. 1999; see also Chapters 18 through 21). In related lines of thinking, concerns for ecological integrity and for social justice have been integrated in examining the rights of indigenous peoples (Westra 2009), the rights of ecological refugees (Westra 2008), and north-south inequities (Westra and Lawson 2001). These schools of ethical thinking may share the most common ground with place ethics in their similar critical stances toward the links between unfettered market economics, excessive consumption in high-income countries, the suppression of civic dialogue that questions global profiteering, and the attendant damage to people and their environments. The most significant distinction between the social justice theorists and place ethics advocates may be the emphasis on human rights in the former lines of inquiry as opposed to the emphasis on ecological obligations in the latter.

The decolonizing aspirations of place ethics also share common *post-colonial* ground with critical theoretical and eco-feminist conceptions of equity and health in contemporary technological societies. For example, there are critical theoretical works in the environmental literature that focus debate on how to democratize and therefore transform the design, uses, and potential benefits of technology in an over-industrialized world (Feenberg 1995; 1999; 2002; 2010; Feenberg and Hannay 1995). There are also critical social analyses within health care that focus on democratizing how we generate and use knowledge within oppressive systems in order to emancipate marginalized groups and generate better health for all (Anderson et al. 2009; 2010; Varcoe and Rodney 2009). In the feminist literature, there are eco-feminists who focus debate on how to recognize and alter oppressive social relationships within patriarchal societies (Chircop 2007; Cuomo 1998; McGuire 1998). In all of these schools of thinking there are shared vital concerns with the problematic linkages between power relations in hierarchical societies, knowledge development and use, and the exploitation of oppressed groups and their environments.

ADVANCING PLACE ETHICS: CHARTING A PATH TO REINHABITATION

Restoration is about accepting the brokenness of things, and investigating the emergent properties of healing. It's the closing of the frontier—ceasing our demand for open land to "develop"—and the reinhabiting of exploited or abandoned places. (Mills 1995, 2)

... what we need to do is help maintain the processes and the elements of the system and they are going to become something new in the future from their own roots, they are the source of their own future. (SSHRC Participant, 2006, Table C, Discussion 1, 11).

The thesis I advance in this chapter is that sustainability issues, along with many of the moral problems and related suffering in health care that currently challenge governments, health professionals, and the communities they serve, are deeply rooted in our persistent neglect of vital connections between our own health and integrity and that of the places we inhabit (Hansen-Ketchum et al. 2009; 2011; Marck 2000; 2004a; in review; Marck et al. 2008). I contend that this neglect represents a collective failure of moral imagination, which results in a deficient communal ethical vision for twenty-first century health systems and for all of the consumptive landscapes that are evident in a technologically over-determined world. The ecological critique that is advanced within place ethics overlaps with several other important schools of ethical thinking that share compatible decolonizing and emancipatory aims. *To counter the impact of our impoverished approaches to both contemporary health systems and ecosystems, we need to enact a communal place ethic that encourages us to reimagine and rebalance the technology and ecology of our endangered world.*

In health systems and in life, it often seems that we act as if our ecological future is something out of our hands, a problem beyond our capacity to effectively address. Yet, as part of nature, we and the complex systems we inhabit are the source of our own future. In a recent editorial about challenges to safety and quality of health care in today's complex health systems, Justin Thomas and Paul Cosford observe that "the issue is not whether health systems throughout the world community can afford to embrace sustainability but whether they can afford not to" (2010, 261). As a way to think about health care ethics and its role in the world, place ethics is not so much a single theory or model for understanding ethical issues in health and health care, as it is a rehabilitated way of seeing, understanding, and being in the world through a recovered connection with nature. As we rehabilitate our relationship with nature, we restore better relations with each other and our world. We can learn again original knowledge that indigenous peoples around the world have handed down through the generations despite successive waves of colonization: the wisdom that this earth is our home, with everything we need to create health, should we be willing to live with it and each other in ways that are more equitable, respectful, and just. This traditional ecological knowledge can help us to resist successive waves of colonization in re-engineered health systems and energize us to question and reimagine what we actually need to do to create health for all.

Summary

As with many schools of ethical thinking, place ethics may be easy to admire, less easy to fully imagine, and much more difficult to practise and critique in our daily work and lives. Enacting a full commitment to place ethics is, like restoration itself, "a work in progress—never finished, never 'corrected'" (Table A, Discussion 1, 1).While many with a stake in health care may be initially drawn to a place ethic by its promise of improving the eco-efficiency and sustainability of tomorrow's health systems, there is a much deeper and even more vital reason to continue exploring the potential for place ethics in the years ahead. That reason is to rediscover more ethical relations with each other as we reestablish more ethically justifiable relations with the places we share.

For Reflection

1. Do you see symptoms of nature deficit disorder in yourself, your fellow students and co-workers, or your community? Do you see evidence of nature deficit disorder in our society or our health system? Can you give some examples?

2. Have you encountered an ethical dilemma in your own practice where you feel that place ethics and related concepts could have helped you with your analysis, decisions, and/or actions? If your answer is yes, describe how you think that this form of thinking could assist your approach. If your answer is no, can you say why?

3. What do you see as the biggest barriers to thinking ecologically in health care? In our society? In our global community?

4. How do you think nurses and other health care professionals can work together with individuals, communities, populations, and institutions to foster place ethics and ecological citizenship in health care? What are the implications for public health? (See also Chapter 20.)

Endnotes

1. The content of this chapter draws on a variety of insights gained during the past nine years while conducting an ongoing program of interdisciplinary research on the ethics, safety, and quality of health care (see Safer Systems research program at http://www.nurs.ualberta.ca/SaferSystems/index.htm). This particular quote and others in this chapter are excerpted from research supported by Social Sciences & Humanities Research Council Grant # 410-2006-2163 HREB#B-220606: *Through the eyes of practitioners: Re-imagining and re-storying medication safety with photographic research* (P.B. Marck, Principal Investigator).

2. For extensive discussions of the Canadian health care system, see Chapters 12, 18, 19, and 20.

3. This participant quote is excerpted from the following research: Grant # N12100032 HREB#121009: *Transforming clinical learning environments for undergraduate nursing students: The piloting and evaluation of a collaborative clinical learning unit (2008–2011).* P.B. Marck (principal investigator) and S. Barton (co-principal investigator); R. Day, S. Gushue, K. Bulmer-Smith, L. Kemp, K. Martin, K. Peterson, J. Worrell (co-investigators). Funding: University of Alberta, Teaching and Learning Enhancement Fund ($147 962.69); University of Alberta Faculty of Nursing & Royal Alexandra Hospital, Alberta Health Services ($67 586.00).

4. For more information on the Interprofessional Clinica Learning Units see http://www.ipclu.ca/.

References

Abassi, K. 1999. The world bank and health. *British Medical Journal, 318,* 1132–1135.

Anderson, J.M., Browne, A.J., Reimer-Kirkham, S., Lynam, M. J., Rodney, P. and Varcoe, C. et al. 2010. Uptake of critical knowledge in nursing practice: Lessons learned from a knowledge translation study. *Canadian Journal of Nursing Research, 42* (3), 106–122.

Anderson, J.M., Rodney, P., Reimer-Kirkham, S., Browne, A.J., Koushambhi, B.K., and Lynam, M.J. 2009. Inequities in health and healthcare viewed through the ethical lens of critical social justice: Contextual knowledge for the global priorities ahead. *Advances in Nursing Science, 32* (4), 282–294.

Association of Canadian Academic Healthcare Organizations, Canadian Association of Physicians for the Environment, Canadian Coalition for Green Health Care, Canadian College of Health Services Executives, Canadian Dental Association, Canadian Health Care Association, Canadian Health Care Engineering Society, Canadian Medical Association, Canadian Nurses Association, Canadian Pharmacists Association, Canadian Public Health Association, David Suzuki Foundation, and National Specialty Society for Community Medicine. 2009. *Joint position statement. Toward an environmentally responsible Canadian health sector.* Ottawa: Author.

Battiste, M. 1996. *Reclaiming indigenous voice and vision.* Seattle, WA: University of Washington Press.

Bellah, R., Madsen, R., Sullivan, W.M., Swidler, A., and Tipton, S.M. 1985. *Habits of the heart.* Berkeley: University of California Press.

Benatar, S.R., Daar, A.S., and Singer, P.A. 2003. Global health ethics: The rationale for mutual caring. *International Affairs, 79* (1), 107–138.

Bergum, V. 2004. Relational ethics in nursing. In J. Storch, P. Rodney, and R. Starzomski (Eds), *Toward a moral horizon: Nursing ethics for leadership and practice* (pp. 485–503). Toronto, ON: Pearson Prentice Hall.

Bergum, V. and Dossetor, J. 2005. *Relational ethics. The full meaning of respect.* Hagerstown, MD: University Publishing Group.

Borgmann, A. 1984. *Technology and the character of contemporary life. A philosophical inquiry.* Chicago: University of Chicago Press.

Brown, T. and Bell, M. 2007. Off the couch and on the move: Global public health and the medicalisation of nature. *Social Science and Medicine, 64* (6), 1343–1354.

Browne, A.J., Smye, V.L., and Varcoe, C. 2005. The relevance of postcolonial theoretical perspectives to research in Aboriginal health. *Canadian Journal of Nursing Research, 37* (4), 16–37.

Buell, L. 1995. *The environmental imagination. Thoreau, nature writing and the formation of American culture.* Cambridge, MA: The Belknap Press of Harvard University Press.

Buell, L. 2001. *Writing for an endangered world. Literature, culture, and environment in the U.S. and beyond.* Cambridge, MA: The Belknap Press of Harvard University Press.

Butler, C.D. and Oluoch-Kosura, W. 2006. Linking future ecosystem services and future human well-being. *Ecology and Society, 11* (1), 30.

Canadian Health Services Research Foundation 2006. *What's ailing our nurses? A discussion of the major issues affecting nursing human resources in Canada.* Ottawa, ON: Author. Available at http://www.chsrf.ca/Migrated/PDF/What_sailingourNurses-e.pdf.

Canadian Nurses Association. 2009. *Position statement: Climate change and health.* Ottawa, ON: Author.

Charon, R. and Montello, M. 2002. *Stories matter: The role of narrative in medical ethics.* New York, NY: Routledge Press.

Chircop, A. 2007. An ecofeminist conceptual framework to explore gendered environmental health inequities in urban settings and to inform healthy public policy. *Nursing Inquiry 15* (2): 135–147.

College and Association of Registered Nurses of Alberta. 2009. *Position statement on the use of restraints in client care settings*. Edmonton, AB: Author.

Cox, D., La Caze, M. and Levine, M, 2008. Integrity, *The Stanford Encyclopedia of Philosophy (Fall 2008 Edition)*, Edward N. Zalta (ed.), URL = <http://plato.stanford.edu/archives/fall2008/entries/integrity/>.

Cuomo, C. 1998. *Feminism and ecological communities*. New York, NY: Routledge Press.

Cypher, J. and Higgs, E.S. 1997. Colonizing the imagination: Disney's wilderness lodge. *Capitalism, Nature, Socialism. A Journal of Socialist Ecology, 8,* (4), 107–130.

Damian, M. and Graz, J.C. 2001. The world trade organization, the environment, and the ecological critique. *International Social Sciences Journal, 53* (170), 597–610.

Dauvergne, P. 2008. *The shadows of consumption: Consequences for the global environment*. Boston, MA: MIT Press.

Edwards, N. and Riley, B. 2006. Can we develop waiting lists for public health? *Canadian Medical Association Journal, 174* (6), 794–796.

Elliott, C. 2005. The soul of a new machine: Bioethicists in the bureaucracy. *Cambridge Quarterly of Healthcare Ethics, 14,* 379–384.

Engel, J.G. 1998. Who are democratic ecological citizens? *Hastings Center Report, 28* (6), S23–S30.

Etzioni, A. 1998. *The essential communitarian reader*. Lanham: Rowman & Littlefield.

Feenberg, A. 1995. *Alternative modernity. The technical turn in philosophy and social theory*. Berkeley, CA: University of California Press.

Feenberg, A. 1999. *Questioning technology*. New York, NY: Routledge Press.

Feenberg, A. 2002. *Transforming technology. Second edition of critical theory of technology*. Cambridge, MA: Oxford University Press.

Feenberg, A. 2010. *Between reason and experience: Essays in technology and modernity*. Cambridge, MA: MIT Press.

Feenberg, A. and Hannay, A. (Eds.). 1995. *Technology and the politics of knowledge*. Bloomington, IN: Indiana University Press.

Gregory, D. 2005. Aboriginal health and nursing research: Postcolonial theoretical perspectives. *Canadian Journal of Nursing Research, 37* (4), 11–15.

Gunderson, L., Folke, C., Lee, M., and Holling, C.S. 2002. In memory of mavericks. *Conservation Ecology, 6* (2), 19.

Gunderson, L.H. and Holling, C.S. 2002. *Panarchy: Understanding transformations in human and natural systems*. Washington, DC: Island Press.

Gunderson, L.H., Holling, C.S., and Light, S.S. (Eds.). 1995. *Barriers and bridges to the renewal of ecosystems and institutions*. New York, NY: Columbia University Press.

Hansen-Ketchum, P., Marck, P.B., and Reutter, L. 2009. Engaging with nature to promote health: New directions for nursing research. *Journal of Advanced Nursing, 65* (7), 1527–1538.

Hansen-Ketchum, P., Marck, P.B., Reutter, L., and Halpenny, E. 2011. Strengthening access to restorative places: Findings from a participatory study on engaging with nature in the promotion of health. *Health and Place, 17* (2), 558–571.

Higgs, E.S. 1999. What is good ecological restoration? *Conservation Biology, 11* (2), 338–348.

Higgs, E.S. 2003. *Nature by design: Human agency, natural processes and ecological restoration.* Boston, MA: MIT Press.

Higgs, E.S. 2005. The two culture problem: Ecological restoration and the integration of knowledge. *Restoration Ecology, 13* (1), 159–164.

Hofmeyer, A.T. and Marck, P.B. 2008. Building social capital in healthcare organizations: thinking ecologically for safer care. *Nursing Outlook, 56* (4), 145.e1–151.e9.

Jones, A.H. 1999. Narrative in medical ethics. *British Medical Journal, 318*, 253.

Kelly, E.N., Schindler, D.W., Hodson, P.V., Short, J.W., Radmanovich, R., and Nielsen, C.C. 2010. Oil sands development contributes elements toxic at low concentrations to the Athabasca River and its tributaries. *Proceedings of the National Academy of Sciences of the United States of America, 107* (37), 16178–16183.

Leibler, J.H., Otte, J., Roland-Holst, D., Pfeiffer, D.U., Soares Magalhaes, R., Rushton, J., Graham, J.P., and Silbergeld, E.K. 2009. Industrial food animal production and global health risks: Exploring the ecosystems and economics of avian influenza. *Ecohealth, 6* (1), 58–70.

Leopold, A. 1949. *A Sand County almanac: With essays on conservation from Round River.* New York, NY: Oxford University Press.

Lewis, S. 2011. *Essays: The ugly Australian.* Longwoods.com. Available at http://www.longwoods.com/content/22093.

Louv, R. 2008. *Last child in the woods. Saving our children from nature deficit disorder.* Chapel Hill, NC: Algonquin Books.

Marck, P.B. 2000. Nursing in a technological world: Searching for healing communities. *Advances in Nursing Science, 23* (2), 59–72.

Marck, PB. 2004a. Ethics in hard places: The ecology of safer systems in modern health care. *Health Ethics Today 14*(1), 2–5.

Marck, P.B. 2004b. Ethics for practitioners: An ecological framework. In J. Storch, P. Rodney, and R. Starzomski (Eds.), *Toward a moral horizon: Nursing ethics for leadership and practice* (pp. 232–247). Toronto, ON: Pearson Education Canada.

Marck, P.B. 2006. Discourse. Field notes from research and restoration in the backcountry of modern health care. *Canadian Journal of Nursing Research Focus on Safety and Risk, 38* (2), 11–23.

Marck, P.B. in review. Towards ecologically emancipated communities: Using research and restoration to re-imagine safe places in a technologically colonized health care world. In L. Hallstrom, N.M. Guehlstorf, and M. Parkes, (Eds.), *Environment, health, and community development.* Vancouver, BC: University of British Columbia Press.

Marck, P.B., Barton, S., Day, R., Bulmer-Smith, K., Gushue, S., Kemp, L., Martin, K., Peterson, K., and Worrell, J. 2010. *Transforming clinical learning environments for undergraduate nursing students: A collaborative clinical learning unit.* Final Report, 23 November 2010. Available at http://www.nurs.ualberta.ca/clu/.

Marck, P.B., Coleman-Miller, G., Hoffman, C., Horsburgh, B., Woolsey, S., Dina, A., Dorfman, T., Nolan, J., Jackson, N., Kwan, J., and Hagedorn, K. 2007. Thinking ecologically for safer healthcare: A summer research student partnership. *Canadian Journal of Nursing Leadership, 20* (3), 42–51.

Marck P.B., Higgs, E.S., Edwards, N., and Molzahn, A. 2006a. *Generating adaptive health systems: An emerging framework of research and restoration for a safer world.* Working Paper #1. Available at http://www.nursing.ualberta.ca/SaferSystems/projects.htm.

Marck, P.B., Higgs, E.S., Vieira, E.R., and Hagedorn, K. 2008. *Through the eyes of practitioners: Adapting visual research methods from ecological restoration to integrate the ethics, science, and practice of safety in health care.* Health Care Systems Ergonomics & Patient Safety International Conference Paper, June 25–27, 2008, Strasbourg, France, pp. 1–8. Available at http://webcache. googleusercontent.com/search?q=cache:http://www.heps2008.org/abstract/data/PDF/Marck_ Patricia. pdf.

Marck, P.B., Kwan, J.A., Preville, B., Reynes, M., Morgan-Eckley, W., Versluys, R., Chivers, L., O'Brien, B., Van der Zalm, J., Swankhuizen, M., and Majumdar, S.R. 2006b. Building safer systems by ecological design: Using restoration science to develop a medication safety intervention. *Quality and Safety in Health Care, 15* (2), 92–97.

Matthew, R. 2000. Educating today's youth in indigenous ecological knowledge: New paths for traditional ways. *World Conference on Science: Science for the twenty-first century, a new commitment,* pp. 439–441. Available at http://unesdoc.unesco.org/images/0012/001207/ 120706e.pdf#121024.

McGuire, S. 1998. Global migration and health: Ecofeminist perspectives. *Advances in Nursing Science, 21* (2), 1–16.

McMichael, A.J, Friel, S., Nyong, A., and Corvalan, C. 2008. Analysis. Global environmental change and health: Impacts, inequalities, and the health sector. *British Medical Journal, 336,* 191–194.

Mills, S. 1995. *In service of the wild. Restoring and reinhabiting damaged land.* Boston, MA: Beacon Press.

Orr, D. 1992. *Ecological literacy: Education and the transition to a postmodern world.* Albany, NY: SUNY Press.

Ostrom, E., Burger, J., Field, C.B., Norgaard, R.B., and Policansky, D. 1999. Revisiting the commons: Local lessons, global challenges. *Science, 284,* 278–282.

Parke, B. and Friesen, K. 2010. Creating elder-friendly acute care hospitals: The physical design dimension. *Perspectives: The Journal of the Gerontological Nursing Association, 34* (1), 5–13.

PEW Commission. 2008. *Putting meat on the table: Industrial farm animal production in America.* Washington, DC: Author.

Pooley, J. and O'Connor, M. 2000. Environmental education and attitudes: Emotions and beliefs are what is needed. *Environment and Behavior, 32* (5), 711–723.

Potter, V.R. 1999. Bioethics, Biology, and the Biosphere. Fragmented Ethics and 'Bridge Bioethics.' *Hastings Center Report, 29* (1), 38–40.

Rodney. P., Varcoe, C., Storch, J.L., McPherson, G., Mahoney, K., Brown, H., Pauly, B., Hartrick, G., and Starzomski, R. 2002. Navigating towards a moral horizon: A multi-site qualitative study of ethical practice in nursing. *Canadian Journal of Nursing Research, 41* (1), 292–319.

Sachs J. 2007. Poverty and environmental stress fuel Darfur crisis. *Nature, 449,* 14–15.

Sandler, R. 2007. *Character and environment: A virtue-oriented approach to environmental ethics.* New York: Columbia University Press.

Sherwin, S. 1999. Foundations, frameworks, lenses: The role of theories in bioethics. *Bioethics, 13* (3/4), 198–205.

Society for Ecological Restoration International Science and Policy Working Group. 2004. *The SER International Primer on Ecological Restoration.* www.ser.org & Tucson: Society for Ecological Restoration International. Available at http://www.ser.org/pdf/primer3.pdf.

Thomas, J.M. and Cosford, P.A. 2010. Editorial: Place sustainability at the heart of the quality agenda. *Quality and Safety in Health Care, 19,* 260–261.

Tuhiwai Smith, L. 1999. *Decolonizing methodologies. Research and indigenous peoples.* New York, NY: Palgrave, St. Martin's Press.

United Nations Educational, Scientific and Cultural Organization. *World commission on the ethics of science and technology. Summary report of the recommendations adopted at the sixth ordinary session.* Kuala Lampur, Malaysia, June 16–19, 2009. Available at http://unesdoc.unesco.org/images/0018/001831/183140e.pdf.

Varcoe, C. and Rodney, P. 2009. Constrained agency: The social structure of nurses' work. In B.S. Bolaria and H. Dickinson (Eds.), *Health, illness and health care in Canada* (4th ed.; pp. 122–150). Toronto: Harcourt Brace.

Waldvogel, F.A. 2004. Infectious diseases in the 21st century: Old challenges and new opportunities. *International Journal of Infectious Diseases, 8,* 5–12.

Westra, L. 2008. *Environmental rights and the rights of indigenous peoples: International and domestic legal perspectives.* London, UK: Earthscan.

Westra, L. 2009. *Environmental justice and the rights of ecological refugees.* London, UK: Earthscan.

Westra, L. and Lawson, B.E. (Eds.). 2001. *Faces of environmental racism: Confronting issues of social justice.* Oxford, U.K.: Rottman & Littlefield Publishers.

Whitehouse, P.J. 1999. The ecomedical disconnection syndrome. *Hastings Center Report, 29* (1), 41–44.

Winner, L. 1977. *Autonomous technology: Technics-out-of-control as a theme in political thought.* Cambridge, MA: MIT Press.

World Medical Association. 2010. *Statement on environmental degradation and sound management of chemicals.* WMA General Assembly. Vancouver: Author.

World Medical Association. 2009. *Declaration of Delhi on health and climate change.* WMA General Assembly. New Delhi, India: Author.

Worster, D. 1984. Thinking like a river. In W. Jackson, W.E. Berry, and B. Colman (Eds.), *Meeting the expectations of the land. Essays in sustainable agriculture and stewardship* (pp. 56–67). San Francisco: North Point Press.

PART 2

Current Applications of Health Care Ethics/Nursing Ethics

CHAPTER 12

Ethics and Canadian Health Care

Bernadette M. Pauly and Janet L. Storch

Our policy decisions are moral decisions. They are issues of care and responsible citizenship. (Kenny 2002, 5)

The provision of health care in any country is influenced by economic, political, social, and cultural forces. While clearly there are many influences on the structure of all social programs, our values as Canadians determine how we frame problems in health care and the solutions we endorse or reject (Kenny 2002). Publicly funded health care in Canada has been a source of pride and is held up as a reflection of Canadian values of equity and solidarity. It involves sharing of burdens and benefits (Beauchamp and Steinbock 1999). As Dickinson (2009) noted,

> As a source of national pride it is widely seen as a central element of our national identity and as something that makes us different from, and more caring and compassionate than, Americans. (23)

In the final report of the Commission on the Future of Health Care (2002), values of universality, equity, and solidarity were identified as enduring and dominant values of Canadians. For Canadians, equity generally means that ". . . all Canadians are equally entitled to access our health system based on health needs, not ability to pay" (Giacomini, Kenny, and DeJean 2009, 64). Solidarity is understood as both "a personal virtue of commitment and a principle of social morality based on the shared values of a group" (Beauchamp and Childress 2001, 233). Equity and solidarity are embedded in the Canadian health care insurance principles of universality, accessibility, and comprehensiveness.

Advocating for health care policies that ensure the funding and delivery of care that supports the provision of safe and quality nursing care is an important aspect of professional nursing practice. Thus, nurses require an understanding not only of Canadian health care but also about nursing values and responsibilities. In the Canadian Nurses Association Code of Ethics for Registered Nurses (2008), nurses are urged to be advocates for quality work environments that "maximize the quality of health outcomes for persons receiving care ". . . where such environments for practice have the resources and structures in place "to ensure safety, support and respect for all persons in the work setting." (5). Registered nurses are viewed as moral agents in their practice and have a role in contributing to improved practice environments. Recognition is given to the reality that ". . . organizations and policy-makers at regional, provincial/territorial, national, and international levels strongly influence ethical practice" (5). This means that nurses in all settings and at all levels of care should be aware of the structures, policies, and underlying values that have shaped and are shaping health care in Canada.

In this chapter, we provide a brief overview of the history, financing, and delivery of Canadian health care, and explicate underlying values, captured in key principles that have driven the development and provision of health care in Canada. Limitations and challenges of publicly funded care in Canada are discussed. We then examine health care financing and delivery through an "ethics lens" and a perspective of ethical theories of justice. Finally, systemic impacts on health care providers and patients, with specific attention to the contributions of nursing and nursing leadership (Canadian Nurses Association 2009c), are then discussed.

At the outset, it is important to make two qualifications. Although many attempts have been made over the years to systemize health care in Canada, it remains an often fragmented collection of policies and programs that are based on Canada's constitution, geography, and political necessity. Nevertheless, Canada's health care policies and programs are often referred to as though they comprised a "system." Thus, we will be using systems language in this chapter, recognizing that there are really multiple systems, particularly since health care is primarily a responsibility of provincial or territorial authorities. A second qualification is that as we begin a discussion of the health care system, including a brief review of its origins and eventual structure and financing, we caution that it is important to acknowledge that Canadians hold multiple and competing values about Canadian health care. Yet, health care in Canada has been founded on a set of values that emphasize fairness and justice in the allocation of health care services. It is these values that we seek to explicate in our discussion.

CANADA'S HEALTH INSURANCE SYSTEM: THE BACKGROUND

When Canada was an emerging nation, its first priorities in health care were public health measures to mitigate or prevent infectious diseases (through quarantine and immunization as preventive knowledge became available), to improve the safety of food and water, and to support the injured and those with communicable disease (Heagerty 1934; Milestones 2010; also see Chapter 20). The *British North America Act* of 1867 (now part of the *Constitution Act* of 1982) assigned major responsibility for health services and education to the provinces, but retained the major share of taxation under federal authority. This left each province to develop its own approach to health care and other provincially mandated services. The province of Saskatchewan moved ahead with plans for universal health insurance that eventually became the foundational pieces of federal programs (Meilicke and Storch 1980). As World War II was ending, plans were being developed in both Canada and the United States—for universal health insurance in the USA and a national health insurance program in Canada. However, both plans failed to launch due to ". . . fears of socialism and government encroachment on individual liberties" in the USA (Feldberg, Vipond, and Bryant 2010, 272) and because of fiscal concerns in Canada (Taylor 1978).

When the Canadian federal government's attempt to mold a comprehensive system of health care in Canada failed, the federal government embarked on a plan to provide the provinces with conditional grants-in-aide (roughly 50:50 funding) to enable them to develop and provide public health services, services for mental health, tuberculosis control, venereal diseases control, cancer care, crippled children, as well as provision for public health research, health survey capability, and grants for hospital construction (Meilicke and Storch 1980, 3–18). But in the end, our current system of health services became focused on acute care delivery. Hospital construction grants quickly lead to the need for hospital operating grants for which funding was made available through the *Hospital Insurance and Diagnostic Services Act* (1957), another cost-shared venture between the federal and provincial governments. In 1967, under the *Medical Care Act*, the medicare program was launched to provide payment for independent physician services, also under a federal-provincial cost share plan (Taylor 1973; Meilicke and Storch 1980). Thus, the "system" of health care financing involved national and provincial governments working together under a set of four principles that included **universality, comprehensiveness, portability**, and **public administration**.

The year 1984 marked a point of departure from more or less shared goals between Canada and the United States when the federal government in Canada developed the *Canada Health Act* (CHA 1989, 2011). This act was designed to replace the *Hospital Insurance and Diagnostic Act* and the *Medical Care Act*, but it also incorporated the four principles of medicare and added one more, **accessibility**, into its mandate. Most importantly, it disallowed "extra-billing" practices, meaning that physicians were no longer allowed to add to the fees they were already receiving from their provincial government's health insurance plan per patient visit. In the end, Canada's system can be described as a "national government sponsored insurance system in which everyone is insured for all medically necessary hospital and physician services through a provincial plan, which is partially underwritten from general revenues of the federal government and partially by the provinces" (Coburn 2010, 83). Coburn notes that

> ". . . the *Canada Health Act* was passed during a period of broad, global rethinking of health care and the determinants of health. The change in name, from the *Medical Care Act* to the *Canada Health Act*, reflected the new approach. (276)

Over the years, the roughly 50:50 cash federal financing to the provinces for health care changed to federal transfers (including both cash and tax-point transfers) to enable the provinces to have more taxation revenue. Whether those additional taxation revenues were actually used for health care in most provinces is debatable, but citizens (including many nurses) perceived federal cutbacks in effect and blamed the federal government for decreased funding. In 2004, the *Canada Health and Social Transfer (CHST) Act* actually *reduced* federal monetary transfers to the provinces (Feldberg et al. 2010, 278).

In early 2000, two studies examining Canada's health care system from differing perspectives regarding how the "system" should be changed were undertaken (The

Standing Senate Committee 2004; Commission on the Future of Health Care 2004). In 2003, the First Minister's Meeting on the Future of Health Care in Canada passed the Accord on Health Care Renewal that reaffirmed their commitment to the five principles of health care insurance in Canada, and called for specific standards of care to address pressing issues, such as wait lists, quality home care, and so forth (Health Canada 2003). This accord, which also determines how much the federal government contributes to health care, will expire in 2014 (Health Canada 2004). As this chapter is being written, there is increasing speculation about how these upcoming negotiations to renew the accord will evolve.[1] (See Chapter 26).

In summary, Canada's national health insurance program can be characterized as a program designed to encourage considerable autonomy of health agencies and physicians while seeking to ensure that there is relatively equal access to health care regardless of an individual's ability to pay (Storch and Meilicke 2006). From the onset, beginning in Saskatchewan, the emphasis was on a collective or shared responsibility to care for all who were sick or injured (solidarity). Thus, the policy-makers held that health (hospital and medical) care should be provided to all (universal), it should be comprehensive in coverage, accessible to all, portable across provinces, and publicly administered (Davidson 2006; Dickenson 2009; Storch 2010). These five principles apply primarily to acute hospital and physician services including hospital stays, physician visits in hospital, laboratory tests, surgeries and treatments, as well as visits to "private" physician offices. In all of Canada's 10 provinces and three territories, funds to support the publicly insured and administered program are covered through taxation. Only three provinces (British Columbia, Alberta, and Ontario) also require payment of health care premiums to supplement this funding.

Across the provinces and territories there is some variation in how this coverage is arranged and in some cases there may be marginal costs incurred for a service that is provided at no cost in an adjacent province. It should also be noted that the provision of health care in Canada is part of a wider network of social security programs (pensions, income assistance, etc.) that have been a critical element of the "social safety net" that, many now observe, is being gradually eroded. These and other challenges highlight some of the limitations of the Canadian health care system.

LIMITATIONS OF THE CANADIAN SYSTEM

Medicare focuses on "medically necessary" services that are understood as primarily hospital and physician services. This means that cohesive funding and delivery of programs such as universal primary *health care*, pharmacare, public health, and home and community care are not assured from one province to another. "Primary care is a medical concept referring to a situation wherein the physician provides diagnosis, treatment and follow-up for a specific disease or problem" whereas "primary *health* care includes health promotion, disease prevention, curative services, rehabilitative, and supportive or palliative care" (Canadian Nurses Association 2000). Most importantly primary health care involves a team of health professionals and continuity of care.

It has been clear for some time that access to medical care, except for the provision of primary health care, is less deterministic of health outcomes than the social determinants of health (Evans 2008; McKeown 1979, Raphael 2009; Starfield, Shi, and Macinko 2005; Starfield 2007). As Bryson (2010) noted,

> Economic and social inequality damages the health of both individuals and populations. The relationships between health and material deprivation, economic relations, social status, social networks, and cultural narratives is complex and multifaceted. It is vital to pursue these questions. . . . Health is much more than healthcare." (2–3)

Many of the social determinants of health that profoundly impact health status—such as assuring access to adequate incomes, affordable housing, food security, and the elimination of poverty—fall outside the health care system (see Chapter 21). In spite of this, there is an important role for the health care system in promoting action on the social determinants of health and the promotion of health equity (Bryant et al. 2010; Health Disparities Task Group 2004; Jones 2008; Patychuk and Seskar-Nencic 2008; Public Health Agency of Canada 2008; Raphael 2009). Public health policy makers, practitioners, and leaders have been key players in this regard. Further, there have been numerous reports highlighting the deficiencies and the need to strengthen the public health system (Federal/Provincial/Territorial Advisory Committee on Public Health 2001; National Advisory Committee on SARS and Public Health 2003; The Standing Senate Committee on Social Affairs, Science, and Technology 2002). Thus, ensuring a strong public health system in addition to provision of illness care services should be a central concern of a publicly funded health care system. In several provinces, restructuring and strengthening of public health services is underway (e.g., Population Health and Wellness 2005; also see Chapter 20).

PUBLIC NEEDS/PROBLEMS: PRIVATE SOLUTIONS?

While the statements above suggest that we should be strengthening public health as part of the Canadian health care system, there have been increasing challenges to the preservation of publicly funded health care itself, with increasing shifts to private funding and private for-profit service delivery. Coburn (2010) notes a continuous strain to privatize almost anything. He states that

> . . . the push toward privatization ranges everywhere from the commodification of knowledge, including knowledge about health, previously commonly held in universities, to privatization of specific human gene pools. All of this has profound implications for provision of health care. It is a daily struggle . . . to preserve any form of collective benefit." (84)

The publicly funded health care system has been under threat of privatization in both funding and delivery of care as a result of shifting neo-liberal values that emphasize markets as the most efficient approach to allocation of resources. These values include a belief that society consists of autonomous individuals motivated primarily by economic considerations, and that competition in the market will yield innovations (Coburn 2000; 2010). An unintended consequence of this value in action is the erosion of social systems including health care.

Many proponents for increasing private for-profit delivery of health services and private funding in health care argue that health care costs are spiraling out of control and that the current publicly funded system is unsustainable. The cuts to health care spending, reducing specific programs, etc., announced by governments at all levels (federal, provincial, and regional) have two main effects. First, people begin to believe that there are no more funds available and that the only answer lies in greater access to private for-profit services and funding. Second, when such announcements ". . . include de-insuring services, governments not only set a boundary on the terrain to be funded by the public purse, but they also establish what could be occupied by privately financed services" (Davidson 2006).

Lewis (2007) suggests that the "sustainability crisis mantra" is traceable to those who suggest that we could barely afford the national health insurance program at is outset, and can no longer afford it now. The evidence of the growth of Canada's GDP (Gross Domestic Product) (21) tells a different story in that health care as a percentage of GDP has not risen substantially.[2] Nevertheless, in Canada, a number of strategies have been introduced that have the potential to shift the balance of public-private funding and delivery of health care. These include imposing user fees on persons seeking care, engaging in public-private partnerships, and increased contracting out of non-clinical services such as housekeeping, dietary, and so on (Romanow 2004).

User fees refer to direct payments for the care received from a physician or a hospital. The basis of the argument for user fees is that such fees will decrease inappropriate use and misuse of the system by patients. However, repeatedly, research has found that people who have the greatest need for care and the least financial resources decrease their use of health care resources when they need care and have to pay a user fee to access care. Despite their needs for care, they are systematically discouraged from seeking care (Canadian Health Services Research Foundation 2001; Evans, Barer, and Stoddart 1993; Kenny 2002, 136; Moorhouse 1993). Yet, as recently as April 2010, the province of Quebec proposed the introduction of user fees to address budget shortfalls in health care.

Public–private partnerships have been embraced in many provinces in Canada as a potential source of capital funding (for buildings or equipment) or for funding a position or a program in health care (Romanow 2004). What is often overlooked is that, unless it is a philanthropic project, the expectation of the private sector is to make a profit. Yet, if money can be borrowed, the public sector is normally able to borrow capital at a cheaper rate than the private sector. Nevertheless, governments have difficulty dealing with multi-year funding commitments in a budgetary model based on single-year funding. Without careful attention to the challenges and the motives for such partnerships, health professionals may well be challenged to promote products or services of the for-profit partner rather than provide services based upon needs.

ETHICS IN PRACTICE 12-1

Public–Private Partnerships

A clinical nurse specialist in a large urban hospital has recently been asked to be part of a chronic disease management program. This program will involve a public–private partnership with a large corporation that produces diabetic medication and equipment. The nurse recognizes that this will provide an important source of funding for an advanced practice position that will provide care to people with diabetes. However, she feels a sense of uneasiness and is concerned that she will be expected to promote the products of this company to her patients.

As Ethics in Practice 12-1 indicates, public–private partnerships have the potential to provide new sources of revenue for developing patient services, building new facilities, and buying much needed equipment. At the level of policy, however, there are few guidelines for how public–private partnerships can be implemented to ensure appropriate and ethical practices. In some areas, public–private partnerships might be workable; in other areas, they might be contraindicated. A constant concern is that for-profit motives might unduly influence clinical advice and decision-making.

Contracting out non-clinical services and/or clinical services is another approach to privatization. Deber (2002) states that for-profit firms have the potential to make profits because of economies of scale and better management, but she raises the following caution:

> Savings frequently arise from more contentious measures including freedom from labor agreements (and different wage levels and skill mixes), evasion of cost controls placed on other providers, sacrifice of difficult to measure intangibles, risk selection or cream skimming, and even dubious practices. (vii)

In 1985, Stoddart and Labelle examined the benefits of contracting out non-clinical services, such as laundry and food services, in an attempt to realize cost savings. They concluded that the cost savings and quality of these strategies were questionable.

Throughout the 1990s, contracting out clinical services, such as laboratory services and surgical services increased without evidence of significant decrease in cost or increase in access to service (Canadian Health Services Research Foundation 2002; Fuller 1998). The SARS (Sudden Acute Respiratory Syndrome) epidemic in 2003 highlighted the importance of maintaining well-trained housekeeping staff; yet contracting out still continues to be portrayed as a cost-saving practice. In 2008–2009, incorrect laboratory results for many women with breast cancer exposed the lack of appropriate regulation in effect for such laboratory services (Commission of Inquiry 2009).

Some analysts also have raised concerns that contracting out has the potential for the activation of potentially irreversible provisions within the North American Free Trade Agreement (NAFTA) and in other world trade agreements that could have the effect of forcing Canada to open our health care system to the market (Crawford 2006; Rachlis 2000; Price, Pollack, and Shaoul 1999). A primary concern related to private contracting out of clinical services includes the potential for creaming (drawing the most profitable clients into the private system), lack of transparency, inappropriate services, and extra-billing (Evans et al. 2000). The net effect is that the most complex and costly care is left to an increasingly overburdened public health care system. In general, those conducting economic evaluations have not found that private-for-profit delivery of services increases efficiency, choice, or quality of care (Romanow 2004). Yet, "enhancing choice" continues to be promoted by some as a rationale for increasing for profit delivery of care.

VALUES IN TENSION IN HEALTH CARE PROVISION

Stone (2001) states that equity, efficiency, liberty, and security are some of the most "enduring values" in policy debates. She argues that policy controversies often turn on these values. A key issue is the framing of policy debates and what values are predominant in the framing of such issues. Evans (1984) noted that ". . . 'need' carries significant ethical overtones; its allegation asserts an obligation on the part of others" (53). He acknowledged that the underlying issue in all modern health care systems is the tension created when those with health and wealth contribute more to the collective than those who are unhealthy and without wealth since the latter group are more likely to access a social system of health care. Evans (2006) has also noted the significant shift in the concentration of wealth in the hands of a few,[3] whose political influence in public policy and health policy has increased. He attributes many of the challenges to public spending on health care, and even challenges to the principles of the Canada Health Act, as a function of the healthy and wealthy resisting government interference and being resentful of principles that oblige them to share their wealth. This reflects an ethical tension between individual rights and freedoms and government intervention, collective interests, and solidarity.

In December 2010, the Health Council of Canada (a body created in 2003 to provide an independent review of health care in Canada) released a report that challenged governments to find "a better balance between investing in the acute care system and investing in the determinants of health" (28). The Council suggested that such a balance can only be accomplished by a "shift in the way governments allocate health care dollars" (28). In doing so, the Council instructed that we need to *decrease health care inequities* to increase sustainability of health care services. Urging us to differentiate between "inequality and inequity" they provide working definitions for each.

> **Inequality** refers to health differences that may be possible to reduce but not eliminate, such as those related to genetics or aging; **inequity** refers to differences that are unfair and preventable. Governments cannot necessarily fix all inequalities, but they can take action to reduce inequities. (5)

This Health Council of Canada (2010) report asked Canadians to make several commitments to equity in health care, including a "willingness to name the difficult problems and barriers that exist, and to provide resources necessary to transcend them" and a "willingness and commitment to ensure a structural approach to placing health projects on the public policy agenda" (25). Differences that are unfair and preventable are rooted in the social conditions that determine health (Whitehead and Dahlgren 2006). Thus, the shift being urged is one that would focus on the health of those with the least power and resources as well as orientating health care services toward the determinants of health. Such a move would further challenge individualistic views of personal responsibility for health and shifts to private for-profit delivery of health care services (Pauly, MacKinnon, and Varcoe 2009).

WHAT IS FAIR?

While values reflect our beliefs, ethics as a discipline is concerned with the normative dimension of decisions and actions. All public policy has a moral dimension because it involves decisions that affect others who may or may not be involved in the process of deciding how a particular problem should be addressed (Malone 1999). As Kenny (2002) observes,

> These moral and ethical dimensions are not always visible in our public policies; health care is a notable exception. Here, our intuitions of vulnerability and our personal experiences of

illness, disease and disability, both for us and for our loved ones, evoke strong convictions that health care policy is about things that really matter. (45)

Theories of distributive justice provide general principles to "determine how social burdens, and goods and services, including health care goods and services, should be distributed—or, as some insist, redistributed" (Beauchamp and Childress 1994, 334; Daniels 1985). Libertarian perspectives generally adopt a free market ideal in the distribution of health care goods and services. In the United States, a libertarian system of health care has predominated, and individual self-reliance and choice are highly valued. Health care is often treated like a commodity (something to be bought and sold in a market) rather than a social good accessible to all and equally distributed (Daniels 1985). Over time, the emphasis on privately funded and private for-profit health care, and the corresponding lack of access to health care by so many, have been identified as a serious ethical concern in the U.S.A. by many American bioethicists (Buchanan 1995; Caplan, Light, and Daniels 1999; Daniels 1985). In 2009, several leading American bioethicists argued that liberty, the basic value of libertarian thinking (that promotes distribution of health care as best left to the marketplace), must be considered more broadly to reconcile liberty and equity (Jennings 2009), that mandating universal participation in health insurance can be just and fair (Menzel 2009), that solidarity is still an American value (Sage 2009), and that stewardship is important for society (Nichols 2009).

Fairness, in an egalitarian sense, assumes that everyone is of equal value or worth and that fairness is achieved by seeking to "reduce the differences in health and health care between groups" (Caplan, Light, and Daniels 1999, 854). In this sense, health care is a public or common good to which everyone should have a right of access. Values embodied in Canadian health care, as discussed previously, are more closely aligned with egalitarian rather than libertarian views of justice and fairness. Although not explored in depth here, theories of social justice support addressing the conditions by which differences in health are shaped (Powers and Faden 2006; Young 1990; also see Chapter 21).

TOWARD INFORMED ETHICAL CHOICES

As Kenny (2002) observed, decisions to embrace certain health care reforms over others reflect ethical choices about how we wish to live together as a society. For example, if we believe that everyone should have access to health care resources, then it is clear that we should continue to embrace a system in which everyone has the opportunity to access health care on the basis of need, not ability to pay. However, if we fundamentally believe that the demand for health care will increase in perpetuity and that health care is a market good (a commodity only those who can afford it should have the privilege to access), then we are much more likely to endorse market reforms that introduce a greater private for-profit role into the funding and delivery of health care (Kenny 2002).

Canadian values, as reflected in the principles of the Canada Health Act, have remained remarkably clear, unchanged, and consistent with an egalitarian approach to justice that is aligned with professional nursing values, and criteria for a just health care system. However, Canadian beliefs about how to *achieve* these values have been strongly influenced by a number of sociopolitical forces and political neoliberal ideologies in which governments' role is deliberately reduced with the unintended consequences of erosion of social programs. Theories of justice seek to examine the ethical basis and consequences of such decisions. From an egalitarian perspective, health is *not* merely a commodity but *is a common good* in which all should share.

TAKE HOME MESSAGE FOR NURSE LEADERS

It is essential that nurse leaders understand the way in which health care is funded and delivered in order to assess the ethical consequences of introducing particular health care reform strategies. There is *no strong economic or ethical evidence* to support moving to greater private funding or private for-profit delivery of health care. There *is good evidence* to support adequate funding for a publicly funded universally accessible system of care, and a need to reorganize and improve the delivery of care (Baylis, Kenny, and Sherwin 2008; Tuohy, Flood, and Stabile 2004), as well as to find a better balance between funds for acute care and investing in reducing health inequities. If we are to maintain a system of health care responsive and available to meet the needs of all, including those experiencing poor health and without financial resources, it is imperative that nurses participate in the health policy process at all levels and advocate for ethical analysis of proposed reforms (Canadian Nurses Association 2008; Canadian Nurses Association 2009b). All registered nurses within the scope of their power and authority have a role to play in maintaining the fabric of a fair and just health care system that meets the needs of Canadians and provides a context for safe, compassionate, competent, and ethical care in nursing (Canadian Nurses Association 2008).

Where Is the Profession of Nursing?

Nurses' work is socially, historically, and contextually situated, and they must understand their practice in relation to organizational and societal forces (Chambliss 1996; Rodney and Varcoe 2001; Varcoe et al 2004; Varcoe and Rodney 2009). Nurses often experience constraints on their practice that are a result of decisions made at other levels of the health care system. For example, nurses continue to attempt to navigate the move to a more corporate, business-oriented approach in which organizational values of efficiency and effectiveness have tended to marginalize values related to quality of care, individual patient good, and societal equity (Varcoe and Rodney 2009; Smedly 2008; Storch et al. 2002). In the context of scarcity, corporatization, and staffing shortages, the ability of nurses to practice ethically and safely is jeopardized (Varcoe et al. 2004; Varcoe and Rodney 2009; also see Chapter 10). Macro decisions force difficult micro-level resource allocations when nurses at the bedside are faced with increasing workloads and pressures as a result of reductions and cutbacks. Rodney and Varcoe (2001) urge that economic evaluation be complemented with ethical inquiry in health care decision-making and health policy development in order to promote a health care system that is humane, effective, and efficient. Further, the endorsement of public–private partnerships in the funding of health care at federal, provincial, and regional levels has meant that nurse leaders are in the position of implementing these directives, often without the legitimate avenues of power or authority to raise questions about the ethical implications of such directives. Yet they are responsible and involved in the implementation of these initiatives that will ultimately shape practice. This means that it is imperative for nurses to be engaged in policy development at all levels and to raise questions about the ethical implications of policies for practitioners and the public.

The Role of Nursing: Individual and Collective Actions

Ethics and politics are inseparable as disciplines concerned with praxis and as "aspects of a unified practice philosophy" (Bernstein 1991, 9). Ethics requires that we think through our political commitments and responsibilities, and such understanding of politics should bring us back to ethics.

Individually and collectively, registered nurses should continue to advocate for health care that promotes a fairer distribution of costs and equitable access to health care; promotes action on health equity and the social determinants of health (Canadian Nurses Association 2009b); supports collaborative research that further explicates the values of Canadians; and fosters the development of ethical frameworks for health policy analysis.

Both national and provincial nursing organizations (colleges, professional associations, and unions) have been active in raising the visibility of nursing issues and concerns at the policy level, and in influencing the development of health policy. At the national level, the Canadian Nurses Association (CNA) uses every opportunity to influence the federal government in maintaining and restoring federal funding for health care to the provinces (Canadian Nurses Association 2009a; Shamian 2010; see Chapter 26). The Canadian Nurses Association has continued to strongly reject greater private for-profit reforms, has embraced moving to a system of primary *health* care as the means for reforming the system, and has urged nurses to advocate for social justice through action on the social determinants of health (Canadian Nurses Association 2008). Professional colleges and associations have been vehicles for bringing the voice of registered nurses into the policy arena at the macro level of health care. As this chapter is being written, more provincial professional associations or colleges across Canada are beginning to redefine their roles as being restricted to registration (licensure) only. Since the Canadian Nurses Association's advocacy stance is not seen by these associations or colleges to align with their goals, some have seen it as necessary for these organizations to separate from CNA, thus weakening nursings' professional voice provincially and nationally.

The Canadian Nurses Association Code of Ethics for Registered Nurses (2008) provides a strong moral basis for supporting reforms that are consistent with social justice. The 2008 Code includes a powerful promotion for attention to broad aspects of social justice including some of the following ethical endeavours, which nurses should seek to fulfill. Examples excerpted from the CNA Code (2008) are listed below.

> iv. Advocating for a full continuum of accessible health-care services to be provided at the right time and right place. This continuum includes health promotion, disease prevention, and diagnostic, restorative, rehabilitative and palliative care services in hospitals, nursing homes, home care, and the community.

> v. Recognizing the significance of the social determinants of health and advocating for policies and programs that address these determinants.

viii. Understanding that some groups in society are systemically disadvantaged, which leads to diminished health and well-being. Nurses work to improve the quality of lives of people who are part of disadvantaged and/or vulnerable groups and communities, and they take action to overcome barriers to health care.

ix. Advocating for health-care systems that ensure accessibility, universality and comprehensiveness of necessary health-care services. (20–21)

To support action on these commitments, the Canadian Nurses Association has endorsed a system of primary *health* care as a strategy that has the capacity to create a more just system of care. Registered nurses need to clearly articulate the definition and principles of primary health care in order to continue to educate politicians, the public, and other health care providers that *primary care* is not the same as *primary health care* (CNA 2005). Further, nurses and nurse leaders can champion nurses as a point of entry into the health care system, the important role of nurse practitioners (Canadian Health Services Research Foundation 2010), and the need to strengthen public health care.

While nursing organizations can clearly articulate values, develop and communicate policy positions, provide key messages, and mobilize nurses, individual nurses have an ethical commitment to be informed and to take action wherever possible. This includes discussion and action at local, provincial, and national levels on health care reform issues in both personal and professional capacities. It is clear that nurses often face ethical challenges in acting politically because of organizational and social constraints (Rodney et al. 2002; Storch et al. 2002; Varcoe and Rodney 2009). While nurses have been called to take up their role in the development of health policy, they often feel unprepared and lacking in the knowledge and skills needed to take on this role. It is critical that nurses, through formal education or involvement in professional activities, develop skills for the ethical analysis of health policy and the ability to articulate their ethical concerns for the benefit of patients, the public, and the profession.

Nursing leaders can monitor their workplaces for changes to care and pay close attention to restructuring that promotes further for-profit privatization. In the face of such proposals, registered nurses can ask what these changes mean for patients/clients, especially those who already face barriers to access because of ethno-cultural diversity, poverty, gender, and age differences. Nurses cannot remain aloof from the politics of the policy process, either professionally or personally, because the result will be health care policy shaped *for* nursing but not *with* nursing (Cohen et al. 1996; Grant 1995; Storch 2010; Whitman 1998). As Grant (1995) observed, the result of not taking action is that nurses remain an invisible, voiceless, and silent majority.

Summary

Although the Canadian health care system is based on values that promote equity and solidarity that have withstood the test of time, and continues to function relatively well by international comparisons, there are trends such as increased private funding and for-profit delivery that have the potential to undermine the system. Greater ethical analysis of health service delivery with attention to health outcomes is needed to promote ethically informed decisions about the impact of private and public funding in the delivery of health care while preserving the principles of the Canada Health Act. These shifts have important implications for nurses as front-line health care providers. Nurses continue to be key witnesses to health delivery that is working and systems that are not working to benefit patient care. Thus, their observations and recommendations for adjustments to the system are important. Further, nurses have an important role to play in supporting trends that promote health equity and action on the social determinants of health within and outside of the health care system, as well as globally.

For Reflection

1. Are Canadian values shifting, and, if so, what is responsible for this shift?

2. What are the ethical tensions associated with greater private for-profit health care funding and delivery in Canada?

3. What are the ethical responsibilities of individual nurses in response to tensions at the various levels of health care (unit, organization, provincial, and national levels)?

4. What constraints or facilitators might nurses experience in taking action consistent with their ethical duties and obligations in the development of health care policy?

Endnotes

1. In May 2011 the Canadian Nurses Association established a National Expert Commission on health system renewal. The mandate of this Expert Commission is to consult and advise on how to accelerate a positive transformation of Canada's publicly funded, not for profit medicare system (Canadian Nurses Association 2011). This information and analysis will be timely for input into the expected Health Care Renewal Accord of 2014.

2. Many Canadian health economists and others have refuted the belief that the Canadian health care system is unsustainable, pointing to the limited change in percentage of GDP allocated to health care over the years. More recently, Chappell and Hollander (2011) have reported on research that supports those who claim Canadian health care is sustainable. In their study they note that it is not the aging population adding to health care costs, as much as technology that is the cost generator.

3. Beginning in September 2011 the 'Occupy Wall Street' movement began to take shape, first in the USA and then in several Canadian cities. According to a report in the *Globe and Mail* on November 8, the "... participants have no official demands, but are advocating for a variety of social justice and economic issues, including nationalizing Canada's banks, closing tax loopholes for the wealthy, and increasing the minimum wage. Most say they are frustrated that a small number of people control most of the world's wealth" (*Globe and Mail*, November 8, 2011, p. A8). A poll conducted by the *Globe and Mail* found most Canadians regard this movement it favorably. (See also Coyne 2011).

References

Austin, W. 2003. Using the human rights paradigm in health ethics: The problems and the possiibilities. In V. Tschudin (Ed.), *Approaches to ethics: Nursing beyond boundaries* (105–114). London: Butterworth Heinemann.

Baylis, F., Kenny, N.P., and Sherwin, S. 2009. A relational account of public health ethics. *Public Health Ethics, 1* (3), 196–209.

Beauchamp, D.E. and Steinbock, B. (Eds.) 1999. *New ethics for the public's health.* New York: Oxford University Press.

Beauchamp, T. and Childress, J. 1994. *Principles of biomedical ethics* (4th ed.). New York: Oxford University Press.

Beauchamp, T. and Childress, J. 2001. *Principles of biomedical ethics* (5th ed.) New York: Oxford University Press.

Bernstein, R.J. 1991. *The new constellation: The ethical-political horizons of modernity/postmodernity.* Cambridge, MA: MIT Press.

Bryant, T. Raphael et al. 2010. *Canada: A land of missed opportunity for addressing the social determinants of health. Health Policy, 101* (1), 44–58.

Bryson, C. 2010. Health as a social phenomenon. *Research News* (Winter 2010), 2–3.

Buchanan, A. 1995. Privatization and just care. *Bioethics, 9* (3/4), 220–239.

Canada Health Act. 1989. Office Consolidation. R.S., 1985, c.C-6. Ottawa: Minister of Justice.

Canada Health Act. 2011, Consolidation, Chapter C-6. Ottawa: Minister of Justice.

Canadian Health Services Research Foundation. 2001. *Mythbusters: User fees would stop waste and ensure better use of the healthcare system.* Ottawa: Author. Available online at www.chsrf.ca.

Canadian Health Services Research Foundation. 2002. *Mythbusters: For-profit ownership of facilities would lead to more efficient health care system.* Ottawa: Author. Avaiable online at www.chsrf.ca.

Canadian Health Services Research Foundation. 2010. *Mythbusters: Seeing a nurse practitioner instead of a doctor is second class care.* http://www.chsrf.ca/mythbusters/pdf/mythbusters_APN_en_FINAL.pdf.

Canadian Nurses Association. 2000. *The primary health care approach.* Fact Sheet. June 2000.

Canadian Nurses Association. 2005. *Primary health care: A summary of issues.* CNA Backgounder. Ottawa: Author.

Canadian Nurses Association. 2008. *Code of ethics for registered nurses.* Ottawa: Author.

Canadian Nurses Association. 2009a. *A healthy population—Key solutions for economic prosperity.* Presentation to House of Commons Standing Committee on Finance, October 20.

Canadian Nurses Association. 2009b. *Determinants of health.* Position Statement. Ottawa: Author.

Canadian Nurses Association. 2009c. *Nursing Leadership.* Position Statement. Ottawa: Author.

Canadian Nurses Association. 2011. *Registered Nurses launch Expert Commission on health system renewal.* .Communique. Ottawa: May 26.

Caplan, R. Light, D., and Daniels, N. 1999. Benchmarks of fairness: A moral framework for assessing equity. *International Journal of Health Services, 29* (4), 853–869.

Chambliss, D. 1996. *Beyond caring.* Chicago: University of Chicago Press.

Chappell, N. and Hollander, M. 2011. Comment: How can we sustain our health-care system?. *Time Colonist,* November 6, D3.

Coburn, D. 2000. Income inequality, social cohesion and the health status of populations: The role of neo-liberalism. *Social Science and Medicine, 51,* 135–146.

Coburn, D. 2010. Health and health care: A political economy perspective. In T. Bryant, D.Raphael, and M. Rioux (Eds.), *Staying alive: Critical perspectives on health and illness* (2nd ed.; pp. 65–92). Toronto: Canadian Scholars' Press Inc.

Cohen, S., Mason, D., Kovner, C., Leavitt, J., Pulcini, J., and Sochalski, J. 1996. Stages of nursing's political development: Where we've been and where we ought to go. *Nursing Outlook, 44* (6), 259–266.

Commission of Inquiry on Hormone Receptor Testing. 2009. Hon. Margaret Cameron, Commissioner. Newfoundland and Labrador: Ministry of Health and Community Services.

Commission on the Future of Health Care in Canada. 2002. *Building on values: The future of health care in Canada.* Roy J. Romanow, Commissioner. Final Report. Ottawa: Author.

Coyne, A. 2011. A phony class war. *Maclean's,* October 31, 24–26.

Crawford, M. 2006. Interactions: Trade policy and healthcare reform after Chaoulli v. Quebec. *Healthcare Policy, 1* (2), 90–102.

Daniels, N. 1985. *Just health care.* Cambridge: Cambridge University Press.

Davidson, A. 2006. Under the radar: Stealth development of two-tier healthcare in Canada. *Healthcare Policy, 2* (1), 25–33.

Deber, R.B. 2002. *Delivering health care services: Public, not-for-profit, or private?* Discussion paper No. 17. Ottawa: Commission on the future of health care in Canada.

Deber, R.B. 2008. Access without appropriateness: Chicken Little in charge. *Healthcare Policy, 4* (1), 23–29.

Dickinson, H.D. 2009. Health care and health reforms: Trends and issues. In B.S. Bolaria and H.D. Dickinson (Eds.), *Health, illness, and health care in Canada* (4th ed.; pp.23–41). Toronto: Nelson Education Ltd.

Evans, R. 1984. *Strained mercy: The economics of Canadian health care.* Toronto: Butterworths.

Evans, R.G. 2006. The world war to class war: The rebound of the rich. *Healthcare Policy, 2* (1), 14–24.

Evans, R.G. 2008. Thomas McKeowan, meet Fidel Castro: Physicians, population health and the Cuban paradox. *Healthcare Policy, 3* (4), 21–32.

Evans, R., Barer, M., and Stoddart, G. 1993. The truth about user fees. *Policy Options, 14* (8), 4–9.

Evans, R.G., Barer, M.L., Lewis, S., Rachlis, M., and Stoddart, G. 2000. *Private highway, one-way street: The deklein and fall of Canadian Medicare?* Centre for Health Services and Policy Research. Available at www.chspr.ubc.ca.

Federal/Provincial/Territorial Advisory Committee on Population Health (2001). *Review of public health capacity in Canada.* Report to the Conference of Deputy Ministers of Health, June 2001.

Feldberg, G., Vipond, R., and Bryant, T. 2010. Cracks in the foundation: The origins and development of the Canadian and American health care systems. In T. Bryant, D. Raphael, and M. Rioux (Eds.), *Staying alive: Critical perspectives on health, illness, and health care* (2nd ed.; pp. 267–286). Toronto: Canadian Scholars' Press.

Fuller, C. 1998. *Caring for profit: How corporations are taking over Canada's health care system.* Vancouver: New Star Books.

Giacomini, M., Kenny, N., and Dejean, D. 2009. Ethics frameworks in Canadian health policies: Foundation, scaffolding, or window dressing? *Health Policy, 89,* 58–71.

Grant, A. 1995. Flex your muscle. *Canadian Nurse, March,* 37–41.

Heagerty, J.J. 1934. The development of public health in Canada. *Canadian Journal of Public Health, 25 (February),* 53–59.

Health Canada. 2003. *First Ministers' Accord on health care renewal.* Available at http://www.hc-sc.gc.ca/hcs-sss/delivery-prestation/fptcollab/2003accord/index-eng.php.

Health Canada. 2004. *First Minister's Meeting on the future of health care 2004: A 10-year plan to strengthen health care.* Available at http://www.hc-sc.gc.ca/hcs-sss/delivery-prestation/fptcollab/2004-fmm-rpm/index-eng.php.

Health Canada. 2010. *Canada Health Act.* Available at http://www.laws-lois.justice.gc.ca.

Health Council of Canada. 2010. *Stepping it up: Moving the focus from health care in Canada to a healthier Canada.* Ottawa: Author.

Health Disparities Task Group of the Federal/Provincial/Territorial Advisory Committee on Population Health and Health Security. 2004. *Reducing health disparities—Roles of the health sector: Recommended policy directions and activities.* Ottawa, ON: Public Health Agency of Canada.

Jennings, B. 2009. Liberty: Free and equal. In M. Crowly (Ed.), *Connecting values to health reform* (pp. 1–3). Garrison, NY: The Hastings Center.

Jones, D. 2008. *Report of the state of public health in Canada.* Ottawa, ON: Public Health Agency of Canada.

Kenny, N.P. 2002. *What good is health care? Reflections on the Canadian experience.* Ottawa: CHA Press.

Lewis, S. 2007. Can a learning-disabled nation learn from healthcare lessons abroad? *Healthcare Policy, 3* (2), 19–28.

Mackreal, K. 2011. The Occupy movement: Most Canadians sympathize with the occupiers, poll shows. *The Glove and Mail,* November 8, A8.

Malone, R. 1999. Policy as product: Morality and metaphor in health policy discourse. *Hastings Center Report, 29* (3), 16–22.

McKeown, T. 1979. *The role of medicine: Dream, mirage or nemesis?* (2nd ed.) Oxford: Basil Blackwell.

Meilicke, C.A. and Storch, J.L. (Eds.). 1980. *Perspectives on Canadian health and social services policy: History and emerging trends.* Ann Arbor, MI: Health Administration Press.

Menzel, P.T. 2009. Liberty: Free and equal. In M. Crowly (Ed.), *Connecting values to health reform* (pp. 1–3). Garrison, NY: The Hastings Center.

Milestones in Canadian Public Health. 2010. *Canadian Nurse, 106* (3), 28–29.

Moorhouse, A. 1993. User fees: Fair cost containment or a tax on the sick? *The Canadian Nurse, 89*, 21–24.

National Advisory Committee on SARS and Public Health. 2003. *Learning from SARS: Renewal of public health in Canada*. Ottawa: Health Canada.

Nichols, L.M. 2009. Stewardship: What kind of a society do we want? In M. Crowly (Ed.), *Connecting values to health reform* (pp. 1–3). Garrison, NY: The Hastings Center.

Patychuk, D. and Seskar-Hencic, D. 2008. *First steps to equity: Ideas and strategies for health equity in Ontario, 2008–2010*. Toronto: Government of Ontario.

Pauly, B.M., MacKinnon, K., and Varcoe, C. 2009. Revisiting "who gets care?" Health equity as an arena for nursing action. *Advances in Nursing Science, 32* (2), 118–127.

Population Health and Wellness. 2005. *A framework for core functions in public health: A resource document*. Victoria, BCBS: Ministry of Health Services.

Powers, M. and R. Fadden. 2006. *Social justice: The moral foundation of public health and health policy*. Toronto: Oxford University Press.

Price, D., Pollock, A.M., and Shaoul, J. 1999. How the World Trade Organization is shaping domestic policies in health care. *Lancet, 354*, 1889–1892.

Public Health Agency of Canada. 2008. *The Chief Public Health Officer's report on the state of public health in Canada*. Ottawa: Health Canada.

Rachlis, M. 2000. *A review of the Alberta private hospital proposal*. Ottawa: Caledon Institute of Social Policy.

Raphael, D. 2009. Social structure, living conditions and health. In D. Raphael (Ed.), *Social Determinants of health: Canadian perspectives* (pp. 20–40). Toronto: Canadian Scholar's Press.

Rodney, P. and Varcoe, C. 2001. Toward ethical inquiry in the economic evaluation of nursing practice. *Canadian Journal of Nursing Research, 33* (1), 35–57.

Rodney, P., Varcoe, C., McPherson, G., Storch, J., Mahoney, K., Brown, H., Pauly, B., Hartrick, G., and Starzomski, R. 2002. Navigating a moral horizon: A multi-site qualitative research study of nurses' enactment of ethical practice. *Canadian Journal of Nursing Research, 34* (3), 75–102.

Romanow, R. 2004. Sustaining medicare: The commission on the future of health care in Canada. In F. Baylis, J. Downie, B. Hoffmaster, and S. Sherwin (Eds.), *Health care ethics in Canada* (pp. 79–100). Toronto: Thomas Nelson.

Sage, W.M. 2009. Solidarity: Unfashionable but still American. In M. Crowly (Ed.), *Connecting values to health reform* (pp. 1–3). Garrison, NY: The Hastings Center.

Shamian, J. 2010. To the editor of the *Vancouver Sun* re: Harper's government ignores the looming health crisis. *Canadian Nurse, 106* (8), 16.

Smedley, B.D. 2008. Moving beyond access: Achieving equity in state health care reform. *Health Affairs (Project Hope), 27* (2), 447–455.

Starfield, B. 2007. Pathways of influence on equity in health. *Social Science and Medicine, 64*, 1355–1362.

Starfield, B., Shi, L., and Macinko, J. 2005. Contributions of primary care to health systems and health. *The Milbank Quarterly, 85* (3), 457–502.

Stoddart, G. and Labelle, R. 1985. *Privatization in the Canadian Health Care System: Assertions, evidence, ideology and options.* Ottawa: Minister of Supply and Services Canada.

Stone, D. 2001. *Policy paradox: The art of political decision-making* (Revised ed.). New York: W.W. Norton and Company.

Storch, J.L. 2010. Canadian healthcare system. In M. McIntyre and C. McDonald, (Eds.), *Realities of Canadian nursing: Professional, practice and power issues* (3rd ed.; pp. 35–55). Philadelphia: Wolters Kluwer/Lippincott Williams & Wilkens.

Storch, J.L. and Meilicke, C.A. 2006. Political, social and economic forces shaping the health care system. In J. M. Hibberd and D. Smith (Eds.), *Nursing leadership and management in Canada* (3rd ed.; pp. 5–28). Toronto: Elsevier.

Storch, J., Rodney, P., Pauly, B., Brown, H., and Starzomski, R. 2002. Listening to nurses' moral voices: Building a quality health care environment. *Canadian Journal of Nursing Leadership, 15* (4), 7–16.

Taylor, M.G. 1973. The Canadian health insurance program. *Public Administration Review, 33 (January–February 1973)*, 31–39.

Taylor, M.G. 1978. *Canadian health insurance and Canadian public policy: The seven decisions that created the Canadian health insurance system.* Montreal: McGill-Queens University Press.

The Standing Senate Committee on Social Affairs, Science and Technology. 2002. *The health of Canadians—The federal role.* Michael Kirby, Chair. Ottawa: Government of Canada.

Tuohy, C.J., Flood, C.M., and Stabile, M. 2004. How does private finance affect public health care systems? Marshaling the evidence from OECD nations. *Journal of Health Politics, Policy and Law, 29* (3), 359–396.

Varcoe, C., Doane, G., Pauly, B., Rodney, P., Storch, J., Mahoney, K., et al., 2004. Ethical practice in nursing: Working the in-betweens. *Journal of Advanced Nursing, 45* (3), 316–325.

Varcoe, C. and Rodney, P. 2009. Constrained agency: The social structure of nurses' work. In B.S. Bolaria and H.D. Dickinson (Eds.), *Health, illness and health care in Canada* (4th ed.; pp.122–151). Toronto: Nelson Education Ltd.

Whitehead, M. and Dahlgren, G. 2006. A discussion paper on concepts and principles for tackling social inequities in health. In *Studies on social and economic determinants of population health,* part 1. Copenhagen: World Health Organization.

Whitman, M. 1998. Nurses can influence public health policy. *Advanced Nursing Practice Quarterly, 3* (4), 67–71.

Young, I.M. 1990. *Justice and the politics of difference.* Princeton, NJ: Princeton University Press.

CHAPTER 13

Working Within the Landscape: Ethics in Practice

Patricia Rodney, Lori d'Agincourt Canning, Gladys McPherson, Joan Anderson, Michael McDonald, Bernadette M. Pauly, Michael Burgess, and J. Craig Phillips

The purpose of inquiry is to achieve agreement among human beings about what to do, to bring about consensus on the ends to be achieved and the means to be used to achieve those ends. (Rorty 1999, xxv)

The ends we want to achieve in ethics include the right, the good, and the fitting action.[1] In Chapter 4 we provided an overview of the history, theoretical underpinnings, and challenges we face in contemporary health care ethics. In Chapter 5, building on Daniels' (1996) argument for theoretical diversity in health care ethics, we sketched out some of the newer theoretical possibilities opened up by cultural, feminist, and relational writings in health care ethics. In this chapter we want to say more about how we might *apply* theory in health care ethics for our practice within complex health care organizations. While other chapters in the text explore the implications of ethical theory for nursing in particular, there are a number of practical insights from health care ethics more generally that we wish to highlight here. This chapter also sets the stage for Chapter 18, A Further Landscape: Ethics in Health Care Organizations and Health/Health Care Policy, where we extend the focus in this chapter to larger organizational and policy questions. Together, Chapter 13 and Chapter 18 take up the call from Sherwin (2011) (cited in Chapter 5) to be "concerned with ethical questions relating to health and life" and also to engage in "critically evaluating the institutional and policy ways in which societies seek to promote and protect health" (78).

Conceptually, throughout the four "landscape" chapters in this text (Chapters 4, 5, 13 and 18) we have been taking direction from Daniels' notion of *wide reflective equilibrium*. Daniels explains that "'[d]oing ethics involves trying to solve very different kinds of problems answering to rather different interests we may have, some quite practical, others more theoretical" (1996, 102). Thus, we have suggested that the ethical theory we adopt, develop, and apply ought to draw on general ethical theories and mid-range ethical principles as well as contextual insights (particularly from cultural, feminist, and relational approaches) (Daniels 1996; Winkler 1996). This means we have been promoting the use of a variety of sources of moral wisdom to solve problems[2] in the real world of practice—in Rorty's (1999) words, above, to figure out "what to do" as well as *how* to do it. In this chapter we will therefore consider how conceptual thinking can be brought to bear for ethical problems in practice.

We start here by taking up the implications of the theoretical challenges we articulated in Chapter 5—that is, how we might actualize the insights generated by cultural, feminist, and relational approaches by using an explanatory framework to address diversity.

Following this we will draw on two practice narratives to help us reflect on interests of persons, particularly those who are made vulnerable through the mediating circumstances of their lives. Having established a theoretical foundation for ethical practice, we will consider the practical dimensions of ethical decision making with and for individuals in health care settings. We close this chapter by looking at the evolution of ethics resources within health care organizations to support ethical practice, with particular emphasis on the importance of resources such as ethics committees and ethics consultants. Because health care ethics simultaneously engages with problems at organizational as well as individual levels, in Chapter 18 we address ethical action for organizations. In Chapter 18 we also explore the policy implications of ethical practice.

ADDRESSING DIVERSITY

Taking up the insights generated by cultural, feminist, and relational approaches requires first coming to grips with notions of diversity. Diversity has become an important concept in health care disciplines, particularly as we negotiate complex ethical decisions with patients, families, and communities who may be considered "different" from the "mainstream" population. The notion of difference can lead to assumptions about the "other" with far-reaching consequences for care (Canales 2010). Yet, we have found in our research related to diversity that it is not only differences in culture that shape how we deal with health, illness, and suffering; in fact, the material circumstances of people's lives, and intersecting social factors (e.g., gender, racialization, ageism) are profound influences (Anderson 2004; Anderson et al. 2009; 2010; Browne et al. 2011; Varcoe, Pauly, and Laliberté in press). This is not to minimize the importance of deep cultural meanings around complex ethical decisions, but rather to recognize that meanings are fluid and embedded in contextual social processes. What has stood out in our studies is that people want to make ethical decisions that will work for them and their families. But difficulties in communicating with health professionals, not fully understanding the consequences of a decision, a feeling of being put down or dismissed by a health professional, being strapped for resources, and the like, often stand in the way. Many people who are seen as different are made vulnerable through the mediating circumstances of their lives.

How, then, might the ethical theory we draw on through the decision-making model we describe later in this chapter be informed by such contextual understandings? We propose an approach that recognizes that *all* patients and their families and health professionals come to the clinical encounter with different *explanatory frameworks.*[3] As health care professionals, we bring our professional knowledge. We also bring our histories; personal, cultural, ethical, and moral perspectives; and prejudices and assumptions, which may be unknown to us, yet operate in ways that influence how we relate to those perceived as the distant other. Patients and families bring their own theories, ethical beliefs, histories, hopes, fears, and the like—often not made explicit to the health professional, partly because the health professional relationship does not provide the space for dialogue. While we expect explanatory frameworks to be different, we know that differences can be negotiated if we can create a space for deep communication (as opposed to speech acts). This kind of engagement goes beyond what is often construed as "respect for difference," which can seem, to those constructed as the distant other, no more than paternalistic/maternalistic "tolerance." *Creating a dialogic space means critical questioning of our own moral and ethical positions and assumptions, which begins by examining on whose grounds taken-for-granted social norms are formed.*

A key question that needs to be confronted is: How receptive are we to viewpoints that are different from our own? Do we see our own ethical positions as located in an unquestionable normative civilizing order (usually grounded in mainstream European epistemologies), to which (non-European or non-mainstream) others should conform, or can we recognize and understand other perspectives through critical reflection? This is not to imply cultural relativism, or a laissez-faire approach that "anything goes" (see Chapter 5). Rather, we argue for the kind of reflective dialogue that goes beyond recognition of power dynamics in health care relationships to addressing them. Such dialogue creates the possibilities for epistemic shifts for the construction of a shared moral agenda.

So, it is not that the health professional or ethicist should draw on ethical theories to make decisions *for* patients/families. Instead, health professionals/ethicists and patients ought to achieve agreement by negotiating ethical decisions in context based on the information at hand. "The problem," therefore, is not identified by the health professional. Rather, the patient/family and health professional identify "the problem" through dialogue, and work through solutions together. Cultural meanings within this dialogic space should be fluid and co-constructed.

The kind of negotiation we are calling for above takes significant theoretical insights and significant interpersonal skills. We address both in the remainder of this chapter. In the next section we offer some reflections on the interests of persons, especially those who are made vulnerable through the mediating circumstances of their lives.[4] In so doing we work with two narrative examples—Ethics in Practice 13-1 about Clarence, a critically ill 14-year-old child, and Ethics in Practice 13-2 about Mr. Johansen, an older adult who has suffered a stroke. Our intent in choosing these narratives (which are fictionalized accounts based on practice and research experiences from McPherson [Clarence] and Rodney [Mr. Johansen]) is not to stereotype children, older adults, or any other group. Rather, we offer what we have learned from our experiences, with the invitation for readers to consider and reflect on how what is being explored might inform ethical practice with other people who have their own unique stories and unique mediating circumstances.

REFLECTIONS ON INTERESTS

The Interests of Persons

As we stated above and in Chapters 4 and 5, in Western health care we are sometimes not very reflective about who does or does not have the opportunity to have meaningful input into their treatment and care—that is, to have their autonomy, including their diversity, respected. As we also noted in Chapter 5, the concept of *relational autonomy* as articulated by Canadian philosopher Susan Sherwin (1998) can help us to appreciate such power dynamics at individual, organizational, and larger systems levels. Relational autonomy directs us to look not at isolated individuals but, rather, at individuals who are always nested within complex interpersonal, organizational, and socio-political contexts (see also Baylis, Kenny, and Sherwin 2008; Hartrick Doane and Varcoe 2005; Yeo 2010, and Chapters 7 and 8 in this text). We see addressing diversity as a cornerstone to respecting relational autonomy.

Further, it is our belief that a better understanding of the interests[5] of all persons—especially those who are unable to act autonomously or who are at risk of having their autonomy overlooked or overridden—can move us toward better appreciating diversity and toward better relational ethical practice. We argue that addressing the interests of persons requires that we understand their *rights, needs, and relationships* (McPherson 2007).[6] Let us start to illustrate what we mean with the story about Clarence in pediatric intensive care (Ethics in Practice 13-1).

ETHICS IN PRACTICE 13-1

Clarence

Clarence was a 14-year-old boy who suffered serious and rare complications of a bacterial respiratory infection. Within days of the onset of the illness Clarence's lungs began to fail and he required artificial ventilation. In addition, he developed bilateral pneumothoraces and pneumomediastinum.[7] In spite of two weeks of aggressive treatment in intensive care, Clarence's condition continued to deteriorate.

Clarence's physicians and parents decided to start ECMO[8] therapy. From that point on, Clarence endured a multitude of complications including persistent bleeding in various sites (including his lungs), periods of low blood pressure, and infection. Many invasive procedures were performed in an effort to save his life. In spite of these aggressive efforts, Clarence died approximately 30 days after the onset of his illness.

As described, Clarence was very sick from early in the course of his treatment. Although Clarence was sedated and received large doses of analgesia, he was conscious some of the time during his hospitalization. Because of the tubes in his airway, he was unable to speak. He could only communicate through gestures and facial expressions. For periods of days, he was pharmacologically paralyzed[9] and consequently unable to communicate in any way. Clarence was never asked if he wanted to proceed with treatment and no one is sure he ever knew the severity of his illness. When not paralyzed there were times when Clarence was obviously dreadfully frightened, and tried to pull at tubes or tried to get up. At those times, he needed to be physically restrained and required additional sedation.

Clarence's parents were at his bedside constantly. Throughout his illness, they spoke on his behalf, seeking to make the Clarence whom they knew visible to the nurses, physicians, and technicians involved in his care. Their wish was that everything possible was done for Clarence, and they provided their consent for every procedure that might offer any hope. When it became evident that Clarence could not survive, his parents stated that they found comfort in their religious faith that led them to believe that this illness was the will of God and that, when Clarence died, he would be going to a better place.

Caring for Clarence was troubling for many nurses. The aggressive nature of the illness, the age of this child, and the experimental nature of the treatment created a tense climate. Staff voiced concerns about the extent to which Clarence could or should be involved in decisions about his care, and questioned the extent to which his parents' interests could reasonably be assumed to truly represent Clarence's interests.[10]

Honouring Rights

Children's Moral Status Claims that children and other persons have certain rights reflect particular beliefs about their moral status (see also Chapter 4 and Chapter 16). Children's and other persons' rights can be considered to include three types: the right to resources, including knowledge; the right to protection from harm or abuse; and the right to autonomy or freedom (McPherson 2007).

In regard to children's participation in decisions about their health care, claims to rights help us to hold in mind the positioning of children within our health care system and heighten our awareness of power differentials between children and adults, as well as between children as health care recipients and nurses and other professionals as health care providers (see also Chapter 16). Thus, the situation in Ethics in Practice 13-1 may cause us to wonder if the (well-intended) power differentials between Clarence, his parents, and the health care providers interfered with Clarence's right to participate in decisions about his treatment. But these claims to rights to participate cannot stand alone. Somehow participation must be appropriate to the patient's capabilities, contextually structured to enhance the particular individual's participation, and considerate with regard to stimulating the patient's growth as a moral agent.[11] While Clarence's active participation in decisions about his treatment might have been appropriate to his age, and might have engaged him as an active agent, the contextual features of the suddenness and cascading severity of his illness made active participation difficult (though not impossible).

The challenge is to look more closely at this issue of children's interests to find a reasonable way to make judgments about "best interests." We need a more nuanced way to think about how to weigh different interests—how to consider the relationship of one person's interests to the interests of others (McPherson 2007). Rights are a *necessary* component of our understanding of children's and other persons' interests, but they are not *sufficient* to provide guidance in complex situations where rights compete with one another and where other needs and relationships come into play. In such situations, rights and rights-based approaches become even more important, especially for people who are made vulnerable by the mediating circumstances of their lives. And in such situations, as we also argued in Chapters 4 and 5, we ought to advocate for the full realization of rights for these persons.

Considering Needs

Thinking about rights may alert us to the critical features that must always be accounted for in the way we treat children and other vulnerable persons. Daniels (1985) suggests that in considerations of health care, theories about needs provide a more intricate means by which to sort out what is fair and just (see also Chapters 4 and 5 and Daniels, Kennedy, and Kawachi 2004). When we look in this direction, another important body of theory and research informs our thinking. For instance, our understanding of children's needs is supported by substantial theory in the field of child development. Reflecting back on Ethics in Practice 13-1, this theory should cause us to ask not only whether Clarence's right to respect was being protected, but also whether his needs were being attended to. Developmental theories would help us to understand his need for privacy, connection to his family, and so forth. These are not unique needs of the individual child; nor are they respect for his autonomy or unique individuality. These are needs based on seeing beyond the technical aspects of health care services to recognize the requirements of children and other persons as human beings. What children need will vary depending on the child's health condition, experience, and unique characteristics (McPherson 2007).[12] For this reason, it would have been relevant to know more about Clarence's previous experiences with health care. This kind of experiential background is also relevant for other persons. For example, research has shown that the experience with illness and the communication of health care providers in complex delivery systems profoundly affects the quality of life of adults and older adults with a chronic illness such as cancer (Thorne, Bultz, and Baile 2005).

Respecting Relationships

Consideration of the rights and needs of children and other vulnerable persons enables us to better appreciate individual characteristics that are important in judgments of their interests. While generally not included in discussions about interests, relationships—who individuals are as members of families and communities—can be seen as important elements in judgments made about benefits for persons, and hence in making ethically sound decisions (McPherson 2007). In Ethics in Practice 13-1, for example, respecting Clarence's relationships leads us to consider the role of his parents in interpreting his interests, and to think about the preservation of his relationships with his parents and others as an important dimension of addressing his best interests.[13]

In summary, *responding to the interests of children and other persons requires that we attend to their rights as well as their needs. Responding to the interests of children and other persons also requires that we understand and promote the family, community, and team relationships that can support and nurture each person.* Further, Clarence's situation shows us that responding to the interests of those who are particularly vulnerable because of the mediating circumstances of their lives makes it important that we develop the skill to attend to their rights, needs, and relationships as fully as possible, and thereby create the possibility for negotiating cultural meanings in a dialogic space. Within health care we require relational approaches to ethical action that can foster this kind of responsiveness (see also Chapters 7, 8, and 16).

ETHICAL ACTION FOR INDIVIDUALS

We commenced this chapter calling for the creation of a dialogic space for ethical action that respects diversity, and used our analysis in Ethics in Practice 13-1 to show that responding to the interests of persons requires that we attend to their rights, needs, and relationships. In our analysis of Ethics in Practice 13-2 we add to the above and put the insights we have explored about rights, needs, and relationships as well as diversity into action through the application of an ethical decision-making framework.

The story in Ethics in Practice 13-2 is based on an advanced practice nurse's account of a practice situation in which a number of morally challenging factors converged for an older adult who had suffered a stroke and for his daughter.

ETHICS IN PRACTICE 13-2

Mr. Johansen

In my role as geriatric clinical nurse specialist, I was asked to see an elderly man who had been living with his daughter, had had a stroke, and had been in hospital on a general medical unit for five days—though he had been held in the emergency [department] for three days before a bed was available on the medical unit or anywhere else in the hospital.

So the nurses on the medical ward are having difficulty, so they call me saying, "He's just not getting any better, the confusion is getting worse, come and see." He had delirium after he came in following his stroke and that seemed to resolve somewhat, but that label of confusion that was placed on him at admission remained firmly attached to him. The nurses told me that he was now worse than he had been originally. Apparently, his daughter [Stephanie] is there every single day. She is very knowledgeable, having read up on stroke, dementia, and delirium. And, by asking many questions she has driven the physicians away—they tend to avoid her like the plague. I go through his chart and see that there are a variety of issues at play here.

The nurses mentioned that their earlier efforts to draw this patient's increasing confusion and delirium to the attention of the attending physician seem to have been ignored. But the attending physician was away and there was an on-call physician taking over for him. I phoned the on-call doc. She was willing to talk to me, so she and I went over some of the facts, including the patient's increasing dehydration, his elevated WBC [white blood cell count], and the nurses' suspicion that he had a UTI [urinary tract infection]. Because the on-call physi-

cian didn't know the patient, she came in right away. When she saw him, he was lying in bed, with his legs over the side rails, picking things out of the air. His daughter was at his bedside, clearly distressed.

As it turns out, this man did have a UTI. When the UTI was treated the delirium disappeared. Although he was still somewhat confused the hallucinations and delirium were gone. The daughter was really relieved. However, when the attending physician returned, he told me that he wouldn't have bothered to treat the patient's UTI if I had called him, saying, "He's just going to die anyway."

But the question I ask is, "What about the daughter's health?" She felt so much better having her father back to somebody she could relate to, even though she knew he would never recover from his stroke. She had been so distressed because in the middle of his delirium he said something like, "I think it's time for the move." To her that meant that he wanted to die. The daughter had tried to say this to the [attending] physician. . . . She would pick out all these threads from his confusion, what he was trying to convey about how he was feeling. . . . She was becoming a thorn in their [the attending physician's and the specialist's] sides.

I had a sense that the daughter felt relieved to have her father back again to somewhat of the person she knew before, even though he'd had this stroke. But to see him and . . . to hear his terror as he verbalized his hallucinations and his delusions . . . that kernel of what was going on inside him, she knew him so well that she could figure it out . . . it was so distressing for her. (Adapted from Rodney 1997)

Rights, Needs, and Relationships

Threats to autonomy are, unfortunately, all too common for older adults such as Mr. Johansen when they experience health challenges. We live in a society where youth and productivity are valued, where ageism is prevalent, and where getting older is seen as a medical problem. Whether they are in their homes, in long-term care facilities, or in acute care hospitals, older adults may experience a lack of respect from care providers, particularly if their level of consciousness is impaired (Agich 1998; 1999; Bužgová and Ivanová 2009; Dahlke and Phinney 2008; Dodds 2005; Penning and Vtova 2009; Randers and Mattiasson 2000; Sellman 2009; see also Suhonen et al. 2010 for a review of related ethics research). Clearly, Ethics in Practice 13-2 raises important issues about the interests of Mr. Johansen, and his daughter, Stephanie. We claimed earlier that responding to the interests of all persons requires that we attend to their rights, needs, and relationships. It will be important to start to understand more about all three categories for Mr. Johansen, Stephanie, and the rest of their family as a prerequisite to engaging in an effective ethical decision-making process. While it will not be possible to do a full analysis, we can make at least a few observations here. Let us start with Mr. Johansen.

First, the *right* of Mr. Johansen to be respected as a unique, self-determining being (founded in the ethical principle of autonomy) was under threat. Indeed, in a fiscally constrained health care system, his basic human rights were, at least to some extent, under threat (see our discussion of human rights in Chapter 5). Whether or not he was dying, he deserved to have some relief of what were treatable symptoms (Jennings et al. 2003; Carstairs 2010; see also Chapter 17.) He did not deserve to have treatment and care withheld because of an assumption that "he was just going to die anyway." Further, he deserved to have his *dignity* protected and to have some choices in his treatment and care. At the time of the story in Ethics in Practice 13-2, Mr. Johansen was no longer competent to enact this right, but his daughter apparently was competent as his proxy (substitute) decision maker.[14] Despite significant progress in *advance directives* over the past few years (see Chapter 17), older adults continue to have little control over how treatment and care decisions unfold throughout their illness trajectories, especially as they approach death (Callahan 2011; Gallagher et al. 2002; Robinson 2011; Rodney and Howlett 2003).

Secondly, the unique *needs* of older persons are often not well attended to in health care delivery. For instance, it took expertise in gerontology to understand that Mr. Johansen's confusion was worsened by his UTI. And it took expertise to understand how much rehabilitation potential he still had post stroke (he may not, in fact, have been close to death). Although gerontology and geriatric medicine have become important new specialties, mainstream health care has a long way to go in understanding and hence addressing the needs of older adults—how they experience pain, social isolation, financial barriers, and a host of other challenges (Gallagher et al. 2002; National Advisory Committee 2000; Penning and Votova 2009). As a society, we have even further to go in understanding capabilities of older adults as well as their needs.

Thirdly, the story in Ethics in Practice 13-2 raises some important questions about Mr. Johansen's *relationships* with the health care delivery system and with his family. As Sherwin (1998) reminds us, relational autonomy should call our attention to organizational as well as interpersonal relationships. Behind the scenes of this account were troubling questions about the allocation of resources for the elderly. The acute medical unit where this patient was placed had many other elderly patients, many of whom were not receiving adequate nursing resources (Rodney 1997). This was by no means atypical at the time of Mr. Johansen's situation, and is a problem that has been steadily worsening

over the past two decades (Austin 2011; Rodney and Varcoe in press). Current gerontological and ethical literature resounds with warnings that the elderly are bearing the
brunt of fiscal policy changes (Dahlke and Phinney 2008; Lachs 2003; Penning and
Votova 2009). That is, they are experiencing a progressive erosion of access to appropriate resources for treatment and care in acute and long-term care facilities, and in-home
care situations (see also Chapters 12 and 19). Older women, and women who must stay
home as caregivers, can be especially vulnerable. These problems should cause us
to wonder, for instance, what kind of home supports Mr. Johansen and Stephanie had
available to them. We will say more about the implications for health care providers in
terms of their organizational and policy responsibilities in Chapter 18.

Interests of Families[15]

One of the most important challenges in contemporary health care ethics is to understand
and attend to our ethical obligations to families—as individual family members, as family
units, and as both connected to and distinct from patients (Blustein 1993/1998; Nelson
1998; Robinson 2011). Attending to families requires that we understand and work with
the community within which families and patients are located (which will be explored
further in Chapters 19 and 20). In Ethics in Practice 13-1, for instance, the family was
very present and was interpreting Clarence's intentions and desires. In Ethics in Practice
13-2, on the other hand, we saw a family member, Stephanie, who was also very much
present yet was not acknowledged. Furthermore, we lacked information about the roles,
relationships, and stories from the rest of Mr. Johansen's family. It appeared that
Stephanie was more vulnerable because she was alone. It would only be through creating
a dialogic space with Stephanie that we could more fully understand her unique material
circumstances, and those of the rest of her family.

It is possible that Stephanie was having her rights as a proxy decision maker ignored.
Unfortunately, this is not uncommon, especially in end-of-life situations. Research tells
us that families have a difficult time having their voices heard on behalf of their family
members at the end of life (Chamber-Evans 2002; Hiltunen et al. 1999; Robinson 2011;
Stajduhar 2003).[16] The sources of this difficulty are multi-faceted, and include lack of
information or advanced discussion about the patient's illness, a failure to address emotions, a lack of understanding of advance directives per se, conflict between family
members, and, perhaps most commonly, communication breakdown between the family,
the patient, and the health care team (Anspach and Beeson, 2001; Charchuk and Simpson
2003; Robinson 2011; Rodney and Howlett 2003; see also Chapter 17). This is not to say
that the rights of the family ought to outweigh the rights of the patient, or that family
members always act in the best interests of patients. But it is to say that we need to
rethink how we involve families in decisions that unfold over time and that have an
impact on family members as well as on patients. As one leading theorist in the field
explained over a decade ago,

> [t]he notion that patients need to be empowered in [health care institutions] is exactly right; the
> mistake is in thinking this is likely to happen if patients are allowed to be alienated from their
> own sources of personal affirmation and authority in the name of giving such authority formal
> protection. (Nelson 1998, 293)

There has been substantial research done on the needs of families in critical care settings. This research tells us that one of the foremost needs of family members such as Clarence's parents in Ethics in Practice 13-1 and Stephanie in Ethics in Practice 13-2 is for access to health care team members—especially physicians—for comprehensible, supportive, and up-to-date information about the patient (Abbott et al. 2001; Anspach and Beeson 2001; Curtis et al. 2001; Heyland et al. 2006; 2010; Vandall-Walker 2002). Research from palliative and chronic care contexts reminds us that family needs include access to adequate resources for treatment and care in the home and/or health care facility (including respite care) as well as access to financial, social, and psychological support (Carstairs 2010; Hayes and McElheran 2002; Rodney and Howlett 2003; Stajduhar 2003; 2011; Wilson 2000). Throughout all of the research there is an implicit or explicit focus on the importance of supportive relationships between patients, family members, community members, and health care team members.

In summary, we can say that attending to family interests requires, at the least,

- respect for family members as individuals and for the family as a unit that has evolved (and will evolve) over time;

- regular communication between the family, the patient, and the health care team based on a dialogic space that is attentive to diversity;

- anticipatory guidance to prepare for expected and unexpected health challenges; and

- careful attention to the resources the family will need to support the well-being of the patient, family members, and the family as a unit—regardless of whether they are in the home, a long-term care facility, an acute care hospital, or any other setting.

It appears that Stephanie would have benefitted from all of the above. In her case, anticipatory guidance would include grief work and making the most of the time she had remaining with her father. In the words of an ethicist who is worried about how the elderly are viewed in our society, "Soon enough, we will no longer be able to walk hand in hand, but it matters deeply that we treasure the companionship while we can" (Lachs 2003, 217).

Ethical Decision Making

Explicit ethical decisions are necessary at those times when value-based questions give rise to difficulties in selecting among health care options or determining respectful care in the course of health care interactions. In particular, ethical decisions are often required because of, or in the context of, uncertainty about important features of the decision. Whether the product of deliberate and considered thinking or not, the decisions made in such moments are ethical in nature because they have an inherent value component. Ethical decisions may have to do with issues such as the type or extent of medical or nursing care, the disclosure of information to patients, the maintenance of patient privacy and confidentiality, interdisciplinary team and family conflict, access to health and social resources, and so on—an infinite range of quandary[17] and everyday issues (Rodney et al. 2002; see also Chapter 1). It is important to note that awareness of the moral dimensions of a particular situation and attentiveness to the possibility of alternate courses of action are prerequisites for ethical deliberation.[18] Ethical decision making *ought* to be a part of all good clinical decision making (Canadian Nurses Association 2008), and may take place through a formal structured process as well as through ongoing, integrated reflection on values in clinical practice. *In our experience, the more complex and conflicted the situation an individual, family, and health care team are experiencing, the greater the benefit of a more formalized and structured ethical decision-making process.*

Ethical decision making can be understood as a structured form of moral deliberation that occurs when an individual confronts an ethical situation (Beyerstein 1993, 422). Over the past two decades or so a number of models of ethical decision making have evolved for clinical practice. Most early models followed a process of rational analysis and drew on a principle-based approach to ethical theory. Ethical principles were applied and weighed, which included explaining the ranking of the principles in each case and providing reasons for preferring one principle over another when they conflicted (Beyerstein 1993, 419). Recently, a more nuanced approach to ethical decision making that is sensitive to context has had increased influence (Rodney et al. 2002). Contextual approaches to ethical decision making encourage us to undertake a careful assessment of the patient's physiological status, personal wishes, cultural and spiritual beliefs, and overall quality of life (Hoffmaster 2001). They also encourage us to consider the patient in the context of his or her family and social environment. *Such models can therefore help us to better appreciate diversity and understand each person's unique interests.* The model we will use here is Michael McDonald's Ethical Decision-Making Framework for Individuals (see Appendix B).[19]

The fundamental concepts we have available for ethical decision making include the traditional principles of autonomy, beneficence/nonmaleficence, and justice as well as more contextual concepts such as fidelity and care (Arras, Steinbock, and London 1999).[20] Moreover, incorporating Sherwin's notion of relational autonomy (1998) can strengthen our use of decision-making models. Approaches to ethical decision making such as McDonald's are therefore consistent with Daniels' (1996) notion of wide reflective equilibrium. A composite approach to theory is taken such that general theories (e.g., deontology, virtue theory), mid-range ethical principles (e.g., autonomy, beneficence/nonmaleficence, and justice), and more experiential/relational concepts (e.g., fidelity, care, and relational autonomy) are implicit in various portions of the model (Rodney and Howlett 2003). Furthermore, some of the models also provide guidance for interpersonal and group processes that can work toward consensus. We have found that McDonald's decision-making framework allows us to do all of this. Referring to Ethics in Practice 13-2, in what follows we look at how we might sort through Mr. Johansen's particular situation using McDonald's Ethical Decision-Making Framework for Individuals. While it is not possible to fully illustrate all the components of the framework, we hope to say enough to promote the application of this framework (or other models or frameworks) to practice.

McDonald's Ethical Decision-Making Framework for Individuals

The details of the story in Ethics in Practice 13-2 bring what might be understood as a typical ethical issue in the care of older persons into a particular context, where the problem—to treat or not to treat—becomes much more complex. The problem depicted in this story could be reduced to a description of a case of "the futility of treating terminally ill elderly persons" or "the problem of power dynamics in nurse–physician relationships." The nurse in the story clearly moves beyond an understanding of this issue as an example of a "generic" ethical case. Within her account of the problem is an array of knowledge that has ethical relevance. Knowledge about the clinical problem, the daughter's experience, and the staff nurses' concerns all entered into her inquiry about this issue.

Effective ethical decision-making models can support description and analysis of the problem in a complex and contextualized way and promote movement toward a negotiated consensus. *Perhaps the greatest asset that models and frameworks such as McDonald's offer us is that they prompt us to ask particular questions of ethically troubling situations, and to take the knowledge gleaned from these questions into our analyses.* McDonald's Ethical Decision-Making Framework for Individuals (Appendix B) consists of five iterative steps: (1) collect information and identify the problem; (2) specify feasible alternatives; (3) use your ethical resources to identify morally significant factors in each alternative; (4) propose and test possible resolutions; and (5) make your choice—live with it and learn from it. It is important to note that this framework is not a linear problem-solving guide or algorithm.[21] As the process unfolds, new information may generate new alternatives for treatment and care.[22]

Furthermore, no model or framework stands alone. What becomes evident is that in addition to the structures for thinking that a model or framework supplies, education in critical thinking, ethical theory, the application of ethical decision-making models, and related ethical issues is also required. In Ethics in Practice 13-2, related ethical issues include contemporary thinking about withholding and withdrawing treatment, controversies about the concept of futility, and the use of advance directives. They also include, as we have argued above, an appreciation of the interests of the patients and family members involved. Similarly, substantive knowledge related to the practice area is beneficial. In Ethics in Practice 13-2 this included, for instance, knowledge of neurology, gerontology, rehabilitation, grief theory, family theory, and conflict resolution theory. Perhaps most importantly, health care professionals and ethicists need the reflective communications skills required to create the dialogic space to address diversity for all involved persons that we called for at the outset of this chapter.

Application of McDonald's Framework to Ethics in Practice 13-2

(1) Collect information and identify the problem.

This step is foundational to the success of the entire decision-making process. In identifying and describing the problem, McDonald suggests that we ought to take into account multiple perspectives. This requires that we seek input from the patient, family, friends, and other health care team members and involve these individuals as much as possible through every step of the process. For Mr. Johansen in Ethics in Practice 13-2, the individual we needed input most from was himself—that is, his prior expressed values and wishes, and/or any hints about his current wishes as they appear to us through his current state. In some instances we might have good reason to think a patient has changed his or her mind, and would want to ask the family whether this would be consistent with a recent trend or some other longstanding values or recent "conversions." We also need input from his daughter, Stephanie, other family members and friends, the nurses on the medical unit, his home care nurses and care aides, his family physician, the medical specialists involved in his care, his attending physicians on the medical unit, his social worker(s), and his rehabilitation therapist(s).

It takes time and communication skill to identify and then gather information from such diverse parties.[23] Indeed, information gathering should be continuous throughout the ethical decision-making process. As we proceed, we ought to ask questions about the patient's physical, psychological, social, cultural, and spiritual status, including changes over time. For instance, more information about Mr. Johansen's symptoms of stroke, and how those progressed, was important. What were his explicit and implicit values in the way he lived his life before the stroke? Did religious faith play an important role in his life? And so on. We also ought to investigate the patient's assessment of his or her own quality of life, and his or her wishes about the treatment/care decisions at hand. This includes determining the patient's competency and determining who is available to speak for him or her. In Ethics in Practice 13-2, this meant finding out if Mr. Johansen had an advance directive and trying to determine what he had told others about his beliefs about life-sustaining treatment, and who he wanted making decisions for him. *A family assessment is crucial, including roles, relationships, and relevant "stories."* We have already raised questions about the apparent isolation of Stephanie. What other family members or friends were available locally? At a distance? How had the decision for her to become her father's caregiver been arrived at? Who did Stephanie define as her family? Further, we ought to identify the health care team members involved and the circumstances affecting them. In this situation, for instance, it appears that the staff nurses believed that they had been disempowered, that their voices had not been heard (or they had not raised them effectively) in previous efforts to address this issue. Why was that? What were the power dynamics in the organization? Had the nurses actually approached the physicians directly to discuss their concerns? And why were the attending physicians apparently so reluctant to treat the patient? Were they under pressure to admit other patients to his acute care bed? Conversely, were they afraid that the daughter was going to launch legal action if they discharged the patient?

As we start to put the information together, we ought to summarize the situation briefly but with all the relevant facts and circumstances, trying to get a sense of the patient's overall illness trajectory. It is also important that we determine what decisions have to be made and by whom. *Thus, a detailed and specific description of the ethical problem—a description that captures the multiple points of view—is crucial to the contextual component of ethical decision making.* Thin descriptions of the problem fail to provide the contextual understanding (see also Chapter 6). The stronger our contextual understanding of the problem, the more effective and relevant the following steps in the process, and the more likely that the resolution will attend to the interests of all involved and be ethically defensible.

Consider the difference between these two descriptions of the problem in the story in Ethics in Practice 13-2:

1. Mr. Johansen, an elderly man who had suffered a stroke, is experiencing increasing confusion. His daughter and the nurses involved in his care believe that he should be

assessed and treated. His attending physician feels this is a waste of scarce resources. Should he be assessed and treated, or not?

2.   Mr. Johansen, an elderly man who recently suffered a stroke, is experiencing increased confusion and is having periods of delirium. His daughter and the nurses who are caring for him have noticed this change and suspect that this increased confusion may be the result of a treatable problem. The attending physicians indicate that because of Mr. Johansen's pre-existing confusion, his age, and his impending death, he ought not receive additional medical treatment. This ethical problem has at least four tracks: (1) What authority should the voices of the daughter and the nurses have in this decision-making process? How are they reflecting Mr. Johansen's interests? (2) Should Mr. Johansen be offered medical assessment and treatment that may well improve the quality of his life even though it will not likely change its duration? What symptom management can be achieved? (3) How can the well-being of Mr. Johansen's family be attended to as they face his uncertain prognosis and possible death? And (4) how can we deal with the interdisciplinary team conflict that has exacerbated this situation?

Notice that the two descriptions of the problem, while related, will lead in quite different directions. The first is much more one-dimensional. It reduces complex issues to two "win–lose" questions: Which patients benefit most when resources are scarce? Who has the final authority here? The second description is more deeply embedded in the context of the particular situation and is, we would argue, more likely to promote ethical practice. It moves significantly beyond simple black-and-white or win–lose choices.

(2) Specify feasible alternatives for treatment and care.

In this second step of the ethical decision-making process, we consider what possibilities exist for action. Although in Ethics in Practice 13-2 we do not have an account of the nurse's reasoning process as she decided on her course of action, important questions about how to treat and care for Mr. Johansen and Stephanie arise for us as we work through the case we are provided. At a juncture such as this, creative and critical thinking are essential, and must be informed by sound clinical judgment. Moral imagination and ongoing self-reflection are also immensely helpful (see also Chapters 6, 8, 9, and 15, as well as Doane 2004; Nortvedt 2004). We should lay out sets of options ("tracks") in accordance with how we have identified the problems.

For Mr. Johansen, this means that we need carefully tailored options to address each of the four tracks. *First*, we need to make a decision about who is best able to speak for Mr. Johansen in accordance with his prior wishes and any advance documentation we are able to find. In doing this it is important for us also to carefully attend to Mr. Johansen's (albeit somewhat confused) expression of his feelings and concerns. *Second*, in this and in most challenging ethical situations, there are more fine-grained alternatives than "treat" or "not treat"—or worse, "heroics" and "no heroics." For example, antibiotics may be appropriate for a palliative patient if they help relieve symptoms of confusion and agitation in an elderly patient. Furthermore, *palliative care ought to be integrated into all levels of care* (Quill 2000; Rocker, Shemie, and Lacroix 2000; Rodney and Howlett

2003; Stajduhar 2011). In other words, even if Mr. Johansen was to be treated with a full range of medical therapy, he and Stephanie should still have the opportunity to benefit from the pain and symptom management, and the personal and social support, that palliative care provides.[24] *Third*, we need options for the personal and social support Mr. Johansen and his daughter will require whether he is discharged home or whether he stays in hospital, and regardless of when he dies. This includes, for instance, home care services, grief counseling, and pastoral care involvement. *Fourth*, we need to identify means by which we can better understand and deal with the intra- and inter-professional team conflict that the various team members are reacting to.[25]

(3) Use ethical resources to identify morally significant factors in each alternative.

Once we have identified sets of alternatives organized around the four tracks in this situation, we need to sort out which alternatives are most ethically defensible. Informed by our understanding of the interests of the patient and family, and also attentive to the interests of the health care team, we should evaluate the alternatives according to ethical principles/concepts, professional standards, and personal judgments and experiences. There may also be a need for a formal ethics case conference, ethics committee meeting, or case consultation in situations that are complex and/or conflicted (Fox et al. 2007; Rodney and Howlett 2003).

To illustrate, for Mr. Johansen in Ethics in Practice 13-2, we might consider a set of alternatives (drawn from each track) that involve (1) formally designating Stephanie as proxy decision maker; (2) medical treatment for his UTI, with a period of more intense physiotherapy and nursing care in hospital and involvement of social work and the family physician to commence planning for his eventual discharge from hospital; (3) referral of Stephanie to the clinical nurse specialist and a pastoral care liaison for ongoing support and grief work; and (4) calling a meeting between medical and nursing staff to discuss the communication challenges they are facing and to help them generate some solutions, including continuing education on end-of-life issues. We would reflect on each of these in terms of ethical principles/concepts, professional standards, and personal judgments and experiences. For example, our understanding of justice and relational autonomy would help us to identify the importance of mobilizing (arguing for) better acute care and eventual home care resources. Our professional standards around palliative care and rehabilitation would help us to come up with a care plan while Mr. Johansen is in hospital and a care plan for his transition home. Our personal judgments and experiences would help us to work out how best to approach Stephanie and recover her trust before helping her with her grief. And our personal judgments and experiences would help us to know how to proceed with getting the health care team together to start to face their own conflict.

(4) Propose and test possible resolutions.

Here we move to select the best alternatives, all things considered—in other words, realizing that we may not achieve either certainty or perfection. The individuals closest to Mr. Johansen, including, for instance, Stephanie, other family members, his family physician, and his spiritual support (if Mr. Johansen identified spiritual support as important for him), will be crucial players here. Proposing and testing possible resolutions includes performing a sensitivity analysis and considering our choices critically: Which factors would have to change to get us to alter our decisions? In Ethics in Practice 13-2, for example, our alternatives would shift if we learned that Mr. Johansen's death was imminent. We also need to think about the effects of our choices upon others' choices: Are we making it easier for others (health care providers, patients, and their families) to act ethically? The fourth set of strategies for Mr. Johansen are targeted explicitly in this direction, as we are hoping to help the members of the team learn from the situation and from each other.

We also need to ask if this is what a compassionate health care professional would do in a caring environment. Here it is helpful to formulate our choices as general maxims for all similar situations. This includes thinking of situations where they do *not* apply as well as where they do. For example, if Mr. Johansen's daughter was estranged from her father, we might be looking elsewhere for a proxy decision maker (see also Chapter 17). Finally, we need to ask if, as decision makers, we are still comfortable with our choices. If there is not reasonable consensus related to this situation, we need to revisit the process.

(5) Make the choice—live with it and learn from it.

This is, perhaps, the most difficult step—to take action on what has been decided. *Making the choice ought to include delineating* how *to implement what has been decided.* In Mr. Johansen's situation, for instance, this would include: (1) following the agency policy to designate Stephanie as proxy decision maker; (2) communicating with the hospital physicians, physiotherapists, nurses, social workers, and family physician(s) who would be involved in Mr. Johansen's treatment and care; (3) arranging for Stephanie to meet with the clinical nurse specialist and a pastoral care liaison; and (4) getting a commitment from medical and nursing staff to discuss the communication challenges they are facing.

Together, all of the steps and actions we have articulated above are consistent with our call at the outset of this chapter to create a dialogic space to address diversity. *Living with* the decision means accepting the responsibility to monitor the outcomes. Most importantly, this includes getting feedback from the patient (if possible), from the family, and from health care team members. Given that ethical decision making is a non-linear process, this may also mean triggering further review or further action.

Learning from the decision should be both informal and formal. Informally, we should talk with colleagues who were involved in the situation, share experiences, and reflect on our feelings. Formally, we ought to have periodic case reviews of situations such as Mr. Johansen's—not to allocate blame, but to be more prepared for the next situation like his that arises, and to recognize when we have made improvements in our ethical practice. Furthermore, our reviews may raise the need for proactive policy work to prevent what otherwise will be or already are recurring problems. In Mr. Johansen's situation, for instance, a review of policies as well as education around end-of-life care and related policies would seem warranted (Stajduhar 2011; see also Chapters 15, 17, and 18). Finally, there is a role for research here to more formally evaluate the outcomes of ethical decision-making processes. For example, a carefully designed qualitative study to explore the experiences of family members such as Stephanie could be beneficial, particularly if it helps us to better understand their diversity and interests (see, for example, Robinson 2011).

In concluding our discussion of Mr. Johansen's story, we can see how the use of an ethical decision-making model helped us to move toward a plan of action that was more ethical than what was occurring prior to the clinical nurse specialist's intervention, and that was closer to supporting all the participants' relational autonomy, including their diversity and their interests.[26] What might otherwise be seen as a case of an older person experiencing the normal course of deterioration toward death was instead understood as an event in which treatment and care could improve the quality of this man's remaining life and the life of his daughter. Further, the members of the health care team who were involved had a much better chance of feeling supported in their practice (see also Chapters 9 and 10).

Toward Consensus

In closing this section of the chapter, we want to elaborate on the notion of consensus that appears at the end of McDonald's Ethical Decision-Making Framework for Individuals. The theoretical landscape of health care ethics has progressed to the point at which we are better able to appreciate the unique interests of individuals, including how those interests change with time and experience. However, it takes negotiation to support individuals and their varied interests within complex and often conflicted family, community, and health care organizational contexts. As we indicated at the outset of this chapter, we therefore wish to advocate for an inclusive and ongoing process of respecting diversity and negotiating consensus as a goal of ethical work. This is not a prescription for an imperialist view of health care ethics; nor is it a descent into ethical relativism (see Chapter 5). Rather, it is meant to be a thoughtful and dialectical process consistent with the concept of wide reflective equilibrium. *We are advocating an approach to reasoning that draws on both deductive and inductive modes of thinking—a contextual approach that does not neglect the wisdom offered by philosophical positions and theoretical perspectives.* We believe that McDonald's Ethical Decision-Making Framework for Individuals offers one means of engaging in both deductive and inductive thinking.

A crucial focal point in a conversation about the application of ethical theory/insights with individuals is to think about who these individual human beings (the persons we refer to as patients) are within their relationships with their family and community, with health care professionals, with the health care system, and with society—a *relational* ethical approach that we have explored in this book in Chapters 5, 7, and 8. As we also argued at the outset of this chapter, it takes many interpersonal skills to come to this understanding and to hear the voices of all those affected by the situation at hand—not just the loudest voices or the voices representing official organizational roles. *Hence, ethical action is as much about process as it is about theory.* What we envision is ethical practice as a dynamic process of building consensus (in contrast to a static group decision)—that is, a "healthy community of open, inclusive moral discovery and growth" (Jennings 1991, 461–462).[27] While this dynamic process is not easy to achieve, it is not impossible to move toward, especially with guidance from effective decision-making models and frameworks and with adequate organizational support. Fortunately, organizational ethics resources have developed well over the past two decades.

ORGANIZATIONAL ETHICS RESOURCES

Ethics Committees

The primary mechanism for addressing ethical issues in health care institutions is the health care ethics committee (HEC) and/or ethics consultation service. Institutional ethics committees date back to the 1970s, but their numbers have increased dramatically in recent years. Spurring this growth has been recognition by accrediting bodies of the essential role that ethics plays in health care delivery. Since 1992, for example, the Joint Committee for Accreditation for Healthcare Organizations in the U.S. has mandated that health care institutions have a standing mechanism for addressing ethical conflicts (Joint Commission on Accreditation of Healthcare Organizations 1992). The majority of hospitals have met this accreditation requirement with an ethics committee. Likewise, Accreditation Canada standards mandate that health care organizations have a comprehensive ethics strategy, which includes processes to handle both clinical and organizational ethics concerns.

Ethics committees support health care institutions with three core functions: (1) deliberation of cases with ethics concerns/consultation; (2) the drafting and review of institutional policy with ethical content; and (3) the education of health care professionals, administration, and other health care staff (Mercurio 2010; Post, Blustein, and Dubler 2007). The membership of the HEC should ensure diverse, interdisciplinary professional (physicians, nurses, social workers, chaplains, and so forth) and lay representation to address the range of ethical issues brought to the committee. The underlying goals of ethics committees are to promote shared decision making between patients (and/or their surrogates) and their clinicians; to help identify, analyze, and resolve ethical problems in an atmosphere of respect and trust; to promote fair policies and procedures with the aim of achieving quality patient care and patient-centred outcomes; and to increase ethics capacity and promote health care practices consistent with high ethical standards (Fox et al. 2007).

The HEC can be helpful when, among other situations, there are questions about respect for patients' (or authorized surrogate) preferences, uncertainty about what is the "right" thing to do, conflict between care providers or between providers and patient/family, and issues concerning institutional policies that have an ethics component. Problems may arise, for example, when the patients or providers in a health care setting have different views of illness and treatment, hold different values in relation to death and dying, use language or decision-making frameworks differently and/or when communication breaks down (Dubler et al. 2009). Ethics committees can provide a forum for respectful discussion, as well as help with the debriefing and education of individual providers and health care teams. Increasingly, HECs are also being asked to consider organizational issues that have ethics implications—for example, resource allocation, clinical priorities, conflicting interests, and community responsibilities (Post, Blustein, and Dubler 2007). Such a resource could certainly have been of assistance in Ethics in Practice 13-1 and 13-2.

A significant culture shift in the realm of health care ethics committees has been an emphasis on collaborative processes that move toward more democratic procedures of deliberation (Dzur 2002). These processes include facilitated dialogue, consensus building; all of which can support the goals for relational autonomy, diversity, and interests as well as family and team well-being we articulated earlier in this chapter. Through programs such as Montefiore-Einstein Center's bioethics mediation paradigm (Dubler and Leibman 2004), and the Veterans Affairs Hospital's Integrated Ethics program (Fox et al. 2010), ethics consultation has taken steps toward utilizing methodologies grounded in conflict management. Rather than assuming an authoritative role, the HEC or ethics consultant seeks to identify ethically viable options and then facilitate deliberation with parties involved to help determine which option is best. This kind of approach respects "the rights of decision maker(s) to decide, within ethically justifiable limits, in accordance with their individual values" (Fox et al. 2007, 35). It contrasts with earlier models, which viewed the HEC or ethics consultant as expert, whose job it was to recommend the single, most ethically preferable course of action.

Ethics Consultants

As is indicated above, ethics consultants are often key components of organizational ethics resources. An ethics consultant is

> someone who has the knowledge, abilities, and attributes of character to facilitate . . . ethical discourse in case consultation on ethical issues in clinical care or clinical research, and in ethics consultation to ethics committees, to research ethics boards (institutional review boards), and to policy formulation committees. (Baylis 1994, 28)

Thus, consultants—who may come from a variety of disciplinary backgrounds—serve as an important adjunct to committees. There is increasing attention being paid in Canada and the United States as to how ethics consultants as well as ethics committee members should be educated and what the core competencies are that ethics consultants should cultivate (American Society for Bioethics and Humanities 2009a; 2009b; 2011; Baker 2009).

Overall, ethics committees and ethics consultants attempt to improve the *moral climate* of health care agencies (Storch, Rodney, and Starzomski 2009). Reflecting back on Ethics in Practice 13-1, for example, an ethics committee and/or an ethics consultant could help Clarence's parents and the members of the health care team to decide how best to involve Clarence in decisions about his treatment and care. Similarly, in Ethics in Practice 13-2, an ethics committee and/or an ethics consultant could help to lead Mr. Johansen's daughter, Stephanie, and the health care team through a structured ethical decision-making process and/or help them to resolve an impasse they may have reached in their decision making. An ethics committee and/or ethics consultant could also help to develop or update policies on end-of-life decision making and advance directives. And they could help with the debriefing and education of members of the health care team for the situations described in Ethics in Practice 13-1 and Ethics in Practice 13-2—each of which will have taken an emotional toll on team members as well as the patients' families.

Evaluating Effectiveness

It is important to note that a substantial evaluative literature has evolved around ethics committees and ethics consultants. While attempting to redress some of the cultural problems that are inherent in health care delivery, both resources are also subject to some of those cultural problems themselves (Fox and Swazey 2008). For instance, they may not be visible, they may function in an autocratic manner, they may be under-resourced, and they may be morally constrained by administration. A key development in the last decade has therefore been the articulation of standards for ethics committees and ethics consultants. In November 2009, the American Society of Bioethics and Humanities (2009b; 2011) released the second edition of "Core Competencies for Health Care Ethics Consultation."[28] Noteworthy were a new section on process standards for consultation and an expanded section on evaluating the quality (i.e., structure, process, and outcomes), access, and efficiency of ethics consultation services. An emerging literature reinforces the importance of developing standards for ethics services/consultation, and the benefits of integrating ethics into the quality improvement culture of health care organizations (Dubler et al. 2009; Fox et al. 2010).

In general, effective ethics consultants and/or ethics committees have the following attributes (Rodney and Howlett 2003):

- a clear focus on the well-being of patients and families;
- a commitment to maintaining the moral integrity of health care team members;
- visibility and accessibility for health care team members, patients, and families;
- strong skills in interpersonal communication, group process, and conflict resolution;
- knowledge of and support from the employing health care organization;
- sensitivity to organizational and professional power dynamics;
- a commitment to an egalitarian approach that fosters trust;
- transparency in decision making and subsequent recommendations; and
- a commitment to education, policy development, and ongoing evaluation of their own effectiveness.

Summary

Achieving wide reflective equilibrium in ethically challenging situations and creating a dialogic space that addresses diversity can be challenging processes. Because it takes place in the context of interactions with an individual or group of individuals, ethical decision making is a complex and nuanced process, as is ethical practice overall. Our goal in this chapter has not been to simplify the complex and contextual nature of ethical decision making, but rather to provide some tools to assist nurses and other health care providers in navigating through the interplay of ethical theories, principles, and contextual features. Decision-making frameworks such as the one explicated in this chapter are intended for this purpose: they are maps to assist in sorting out the terrain when ethical questions arise. As authors, our experiences in ethics consultations, policy work, and education have convinced us that such maps *can* make a difference in the turbulent and challenging world of practice, and *can* help us attend to relational autonomy, including the diversity and unique interests of the people whom we serve.

For Reflection

1. How does Sherwin's (1998) notion of relational autonomy strengthen the traditional ethical principle of autonomy when used in an ethical decision-making model?

2. We have argued that understanding the interests of persons requires understanding their rights, needs, and relationships. Sketch out what you would consider in understanding the rights, needs, and relationships of persons with disabilities. What about persons who are gay/lesbian, bisexual, transgendered, or questioning (LGBTQ)?

3. Compare the McDonald (Appendix B) and Storch (Appendix A) models of decision making. What are their similarities? Their differences?

4. Organizational ethics resources such as ethics committees and ethics consultants are often under-utilized. How can health care providers, patients, and families be made more aware—and trusting—of such resources?

5. How might research about diversity from nursing and other disciplines continue to inform our understanding of relational autonomy?

Endnotes

1. We wish to thank an anonymous reviewer of the first edition of this chapter for this phrasing.

2. We are using the term ethical *problems* quite broadly. We consider ethical problems to involve questions about what is right or good at individual, interpersonal, organizational, and even societal levels.

3. We acknowledge the work of Dr. Arthur Kleinman (1988), who introduced the notion of *explanatory models*. While we draw on this notion, we develop a method of inquiry that has arisen from our research.

4. Mediating circumstances can include, for example, age, sexual orientation, language fluency, chronic illness, income, availability of family support, ethnocultural stereotyping by others, rural or remote geographic location, and so forth.

5. We are using the term *interests* to reflect what persons as unique individuals situated in multi-faceted relational contexts require for their well-being. This is in contrast to an objective reasonable person standard, where we make assumptions about what an "average prudent person" would want.

6. This conceptual approach to interests has been developed by one of the authors of this chapter (McPherson).

7. Pneumothoraces and pneumomediastinum are both types of air leakage from the lungs into the chest cavity. They are the result of severe injury to the lung tissue, and cause further deterioration in lung function.

8. ECMO is an acronym for Extra-Corporeal Membrane Oxygenation. This is a highly technical procedure in which a heart–lung machine takes over the work of the heart and lungs for a period of days in order (as in Clarence's case) to give the patient's lungs time to heal.

9. Pharmacological paralysis makes a child or any other person unable to move or breathe, but has little effect on sensory experiences and cognition unless sedatives and/or analgesics are added.

10. Ethics in Practice 13-1 is adapted (and fictionalized) by McPherson from the clinical experiences of she and her colleagues.

11. See Chapter 9 and Chapter 16 for related discussions of moral agency.

12. Unique characteristics are often addressed through terms such as "personality" and "temperament."

13. It also possible that parents and other family members are *not* acting in patients' best interests. Based on our experiences this is not common. Actions of family members that seem to go against patients' best interests are usually a response to unresolved grief, and/or conflict and lack of trust within and between family members and the health care team, and should be addressed as such. Nonetheless, there are times when family members may be jeopardizing patients' autonomy and well-being. Such situations call for expert clinical, ethical, and legal assessments and interventions.

    Further, an anonymous reviewer of the first edition of this chapter quite correctly pointed out that this level of family involvement presupposes that the (capable) patient has chosen to have his or her family engaged in his or her treatment and care. Some patients may want to circumscribe the level of their family's involvement. Other patients are estranged and/or isolated from their next of kin, and may choose to define their friends or neighbours as family.

14. See also Chapter 17. Advance directives include an *instruction* directive, which "allows the person to specify which life-sustaining treatments he or she would not wish in various situations" as well as a *proxy* directive, which "allows individuals to identify a substitute decision maker should they ever be rendered incompetent" (Keatings and Smith 2010, 240). It would be important to conduct a family assessment and try to ascertain Mr. Johansen's prior wishes to ensure that Stephanie was, in fact, whom he would choose as his proxy decision maker.

15. Within this chapter, we are using the term "family" quite broadly (Rodney 1997). We agree with family theorists that "it is quite possible for people to have a family experience (including the feelings of intimacy, connectedness, commitment, and so forth) with people who are not in one's actual family" (Hartrick and Lindsey 1995, 154). Therefore, we take it that the "most useful definition of family [is] "Who the family says it is." Furthermore, who "counts" as family may vary depending on the health concern" (Robinson 1995, 119; see also Robinson 2011).

16. See also Burgess and Brunger (2000) for a relational approach to autonomy that extends to family and community.

17. By quandary we mean "high profile" life or death decisions, such as treatment withdrawal, euthanasia, abortion, and cloning.

18. This has implications for basic and continuing ethics education. As people who engage in ethics education and ethics consultation, we authors find it useful to start by asking people to notice "when their gut is in a knot." See also Doane (2004) and Nortvedt (2004) about the role of emotion in ethics, as well as Hartrick Doane (2002a; 2002b) and Doane et al. (2004) about moral identity and ethics education. See also Chapter 6 and Chapter 15.

19. There are, of course, a variety of effective ethical decision-making models or frameworks available to choose from. We have made an alternate model available in Appendix A, Storch's Model for Ethical Decision Making for Policy and Practice.

20. See also Chapter 5. *Fidelity* is a concept that directs our attention to trust (including, but not limited to, truthtelling), while *care* directs our attention to enhancing patient/family/team relationships (in the present and over time).

21. Storch's Model for Ethical Decision Making for Policy and Practice (Appendix A) is for this reason constructed as a circle.

22. In our experience, linear approaches or algorithms do not work well in the real world of practice, where we are often dealing with uncertainty and where new information generates new alternatives. We usually have to cycle back and forth between information, reflection, and alternatives. Furthermore, one of the challenges we face with most models or frameworks (including McDonald's) is to

try to capture a process that changes over time as the patient's illness trajectory unfolds (see also Rodney et al. 2002).

23. For patients and family members for whom English (or French in francophone communities) is not a first language, the availability of trained interpreters throughout the process is crucial (Anderson et al. 2010; Kaufert and Putsch 1997).

24. In fact, there are a growing number of research studies and practice guidelines promoting the integration of palliative care interventions within critical care (Heyland et al. 2006; 2010; Quill 2000; Rocker 2002; Rocker, Shemie, and Lacroix 2000; Rodney and Howlett 2003).

25. See also Chapter 9 and Chapter 10. We ought to proceed with the understanding that the well-being of the team is linked to the well-being of the patient and family.

26. In the story recounted by the clinical nurse specialist in Ethics in Practice 13-2, the clinical nurse specialist, the physician on call, and the nursing staff implemented an ethical decision-making process, although not necessarily with the use of a formal model or framework. They were able to work out and implement a number of ethically sound alternatives. In other words, a formal model/framework and consultation process were not required. In more complex or conflicted situations, though, the use of a formal model or framework is beneficial. Calling for an interdisciplinary team meeting and possibly a formal ethics consultation *as early as possible* can prevent deteriorations in patient/family care and escalations in family/team conflict.

    It is important to note that a follow-up case review with staff involved in Ethics in 13-2 (as well as 13-1) would have been beneficial. Such follow-up is helpful in any situation where there has been conflict and uncertainty.

27. For more information about egalitarian and practical approaches to group process that foster consensus, see Chinn (2008), DeRenzo and Strauss (1997), and Pangman and Pangman (2010). It is important to note that in using the word "consensus" we are talking about processes that work toward an equalization of power, respect a diversity of perspectives, and generate a range of carefully crafted options. We are *not* talking about processes in which the majority rules, where there is "groupthink," or where dissent is silenced. The latter three processes are too often (incorrectly, we believe) attributed to consensus.

28. The Canadian Bioethics Society (CBS) is the national interdisciplinary group of people doing work in health care ethics in Canada, The CBS (http://www.bioethics.ca/index-ang.html), has been playing a significant role in advancing the professional status of bioethicists. See Baker (2009) for some shared Canadian and American history.

References

Abbott, K.H., Sago, J.G., Breen, C.M., Abernethy, A.P., and Tulsky, J.A. 2001. Families looking back: One year after discussion of treatment withdrawal or withholding of life-sustaining support. *Critical Care Medicine, 29* (1), 197–201.

Agich, G.J. 1998. Respecting the autonomy of elders in nursing homes. In J.F. Monagle and D.C. Thomasma (Eds.), *Health care ethics: Critical issues for the 21st century* (pp. 200–211). Maryland: Aspen.

Agich, G.J. 1999. Ethical problems in caring for demented patients. In S. Govoni, C.L. Bolis, and M. Trabucchi (Eds.), *Dementia: Biological bases and clinical approach to treatment* (pp. 297–308). Milano: Springer–Verlag Italia.

American Society for Bioethics and Humanities. 2009a. *Improving competencies in clinical ethics consultation: An education guide.* Glenview, IL: American Society for Bioethics and Humanities.

American Society for Bioethics and Humanities. 2009b. *Task Force on Standards for Bioethics and Consultation, Core Competencies for Health Care Ethics Consultation*. Glenview, IL: American Society for Bioethics and Humanities.

American Society for Bioethics and Humanities. 2011. *Core competencies for healthcare ethics consultation* (2nd ed.). Glenview, IL: American Society for Bioethics and Humanities.

Anderson, J.M. 2004. Lessons from a postcolonial-feminist perspective: Suffering and a path to healing. *Nursing Inquiry, 11* (4), 238–246.

Anderson, J., Reimer, J., Basu Khan, K., Simich, L., Neufeld, A., Stewart, M., and Makwarimba, E. 2010. Narratives of dissonance and repositioning through the lens of critical humanism: Exploring the influences on immigrants and refugees health and well-being. *Advances in Nursing Science, 33* (2), 101–112.

Anderson, J.M., Rodney, P., Reimer Kirkham, S., Browne, A.J., Khan, K.B., and Lynam, M.J. 2009. Inequities in health and health care viewed through the ethical lens of critical social justice: Contextual knowledge for the global priorities ahead. *Advances in Nursing Science, 32* (4), 282–294.

Anspach, R.R. and Beeson, D. 2001. Emotions in medical and moral life. In B. Hoffmaster (Ed.), *Bioethics in social context* (pp. 112–136). Philadelphia: Temple University Press.

Arras, J.D., Steinbock, B., and London, A.J. 1999. Moral reasoning in the medical context. In J.D. Arras and B. Steinbock (Eds.), *Ethical issues in modern medicine*. Toronto: Mayfield.

Austin, W.J. 2011. The incommensurability of nursing as a practice and the customer service model: An evolutionary threat to the discipline. *Nursing Philosophy, 12,* 158–166.

Baker, R. 2009. The ethics of bioethics. In V. Ravitsky, A. Fiester, and A.L. Caplan (Eds.), *The Penn Centre guide to bioethics* (pp. 9–20). New York: Springer Publishing.

Baylis F.E. (Ed.). 1994. *The health care ethics consultant*. Totowa, NJ: Humana Press.

Baylis, F., Kenny, N.P., and Sherwin, S. 2008. A relational account of public health ethics. *Public Health Ethics, 1* (3), 196–209.

Beyerstein, D. 1993. The functions and limitations of professional codes of ethics. In E.R. Winkler and J.R. Coombs (Eds.), *Applied ethics: A reader* (pp. 416–425). Oxford: Blackwell.

Blustein, J. 1998. The family in medical decision making. In J.F. Monagle and D.C. Thomasma (Eds.), *Health care ethics: Critical issues for the 21st century* (pp. 81–91). Maryland: Aspen.

Browne, A.J., Smye, V.L., Rodney, P., Tang, S.Y., Mussell, B., and O'Neill, J. 2011. Access to primary care from the perspective of Aboriginal patients at an urban emergency department. *Qualitative Health Research, 21* (3), 333–348.

Burgess, M. and Brunger, F. 2000. Collective effects of medical research. In M. McDonald et al. *The governance of health research involving human subjects*. Ottawa: Law Commission of Canada. Available at www.lcc.gc.ca/en/themes or www.ethics.ubc.ca/people/burgess/lccburgess.pdf.

Bužgová, R. and Ivanová, K. 2009. Elder abuse and mistreatment in residential settings. *Nursing Ethics, 16* (1), 110–126.

Callahan, D. 2011 End-of-life care: A philosophical or management problem? *Journal of Law, Medicine and Ethics,* (Summer), 114–120.

Canadian Nurses Association. 2008 *Code of ethics for registered nurses*. Ottawa: Authors.

Canales, M.K. 2010. Othering: Difference understood?? A 10-year analysis and critique of the nursing literature. *Advances in Nursing Science, 33* (1), 15–34.

Carstairs, S. 2010. *Raising the bar: A roadmap for the future of palliative care in Canada.* Ottawa: The Senate of Canada.

Chambers-Evans, J. 2002. The family as window onto the world of the patient: Revising our approach to involving patients and families in the decision-making process. *Canadian Journal of Nursing Research, 34* (3), 15–32.

Charchuk, M. and Simpson, C. 2003. Loyalty and hope: Keys to parenting in the NICU. *Neonatal network, 22* (4), 1–7.

Chinn, P.L. 2008. *Peace and power: Creative leadership for building community* (7th ed.). Boston: Jones and Bartlett.

Curtis, J.R., Patrick, D.L., Shannon, S.E., Treece, P.D., Engelberg, R.A., and Rubenfeld, G.D. 2001. The family conference as a focus to improve communication about end-of-life care in the intensive care unit: Opportunities for improvement. *Critical Care Medicine, 29* (2, supplement), N26–N33.

Dahlke, S. and Phinney, A. 2008. Caring for hospitalized older adults at risk for delirium: The silent, unspoken piece of nursing practice. *Journal of Gerontological Nursing, 34* (6), 41–47.

Daniels, N. 1985. *Just health care.* Cambridge: Cambridge University Press.

Daniels, N. 1996. Wide reflective equilibrium in practice. In L.W. Sumner and J. Boyle (Eds.), *Philosophical perspectives on bioethics* (pp. 96–114). Toronto: University of Toronto Press.

Daniels, N., Kennedy, B., and Kawachi, I. 2004. Health and inequality, or, why justice is good for our health. In S. Anand, F. Peter, and A. Sen (Eds.), *Public health, ethics, and equity* (pp. 63–91). Oxford: Oxford University Press.

DeRenzo, E.G. and Strauss, M. 1997. A feminist model for clinical ethics consultation: Increasing attention to context and narrative. *HealthCare Ethics Committee Forum, 9* (3), 212–227.

Doane, G. 2004. Being an ethical practitioner: The embodiment of mind, emotion, and action. In J. Storch, P. Rodney, and R. Starzomski (Eds.), *Toward a moral horizon: Nursing ethics for leadership and practice* (pp. 433–446). Toronto: Pearson-Prentice Hall.

Doane, G., Pauly, B., Brown, H., and McPherson, G. 2004. Exploring the heart of ethical nursing practice: Implications for ethics education. *Nursing Ethics, 11* (3), 240–253.

Dodds, S. 2005. Gender, ageing, and injustice: Social and political contexts of bioethics. *Journal of Medical Ethics, 31*, 295–298.

Dubler N. and C. Liebman. 2004. *Bioethics mediation: A guide to shaping shared solutions.* New York, NY: United Hospital Fund.

Dubler, N., Webber, M., Swiderski, D., and the Faculty and the National Working Group for the Clinical Ethics Credentialing Project. 2009. Charting the Future: Credentialing, Privileging, Quality, and Evaluation in Clinical Ethics Consultation. *Hastings Center Report, 39* (9), 23–33.

Dzur, A.J. 2002. Democratizing the hospital: Deliberative-democratic bioethics. *Journal of Health Politics, Policy and Law, 27* (2), 177–211.

Fox, E., Bottrell, M., Berkowitz, K., Chanko, B., Foglia, M., and Pearlman, R. 2010. Integrated ethics: An innovative program to improve ethics quality in healthcare. *The Innovation Journal, 15* (2), article 8.

Fox, E., Bottrell, M., Foglia, M.B., Chanko, B.L., and Stoeckle, R. 2007. *Ethics consultation: Responding to ethics concerns in health care.* Washington: National Center for Ethics in Health Care of the Veterans Health.

Fox, R.C. and Swazey, J.P. 2008. *Observing bioethics.* Oxford: Oxford University Press.

Gallagher, E., Alcock, D., Diem, E., Angus, D., and Medves, J. 2002. Ethical dilemmas in home care case management. *Journal of Healthcare Management, 47* (2), 85–96.

Hartrick Doane, G.A. 2002a. In the spirit of creativity: The learning and teaching of ethics in nursing. *Journal of Advanced Nursing, 39* (96), 521–528.

Hartrick Doane, G.A. 2002b. Am I still ethical? The socially-mediated process of nurses' moral identity. *Nursing Ethics, 9* (6), 623–635.

Hartrick, G.A. and Lindsey, A.E. 1995. The lived experience of family: A contextual approach to family nursing practice. *Journal of Family Nursing, 1* (2), 148–170.

Hartrick Doane, G. and Varcoe, C. 2005. *Family nursing as relational inquiry: Developing health promoting practice.* Philadelphia: Lippincott, Williams and Wilkins.

Hayes, V.A. and McElheran, P.J. 2002. Family health promotion within the demands of pediatric home care and nursing respite. In L.E. Young and V. Hayes (Eds.), *Transforming health promotion practice: Concepts, issues, and applications* (pp. 265–283). Philadelphia: F.A. Davis.

Heyland, D.K., Cook, D., Rocker, G., Dodek, P., Kutsogiannis, D.J., Skrobik, Y. et al. 2010. Defining priorities for improving end-of-life care in Canada. *Canadian Medical Association Journal, 182* (16), E747–752.

Heyland, D.K., Dodek, P., Rocker, G., Groll, D., Gafni, A., Pichora, D. et al. 2006. What matters most in end-of-life care: Perceptions of seriously ill patients and their family members. *Canadian Medical Association Journal, 174* (5), online1–9. Available at www.cmaj.ca.

Hiltunen, E.F., Medich, C., Chase, S., Peterson, L., and Forrow, L. 1999. Family decision making for end-of-life treatment: The SUPPORT nurse narratives. *The Journal of Clinical Ethics, 10* (2), 126–134.

Hoffmaster, B. 2001. Introduction. In B. Hoffmaster (Ed.), *Bioethics in social context* (pp. 1–11). Philadelphia: Temple University Press.

Jennings, B. 1991. Possibilities of consensus: Toward democratic moral discourse. *The Journal of Medicine and Philosophy, 16*, 447–463.

Jennings, B., Ryndes, T., D'Onofrio, C., and Baily, M.A. 2003. Access to hospice care: Expanding boundaries, overcoming barriers. *Hastings Center Report (Special Supplement), 33* (2), S3–S59.

Joint Commission on Accreditation of Healthcare Organizations. 1992. *Comprehensive accreditation manual for hospital.* Oakbrook Terrace, IL: Authors.

Kaufert, J.M. and Putsch, R.W. 1997. Communication through interpreters in healthcare: Ethical dilemmas arising from differences in class, culture, language, and power. *The Journal of Clinical Ethics, 8* (1), 71–86.

Keatings, M. and Smith, O. 2010. *Ethical and legal issues in Canadian nursing* (3rd ed). Toronto, ON: Mosby Elsevier.

Kleinman, A. 1988. *The illness narratives: Suffering, healing, and the human condition.* New York: Basic Books.

Lachs, J. 2003. Dying old as a social problem. In G. McGee (Ed.), *Pragmatic bioethics* (2nd ed; pp. 207–217). Cambridge, MA: MIT Press.

Mercurio, B. 2010. Pediatric ethics committees. In G. Miller (Ed.), *Pediatric bioethics* (p. 87–110). New York: Cambridge University Press.

McPherson, G. 2007. *Children's participation in chronic illness decision-making: An interpretive description.* Unpublished doctoral dissertation, University of British Columbia School of Nursing, Vancouver, BC.

National Advisory Committee. 2000. *A guide to end-of-life care for seniors.* Ottawa: Health Canada.

Nelson, J.L. 1998. Death, medicine, and the moral significance of family decision making. In J.F. Monagle and D.C. Thomasma (Eds.), *Health care ethics: Critical issues for the 21st century* (pp. 288–294). Maryland: Aspen.

Nortvedt, P. 2004. Emotions and ethics. In J. Storch, P. Rodney, and R. Starzomski (Eds.), *Toward a moral horizon: Nursing ethics for leadership and practice* (pp. 447–464). Toronto: Pearson-Prentice Hall.

Pangman, V.C. and Pangman, C. 2010. *Nursing leadership from a Canadian perspective.* Philadelphia: Wolters Kluwer, Lippincott Williams & Wilkins.

Penning, M.J. and Votova, K. 2009. Aging, health, and health care: From hospital and residential care to home and community care. In B.S. Bolaria and H. Dickinson (Eds.), *Health, illness, and health care in Canada* (4th ed.; pp. 349–366). Toronto, ON: Nelson Education.

Post, L., Blustein, J. and Dubler, N. 2007. *Handbook for health care ethics committees.* Baltimore: Johns Hopkins University Press.

Quill, T.E. 2000. Perspectives on care at the close of life. Initiating end-of-life discussions with seriously ill patients: Addressing the "elephant in the room." *Journal of the American Medical Association, 284* (19), 2502–2507.

Randers, I. and Mattiasson, A.C. 2000. The experiences of elderly people in geriatric care with special reference to integrity. *Nursing Ethics, 7* (6), 503–519.

Robinson, C.A. 1995. Beyond dichotomies in the nursing of persons and families. *Image, 27* (2), 116–120.

Robinson, C.A. 2011. Advance care planning: Re-visioning our ethical approach. *Canadian Journal of Nursing Research, 43* (2), 18–37.

Rocker, G. 2002. End-of-life care: An update. *Critical Care Rounds, 3* (5).

Rocker, G.M., Shemie, S.D., and Lacroix, J. 2000. End-of-life issues in the ICU: A need for acute palliative care? *Journal of Palliative Care, 16* (supplement), S5–S6.

Rodney, P.A. 1997. *Towards connectedness and trust: Nurses' enactment of their moral agency within an organizational context.* Unpublished doctoral dissertation, University of British Columbia, Vancouver, BC.

Rodney, P. and Howlett, J. 2003. Elderly patients with cardiac disease: Quality of life, end of life, and ethics. Paper in unpublished *Canadian Cardiovascular Society Consensus Document on the Elderly and Cardiac Disease.* Available at http://www.ccs.ca/download/consensus_conference/consensus_conference_archives/2002_11.pdf.

Rodney, P. and Varcoe, C. in press. Constrained agency: The social structure of nurses' work. In F. Baylis, J. Downie, B. Hoffmaster, and S. Sherwin (Eds.), *Health care ethics in Canada* (3rd ed.). Toronto: Nelson. (rev. of Varcoe, C. and Rodney, P. 2009 Constrained agency: The social structure of nurses' work. In B.S. Bolaria and H.D. Dickinson [Eds.], *Health, illness, and health care in Canada* [4th ed.; pp. 122–151]. Toronto: Nelson Education.)

Rodney, P., Varcoe, C., Storch, J.L., McPherson, G., Mahoney, K., Brown, H., Pauly, B., Hartrick Doane, G., and Starzomski, R. 2002. Navigating toward a moral horizon: A multi-site qualitative study of ethical practice in nursing. *Canadian Journal of Nursing Research, 34* (2), 75–102.

Rorty, R. 1999. *Philosophy and social hope.* London: Penguin.

Sellman, D. 2009. Editorial: Ethical care for older persons in acute care settings. *Nursing Philosophy, 10,* 69–70.

Sherwin, S. 1998. A relational approach to autonomy in health care. In S. Sherwin and Canadian Feminist Health Care Research Network (Eds.), *The politics of women's health: Exploring agency and autonomy* (pp. 19–47). Philadelphia, PA: Temple University Press.

Sherwin, S. 2011. Looking backwards, looking forward: Hopes for bioethics' next twenty-five years. *Bioethics, 25* (2), 75–82.

Stajduhar, K.I. 2003. Examining the perspectives of family members involved in the delivery of palliative care at home. *Journal of Palliative Care, 19* (1), 27–35.

Stajduhar, K.I. 2011. Discourse: Chronic illness, palliative care, and the problematic nature of dying. *Canadian Journal of Nursing Research, 43* (3), 7–15.

Storch, J., Rodney, P., and Starzomski, S. 2009. Ethics in health care in Canada. In B.S. Bolaria and H. Dickinson (Eds.), *Health, illness, and health care in Canada* (4th ed.). Toronto: Nelson Education.

Suhonen, R., Stolt, M., Launis, V., and Leino-Kilpi 2010. Research on ethics in nursing care for older people: A literature review. *Nursing Ethics, 17* (3), 337–352.

Thorne, S., Bultz, B., and Baile, W. 2005. Is there a cost to poor communication in cancer care? A critical review of the literature. *Psycho-Oncology, 14,* 875–884.

Vandall-Walker, V.A. 2002. Nursing support with family members of the critically ill: A framework to guide practice. In L.E. Young and V. Hayes (Eds.), *Transforming health promotion practice: Concepts, issues, and applications* (pp. 174–189). Philadelphia: F.A. Davis.

Wilson, D.M. 2000. End-of-life care preferences of Canadian senior citizens with caregiving experience. *Journal of Advanced Nursing, 31* (6), 1416–1421.

Winkler, E. 1996. Moral philosophy and bioethics: Contextualism versus the paradigm theory. In L.W. Sumner and J. Boyle (Eds.), *Philosophical perspectives on bioethics* (pp. 50–78). Toronto: University of Toronto Press.

Yeo, M. 2010. A primer in ethical theory. In M. Yeo, A. Moorhouse, P. Khan, and P. Rodney (Eds.), *Concepts and cases in nursing ethics* (3rd ed.; pp. 37–72). Peterborough, ON: Broadview Press.

CHAPTER 14

Research Ethics and Nursing

Kathleen Oberle and Janet L. Storch

Research ethics is particularly important in nursing research for several reasons. Researchers often approach people at vulnerable times in their lives. Participants contribute both time and effort, and sometimes even divulge the innermost secrets of their lives, despite the fact that they often gain little or no direct benefit from the research. The performance of research sometimes conflicts with the practice of care, and ethical dilemmas may occur when researchers attempt to design studies that are both ethical and methodologically rigorous. (Kjellstrom and Fridlund 2010, 383)

Roles for nurses relative to research ethics are multiple and diverse, and include important responsibilities. Our purpose in this chapter is to enhance nurses' knowledge about the broad range of ethical issues that can arise in the context of human health research so that they can develop the skills and sensitivities needed to fulfill their obligations as part of ethical practice. We offer a review of

- the evolution of research ethics;
- central guiding principles for research ethics in Canada;
- responsibilities of research ethics boards;
- details about roles for nurses in research ethics; and
- responsibilities of nurses as leaders in research ethics.

We begin with a focus on the evolution of research ethics using an example of research ethics abuse that stimulated the development of research ethics guidelines in the U.S. and subsequently in Canada (Ethics in Practice 14-1).

ETHICS IN PRACTICE 14-1

The Tuskegee Study

In 1932, a study on the effects of untreated syphilis was begun as part of a broader U.S. government public health initiative. Research subjects were impoverished African-American men living in Alabama; the researchers were from a branch of the U.S. Public Health Services that would later become the Center for Disease Control. The Tuskegee Institute was utilized as the site of the research because of its position of trust in the local community. Since at the time there was no known effective treatment for syphilis, the researchers believed that basic medical care offered as part of the study would be sufficient compensation for subjects' involvement. The men were encouraged to participate in the study and consented to do so to receive health benefits. A number of non-therapeutic interventions, including lumbar punctures, were performed on subjects, but they were not informed that these were not part of the study as such, and no consent was sought. In 1943, penicillin was confirmed as an effective treatment for syphilis, but subjects were not told about this medical break-through and penicillin was not offered to them. A local nurse named Eunice Rivers (trained at the Tuskegee Institute) was engaged to be the on-site representative (or local coordinator) of this study. Ms. Rivers had a significant role in recruiting subjects and administering the research protocol. She did not speak against the study even when it became evident that participants were being seriously disadvantaged by their involvement. The study was stopped in 1973 only after journalists exposed the lack of ethical attention to study subjects (Dunn and Chadwick 2004; MacNeill 2009; Meslin and Dickens 2008; Smith 1996).

Why did nurse Eunice Rivers not speak up to try to stop this study? The reason she offered for her support of the study was that the men involved were able to access better medical care by being included in the study (Smith 1996).[1] There might have been many other reasons for not withdrawing her support, including feelings of powerlessness.

Could the Tuskegee study happen today? Our understanding of the ethical aspects of research has developed markedly since that study began, and there are many more protections in place, but in the process of conducting investigations there is always a potential for harm to research subjects. How might individuals and groups involved as human participants in research be better protected? What do nurses need to know in order to feel empowered and better serve patients and research participants in this regard?

BACKGROUND: EVOLUTION OF RESEARCH ETHICS IN CANADA

Understanding some of the historical research violations is important to try to minimize the possibility that they be repeated under a different guise. When the topic of ethical violations in research arises, it is not uncommon to cite the Nazi experiments conducted during World War II as the most egregious examples. These experiments, carried out in the name of medical science, included deliberately infecting people in prison camps and elsewhere with pathogens, exposing individuals to harmful gases, placing others in high-altitude chambers until they became unconscious, and severely chilling or freezing and then reviving victims (Dunn and Chadwick 2004; Luna and Macklin 2009; MacNeill 2009). Nurses were involved in selection of non-voluntary subjects and assisted with these experimental procedures in much of this research (see for example, Steppe 1992; 1996).[2]

The war crimes trials following exposure of Nazi atrocities led to the development of the famous Nuremberg Code of research ethics in 1949. Later the Helsinki Declaration on Medical Research (1964) was developed by the World Medical Association to delineate clear rules for clinical trials. Both the Nuremberg Code and the Declaration of Helsinki were influential in the development of research ethics guidelines and both have been revised frequently, most recently in 2000 for the former and 2008 for the latter.

However, despite the development of such guidelines, unethical conduct is not confined to the past. There have been numerous examples of unethical research since Nuremberg, of which the Tuskegee syphilis experiments are but a single notorious example. McNeill (2009) provides a rich discussion of numerous more recent studies from many countries, and as this paper was being prepared, an unethical study from Guatemala involving U.S. researchers surfaced.[3]

In the mid-1970s the United States Department of Health, Education, and Welfare, partly in response to the public outcry from the Tuskegee syphilis study, established a commission to develop U.S.-generated guidelines for research ethics. The result was the Belmont Report, released in 1979. The report built on earlier documents and established ethical principles that would not only inform research ethics but also form the basis of the newly emerging field of bioethics (see Chapter 4 in this text). The principles included respect for persons (therefore the need for informed consent), beneficence and non-maleficence (thus, the requirement to assess both the benefits and risks of any pro- posed research), and justice (therefore fair selection of subjects and fair processes in recruitment). After release of the report academic and clinical institutions in the United States began the process of appointing Institutional Research Boards (IRBs) to review the ethics of proposed research and enacted a number of laws to ensure that researchers adhered to the stated ethical principles.

In Canada no such legislation was put in place and none exists today. However, Canadians have adopted some unique ways of approaching ethics and establishing means to promote conformity with principles. Research ethics guidelines in Canadian health research were first developed by the Medical Research Council (MRC), a government research granting agency, and released in 1978. In the mid-1980s, as medical research progressed, MRC began to revise its guidelines and became sensitive to the need for some kind of oversight to ensure that institutions were following the guidelines. To meet this need, the National Council on Bioethics in Human Research (NCBHR) was founded in 1989 with financial support from MRC and Health Canada. Council staff and board volunteers provided research ethics education and assessed operation of Research Ethics Boards (REBs—the equivalent of the U.S. IRBs) across the country. Later NCBHR replaced "bioethics" with "ethics" in its title to become the National Council on Ethics in Human Research (NCEHR).

Throughout this period research with human subjects was expanding to involve pro- fessionals outside of medicine (including many nurse researchers) and researchers out- side of health care. Three main bodies were responsible for the public funding of research: MRC (which in 2000 was transformed into the Canadian Institutes of Health Research—CIHR), the Social Sciences and Humanities Research Council of Canada (SSHRC), and the Natural Sciences and Engineering Research Council of Canada (NSERC). It became evident that lack of a common Canadian standard for research eth- ics was resulting in differences across disciplines and across jurisdictions. CIHR, SSHRC, and NSERC therefore combined their efforts to form the group known as the Tri-Council. This joint effort resulted in the *Tri-Council Policy Statement: Ethical Con- duct for Research Involving Humans* released in 1998. Few other countries had attempted such a comprehensive coverage of fields involving human participants in research and requiring research ethics scrutiny.

Upon the release of the Tri-Council Policy Statement (TCPS) the three councils announced that every institution receiving funding from one of the three councils must be in compliance with the policy statement; if not, funding could be withdrawn and researchers in institutions (universities and health agencies) could no longer receive research funds until they and their institution were compliant with the guidelines. "Compliance" in this case meant that every research protocol (even those not funded directly by one of the Tri-Council agencies) had to be approved by an REB constituted according to the TCPS, and all studies were to adhere to the policy in every aspect. That resulted in major changes in procedure in some institutions as researchers in all disciplines were suddenly expected to adhere to the common national standard. REBs sprang up across the country.

In its first decade the TCPS served as a useful tool for researchers and REBs, but it soon became clear that the policy was lacking in some important aspects. In December 2010, following national consultation with researchers, the second edition of the TCPS, known as TCPS-2, was released.[4] Major changes included a complete reorganization and extension of existing chapters, reworking of the philosophical foundations, new chapters on qualitative and multi-jurisdictional research, and an extended section on research with First Nations, Inuit, and Métis communities. There is no single body providing oversight of REBs and research ethics in Canada, but there is considerable discussion to how such oversight can and should be effected. Clearly, research ethics in Canada is dynamic and evolving.

Guiding Principles in Canada

Core principles of respect for persons, concern for welfare, and justice form the foundation of the revised TCPS now titled TCPS-2 (Tri-Council 2010). These are similar to, but not the same as, the foundational concepts of the Belmont Report and the first TCPS. *Respect for persons* in TCPS-2 is first reflected in the use of the word "participant" rather than "subject" to denote "an individual whose data, or responses to interventions, stimuli, or questions by a researcher are relevant to answering a research question" (194). The change was made in an effort to emphasize "that individuals who choose to participate in research play a more active role than the term 'subject' conveys" (16). Respect for persons also "incorporates the dual moral obligations to respect autonomy and to protect those with developing, impaired, or diminished autonomy" (49). Respecting autonomy in the research context includes seeking informed consent from participants before collecting data about them. While it is recognized that some individuals such as young children, the mentally challenged, those suffering from dementia, and so on may not be able to provide fully informed consent because of their cognitive incapacity, they must always be involved in decision making to the extent that they are able. If they are unable, consent must be sought from others who are responsible for decision making and who are likely to know and respect the individual's wishes. To demonstrate *concern for welfare* "researchers must ensure that participants are not exposed to unnecessary risk [and] . . . should attempt to achieve the most favourable balance of risks and potential benefits in a proposed research study" (Tri-Council 2010, 50). *Justice* "refers to the obligation to treat people fairly and equitably. Fairness entails treating all people with equal respect and concern. Equity requires distributing the benefits and burdens of research participation in such a way that no segment of the population is unduly burdened by the harms of research or denied the benefits of the knowledge generated from it" (51).

RESPONSIBILITY OF RESEARCH ETHICS BOARDS

It has become a Canadian requirement that anyone wishing to conduct research with human subjects submit their research proposal to an REB for review and approval prior to commencing collection of data. According to the TCPS-2 (2010), an REB must have a minimum of five members, "including both men and women, of whom

- at least two members have expertise in relevant research disciplines, fields, and methodologies covered by the REB;

- at least one member is knowledgeable in ethics;

- for biomedical research, at least one member is knowledgeable in the relevant law (but that member should not be the institution's legal counsel or risk manager). This is advisable but not mandatory for other areas of research;

- and at least one community member who has no affiliation with the institution" (111).

Customarily, institutions develop their own forms to be used by the researcher in submitting an application for review. The REB examines the proposal for evidence of compliance with the TCPS, as well as other international documents, where relevant.[5]

The REB examines each element of the proposal in detail and normally provides feedback to the researcher when changes are required. Typical areas of scrutiny and associated questions are outlined in Table 14-1. If the REB membership does not have the necessary expertise to review a project (based on method or substantive content area), then it must seek assistance from an external reviewer. If the study involves more than minimal risk, it generally undergoes review by the entire REB; if it involves minimal risk, then review may be delegated to a smaller number of reviewers. Rarely is a proposal rejected outright. The researcher receives feedback and submits requested changes, or may request clarification or reassessment. Once both researcher and REB are satisfied with the changes, a certificate of ethics approval is issued. If the proposal is rejected the researcher may request an appeal, which will be binding.

Some researchers consider the process of ethics review to be cumbersome and unnecessarily restrictive.[6] Nonetheless, oversight is required to reduce risk to participants. REBs are expected to do everything they can to complete the process expeditiously and not hinder or delay the conduct of good research, as that, in itself, would be unethical. A certain amount of flexibility is required, for seldom is it possible to ensure that there is no risk to participants; rather, risk must be mitigated to the extent possible, and benefit maximized. Excellence in the informed consent process is essential to ensure that individuals are offered and understand choices regarding participation (Emanuel, Wendler, and Grady 2000). Ideally, researchers who wish to involve human participants in their research should develop their research proposal and their research ethics review applications in a parallel manner. This means they would keep research ethics guidelines at the forefront of their thinking. In that way there are few or no surprises arising from the REB review.[7]

TABLE 14-1	Key Considerations for REBs in Proposal Review
TOPIC	**RELATED QUESTIONS**
BACKGROUND AND RATIONALE To ensure that the study is important, merits participants' time, and generates important knowledge	• Is there evidence that the study is necessary and important? • Is there evidence that the right questions are being asked? • Is there evidence that the approach used is appropriate?
STUDY OBJECTIVES To ensure that the study is feasible and reasonable	• Are the objectives of the study reasonable and manageable given previous work in the area?
METHOD To ensure that results are valid and meritorious, as conduct of an ill-designed study is a waste of time and funding dollars, and is therefore unethical	• Does the research method seem appropriate to the question? • Is the study likely to produce valid results?
SAMPLE/RECRUITMENT	• Is the sample appropriately delineated? Are appropriate inclusion criteria present? Is any population excluded inappropriately (e.g., pregnant women, children)? • Are people in the sample vulnerable in any way? What has been done to protect potential participants from harms? From feeling coerced? Is there evidence of undue inducement to accept more than minimal risk?
CONSENT	• Is there evidence that elements of informed consent (voluntariness, capacity, and comprehension) will be present? • Are alternatives to participation outlined (for therapeutic studies)? • Are the required elements of the consent (as outlined by TCPS and institutional policy) present? Will consent be oral or written? • Is there a justified request for waiver of consent if appropriate?
HARMS AND BENEFITS	• Are potential harms adequately described? • Are possible benefits described appropriately (i.e., not overstated) • Have appropriate measures been taken to maximize benefit and minimize harm?
BUDGET	• Is the budget appropriate? Are expenses of the study clearly laid out? • Are expenses to be assumed by appropriate bodies? (e.g. Who pays for extra diagnostic tests?) • Are participants to be compensated for out-of-pocket expenses? • Is there evidence that the investigator might benefit inappropriately (i.e., Is there a suggestion that the researcher is paid to recruit participants, and could this then lead to inappropriate recruitment?)

ROLES FOR NURSES IN RESEARCH ETHICS

The core principles of research ethics align well with core values in the Canadian Nurses Association (CNA) Code of Ethics for Registered Nurses (2008): providing safe, compassionate, competent and ethical care; promoting health and well-being; promoting and respecting informed decision making; preserving dignity; maintaining privacy and confidentiality; promoting justice; and being accountable. Respect for persons is a key element in all the values outlined in the CNA Code of Ethics, particularly promoting and respecting decision making and preserving dignity; concern for welfare is inherent in nurses' obligation to promote safe, compassionate, competent, and ethical care; and promoting justice is a core value for nurses. Nurses are ideally situated to examine and support the ethics of research being conducted in the health care environment, and have a clear mandate to do so through a variety of roles and responsibilities (Grady and Edgerly 2010).

Nurses may be direct care providers for patients who are research subjects, managers of units where research is conducted, research assistants or research coordinators for medical research, principal investigators or co-investigators in their own studies, and members of REBs or the manager responsible for the REB. An ethical responsibility for nurses is to "support, use and engage in research and other activities that promote safe, competent, compassionate and ethical care, and . . . use guidelines for ethical research that are in keeping with nursing values" (Canadian Nurses Association 2008, 9). Consequently nurses need a good working knowledge of how ethical principles apply in the research context. To aide them in this the Canadian Nurses Association released "Ethical Research Guidelines for Registered Nurses" in 2002. The document contains a clear statement about the breadth of research ethics roles nurses should take and how the core values in the CNA Code of Ethics are operationalized by nurses in their research-related responsibilities. It also provides details about problems and cases, offers analysis of typical ethical conflicts around research, and suggests ways for nurses to approach these conflicts. This CNA document is a valuable resource since nurses' roles in research are varied and they need a more detailed account of ethics in research if they are to act in an advocacy role. Concerns related to nurses' unique research-related experiences are highlighted below. Ethics in Practice scenarios serve to illustrate the points.

ETHICS IN PRACTICE 14-2

Withdrawing from a Clinical Trial

Mr. Chen was a 52-year-old man with acute myelocytic leukemia. I was looking after him the day his doctor came to ask him if he would consent to being in a clinical trial. The doctor explained that they wanted to try a combination of drugs that might have a better chance of putting him into full remission. A new, experimental drug was to be added to the usual medications. The study was a placebo-controlled trial, so Mr. Chen would have a 50-50 chance of getting the experimental drug. He would not know whether he was in the experimental arm of the study, because either way he would be getting an extra pill once a day, and it could be either the placebo or the experimental drug. The doctor explained all the side effects of the usual chemotherapy protocol, and added a list of side effects that were possible from the new drug. Mr. Chen signed the consent form saying he would give it a try—anything that might help him and others get better.

The next morning Mr. Chen started on his treatment regimen. Later that day he experienced severe nausea, vomiting and diarrhea, a blinding headache, and awful itching. He was so weak he could hardly lift his head from the pillow except to vomit. I was quite certain these were side effects of the trial drug but I was surprised that they came on so fast. He was suffering terribly. Each day when I gave him his meds he asked me if I thought it was worth it. On the fourth day he told me that he was pretty sure the problems were side effects of the study drug, and that he wouldn't take the new pill. He said it wasn't worth it to him to be in the trial anymore—he wanted to drop out. I tried to reach his doctor but she was unavailable. I didn't know what to do, because the drugs were to be given together, and at the same time every day. Should I honour Mr. Chen's choice or try to talk him into taking the pill?

Nurse as Care Provider

As care providers, nurses are expected to protect their patients or clients from harm and to promote their well-being, but in the research context it may be unclear exactly what nurses should do to act ethically (Connelly 2009). For example, in a blinded placebo-controlled trial where neither patient nor caregiver know if the patient is on placebo or experimental treatment, nurses may question whether a patient is receiving adequate treatment or is being harmed by the research. They may feel reluctant to give a medication when they do not know what it is or what side effects might be expected, yet they may feel obligated to give it. Or they may be unclear what their action should be if a patient is dissatisfied with participation in the study. In Mr. Chen's case the nurse was concerned about the side effects the patient was experiencing, but the study was blinded so she did not know if he was receiving the experimental treatment. She felt obligated to support the research, but also wanted to honour the patient's right to withdraw from the study. She felt compromised in her obligations to Mr. Chen (i.e., she felt moral distress).

Other issues that can arise for nurses in the context of research raise important questions. For instance, research has shown that many patients have little understanding of the nature of research and the study in which they are enrolled (Henderson et al. 2007; Lidz et al. 2004; Miller and Brody 2003). Clinical care aims to give the best possible treatment to an individual patient, whereas clinical research aims to answer scientific questions in the interests of future patients. At times, the boundary between clinical care and clinical research is blurred, for example, in cancer care. In a research study there is no guarantee that the experimental treatment will be effective, and in a placebo-controlled trial the patient may not be given active treatment at all. Yet numerous researchers have shown that even after having a study explained to them, many patients still believe that they are getting the best care possible. Failure to distinguish between the goals of clinical care and clinical research has been labelled *therapeutic misconception* (Appelbaum, Lidz, and Grisso 2004; Henderson et al. 2007; Miller and Brody 2003; TCPS-2 2010). This can have serious ramifications for a truly informed consent (King and Churchill 2008). Also, when participants discover that they received experimental treatment or a placebo, their trust in their care providers and research in general can be undermined. What obligation do nurses have to be sure patients understand their involvement in a trial? Similarly, what should nurses do if they perceive that patients have been coerced or pressured into taking part in a study?

Another professional issue arises around requirements of nurses to carry out research protocols. If the protocol conflicts with the nurse's professional judgment about what the patient needs at any given time, the nurse may experience moral conflict. What action should a nurse take in this situation? Further, if nurses are held accountable for the care provided to their assigned patients, what is their responsibility for interventions provided by researchers? If the requirements of the research project are impacting workload to the extent that other patients are not receiving adequate care, what is the nurse's responsibility to take some action?

The CNA Code of Ethics (2008) states: "Nurses advocate for persons in their care if they believe that the health of those persons is being compromised by factors beyond their control, including the decision-making of others" (11). According to the research ethics principle of respect for persons, decision making about research participation must be free and informed. To meet this criterion, three elements must be present: capacity, comprehension, and voluntariness. In other words, the potential participant must have the ability to understand (capacity), and must demonstrate understanding (comprehension). The decision must be made free of coercion or pressure, and without undue inducement or promise of reward or benefit (voluntariness). A nurse who perceives that a patient is lacking comprehension about his or her involvement in a research study (whether due to limited cognitive capacity or merely insufficient explanation and/or inadequate time to consider his or her involvement) has a moral obligation to ensure that the patient's participation is, indeed, fully informed and voluntary. This involves assurance that the patient understands the relative risks and benefits of the study, is able to weigh them in making a decision about participation, and in no way feels pressured to participate. If the patient lacks cognitive capacity, consent from an appropriate proxy must be sought, and the proxy must, likewise, be fully informed of risks and benefits and equally free from pressure. If a nurse believes that a patient (or proxy) does not have full comprehension, yet is being asked to consent for research, this lack of comprehension must be addressed with the investigator. If it is not resolved to the nurse's satisfaction the REB should be informed (Dunn and Chadwick 2004, Chapter 9; Emanuel, Wendler, and Grady 2000; CNA Guidelines 2002; see also Chapter 4).

Research ethics principles of respect for persons and concern for welfare require that participants be assured that they have a right to withdraw from studies, and the conditions with respect to withdrawal (e.g., time limits or whether or not data will be retained) must be detailed in the consent form. Nurses are expected to advocate for patients who wish to withdraw by contacting the researcher and facilitating a discussion between participant and researcher as needed. Provisions for a patient to withdraw from a study should be discussed at the time consent is given (i.e., before the study commences). Researchers and research coordinators should make all necessary information available to staff nurses, including contact numbers where the researcher can be reached around the clock. If such information is not available, nurses should contact the researcher or the REB to request this information and report any concerns.

Nurses require adequate information about research studies to enable them to assess the level or standard of care being administered as part of a study. If nurses find elements of the research troubling, these concerns should be made clear to researchers, nursing managers or the REB, as it is the nurse who is accountable for her practice. If the nurse believes that demands of a research protocol impinge on the care needed by non-study patients, this concern should be discussed with the nurse manager, and potentially the researcher. Obedience and loyalty to outside authorities or higher authorities (e.g., medical researchers or organizational executives) should not constrain a nurse from raising questions, as may have been the constraints on Ms. Rivers in the Tuskegee study. That is not to suggest that is easy; it requires considerable moral courage and excellent communication skills to speak up.

Nurse as Manager

Front-line nurse managers and leaders are responsible for assessing and managing nursing workload and quality of care on nursing units, for ensuring a positive work environment, and for managing unit budgets. Research can have an impact on all of these, and in many institutions, the signature of the nurse manager is required before a researcher is permitted to bring a study onto a nursing unit. Before providing that signature, the manager has a responsibility to become familiar with the protocol, ask any questions that arise, and await satisfactory answers provided by the researcher. Only then should the manager sign the permission form. If there is no signature requirement for research within an institution, managers should be prepared to seek a change in institutional policy. Part of that policy should include an outline of responsibilities of staff nurses vis-à-vis research, statements about workload and funding issues, and requirements for nursing support. Institutions should not be silent on such matters, as failure to address such issues can put both patients and nurses at unnecessary risk, or cause them undue stress.

Senior nurse managers may be responsible for making provisions for, and providing oversight of, the Research Ethics Board. Therefore, it is critical that those managers (and their superiors) are aware of the TCPS-2, including the provisions required to establish an REB in compliance with specifications about who shall sit on the REB and how the REB shall function. Providing sufficient resources for the REB to do its job is vital to its effectiveness.

Nurse as Research Assistant/Coordinator

The role of nurse as research assistant or project coordinator (research nurse) can entail significant ethical challenges. Nursing ethics is founded in relationships and caring (Bergum and Dossetor 2005; Doane and Varcoe 2007; Oberle and Raffin 2009) and is focused on the individual good of the patient (Canadian Nurses Association 2008; see also Chapters 7, 8, and 9). By contrast, the goals of science are, essentially, furthering the greater good. Thus, when a research nurse assistant or coordinator encounters a situation where the goals of science appear to be at odds with the individual good, he or she may experience a conflict between obligations to the employer (researcher or research organization) and to the patient (Poston and Bueshcer 2010). For example, in Mr. Chen's case, the research nurse assistant or coordinator was likely to be the first to be contacted by the staff nurse when Mr. Chen decided he wanted to leave the study. As an employee of the principal investigator, the research nurse might experience some degree of conflict as well. The research nurse might be more aware of the elements of blinding and placebo, as well as the importance of sample size, and might be tempted to try to convince the patient to continue in the study. Nonetheless, the research nurse assistant or coordinator must be alert to the point at which attempts to explain or reinterpret the study to the patient become harassment or coercion, and be prepared to alter the approach to ensure that continued participation is truly voluntary (TCPS-2; CNA Guidelines 2002).

Inclusion and exclusion criteria (who gets into the study) are also matters of research ethics. Research ethics principles and nursing ethics values include promoting justice, which incorporates fair distribution of benefits and burdens of research. Research nurses need to be prepared to speak up when they believe potential participants, for example, pregnant women, are unfairly excluded from a research protocol. They must also be aware of burdens that a study might place on participants, such as the frail elderly who might have difficulty coming for follow-up visits. Burdens of the study should be outlined clearly to avoid therapeutic misconception and coercion when seeking consent (TCPS-2, see also Chapter 11).

Even seasoned researchers may be driven by their interest in a valid research outcome (e.g., the need to have sufficient numbers of participants in a study for purposes of validity) and be blind to their violations of research ethics. Sometimes researchers may be unaware of research ethics, a gap that the Council of Canadian Academies and other agencies have tried hard to fill through publication of documents on research integrity.[6] Nurses cannot assume that all researchers have sufficient knowledge about research ethics. Thus, when research nurses are requested to participate in what they regard as breaches of ethical conduct, they need to voice their concerns to the researcher. This can be difficult, especially if their concerns are not heeded. In extreme cases the nurse may need to become a **whistle-blower**, that is, the person who reports a perceived wrongdoing. When nurses' employment is threatened, or when they feel obligated to "betray" an employer for whom they have had respect, considerable moral courage is required to act according to their conscience (Ahern and McDonald 2002). Ethical practice demands that the first duty is to the patient. Careful documentation of concerns and processes followed is very important. Action strategies could include calling for a meeting of like-minded people to discuss the issue and thereby check out a nurse's perceptions and calling upon an REB or a clinical ethics committee for assistance.[8]

In summary, nurses as research assistants or project coordinators may experience a variety of moral problems in the conduct of the research. Despite difficulties, the nurse as professional is required to act ethically. When the nature of the obligation is not clear, as during recruitment of participants/subjects, these problems should be discussed with the principal investigator. The nurse should be aware that some conflicts may remain unresolved; however raising ethical concerns is still important to minimize harm to the patient and to protect the nurse's integrity. A cultivated ethics awareness and active reflection on practice are necessary to ensure that nurses have a clear sense of how they ought to act. They then must find the moral courage to follow through on that "ought."

Nurse as Researcher

Nurses as researchers are subject to the same ethical guidelines as any other researcher, but may experience some unique problems because of the nature of their research and their relationship with patients. It is important that potential problems be anticipated and avoided to the extent possible at the proposal development stage. That is why developing an ethics application parallel to developing a proposal can be helpful. Some issues may be difficult to predict (see for example, Clancy 2011), and nurse researchers need to think ahead about protection of human participants to develop sensitivity to ethics issues in their research.

Sometimes constraints imposed by the Health Agency or the REB may present nurse researchers with difficulties in accessing research subjects in clinical settings. To uphold the principle of respect for persons and to protect confidentiality, most REBs require participant recruitment to follow one of two pathways: self-selection, in which the participant responds to advertisements or word-of-mouth contacts by approaching the researcher directly; or face-to-face recruitment, in which the initial approach is made by a direct caregiver or a third party on behalf of the caregiver. Most REBs require a researcher who is a direct caregiver for potential participants to have others make the first contact to reduce the potential for coercion. For example, the researcher might ask staff nurses to identify potential participants and request the patients' permission to have the researcher approach them to explain the study. Even if the organization's ethics review allows nurses simultaneously to assume a role as caregiver and as researcher, they should recognize the importance of third-party assistance in subject recruitment. No patient should be placed in the position of agreeing to be part of a study to please a caregiver. Although third-party involvement makes recruitment more laborious, it is necessary to protect participants from coercion and perhaps from therapeutic misconception (King and Churchill 2008). In some organizations there may be a requirement that nurses seek permission from the physician before a patient is contacted. Nurses might well disagree that the doctor has a right to control nursing research and to prevent their patients from enrolling in studies; however, this is standard practice in some institutions. Therefore, nurses considering recruitment of a clinical population would be well advised to seek advice from the nurse manager or the REB before proceeding. When nurse researchers are wishing to conduct research on a group of individuals they also supervise in clinical practice or education, they need to be thoughtful about how to ensure potential participants are given a free choice about their involvement in the study. In educational programs, the nurse researcher will seek a third "disinterested party" to explain the project and obtain consent from students.

Research design may also pose ethical challenges for nurse researchers. Many nurse researchers use qualitative methods (Dierckx de Casterle et al. 2011; Epstein 2010; Ersoy and Akpinar 2010; Lohne et al. 2010) that require particular ethics sensitivities. One of the most important of these is a function of the relationship that a qualitative nurse researcher develops with the participant, and the possible blurring of roles between nurse researcher and nurse caregiver (Morse 2007), particularly when the study involves a population with health problems in the nurse's area of expertise. Nurse researchers must be very clear at the outset about the dual role in these relationships, indicating to the participant the differences between research and care (CNA Guidelines 2002; Shaw 2008). Ethics in Practice 14-3 provides a practical example of the conflicts arising within a dual role, and the danger of therapeutic misconception.

ETHICS IN PRACTICE 14-3

Recruiting Participants Who Need Care

As a master's student undertaking thesis research, Millie went to her supervisor with a problem. She was having some difficulty recruiting participants for her study. What she wanted to do was go to patients' homes after they were discharged from surgery to provide a type of supportive care she believed would enhance their healing, reduce the number of visits to the emergency and/or the physician after surgery, reduce complications such as infection, and enhance well-being. First, she had trouble getting the nurses to remember that they were to ask patients if she could come in and talk to them.

Secondly, the nurses kept suggesting that she simply look over the OR slate each day and find the patients herself, which would make it much easier for them. Also, when she did talk to patients, they seemed very reluctant to sign the consent. Many indicated that they wanted to ask their doctor if he thought it was a good idea. Others said they didn't think they wanted to be bothered at home. Millie was quite convinced that patients would do better if they had her support, but she was reluctant to try to talk them into being in the study because she was afraid that she was pressuring them too much.

Other important issues arise in the context of informed consent. In a qualitative study it may be difficult to anticipate risks, and one must question just how informed a consent can be if risks cannot be disclosed prior to in-depth interviews. The reporting of data also generates special concerns about engagement and confidentiality. Nurses' skills in relational communication make them especially effective interviewers and this same effectiveness may lead to research subjects revealing more than they anticipated. Patients may feel damaged in some way by having disclosed highly personal information. Further, in reporting data qualitative researchers often use verbatim portions of interviews to illustrate key points of the person's perceptions. If the research participants recognize themselves in the report, they may experience even more distress. Verbatim reports combined with detailed demographic data may make participants identifiable to those who know them, which make promises of confidentiality suspect (Shaw, 2008). Researchers should carefully consider whether demographic data are necessary to the integrity of the project, particularly when findings are reported, and whether the quotations they use are too revealing (Morse 2007). Purposefully masking biographical details in publication or verbal reporting and letting the reader or listener know this is the case is one way of protecting confidentiality.

How can researchers minimize other harms they cause to participants? Part of the answer is to approach informed consent as **process consent**, in which the researcher frequently seeks permission to proceed as the study progresses (Beebe and Smith 2010). Although a process consent cannot overcome the problem of raising unexpected emotions or memories, it is important that the nurse researcher "expect the unexpected" and have a plan in place for such eventualities. This might include the provision of counselling support if necessary. Ideally process consent should extend, not just to the data collection phase of the study, but also to the reporting phase. Further to this point the issue of "who owns the story" often arises. Qualitative research is often portrayed as an egalitarian endeavour designed to present the participant's viewpoint—the so-called "emic perspective." What happens, then, when the researcher and participant disagree with the findings? Whose interpretation is to be respected? Morse (2007) suggests that these and related questions must be discussed with participants as part of the process of informed consent. This implies that the researcher must think these matters through before seeking consent, and by extension, requires the researcher to have examined the philosophical premises on which the research is based.

Nurses occupy a special position of trust with people in their care, and, while research is essential to the improvement of care, nurses should never allow their enthusiasm for a study to overshadow their obligation to fulfill that trust. An awareness of the kinds of issues that can arise is an essential part of the research process, and the CNA (2002a) document on ethics in research can be invaluable in helping the nurse to gain the necessary sensitivity.

Nurse as a Member of Review Boards

A research role growing in importance for nurses is their membership on research review boards, including research ethics boards (REBs). Nurses are accustomed to acting in an advocacy role, and their perspectives on how studies might affect patients means their voices are exceptionally important. They are often more aware than other health care providers of the kinds of worries patients have because patients frequently confide in nurses more than anyone else. As patients themselves are seldom consulted in developing research proposals, the nurse has a greater obligation to reflect the patient viewpoint (Pringle 2008).

It is important that nurses be present at the table when decisions are being made about which studies may proceed. REBs generally consider scientific merit of the study in their deliberations, based on the premise that conducting scientifically unsound research is inherently unethical (Emanuel, Wendler, and Grady 2000). A problem may arise if the REB does not have sufficient knowledge of the kinds of methods nurses use to make an accurate assessment of the scientific merit of a study. For example, researchers schooled in experimental design may have difficulty seeing the worth of a qualitative study that has no control group, no hypotheses, and no calculation of sample size. This raises a danger that valuable qualitative nursing studies (e.g., Dierkx de Casterle et al. 2011) could be blocked on the basis of inadequate method, which could translate into inappropriate controls on the development of nursing knowledge. Nursing membership on the REB can provide the necessary expertise, but this is only valuable if the nurse is knowledgeable, prepared to speak up, and willing to champion well developed nursing proposals.

Despite recent advances, the possibility still exists that some areas do not have REBs for the review of research protocols. This could be the case, for instance, in rural settings (such as the Ethics in Practice 14-4) or in private clinics. Nursing expertise may then be required to assess the merit of a protocol, as in remote northern communities where the nurse may be the only person available with advanced education. Community leaders might request the nurse's advice regarding the impact of the study and whether the researcher should be allowed to collect data. Clearly, it is incumbent on the nurse to have a good working understanding of research methods, sensitivity to ethics issues, and a defined route for seeking further advice. This means that nurse educators need to know and sensitize students to research ethics, including knowing whom to call if advice is needed.

ETHICS IN PRACTICE 14-4

Voicing Concerns about a Protocol

Marit was a nurse manager of a public health unit in a remote rural area. She contacted me because she knew I chaired the research ethics board of a large city hospital. She told me that a research protocol had been submitted to her chief medical officer (CMO) by a psychologist who was also the CMO's close friend. The CMO read the proposal, approved it, and forwarded it to Marit for nursing approval. When Marit reviewed the proposal she became concerned that the study would create problems for the nurses and the community. The topic was elder abuse, and the nurses were expected to collect the data using a questionnaire that they would fill in after visiting homes in which there were dependent elders. In Marit's estimation the questionnaire was badly designed, and the questions decidedly biased. In fact, Marit felt that if the nurses were to fill out the

questionnaires, it was almost a guarantee that the community would be revealed as having a high incidence of elder abuse, even though she believed that to be incorrect. Her worry was that the community could be harmed by faulty study results, and that the trust relationship between the nurses and the community would be badly damaged. Consequently, she informed her CMO that she would not sign off on the protocol until it had been reviewed by an ethics board, and she made a written request to me as REB chair. Her CMO was annoyed, but had little choice but to accept her decision. When our REB reviewed the protocol we agreed with Marit's assessment, and sent her a written statement that the study would not have received approval from our REB. When faced with this response, the CMO rescinded his approval and the study was stopped.

RESPONSIBILITY OF NURSES AS LEADERS IN RESEARCH ETHICS

According to Pringle (2008), nurses have had little involvement in setting national research ethics standards, despite the fact that they are front-line caregivers for patients in clinical studies, and increasingly are themselves researchers. By contrast, physicians have taken leadership in this area. This situation Pringle believes is "not acceptable" (4). If nursing is to become "a major player in this national drama" (4) nurses require a deeper understanding of and involvement in research ethics.

Fortunately, nurses are taking leadership in several areas of national research ethics. Both authors of this chapter, for example, serve on the Research Ethics Board of Health Canada and the Public Health Agency of Canada, one author previously served as president of the National Council on Ethics in Human Research, and the other sits as current member of the Canadian Institutes of Health Research Standing Committee on Ethics.

Other nurses are taking leadership in setting research agendas individually, through the Canadian Association of Schools of Nursing, through the Canadian Nurses Association, and through other national and provincial bodies.

Nurses also have an important role in "research in ethics," that is, research about ethics. Until fairly recently, there was little nursing research in this area. In the past most undergraduate nursing research textbooks suggested that questions of ethics, as value questions, were inherently "unresearchable," but nurses are now turning to research to help them define nursing ethics and the kinds of ethical issues nurses encounter in their practice and in their research (Gustafsson et al. 2010; Lutzen et al. 2010; Pauly et al. 2009). The journal *Nursing Ethics,* established in 1994, is an important vehicle for dissemination and discussion of international nursing ethics scholarship. It includes both conceptual and research articles about ethics in nursing practice, many from an international perspective. Its influence is growing, as evidenced by the increasing "impact factor," which is a measure of how often articles in the journal are cited by others.

Nurses also conduct studies on research ethics (see for example, Beebe and Smith 2010), although the numbers of studies are relatively small to date. That is unsurprising, given that few researchers from any discipline have undertaken research in this area. Nurses are making a large contribution to understanding of research ethics by writing philosophical papers in which they discuss key issues, particularly from a feminist perspective. They have called for new ways of looking at the influence of power and social justice on the kinds of research questions that are asked, on research design, on notions of informed consent, and on understanding of benefit and burdens of research (see for example, Kagan et al. 2010; Reimer-Kirkham and Anderson 2010).

Being at the front line of care, nurses have an obligation to support research and knowledge development for clinical practice, but at the same time, their role as patient advocate places them in a position to ensure that participants in health research are protected from harm. It is essential that this perspective be brought to light through research and scholarly writing. Nurses, as caregivers and researchers, are ideally situated to be leaders in this area. This could be interpreted as a moral obligation to strive for growing ethical sensitivity around research and its conduct.

Summary

In this chapter we have underscored important roles nurses play in the promotion of ethical research and the protection of human participants. We have demonstrated that nurses are key contributors to research ethics through their own practice and research, their participation on REBs, their engagement in setting fair research agendas, and their leadership in developing structures to attend to research ethics review where none currently exist. We have reviewed key documents and structures in research ethics in Canada as a reminder to nurses (and others) of past history and the present guidance available and in continuing development. While we recognize that research is important, we also note that it takes significant energy and moral courage to support research while at the same time protecting human participants. Nurses with an awareness of ethical issues are ideally positioned to meet this difficult challenge.

For Reflection

1. What kinds of guidelines are in place in your institution to guide nurses' involvement in research?

2. Why might there be a gap between what nurses believe they ought to do in research-related situations involving another's research, and what they actually do?

3. Why might there be a gap between what nurses believe they ought to do in research-related situations involving their own research, and what they actually do?

4. What kinds of research-related issues have you encountered in your practice, and what action have you taken?

Endnotes

1. Smith (1996) provides an intensive review of the context surrounding the Tuskegee Institute Study pointing out the economic, political, and social motivations of the researchers and research staff. For example, Rivers needed a day job that paid well, the Institute stood to benefit through political attention bringing status and increased funding, and Rivers (whose public health nurse positions over the years endeared her to her clients) was highly trusted by the male subjects. Smith also found that the movement to "professionalization" of all health professionals at the time seemed to play a part in their decisions to maintain the status quo. As professions were developing the tendency to support each other, by standing by and not disagreeing with each other was more common.

2. Less well known about world-wide ethics violations is that from 1932 to the end of World War II there were similar, and potentially more degrading and deadening, Japanese medical experiments largely on Chinese residents and prisoners (MacNeill 2009).

3. Another violation of research ethics in research on vulnerable populations in Guatemala has recently been disclosed. While pursuing research on another topic, Susan Reverby discovered that in 1946–1948 U.S. government researchers had deliberately infected nearly 700 Guatemalans with venereal disease to test the effectiveness of penicillin. On learning of this violation, the U.S. government apologized publicly to Guatemala (Frieden and Collins 2010; *The New York Times,* October 1, 2010).

4. The interested reader can find the original and revised versions of the TCPS online (http://pre.ethics. gc.ca/eng/policy-politique/tcps-eptc/readtcps-lireeptc/).

5. Other research guidelines pertinent to Canadian researchers conducting clinical research are the *Good clinical practice: Consolidated guidelines* published by Health Canada as an ICH harmonized Tripartite Guideline (International Conference on Harmonization of Technical Requirements for the Registration of Pharmaceuticals for Human Use); *Canada Gazette, Part II,* June 20, 2001, Statutory Instruments, that paved the way for phase 1 trials; *Operational guidelines for ethics committees that review biomedical research,* World Health Organization, 2000.

6. Many researchers are frustrated by the need to apply to many research ethics boards when doing province-wide or nation-wide research. Attempts are underway to find ways to reduce the time and complexity of these multiple applications, for example, establishing one REB in Newfoundland; REB harmonization in Alberta; and projects' to develop a multi-site review processes in the U.S. and Canada (Greene et al. 2010).

7. An additional resource titled *Honesty, Accountability and Trust: Fostering Research Integrity in Canada* was released by the Expert Panel on Research Integrity in 2010. This resource can be

particularly useful for nurses and others involved in research, and particularly those serving on (or responsible for) research ethics boards.

8. Some Canadian nurse research assistants and coordinators recommend SOCRA (the Society of Clinical Research Associates), a helpful group for developing greater knowledge and skills in clinical research (http://www.socra.org/).

References

Ahern, K. and McDonald, M. 2002. The beliefs of nurses who were involved in a whistleblowing event. *Journal of Advanced Nursing, 38*, 303–309.

Appelbaum, P.S., Lisz, C.W., and Grisso, T. 2004. Therapeutic misconception in clinical research: Frequency and risk factors. *IRB: Ethics and Human Research, 26* (2), 1–8.

Beebe, L.H. and Smith, K. 2010. Informed consent to research in persons with schizophrenia spectrum disorders. *Nursing Ethics, 17* (4), 425–434.

Bergum, V. and Dossetor, J. 2005. *Relational ethics: The full meaning of respect.* Hagerstown, MD: University Publishing Group.

Canadian Nurses Association. 2008. *Code of ethics for registered nurses.* Ottawa: Author.

Canadian Nurses Association. 2002. *Ethical research guidelines for registered nurses.* Ottawa: Author.

Clancy, A. 2011. An embodied response: Ethics and the nurse researcher. *Nursing Ethics, 18* (1), 112–121.

Connelly, L.M. 2009. Staff nurses' responsibilities when caring for patients in a research study. *Medsurg Nursing, 18*, 385–386, 388.

Declaration of Helsinki. 2008. Available at http://www.wma.net/en/30publications/10policies/b3/index.html.

Dierckx de Casterle, B., Verhaeghe, S., Kars, M., Coolbrandt, A., Stevens, M., Stubbe, M., Deweirdt, N., Vincke, J., and Grypdonck, M. 2011. Researching the lived experience in health care. *Nursing Ethics, 18* (2), 232–242.

Doane, C. and Varcoe, C. 2007. Relational practice and nursing obligations. *Advances in Nursing Science, 30*, 192–205.

Dunn, C.M. and Chadwick, G.L. 2004. *Protecting study volunteers in research* (3rd ed.). Boston: Thomson Centerwatch.

Emanuel, E.J., Wendler, D., and Grady, C. 2000. What makes clinical research ethical? *Journal of the American Medical Association, 283* (20), 2701–2711.

Epstein, E.G. 2010. Moral obligations of nurses and physicians in neonatal end-of-life care. *Nursing Ethics, 17* (5), 577–589.

Ersoy, N. and Akpinar, A. 2010. Turkish nurses' decision making in the distribution of intensive care beds. *Nursing Ethics, 17* (1), 87–98.

Expert Panel on Research Integrity. 2010. *Honesty, accountability and trust: Fostering research integrity in Canada.* Ottawa: Council of Canadian Academies.

Frieden, T.R. and Collins, F.S. 2010. Intentional infection of vulnerable populations in 1946–1948: Another tragic history lesson. *Journal of the American Medical Association,* Commentary. Published online, October 11, 2010.

Grady, C. and Edgerly, M. 2009. Science, technology, and innovation: Nursing responsibilities in clinical research. *Nursing Clinics of North America, 44,* 471–481.

Greene, S.M., Braff, J., Nelson, A., and Reid, R.J. 2010. The process is the product: A new model for multisite IRB review of data-only studies. *IRB Ethics and Human Research, 32* (3), 1–6.

Gustafsson, G., Eriksson, S., Stranberg, G., and Norberg, A. 2010. Burnout and perceptions of conscience among health care personnel: A pilot study. *Nursing Ethics, 17* (1), 23–38.

Henderson, G.E., Churchill, L.R., Davis, A.M., Easter, M.M., Grady, C., Joffe, S., Kass, N., King, M.P., Lidz, C.W., Miller, G.F., Nelson, D.K., Peppercorn, J., Rothschild, B., Sankar, P., Wilfrond, B., and Zimmer, C.R. 2007. Clinical trials and medical care: Defining the therapeutic misconception. *Public Library of Science, Medicine, 4,* 1735–1738.

Kagan, P.N., Smith, M.C., Cowling, W.R. III, and Chinn, P.L. 2010. A nursing manifesto: An emancipatory call for knowledge development, conscience, and praxis. *Nursing Philosophy, 11* (1), 67–84.

King, N. and Churchill, L. 2008. Clinical research and the physician–patient relationship: The dual roles of physician and researcher. In P. Singer and A.M. Viens (Eds.), *The Cambridge textbook of bioethics* (pp. 214–221). Cambridge: Cambridge University Press.

Kjellstrom, S. and Fridlund, B. 2010. Status and trends of research ethics in Swedish nurses' dissertations. *Nursing Ethics, 17,* 383–392.

Lidz, C.W., Appelbaum, P.S., Grisso, T., and Renaud, M. 2004. Therapeutic misconception and the appreciation of risks in clinical trials. *Social Science and Medicine, 58,* 1689–1697.

Lohne, V., Aasgaard, T., Caspari, S., Slettebo, A., and Naden, D. 2010. The lonely battle for dignity: Individuals struggling with multiple sclerosis. *Nursing Ethics, 17* (3), 301–311.

Lutzen, K., Blom, T., Ewalds-Kvist, B., and Winch, S. 2010. Moral stress, moral climate and moral sensitivity among psychiatric professionals. *Nursing Ethics, 17* (2), 213–224.

MacNeill, P.U. 2009. Regulating experimentation in research and medical practice. In H. Kuhse and P. Singer (Eds.), *A companion to boethics* (2nd ed.; pp. 469–486). Oxford, UK: John Wiley-Blackwell.

Medical Research Council of Canada. 1978. *MRC Report No. 6, Ethics in human experimentation.* Ottawa: Author.

Medical Research Council of Canada. 1987. *Guidelines on research involving human subjects.* Ottawa: Author.

Meslin, E.M. and Dickens, B.M. 2008. Research ethics. In P.A. Singer and A.M. Viens (Eds.), *The Cambridge textbook of bioethics* (pp. 187–193). Cambridge: Cambridge University Press.

Miller, F.G. and Brody, H. 2003. A critique of clinical equipoise: Therapeutic misconception in the ethics of clinical trials. *Hastings Center Report, 33*(3), 19–28.

Morse, J. 2007. Ethics in action: Ethical principles for doing qualitative health research. *Qualitative Health Research, 17,* 1003–1005.

National Commission for the Protection of Human Subjects of Biomedical and Behavioral Research. 1979. *The Belmont report. Ethical principles and guidelines for the protection of human subjects of research.* Publication No. OS 78-0012. Federal Register Document 79–12065. Washington, DC: US Department of Health, Education and Welfare. Available at http://ohsr.od.nih.gov/guidelines/belmont.html#top.

Nuremberg Code. 1947. Available at http://ohsr.od.nih.gov/guidelines/nuremberg.html.

Oberle, K. and Raffin, S. 2009. *Ethics in Canadian nursing practice: Navigating the journey.* Toronto: Pearson.

Pauly, B., Varcoe, C., Storch, J., and Newton, L. Registered nurses' perceptions of moral distress and ethical climate. *Nursing Ethics, 16* (5), 561–573.

Poston, R.D. and Buescher, C.R. 2010. The essential role of the clinical research nurse (CRN). *Urologic Nursing, 30* (1), 55–63, 77.

Pringle, D. 2008. How well protected are Canadian research participants? Who knows? *Nursing Leadership, 21*, 1–5.

Reimer-Kirkham, S. and Anderson, J.M. 2010. The advocate-analyst dialectic in critical and postcolonial feminist research: Reconciling tensions around scientific integrity. *Advances in Nursing Science, 33*, 196–205.

Shaw, I. 2008. Ethics and the practice of qualitative research. *Qualitative Social Work, 7*, 400–414.

Smith, S.L. 1996. Neither victim nor villain: Nurse Eunice Rivers, the Tuskegee experiment and public health work. *Journal of Women's History, 8* (1), 95–113.

Steppe, H. 1992. Nursing in Nazi Germany. *Western Journal of Nursing Research, 14* (6), 744–753.

Steppe, H. 1996. The war and nursing in Germany. *International History of Nursing Journal, 1* (4), 61–71.

Tri-Council Policy Statement. 1998*: Ethical conduct for research involving humans.* Available at www.nserc.ca/program/ethics/english/policy.htm.

Tri-Council Policy Statement. 2010. *Ethical conduct for research involving humans.* Available at http://pre.ethics.gc.ca/eng/policy-politique/tcps-eptc/readtcps-lireeptc/.

CHAPTER 15

Educative Spaces for Teaching and Learning Ethical Practice in Nursing

Helen Brown and Gayle Allison

No matter what kind of relationships we enter into, nurse–patient, teacher–student, the relational space between needs as much care and development as the theoretical and abstract knowledge of nursing science, and the practical development of skills and techniques. (Bergum 2003, 125)

INTRODUCTION

The call for reflexive and critical pedagogies in nursing has placed the importance of continual scrutiny on our practices and commitments in our shared educational agenda (Diekelmann 2005; Ewashen and Lane 2007; Hartrick Doane and Brown 2011; Ironside 2001). The complexity of contemporary nursing practice demands that nurse educators continually engage in efforts to reflect upon and enact educative moments in ways that will ultimately contribute to ethical practice in nursing (Brown and Rodney 2007; Ewashen and Lane 2007; Hartrick Doane and Varcoe 2005). Critical, narrative, and feminist pedagogy, where social justice, co-operation, and transformation are emphasized, are influencing both learning in nursing (Ironside 2001) and nursing ethics education. Therefore, considering how we educate toward ethical practice is not a separate topic from how it is that nurses think about, engage in, and develop knowledge for ethical practice within everyday moments and contexts of practice. It is in this very place that our educative practice is considered. In this chapter we explore the ethical dimensions of the nurse educator role through reflection on our experiences in teaching/learning relationships and our educative practice, acknowledging that our approach implies that ". . . the meaning of what is good is found in nursing practice and that the notion of ethics is embedded in practice" (Brown et al. 2004, 131).

We join the many voices in nursing that theorize that ethical practice is both a personal and contextual process of engaged and responsive action. Such calls for the "re-personalization of ethics" (Doane 2004) challenge the dominance of rationalist approaches to moral truth and ethical decision-making processes. Rationalist approaches take the role of reason in moral deliberation and ethical decision making as primary. There now exists a surge of writing in nursing ethics theorizing how ethical practice is imbued with the everyday complexities of nursing work, where values, emotion, experience, and relationships intersect to underpin ethical challenges and moral deliberations in contemporary health care contexts (see Chapters 6–11). Learning to "be" ethical requires that as educators we carefully and critically consider how to create educative spaces imbued by similar complexities. We believe that teaching/learning relationships are another site where ethical nursing practice is lived and learned. We focus our attention in this chapter on exploring how to create educative spaces that contribute to this overall goal.

OUR INTENT

Our intent is to consider ways to create educative spaces that align the teaching and learning of ethics with ethical nursing practice. Our inquiries and analyses are guided by our experiences as teachers within both academic and clinical contexts, our reading and critical analysis of theoretical work in nursing ethics and nursing ethics education literature, and our view of the importance of the relational moment where teaching and learning occur. Because students and teachers together shape possibilities for knowing through their ways of engaging and by exploring the context of their engagement, our focus is on enhancing relational experiences and spaces within which ethical nursing practice is both taught and learned.

We begin by describing our understanding of what underlies dominant approaches to nursing ethics education and by drawing attention to what is overlooked or taken for granted in such approaches. Rather than exploring the existing game for a new move, we propose a "new game"; one that describes strategies for creating ethical educative spaces that can contribute to the goal of enhancing ethical practice in nursing. We elucidate what has typically guided ethics education, what is taken for granted in such approaches, and we make some proposals for expanding and evolving possibilities for creating educative spaces to support ethical practice in nursing.

NURSING ETHICS PEDAGOGY IN CONTEXT

We propose the evolution of the three approaches that have typically guided nursing ethics education. These approaches are based on several assumptions: that ethics education is (1) an epistemological activity, (2) behaviourist in orientation, and (3) guided by collective ethical values and moral obligations. We discuss each of these and outline both limits and possibilities for evolving our educative practices.

Ethics Pedagogy as an Epistemological Activity

As a clinical nurse educator, I (Gayle) have been asked to support nurses whose practice is deemed by others as "unethical." For example, we may be called upon when a nurse's action threatens a patient's physical or emotional safety. Unethical practice in a clinical context will span a variety of situations, from a medication error to concerns about a lack of cultural competence. Nurses often feel anxiety and fear when advised that their knowledge is not up to the required standard, and that ethical practice was compromised as a result. When staff nurses' knowledge is considered to be "underdeveloped," "lacking," even "wrong," it is commonly believed that it is their lack of knowledge that is constraining their capacity to be ethical in practice. The proverbial bucket isn't full enough. When unethical practice is framed as a lack of knowledge, the solution is often to call upon the educator to fix this so-called "problem of knowledge." Yet, how we are with learners when a judgment is made and the problem is defined is a critical educative moment. In entering into critical educative moments such as this, we must also engage in a critical reflection of our role and our approach to teaching/learning. Is our role to impart knowledge to create an ethical nurse? Will more knowledge be the solution to engaging with patients/clients ethically? Might the very ways we engage with learners in these educative moments also teach them to how to "be" ethical in the everyday ethical complexities and challenges of nursing?

In considering these questions it is essential to question the assumptions underlying the tendency to frame unethical practice as a "problem of knowledge." In practice "knowledge" is considered the essence of all good, safe, ethical nursing practice. Knowledge is the marker or symbol of excellence in nursing care. When a nurse is determined to be practicing in ways that are not consistent with ethical standards, one assumption too readily made is that he or she lacks knowledge or the capacity to "apply" particular theories to concrete situations. The perceived solution to such a lack of knowledge is education. Education, in this context, is then generally interpreted to mean that the teacher will step in and correct the problem of insufficient knowledge. Working from an "epistemologies' grasp" (Diekelmann 2002, 469) the teacher provides the learner with the "right" content (Brown and Doane 2007; Hartrick Doane and Brown in press).

Thus, the uptake of knowledge is perceived to be the solution to the problem of unethical practice. For example, teaching ethical theory and principles as prescriptive guides that nurses apply implies that ethical comportment is something that is infused into a nurse's conduct. The underlying assumption is that the learner needs only to be given the right content to improve their practice, and within the context of ethics education, become more ethical. The dominant rationalist view of knowledge at play is just teach her so she will "know." Yet, contemporary writers in nursing ethics indicate that knowledge for ethical practice requires seeing how knowing is inseparable from the personal, embodied, and experiential moments of practice. Sellman (2009) notes, ". . . teaching *for* ethical practice is, pedagogically speaking, of a different order from the teaching *of* ethics to prospective practitioners" (90). Bergum (2003) claims that for students to learn ethical practice, they require ". . . knowledge of the subject matter but without the ability to connect the information to the lived life (organic nature, own bodies) of students, the information is merely technical, rather than whole" (125).

The challenge in nursing has been to focus on the knowledge required to discern moral truths, engage in ethical deliberation, and to recognize that knowing in nursing is personal and contextual. Ethics in nursing practice has been described as relational and highly contextual; being ethical has been described as a way of engaging with self, others, and contexts that brings values, emotions, intuitive thought, and bodily experience in each moment of ethical deliberation (Varcoe et al. 2004, 319). The concomitant challenge for educators is to facilitate ethical reasoning, knowledge, and action in ways that are both personal and contextual. This implies that our educative strategies must become oriented to providing the requisite knowledge so that nurses know how to apply theory to enact their ethical duty and moral obligations in specific situations.

Being ethical in nursing involves knowledge, but cannot be reduced to a simplistic and inaccurate dichotomy of knowing and not knowing. The challenge for teaching ethical practice in nursing is to engage learners in an exploration of ethical knowledge as developed through reasoned deliberation and through experiences that are shaped by relationships and contexts. For example, a nurse who does not know the concept of cultural competence as it relates to ethical engagement might very well have had experiences of relating to others where differences exist. Thus, the practice of ethical engagement becomes known through theorizing practice to develop knowledge into the future.

What is taken for granted and/or overlooked when ethics education is framed primarily as an epistemological activity? We propose that the tendency to focus our teaching practice on facilitating knowledge development (the epistemological) and moral truth without equal attention to *being* (the ontological)—that is how a nurse engages with others—reduces our capacities as educators and learners to see how being itself is a fundamental condition for knowing anything. Heidegger (1962) advances the important idea that knowledge and knowing are fundamentally ontological; that is, knowledge is not a set of correct axioms or descriptions that relate to an external world, but rather a series of interpretations that can be contingent, inconsistent, and fluctuating amidst experiencing individuals. Thus, experiences of being-in-the-world create the conditions through which knowledge and truth become known and the creating of knowledge is fundamentally experiential. Within the context of ethical knowledge then, facilitating the learning of ethical practice requires engaging learners in tuning in to the personal and contextual experiences of *being ethical* in everyday moments of practice. Pedagogical strategies and principles are to "reflect the primacy of the pedagogic relationship premised on lived experience, experiential and personal knowing, and the critical consciousness required for honoring the values of equality, justice and freedom" (Ewashen and Lane 2007, 258).

Evolving the tendency to approach nursing ethics pedagogy with an exclusive focus on knowledge development also requires us to reconsider the behaviourist orientation embedded in conceptualizations of ethical practice.

A Behaviourist Orientation

In our undergraduate program, faculty meet to discuss students in need of learning contracts to transition from one clinical course to the next. One aspect of reporting on students consists of an effort to assess their capacities for learning and enacting safe, competent, and ethical care. While the criteria for safe and competent practice appear unambiguous, the question of judging students' ethical comportment reveals to me (Helen) several problematic assumptions. First, descriptions of "weak" students in terms of ethical comportment focus on aligning moral development and comportment with rational processes of moral reasoning and/or questions of "enough" or "not enough" knowledge applied in practice. Faculty discussions focus on supporting students to become aware of how their own values, insights, and emotional responses are knowing places; that is, the existence of any value-free "right" action in a given moment of practice or case study can only be known by seeing its connection to personal knowledge and experience. The student's achievement of the clinical competencies and acquisition of ethical knowledge and decision-making skills is best served by helping him or her see these connections. Our educational objectives ought to be aligned with the inseparability between ethical knowing and being in pursuit of learning outcomes. Helping students see the connections among what they know and what they can learn from ethical theory underscores how ethical comportment is a living and dynamic process that is enacted within particular contexts of care.

Conventional pedagogy, the predominant pedagogy used in nursing education, emphasizes the efficient and effective provision of information on what it is learners need for practice (Ironside 2004). Considering the reflections above, it is worth considering how ethics education may be limited from a behaviourist orientation to learning. Ethics education ought to be action-oriented without being exclusively behaviourist. And, ethical theory can inform ethical comportment; there is a need to also adapt and evolve such roles for the relational and contextual complexities of practice. Caputo claims ". . . the singular situations of life fly too close to the ground to be detected by the radar of ethical theory" (Caputo 2000, 173).

Traditional institutional attachment to roles such as the educator role or the learner role is often framed in behaviourist terms. The traditional view of teacher-learner roles understands the moral development of the educator within the rationalist tradition where the focus is on what one should do, or the codes and principles one should follow, rather than how one might be in the educational space. In framing the teacher-learner relationship in behaviourist terms the important question of how nurse educators engage in educative moments is made less visible. How nurse educators live out their own moral commitments while also educating toward a particular end in view necessarily engages questions of being.

In each classroom interaction, it is tempting to be able to see what will unfold by asking: Who is this student? Who is this teacher? And, yet, engaging in the learning and practice of ethics relies equally on non-knowing and curiosity (Caputo 2000). In a condensed 22-month BSN (Bachelor of Science in Nursing) program, educators' efforts to know a nursing student and to establish a sense of their prior knowledge are traditional approaches to entering into the learning relationship. When the learner is someone of advanced standing (already possessing an undergraduate degree), it is critical to stay open to who the learner will become through socialization into nursing while also building upon previous experiences of engaging in moral deliberation. The notion of individual trajectories of moral development are relevant to nursing, however, we suggest that the very experiences of teaching and learning about ethics are the site where learners see their personal involvement in developing the skills of responsiveness, curiosity, moral imagination, and enlisting emotive experience. Considering this intent, it is worth examining how we teach ethical practice as being prepared for, as Derrida states, the unknown in relation to the "coming of the other." This implies that it is problematic to cast our gaze toward teachers or students as individual beings requiring moral development without accounting for the insight that all knowing-being is relational; that is, without simultaneously considering learners and the construction of teaching/learning moments. It is "the lived space between teacher and learner, nurse and patient, where new knowledge is constructed. Such knowledge 'resounds bodily' and is always under construction" (Bergum 2003, 121).

We now turn toward another feature of ethics pedagogy in nursing that may warrant closer scrutiny as we describe possibilities for evolving educative space for nursing ethics education; that is, the necessity and complexity of teaching toward nursing values and ethical obligations.

Teaching Toward Nursing Values and Ethical Obligations

A student nurse reflected after a home visit to a pregnant woman who arrived in Canada with refugee status one year ago. Her client's partner was present in the home but the learner was uncertain as to how he was doing or the level of support he was able to offer. There was no other family in Canada. The community health nurse (CHN) preceptor explained to the student prior to the home visit that women are screened for depression during the antenatal period using a standardized scale. The screening allows CHNs to identify women at risk for postnatal depression so that resources and support can be arranged. An interpreter accompanied the CHN and student on the visit since the screening tool was only available in English and the woman spoke and understood limited English. As the screening progressed, the student described becoming uncomfortable. She understood the degree of poverty the woman was experiencing by noticing her living circumstances and when recalling the social assessment on the chart. When she returned to class the following week, the student expressed feeling as though her home visit and follow-up care for the pregnant client did little to meet this client's needs. She recounted that although an interpreter was present, it was evident that several forces beyond the student's control complicated any conclusion about risk for postnatal depression and her efforts to provide ethical care. I (Gayle) find it challenging to educate nurses to work toward the ethical values of the profession knowing how nurses' agency and moral actions can work against particular ideologies. In this case, the assessment focus and risk analysis did little to reveal how poverty was undermining the woman's mental and physical health in the antenatal period. As a consequence, the student felt she did very little to achieve the goal of effective, respectful, and responsive care. In this example, it is one thing to teach toward the values of justice and equity, however, it is quite different to facilitate students' learning about ethical practice within the structural contexts where such values are challenging to uphold.

The question of purpose—what are we teaching toward in nursing ethics education—has generated important and lively dialogue within curricular discussions. Sellman (2009) claims, "The teaching of ethics to nurses is generally assumed to be a professional requirement although the purpose of this activity remains both poorly articulated and fraught with conceptual and logical difficulties" (90). In addition, the question of how to teach nursing ethics accompanies such deliberations, for example, the advantages and disadvantages of discrete ethics courses or ethics threaded throughout the curriculum. Our educative strategies may benefit from bringing some clarity to the challenges of teaching toward particular ends in view of ethical practice. We propose that scrutinizing our educative practices in light of our intentions and our "ends in view" may indicate possibilities for learning ethical practice shaped by current health care contexts.

In the above example, the educator's response to the student's distress about feeling unable to uphold ethical values requires educative practices that can hold values and context in each pedagogical moment. Teaching toward ethical values requires that our pedagogical practice evolve in order to help learners navigate the tensions inherent in grasping both normative values and particularities of contexts all at once. Hartrick Doane and Varcoe (2007) claim that

". . . as social inequities deepen and neoliberal ideologies hold individuals responsible for their own health and well-being regardless of how poverty, disability, remote geographical locations, or other inequities determine health; notions of obligation, responsibility, accountability and efficiency are vital to nursing relationships as are notions of compassion, responsiveness, trust, and respect." (194)

We propose that an inherent difficulty exists in teaching toward nursing values and ethical obligations within the complexities of practice and the diversities of peoples' lives (nurses and clients). This difficulty is not to be ignored but ought to be taken up in teaching/learning moments and relationships. Standing amidst difficulties associated with knowing how to enact ethical values and obligations whilst attending to the complexities of context and constraints pressing upon nurses' ethical practice has the potential to enhance and evolve the instructiveness of ethical values and nursing obligations. In this way, it may become possible to evolve understandings of nursing obligations as externally derived and sanctioned entities. To evolve more complex understandings of nurses' ethical practice and to infuse nursing ethics pedagogy with ideas and strategies that expand simplistic notions of "right" responses requires the intentions of educators to focus on the ethical being and knowing required to enact nursing values and ethical obligations in everyday practice (Hartrick Doane and Varcoe 2007; Patterson 2001; MacDonald 2007). The difficulty inherent in teaching toward nursing values and ethical obligations is manifested when learners' personal and professional values are conflicted or they face conflicting obligations. In fact, Patterson (2001) suggests that the very adherence to obligations may thwart nurses' capacities, and those who are teaching and learning nursing need to develop "active independent critical judgment and discernment" (8). When learning ethical practice, we might consider how to create educative spaces that open up questions, possibilities, and scrutiny of the consequences of action rather than prescribing specific values and obligations.

PRINCIPLES AND PRACTICES: CREATING EDUCATIVE SPACES FOR NURSING ETHICS PEDAGOGY

Releasing Epistemologies' Grasp

In order to understand and honour the complexity of nursing practice "we must be aware of who and what we bring to the here and now of any nursing moment . . . being aware of and reflexively scrutinizing our emotional and embodied knowing in our everyday nursing work" (Hartrick Doane and Varcoe 2005, 155). The embodiment of ethical action requires attention at the level of being, at the level of ontology: Who am I? How am I compelled to act? How are the complexities of practice shaping my capacity to be ethical? How are the forces acting upon me shaping my capacity for moral agency? Oriented to the ontological, we move toward the rightful place of knowing in our teaching and learning of ethical practices in nursing.

As nurse educators it is our moral responsibility to explore and reflect on the relationship between who we are and our beliefs and assumptions in teaching and learning. Ontology shapes educator knowledge of learning and learners, and it shapes how educators and learners come to understand who they are as knowers. Our knowledge is never separate from who we are (Hartrick Doane and Varcoe 2008). The importance of attending to ontological experience is integral to a relational view of the educative space. It is who the educator is that "opens the possibility of relation between teacher and student where teaching is understood as a watchfulness, trust of the student, letting the student learn, with the goal of opening the space for the student to 'come into one's own'" (Bergum 2003, 121).

Educators may find themselves turning away from rather than toward the vulnerability inherent within being cast as knowledge "expert." If ethical knowledge is considered to be the property of the teacher, then there is little space for learning about how ethical practice is contextual and personal. Teaching ethics is the priority over teaching *for* ethical practice. Seeing knowledge and experience as separate entities implies that knowing is somehow distinct from being. Yet, the complexities of nursing practice require nurses to enlist experience as they theorize ethical practice (Rodney, Brown, and Liaschenko 2004).

Nurse educators teaching for ethical practice can consider where they position themselves philosophically and pedagogically and assess the effects of these values on their relationships with students (Ewashen and Lane 2007). In moving away from our positions as knowledge experts we have the opportunity to enter into an educative space where learning and engagement is a shared experience. Here educators may join learners by inviting thinking and questioning (Diekelmann and Smythe 2004). For example, educators are often involved in teaching new protocols. Checklists of what nurses know or do not know about the protocol accompanies the protocol. As educators, we are focused on getting them up and running as soon as possible, leaving little time to fully explore the ethical challenges associated with protocol implementation and the deliberations and nuances that accompany effective protocol implementation. In some public health situations, the protocol takes precedence over the focus on relationship building that ensures protocol adherence. In nursing education we have the ethical obligation to engage learners in critical exploration of how practice-based tools influence the ways nurses engage with patients and clients to promote health, however, we also are obligated to responsive and individualized care—two elements that can be compromised by protocol-driven care.

Teaching for Ethical Being

What is essential in any discussion of knowledge is the educator's moral responsibility to reflect on what is knowledge and how new knowledge is created. Nursing educators recognize that knowledge is not fixed or certain, and that "truth" may never actually be determined (Polifroni and Welch 1999). In moving away from privileging a rationalist view of knowledge, we invite students into learning ethical practice through the view that multiple realities exist and that knowledge is co-created and contextually shaped (Hartrick et al. 2004).

Learning nursing ought to involve seeing how each moment of being is inseparable from knowledge development. This engagement with knowledge is created through a relationship to knowledge (Brown and Doane 2007). Knowing for each individual nurse is unique as it is the result of knowledge gained through personal and professional nursing experience. In considering the intricate relationship between knowledge and knower, educators have an ethical responsibility to enact pedagogies where learners are invited to enter into a relationship with the educator and the living process of knowledge creation.

> Emerging pedagogies such as narrative pedagogy . . . reflect the primacy of a pedagogic relationship premised on shared lived experience, experiential and personal knowing, transformative interpersonal and caring connection inclusive of critical consciousness-raising, co-learning with active teacher–student participation, and the engendering of community honoring the humanist values of equality, justice and freedom. (Ewashen and Lane 2007, 258)

We believe that it is an educator's moral responsibility to consider how both episte-mology and ontology shape nursing knowledge and ethical nursing action. What may be "interpreted as inadequate knowledge or inadequate application of knowledge may from an ontological view be more related to how, as situated beings, we have come to be" (Hartrick Doane and Varcoe 2008, 288). When I am asked to consult with a nurse seen to have a "problem with knowledge" an ethical response would be to be present, caring, and curious about her situatedness and how she has made meaning of her learning experiences. "Ontology and ontological motivation are central to how we live/translate/enact knowledge in complex moments of practice" (Hartrick Doane and Varcoe 2008, 284).

As a nurse educator, my (Gayle) goal is to move away from a focus on acontextual knowledge and behavioural approaches to supporting learner-centered approaches where nurses have opportunities to expand their capacity for learning in relationship with oth-ers. It is in this process of guided reflection and meaning-making that new knowledge is created. It is in this process that nurses have the opportunity to see themselves in new ways. In supporting learners deemed to lack knowledge our ethical response to the learner–educator relationship becomes one of empowerment and of supporting learners in their own learning. When a nurse is advised she lacks knowledge in practice she may be vulnerable and defensive, sensitized to the gaze of authority. Mutual respect, trust, and fidelity are foundational ethical dimensions of relationships between nurse educators and learners and learning organizations (Brown et al. 2004).

Learning How to Learn

I (Gayle) recently supported a nurse new to a unit. She was identified as having diffi-culty with family assessment; that is, lacking knowledge of how to conduct a family assessment. My first priority was to build a trusting relationship with the learner. It was through this trusting relationship that I was able to invite the nurse to reflect on her prac-tice. As reflection on practice was a new concept to her, there was a tentative space between us where this suggestion could have become simply another expectation rather than something that had meaning for her. After several reflective conversations this nurse shared with me that she felt as though she was "learning how to learn." Learning to become a reflective practitioner is foundational for ethical nursing practice—therein lay the opportunity to blend conventional approaches to learning and those derived from strategies that engaged her in the active process and personal experience of knowledge development.

When nurses experience caring collaborative partnerships with educators they have the potential to carry this with them into practice. The significance of ethical decision-making with respect to epistemology, ontology and pedagogy is in promoting the development of ethical and responsive practitioners. By recognizing the place of ontology in knowledge development, nurse educators are better able to promote relevant ethical knowledge development within complex moments of nursing practice. The spaces where student can both be and become ethical practitioners expand beyond learning situations to situations in nursing practice.

Teaching Toward Values and Obligations in Relational Moments

Teaching toward nursing values and ethical obligations may be achieved by explicitly exploring and accounting for the way those relational moments of nursing practice shape possibilities to uphold such values and obligations. Educative spaces where teachers and learners can expand possibilities for knowing require that opportunities where the complexity of enacting values and obligations is considered. Engaging with learners in the difficulty of knowing and not knowing how to "be" and "do" may provide learners with the skills of attunement, intentionality, and reflexivity so that they can consider multiple courses of action across diverse circumstances. Thus, the skills together can enhance the self-authorship critical for ethical being and knowing to enact values and obligations in relational moments.

Using social justice as an example, we suggest that understanding the meaning of socially just care cannot be taught solely from its place in a nursing code of ethics, as it prescribes the ethical endeavours of ethical nursing practice (Canadian Nurses Association 2008). Social justice is embedded in many facets of health care (values of equity, fairness, and justice pervade public health, health policy, and issues related to access to care), yet there are varying interpretations, in both theory and practice, of what social justice entails (Reimer Kirkham and Browne 2006; see also Chapter 21). Therefore, we propose carefully considering how teaching toward social justice can evolve in nursing ethics pedagogy. By using social justice as an illustration, we suggest that particular values, obligations, and goals can be taught and learned in ways that help students analyze and attend to the ways that justice and injustices are sustained through social institutions and social relationships. By reflecting on personal experiences students can better appreciate that the meaning of socially just care is only partially known beyond specific situations. Students can be guided to be both knowers and non-knowers in each moment of ethical practice. Being amidst knowing and not knowing provides the impetus for the development of consciousness fundamental to social justice and ethical action.

Teaching Toward Social Justice

Teaching toward social justice, educators can consider creating the space for students to experience the importance of several critical lenses, one of which is a critical cultural lens. Despite an expanding critical scholarship in nursing, cultural perspectives continue to be applied in ways that diminish the significance of multiple ways of knowing and power relations and structural constraints on health and health care (Browne and Varcoe 2006; Duffy 2001). We must be critically aware of how we teach nurses about culture, so that our teaching does not contribute to racialization (Varcoe and McCormick 2007). A social justice theoretical perspective in nursing education requires us to move beyond the traditional view of cultural education to the creation of spaces for reflection on the power relations in caring for others. Risk taking and critical self-reflection are central in transformative educational approaches (Duffy 2001). Social justice in nursing education requires the conscious awareness of the nurse educator in engaging learners in critical reflection of moral questions within the larger societal context. Issues of social justice cut across different contexts of practice. It is through critical reflection that nurses at all levels of practice may begin to notice and understand the presence of an essentializing and racializing gaze in practice, and to find the moral courage to disrupt this (Anderson et al. 2009).

Teaching toward nursing values and ethical obligation within relational moments requires the practice of inquiry. When entering into nursing practice as an inquirer, bringing ethical knowledge to practice can be viewed as "a process of reshaping our ways of being, knowing, relating and acting" (Hartrick Doane and Varcoe 2008, 292). Such ways of being, knowing, and acting within relational moments is also shaped by the discursive contexts within which education and practice take place. We cannot fully understand the nature of educator–learner relationships ". . . without also accounting for the often taken for granted discourses and ideologies in the larger sociopolitical contexts" (Brown et al. 2004, 133). Thus, educative spaces ought to also be created in ways that facilitate dialogue and questioning to support learners to voice opinions that may have been silenced with a more traditional classroom approach (Arhin and Cormier 2005). "Like scientific inquiry, inquiry-based practice involves picking out clues that seem relevant to the present moment, examining what it is they appear to indicate while simultaneously responding with possibilities for action" (Hartrick Doane and Varcoe 2008, 291). Teaching toward enacting values and obligations within relational moments can optimize learners' capacities to be ethically responsive to families.

Summary

In this chapter we have offered ideas for how to create educative spaces that facilitate nursing ethics education. We have drawn on the voices of nursing scholars who call for expanded pedagogies to explore the complexity of ethical practice, to appreciate the significance of teaching/learning relationships, and to describe ways that educators can engage learners in educative spaces. We invite you to see educative spaces—classrooms, clinical practice courses, or educational development opportunities—as always in the making, where fixed practices can be questioned, and new possibilities imagined.

For Reflection

1. How is teaching *for* ethical practice different than ethics education in nursing?
2. Reflect on the relationship between epistemology and ontology in ethics education. What stands out for you in your teaching practice?
3. What is it like for you to reconsider your teaching practice and related assumptions?

4. How would you as a nurse educator support a learner who encountered marginalizing or dismissive care? What kind of educative space would you create to invite the learner?

References

Anderson, J., Rodney, P., Reimer-Kirkham, S., Browne, A., Khan, K., and Lynam, M. 2009. Inequities in health and healthcare viewed through the ethical lens of critical social justice: Contextual knowledge for the global priorities ahead. [Electronic version] *Advances in Nursing Science, 32* (4), 282–294.

Arhin, A.O. and Cormier, E. 2005. Using deconstruction to educate Generation Y nursing students. [Electronic version] *Journal of Nursing Education, 46*, 562–567.

Bergum, V. 2003. Relational pedagogy, embodiment, improvisation, and interdependence. [Electronic version] *Nursing Philosophy, 4*, 121–128.

Browne, A.J. and Varcoe, C. 2006. Critical cultural perspectives and health involving Aboriginal peoples. [Electronic version] *Contemporary Nurse, 22*, 155–167.

Brown, H. and Doane, G. 2007. From filling a bucket to lighting a fire: Aligning nursing education and nursing practice. In L. Young and B. Patterson (Eds.), *Teaching nursing: Developing a student-centered learning environment* (pp. 97–118). Philadelphia: Lippincott, Williams and Wilkins.

Brown, H. and Rodney, P. 2007. Beyond case studies in practice education. Creating capacities for ethical knowledge through story and narrative. In L. Young and B. Patterson (Eds.), *Teaching nursing: Developing a student-centered learning environment* (pp. 141–163). Philadelphia: Lippincott, Williams and Wilkins.

Brown, H., Rodney, P., Pauly, B., Varcoe, C., and Smye, V. 2004. Working within the landscape: Nursing ethics. In J. Storch, P. Rodney and R. Starzomski (Eds.), *Toward a moral horizon: Nursing ethics for leadership and practice* (pp. 126–153). Toronto: Pearson Education Canada Ltd.

Caputo, J. 2000. *More radical hermeneutics.* Bloomington, IN: Indiana University Press.

Canadian Nurses Association. 2008. *The code of ethics for registered nurses.* Ottawa, ON: Author.

Diekelmann, N. 2002. "Too much content . . .": Epistemologies' grasp and nursing education. *Journal of Nursing Education, 41* (11), 469–470.

Diekelmann N. 2005. Keeping current: On persistently questioning our teaching practice. *Journal of Nursing Education, 40*, 485–488.

Diekelmann, N. and Smythe, E. 2004. Covering content and the additive curriculum: How can I use my time with students to best help them learn what they need to know? [Electronic version] *Journal of Nursing Education, 43*, 341–344.

Doane, G. 2004. Being an ethical practitioner: The embodiment of mind, emotion and action. In J. Storch, P. Rodney, and R. Starzomski (Eds.), *Toward a moral horizon: Nursing ethics for leadership and practice* (pp. 433–446). Toronto: Pearson Education Canada Ltd.

Duffy, M. 2001. A critique of cultural education in nursing. [Electronic version] *Journal of Advanced Nursing, 36* (4), 487–495.

Ewashen, C. and Lane, A. 2007. Pedagogy, power and practice ethics: Clinical teaching in psychiatric/mental health settings. [Electronic version] *Nursing Inquiry, 4* (3), p. 255–262.

Hartrick Doane, G. and Brown, H. 2011. Recontextualizing learning in nursing education: Toward an ontological turn. *Journal of Nursing Education, (50)* 1, 21–26.

Hartrick Doane, G. and Varcoe, C. 2005. *Family nursing as relational inquiry. Developing health promoting practice*. Philadelphia: Lippincott, Williams and Wilkins.

Hartrick Doane, G. and Varcoe, C. 2007. Relational practice and nursing obligations. [Electronic version] *Advances in Nursing Science, 30*, 192–205.

Hartrick Doane, G. and Varcoe, C. 2008. Knowledge translation in everyday nursing, from evidence-based to inquiry based practice. [Electronic version] *Advances in Nursing Science, 31*, 283–295.

Hartrick G., Pauly, B., Brown, H., McPherson, G. 2004. Exploring the heart of ethical nursing practice: Implications for ethics education. [Electronic version] *Nursing Ethics, 11*, 240–253.

Heidegger, M. 1962. *Being and time*. Oxford: Blackwell.

Ironside, P. 2001. Creating a research base for nursing education: An interpretive review of conventional, critical, feminist, postmodern, and phenomenologic pedagogies. [Electronic version]. *Advances in Nursing Science, 23*, 72–87.

Ironside, P.M. 2004. "Covering content" and teaching thinking: Deconstructing the additive curriculum. [Electronic version] *Journal of Nursing Education, 41*, 5–12.

MacDonald, H. 2007. Relational ethics and advocacy in nursing: Literature review. *Journal of Advanced Nursing, 57* (2), 119–126.

Patterson, S. 2001. Are nursing codes of practice ethical? [Electronic version] *Nursing Ethics, 8* (1), 4–18.

Polifroni, E.C. and Welch, M. (Eds.). 1999. *Perspectives on philosophy of science in nursing, a historical and contemporary anthology*. Philadelphia: Lippincott, Williams and Wilkins.

Reimer Kirkham, S.R. and Browne, A.J. 2006. Toward a critical theoretical interpretation of social justice discourses in nursing. *Advances in Nursing Science, 29* (4), 324–339.

Rodney, P., Brown, H., and Liaschenko, J. 2004. Moral agency: Relational connections and trust. In J. Storch, P. Rodney, and R. Starzomski (Eds.), *Toward a moral horizon: Nursing ethics for leadership and practice* (pp. 154–157). Toronto: Pearson Education Canada Ltd.

Sellman, D. 2009. Practical wisdom in health and social care: Teaching for professional phronesis. *Learning in Health and Social Care, 8* (2), 84–91.

Varcoe, C., Doane, G., Pauly, B., Rodney, P., Storch, J.L., Mahoney, K., McPherson, G., Brown, H., and Starzomski, R. 2004. Ethical practice in nursing: Working the in-betweens. *Journal of Advanced Nursing, 45*, 316–325.

Varcoe, C. and McCormick, J. 2007. Racing around the classroom margins: Race, racism and teaching nursing. In L.E. Young and B. Patterson (Eds.), *Teaching nursing: Developing a student-centred learning environment* (pp. 437–466). Philadelphia: Lippincott, Williams and Wilkins.

CHAPTER 16

Listening Authentically to Youthful Voices: A Conception of the Moral Agency of Children

Franco A. Carnevale

. . . [W]e ought to listen to the moral voices of children in a deeply engaged manner, and not trivialize them.

In this chapter, I examine one of the most vexing issues in pediatrics: What significance should be accorded to the voice of children in decisions about their medical care? My aim is to (1) highlight the limitations of the prevalent adult-centred modes of construing the experiences of children, (2) outline a child-centred conception of moral agency, and (3) briefly discuss some of the corresponding implications for the clinical care of children.

The six Ethics in Practice cases I present below, drawn from my clinical experience, help me focus the discussion throughout the remainder of the chapter. They allow me to demonstrate a range of encounters lived by children that are commonly under-recognized as *moral* experiences.[1] Such stories are frequently interpreted within adult-centred psychological frameworks that minimize the moral experiences of children as expressions of immaturity.

NARRATIVES OF MORAL EXPERIENCE

ETHICS IN PRACTICE 16-1

Coercive Moral Language

William is a five-and-a-half-year-old boy who has come in for day treatment requiring the administration of an intravenous antibiotic. His parents have indicated that he has been seriously dreading coming to the hospital to have this needle put into him. He has shed a lot of tears in the couple of days leading up to this treatment. As the nurse very gently approaches him to start the intravenous, he becomes very pale and silent. He readily co-operates with every instruction that the nurse gives him, holding out his arm, making a fist, and taking a deep breath as the needle goes in. Every step of the way, each time little William co-operates with an instruction, the nurse very warmly tells him, "Good boy, William—you're such a good boy—what a big boy you are."

ETHICS IN PRACTICE 16-2

Unspoken Diagnosis

Benjamin is a twelve-and-a-half-year-old boy with a metastasized inoperable abdominal tumour. His parents have been asking for help because he has been frequently crying at home—seeming to be discouraged about all the time he has to spend at the hospital, while missing his friends so much.

His parents have also indicated that they do not want Benjamin to know his diagnosis because that would discourage him too much. They have been telling him that the intravenous chemotherapy he was receiving was actually antibiotics to help fight an infection.

ETHICS IN PRACTICE 16-3

Anticipating Suffering

Gloria is a six-year-old girl with a degenerative neuromuscular disorder. She has been admitted to hospital with respiratory failure that has been judged to be an end-stage manifestation of her neuromuscular disorder. She will require long-term mechanical ventilation. Her parents, who have always been by Gloria's side providing her exceptional care and love, are devastated by the fact that she will never be able to breathe on her own

again. They have decided that they would like to have her life-support terminated in order to let Gloria die and prevent the long life of suffering that they foresee for her. Meanwhile, when most of the health care professionals (HCP) look at Gloria, they see a playful girl who loves loud music and celebrities and frequently laughs out loud as she watches videos with her parents or her favourite nurses. She seems to enjoy life.

ETHICS IN PRACTICE 16-4

Protective Secrets

Nine-year-old Marianne has been in the intensive care unit for two days for the care of severe injuries following a major car accident that took her father's life. Following two days of unconsciousness, she is awakening rapidly despite her ongoing need for support of numerous vital functions (such as mechanical ventilation). She is clearly very

agitated and is mouthing many questions about the accident and asking for her father. Her mother and the clinicians caring for her are torn over whether it is better to immediately tell her the truth about her father's death or invent a less painful account to tell her for now, and wait to tell her the truth at a later time.

ETHICS IN PRACTICE 16-5

Hurt in the Crossfire

David is an eight-year-old boy who frequently comes to hospital for the management of recurrent back pain. Over the past year, he has increasingly become more involved in identifying ways to manage his pain. Despite this, the frequency and intensity of his pain has increased significantly in recent months. One day he discloses that he is very upset inside over how much his divorced mom and dad fight over him. He believes that "they're so busy fighting all the time that they don't think that maybe it hurts me so much to see my mom and dad fighting about me. Sometimes I wish I wasn't there so they wouldn't have to fight so much. What good am I? I wish that some days they would just play with me or just think about *me*."

ETHICS IN PRACTICE 16-6

Struggling to Escape

Robbie is a fourteen-year-old boy who has recently survived a four-week stay in an intensive care unit for the care of severe burns that he sustained through a supposed accident while manipulating a heating stove. He has just been weaned off the ventilator and had his endotracheal tube removed so that he can once again use his voice. During a particularly intense conversation, talking about the painful ordeal he has just been through, he says that the incident that caused his burns was not an accident. He tried to kill himself. He wanted to die because he could no longer bear to see his father physically beat his mother every evening after he got drunk.

EXAMINING THE CONVENTIONAL FRAMEWORK

The clinical care of children entails a number of complex ethical issues as illustrated in the opening narratives (Ross 1998).[2] One of the most challenging and least resolved issues is the extent and type of involvement that children should have in decisions relating to their care. As with adults, informed consent is required for the medical treatment of children. If a patient has the required mental capacity to do so, consent must be provided by the patient based on the provision of all relevant information and be free of any undue influence or coercion.

Some Canadian provinces have legislated a specific age of consent for medical treatment, below which a minor cannot autonomously provide legally valid consent. For example, in Quebec, minors have the right to provide consent for treatment required by their state of health—with some limitations—starting at the age of 14 years. In many other jurisdictions throughout North America, no specific age threshold is legislated. The child's capacity should be assessed on a case-by-case basis, although it is largely agreed in practice that this capacity should be recognized at about 14 years in general, allowing for younger children on the basis of their demonstrated capacities.

The Canadian Pediatric Society (CPS) has published an important statement regarding medical treatment decisions involving children (CPS 2004). This reflects the legal and ethical norms that are widely agreed upon throughout North America (AAP 1994; 1995).

The CPS states that "Capacity is not age- or disease-related, nor does it depend on the decision itself, but is a cognitive and emotional process of decision making relative to the medical decision . . . Children who have partial skills to make decisions should be recognized as having some authority over their own health care . . . Children and adolescents should be appropriately involved in decisions affecting them. Once they have sufficient decision-making capacity, they should become the principal decision maker for themselves" (CPS 2004, 100–101).

The CPS highlights that some pre-adolescent children, particularly those with more experience with illness, may have greater capacities to make medical decisions than other children their age, as demonstrated by eight-year-old David's pain management in Ethics in Practice 16-5. Alderson and associates (2006) demonstrated that children with juvenile (Type 1) diabetes, who had medical decision-making experience, were subsequently more capable of making decisions regarding their own care. Age was not found to be a distinguishing factor in the determination of capacity. McPherson's (2007) examination of children's participation in chronic illness decision making challenged the prevalent view of decision making as a discrete, autonomous, decontextualized process. This researcher uncovered the contextual basis of children's participation: relational processes indistinguishable from everyday decisions, embedded in children's relationships with parents, teachers, friends, and health care providers (HCP). Children's participation involved two domains: (1) resonance of children's voices (i.e., opportunities and abilities to formulate and express their views) and (2) relevance of children's voices (i.e., the standing children achieved within decisional processes).

In short, children's decisional capacities vary widely. Prior decision-making experience can significantly enhance a child's capacities. Thus, individualized assessment of a child's participation in decision making is important both in terms of properly recognizing the child's current capacity as well as promoting the child's ongoing capacity development.

Although there is some recognition of minors' capacity to consent, the prevalent bioethical and legal framework for medical treatment decisions involving children is centred on the best-interests standard (American Academy of Pediatrics 1994; 1995; CPS 2004). This requires a weighing of the burdens and benefits associated with each treatment option—this weighing is performed by legally authorized surrogate decision makers. However, many cases present a complex scenario whereby the benefits and burdens are difficult to judge because they relate to goods that cannot be ranked according to any universally agreed upon criteria. For example, in Ethics in Practice 16-3, the various adults in Gloria's life cannot agree on whether the burdens in her life render it unworthy of ongoing support. Furthermore, how can the significance of quality of life be ranked in relation to the sanctity of life as a good in itself? Some members of diverse cultural communities argue that the preservation of life is mandatory regardless of the quality of that life, whereas others argue that life is only valuable in terms of the quality of life that can be achieved (Carnevale 2005a).

In light of the difficulties inherent in reconciling such dilemmas, the most widely accepted view is to recognize parents as the surrogate decision makers for minors (American Academy of Pediatrics 1994; 1995; CPS 2004). This can be traced to the modern Western value assigned to the autonomy of families. It is largely held that families should be enabled to establish their own respective moral norms because such judgments should be based on the loving intimacy that is commonly inherent in familial relationships (Nelson and Nelson 1995).[3]

It is also recognized that the cultural and religious freedom of families should be respected (Canadian Charter of Rights and Freedoms 1982). Here too, the state imposes some limitations in situations where such freedoms conflict with some more fundamental rights. For example, in cases where a minor has a life-threatening medical condition that can be effectively corrected with a blood transfusion, the courts have commonly overruled the objection to such transfusions by Jehovah's Witnesses families, declaring that the child's right to have his or her life preserved overrides the family's religious freedom.[4]

FROM MORAL SUBJECT TO MORAL OBJECT

Throughout this chapter, I argue that children should be regarded as moral subjects—agents who are highly capable of moral awareness. However, a significant body of literature has demonstrated that children are frequently exploited as moral objects; that is, they are regarded as means to the moral pursuits of the more powerful adults in their lives.

The moral worthiness of the lives of individual children has not consistently held a universal value. Wright's (1988) historical analysis of the medicalization of infant mortality in turn-of-the-century England (from nineteenth to twentieth century) highlights that the turn to medicine to combat the high prevalence of infant deaths corresponded with a period of urbanization and diminution of family size, increasing each child's worth as a future source of labour and revenue.

The moral objectification of children is critically examined by Nancy Scheper-Hughes and Carolyn Sargent (1988) in *Small Wars: The Cultural Politics of Childhood*. Children are construed socially as both material possessions and as "selfish" burdens on their surrounding adults.

The moral objectification of children can also be traced within the contemporary North American clinical encounter. Parents commonly speak of the enormous burden they feel toward doing right by their children, ensuring that they get the kind of care they deserve (Carnevale 1998; 2002; Carnevale et al. 2006; 2007). Parents are often overwhelmed by their sense of duty toward being a good parent.[5] They also struggle with profound apprehensions about the possibility that their child may die. Although parents are commonly the most suitable advocates for a child's interests, the child's interests are intertwined with the parents' self-interests.

Further, conscientious HCP may be authentically concerned about a child-patient's interests. However, these interests are sometimes difficult to distinguish from the HCP's own interests in attending to the interests of other patients, having a reasonable quality of work-life while pursuing opportunities for clinical innovation that may be beneficial for the child but could also yield some professional recognition. Similarly, health care institutions (e.g., hospitals) may be interested in ensuring that patients get the care they require while balancing such care with their interests in containing costs or pursuing politically meaningful goals.

Thus, although an ill child may be surrounded by various adult moral agents claiming to advocate for the child's best interests, these adults are also pursuing their own interests. Given the significant power imbalance between these adult-centred agents and the largely silent, morally subordinated children, the latter run a significant risk of moral objectification.

WHAT ABOUT THE VOICE OF THE CHILD?

The "best-interests model" for examining ethical issues related to children casts the child in a highly passive role. The voice of the child is essentially muted. I attribute this problem to two phenomena: (1) underestimation of the "maturity" of children's moral reasoning, and (2) the "adult-centredness" of the best-interests model. I discuss these separately.

Recognizing the "Maturity" of Moral Reasoning in Children

Children (or legal minors) are more capable of engaging in what is regarded as mature adult moral reasoning than is typically recognized. In a 1990 brief submitted by the American Psychological Association (APA) in the *Hodgson v. Minnesota* case, the APA stated:

> [By] age 14 most adolescents have developed adult-like intellectual and social capacities including specific abilities outlined in the law as necessary for understanding treatment alternatives, considering risks and benefits, and legally competent consent. (Schneider, Bersoff, and Podolsky 1989, 8–20, cited in Melton 1999)

Christine Harrison and colleagues (1997) outlined three groups of children with respect to their decisional capacities: (1) preschool children who cannot provide their own consent because they have no significant decision-making capacity; (2) primary-school children who do not have full decision-making capacity, so parents should authorize or refuse treatments although the child's assent should be sought and sustained dissent should be taken seriously; and (3) adolescents who can have the decision-making capacity of an adult although this capacity will need to be assessed specifically for each child.[6] An inference that can be drawn from this work is that it is wrong to tell Benjamin, the adolescent boy in Ethics in Practice 16-2, that his chemotherapy is an antibiotic.

No universally accepted standard exists for determining when the child's voice is to be regarded as a sufficiently competent expression of an autonomous will. The child's voice matters, but when and how it matters is subject to a case-by-case interpretation of the child's "maturity." This may imply that six-year-old Gloria in Ethics in Practice 16-3 is too immature to meaningfully express preferences regarding life-support decisions. This view was extended to the withholding of a grave prognosis from Benjamin in Ethics in Practice 16-2, on the basis of his parents' belief that he would be unable to deal with such news.

Confronting the Adult-Centredness of the Best-Interests Model

The best-interests model is premised on an adult-centred conception of moral agency. This model corresponds with the doctrine of self-determination underlying ethical decision making in adults. This regards adults as self-determining agents capable of independently judging their respective moral interests. Furthermore, persons should not be impeded in their pursuit of these interests.[7]

This ideal of autonomy is further expressed through the leading psychological frameworks "explaining" moral development (Erikson 1950; Levinson 1978). These establish a moral norm for mature adults as highly rational and autonomous. Children are consequently regarded as less mature—or immature—and therefore as not worthy of a comparable recognition as moral agents.[8] Consequently, these immature agents, construed as incapable of rationally discerning their own moral interests, are classed as moral minors who are dependent upon adult custodians for the care of their interests. However, the cases of David and Robbie in Ethics in Practice 16-5 and 16-6, wherein both boys conceal their diminished sense of self-worth, demonstrate how adult custodians can be highly mistaken in their understanding of their children's moral lives.

Jean Piaget, a pioneer in the formulation of such psychological frameworks, characterized moral development in terms of three stages (1932/1965); constraint, co-operation, and generosity. Lawrence Kohlberg (1981) drew on this Piagetian model to develop his own three-level framework for moral judgment in adolescents and adults; preconventional, conventional, and postconventional levels. The preconventional level is self-centred; the individual formulates moral norms in terms of his or her own needs and is essentially incapable of construing socially shared views. Conventional morality (associated with the preadolescence-adolescence juncture) relates the "good or right thing to do" with the surrounding social values and moral norms that serve to sustain relationships, communities, and societies. The postconventional level involves a reflective view that transcends the conventional, seeking to discover—through a process of personal enlightenment—a universal construal of morality.

Kohlberg's framework is differentiated along a six-stage (three-level) model of moral development. The child is characterized by Kohlberg as developing from an ego-centric and individualistic view of rightness based on avoidance of punishment and individual need (stages one and two), to an understanding based on "The Golden Rule" (putting oneself in the shoes of the other person) and shared conventions of societal agreement (stages three and four). Finally, the child develops a principled understanding of morality that upholds the basic rights and values of a society and a free-standing logic of universal principles that all humanity should follow (stages five and six) (Kohlberg 1981). For Kohlberg, the ultimate morally mature person is capable of engaging in rational reasoning (drawing on a highly deductive logic) to arrive at an ethically principled conception of justice.

The conceptual soundness of these leading theories of moral development is challenged by Carol Gilligan (1982) through her study of moral experience among girls and women. She argues that the Piaget and Kohlberg models are based on studies of boys and men and consequently give rise to a male-centred conception of moral development.[9] Whereas Piaget and Kohlberg argue that humans (i.e., men) strive to become *independent* moral agents, Gilligan reported that girls and women strive to be *interdependent*. Her research findings suggested that females speak of moral matters "in a different voice."

Gilligan's moral orientation toward care and responsibility distinguishes the moral agency of women from men; the latter are primarily concerned about justice and the preservation of the rights of individuals with an entitlement to freedom from interference in their pursuit of self-fulfillment. This feminist challenge to the conventional (male-centred) view of human morality suggests that women employ a different moral framework and raises the plausibility that additional distinctive moral frameworks can exist. In the next section, I argue that although children may not reason according to the prevailing adult, male-centred Kohlbergian morality nor the female-oriented framework of Gilligan, there exists a significant body of evidence indicating that children are capable of a rich degree of moral awareness. The moral viewpoints of children should not be judged in terms of how they might resemble or approximate adult moral reasoning, but instead warrant recognition on their own merits.

The Moral Awareness of Children

Numerous works have highlighted that children have a greater awareness of morally significant matters than is commonly granted. Psychiatrist Irwin Yalom (1980) has asserted that children's first awareness of death can emerge as early as three years of age. Anthropologist Myra Bluebond-Langner (1978) conducted a highly respected ethnographic study of three- to nine-year-old children's encounters with leukemia. She poignantly voiced the silent experiences of children's struggles with sickness and dying, demonstrating a depth and richness in the children's comprehension that far surpassed the understandings attributed to them by the adults in their lives. Particularly remarkable was how these children wilfully complied with social taboos and respected the silence that adults seemed to prefer in relation to the children's foreseen mortality. This finding corresponds with Benjamin's case in Ethics in Practice 16-2. This invites us to scrutinize children's silence, which may express their motivation to conform to socially desired behavioural norms for children, rather than demonstrate moral immaturity.

Psychologist Barbara Sourkes (1995) has reported (1) accounts of anticipatory grief among children facing their own deaths; (2) children's temporal understanding of death, with a comprehension of contributory causes and consequences; and (3) children's abilities to reflect on matters pertaining to a broad moral order. In the cases of Benjamin and Gloria (Ethics in Practice 16-2 and 16-3), both appear to have a highly limited awareness of their situation. This can be partially attributed to restrictions in the information that was available to them. In light of Bluebond-Langner's (1978) findings, they may have also realized that the adults in their lives prefer that they inhibit particular expressions of their moral experience.

Philosopher Thomas Attig (1996) has argued that children are able to anguish existentially, wondering about how they view their "finite existence, the nature and purpose of life, God, punishment, fate, what is fair, and the meanings of suffering and death" (21). David, in Ethics in Practice 16-5, described himself as a cause of his parents' fighting while also expressing moral outrage toward the unfairness of their spending insufficient "quality time" with him.

Psychiatrist Robert Coles (1986) examined the moral experiences of children in detail in his acclaimed text *The Moral Life of Children*. He relates accounts from poor families in the American South to convey that children do not simply express parental views, but are capable of formulating and asserting their own independent sense of how the world should be. He explains that the moral life of children can be character-ized as charitable but also "by extended stretches of moral stinginess, amoral self-absorption, even a persistent immorality that takes the form of spitefulness, rudeness, assaultiveness" (44).

In my own work with critically ill children and their siblings, I have witnessed rich expressions of children's moral lives (Carnevale 1997; 1998). Bereaved siblings, ranging from 5 to 19 years of age expressed feelings of guilt about the ways they may have acted toward their deceased sibling, demonstrating a capacity for moral contemplation. Many siblings commonly expressed outrage toward the attention accorded to their seriously ill or deceased sibling. Although their parents may regard such sentiments as amoral, they nonetheless express the child's sense of right and wrong. David, in Ethics in Practice 16-5, expressed outrage toward his father because he frequently did not follow through on his promises to make time for him: "He thinks only about himself. He's selfish! I feel like I'm useless to him—just a bother for him." David condemns what he perceives as morally wrong parenting.

Although the demeanour of children may sometimes fall short of what adults might consider virtuous, it nonetheless expresses a moral stance toward their world. Children are morally aware, sometimes with rich sophistication, at other times with a simplistic matter-of-factness. Although the moral values children subscribe to may sometimes cor-respond with those commonly held by adults, their moral awareness should not be judged according to such an adult-centred standard. Given their unique perspectives on the world, it is understandable that children will hold some distinctive moral outlooks. Rather than construing these as immature forms of what is to follow later in their devel-oping lives, based on adult-centred moral development models, the moral views of chil-dren merit recognition in their own right. The works outlined above help justify a call for the recognition of the moral voice of children—a further "different voice."[10]

WHAT ABOUT MORAL RESPONSIBILITY?

Some may argue that it is a mistake to speak of moral agency in children without a direct implication of moral responsibility. It can be argued that the moral agency of children should be construed narrowly because of the limited formal responsibility that can be assigned to their actions, given the limits of their understanding of the world that sur-rounds them. On the other hand, it could be argued that if we want to grant children a broad measure of moral agency in light of the depth of their moral awareness, then we ought to assign them a proportional degree of responsibility.

This relating of responsibility with moral agency can be traced to Aristotle's *Nichomachean Ethics* (350 BCE/1985).[11] Aristotle rooted moral responsibility in the voluntariness of human action. He further elaborated on two conditions that excuse the voluntariness of an act: ignorance or compulsion.[12] Perhaps some children's actions could be considered morally involuntary in light of their variable degrees of ignorance with regard to the morally significant particulars in their surrounding world and their compulsive urges to seek immediate gratification of emerging needs—which may both be manifested, for example, in an act of running across a highly dangerous street to chase after a ball.

Following Aristotle's framework, it can be argued that the degree of moral responsibility that ought to be assigned to children's actions should vary according to the genuine voluntariness of their actions. Although there may be grounds for limiting their responsibility for the consequences of their actions, this should not imply a diminution of their moral agency. Considering the depth of moral awareness of which children are capable, they can experience moral distress, guilt, remorse, indignation, and pride—a full range of conscientious sentiments. Therefore, they should be accorded significant recognition as moral agents. That is, children's voices should merit genuine attention—not curious "listening to" the perspective of an immature moral inferior. Children's voices should not be discounted by adults wanting to accomplish what they consider required, using coercion as they judge necessary (e.g., as with William in Ethics in Practice, 16-1).

AGENCY WITHIN A MORAL WORLD

I have argued throughout this analysis for a maximization of our attentiveness to the moral voices of children. I should add that attending to the moral lives of children consists of more than solely recognizing their individual moral experiences. In light of their relative position of disempowerment, consideration should also be given to the fragility of their "moral worlds." Given their limited capacities to shape their own particular worlds, children rely on the significant adults in their lives (who model enactments of "right and wrong" ethical comportment) to help build and sustain their world's *moral order*. Moral order refers here to the ways right/wrong, good/bad, and just/unjust are defined by the child's social and cultural context (Carnevale 2005a; Carnevale and Rafman 1998).

Children also form their own moral outlooks, in the manner outlined in this chapter. They forge modes of coexistence, continually negotiating co-operation with their significant adults. Co-operation enables children to develop their particular moral character that they can express and cultivate within their adult-powered moral order. Some traumatic experiences for children may rupture their moral order resulting in extreme moral distress (Carnevale 1997; 1998; Carnevale and Rafman 1998). To understand moral order, consider Robbie, in Ethics in Practice 16-6; life seemed meaningless in light of his repeated experiences of witnessing his mother's beatings by his father. His distress can be traced to the disruption in his moral order. He experienced profound discontinuities in the everyday web of relationships that constituted his social world and moral order. Such profound experiences as his can disrupt children's socially mediated moral order: their ability to rely on significant adults as (1) sources of comfort and security who can protect them from the multitude of threats perceived within the everyday lives of children, as well as (2) important sources of moral inspiration and support for the constitution and maintenance of the children's own moral systems. Significant disruptions in children's moral orders can give rise to profound distress. In turn, preservation or restoration of such moral orders can serve as vital sources of comfort.

Therefore, attending meaningfully to the moral lives of children ought to consist of not only authentic listening but also devoting genuine consideration toward securing children's moral order—their moral world. Within the clinical context, this implies the enactment of strategies that optimize the stable maintenance of relationships that are morally significant for the afflicted children.

Toward a Broad Conception of Assent

The position I argue for in this chapter raises questions about how we ought to genuinely attend to the moral voices of children, while recognizing the limits to the degree of responsibility that can be assigned to their actions.

The genuine attention I am implying here resembles the "authentic listening" advocated by Carl Rogers (1951) in his client-centred therapy framework, where the clinician seeks a profoundly empathic attunement to the experiential perspective of the patient.[13] This can be managed by interpreting the current standard of child *assent* more broadly. Obtaining assent implies seeking the child's willingness to accept the proposed care based on his or her developmentally adapted understanding of the condition, proposed tests, and treatments. The American Academy of Pediatrics (AAP) recommends that for children who cannot give consent themselves, parents should be responsible for giving permission for treatment while giving great weight to the clearly expressed views of the child. Situations involving older children and adolescents should also include the assent of the child, to the greatest extent possible (AAP 1995).

The foregoing discussion of the moral awareness of children implies that this AAP recommendation ought to be applied with an *a priori* valuation of the richness of the moral lives of children. What children say should be regarded as morally meaningful, and the adults in their lives (e.g., parents and/or HCP) should genuinely seek to reconcile any matters that seem to be causing the child moral distress. This would involve attending meaningfully to their questions, objections, contestations, and possible protests.

Some clinical situations can involve a complexity of phenomena—clearly oriented toward the child's long-term good—that a child may not be able to grasp fully (e.g., emergency surgery for a four-year-old with appendicitis). Although the responsible adults in such a situation (typically the parents) might authorize surgery despite the child's objections, such an authorization should follow the adults' best efforts to foster the child's understanding and acceptance of such an intervention. In the end, if it is judged that some interventions may be warranted despite the child's objections, such a coercive overriding of the child's moral voice should still be regarded as a source of moral distress. Although such a situation may be considered excusable, it should still carry the moral significance of a harm—a consequence that should be prevented and ameliorated as much as possible.[14] This scenario can be distinguished from the approach used by Benjamin's parents in Ethics in Practice 16-2. Here, morally significant information that would help Benjamin to understand what is happening to his body and enable him to express his own preferences toward his care is withheld by his parents, requiring him to undergo chemotherapy without his consent or his assent. In light of the arguments I present in this chapter outlining (1) the depth of children's moral capacities and (2) the moral harms that can be attributed to a neglect of their moral agency, the withholding of morally significant information from Benjamin is difficult to justify.

Implications for Clinical Care

The narratives I presented at the beginning of this chapter highlight a diversity of moral dilemmas that can be experienced by children in clinical settings. The occurrence of such dilemmas suggests the potential for children's moral experience to be under-recognized by adults, including their families and HCP. Some implications for clinical care can be inferred from this analysis of moral agency.

First, this discussion calls for an authentic recognition of the moral voices of children. The views and sentiments of children have moral worth and ought to be treated as such. For example, there exists a significant body of evidence justifying the requirement of consent for treatment decisions from young adolescence onward (AAP 1995; CPS 2004; Harrison et al. 1997; Melton 1999; Schneider, Bersoff, and Podolsky 1989). Second, HCP should seek to maximally apply the standard of assent, with a genuine stance toward the (spoken and bodily) voices of children. HCP should regard children's views as worthy in their own right and not just as immature expressions requiring attention and pacification—the latter arising from an adult-centred conception of moral agency.

Toward the increased recognition of children's participation in treatment decisions, Kenny and associates (2008) have proposed a framework for the "respectful involvement of children in medical decision making." They argue for the "participative assessment" of (1) what the child wants to know, (2) what the child can understand, (3) the extent of the child's decision-making capacity, and (4) what the child needs to know to participate appropriately.

Finally, HCP should also attend to children's moral order, predominantly constituted and sustained by the web of significant relationships in their social world. This would require (1) identifying the persons who matter (morally) in each child-patient's life, (2) seeking to understand how these persons matter, and (3) striving to find ways to help preserve the continuity of such relationships within the context of clinical care. To illustrate, hospital policies should facilitate the presence of significant adults for children (Brinchmann, Forde, and Nortvedt 2002). In addition to serving the psychological needs of these adults, these policies can be fundamentally important toward minimizing the traumatization of children. So-called hospital "visiting policies" imply a subordination of the significance of families (Carnevale 1998; 2005b). When parents tend to their hospitalized children, they are "parenting" not "visiting." Characterizing significant family members as visitors serves to marginalize their importance, helping to justify limiting their presence through restrictive policies. Given children's complex interdependencies within their families and how children's well-being is interrelated with their families' well-being, clinical practices should commonly involve ongoing family assessment and the promotion of required family supports (Carnevale 1998; 2003). Moreover, HCP should seek to understand the cultural outlooks of children and families, which commonly underlie children's moral orders, and strive to adapt their practices accordingly (Carnevale 2005a).

Finally, the care of children requires many complex, overlapping areas of expertise. Their care is therefore optimized when diverse interdisciplinary teams can be adapted to each child's particular needs, drawing broadly on experts in nursing, medicine, social work, child psychology and psychiatry, child life, childhood education, pastoral care, and clinical ethics, among others, as well as subspecialists within these disciplines (Carnevale 2003; CPS 2004).

REVISITING THE ETHICS IN PRACTICE NARRATIVES

I end this chapter by returning to the Ethics in Practice narratives at the beginning of the chapter to discuss corresponding implications for clinical care. Space constraints permit only a brief treatment of each situation. An authentic approach to these requires a commitment to examining the particularities of each narrative to uncover the specific moral phenomena and corresponding circumstances at issue within each case. It should also be noted that the discovery of the moral angst reported in each narrative required a child-centred attunement to moral experience in itself.

One of the most profound messages that runs through every one of the Ethics in Practice narratives (taken from experiences within my practice) is that we ought to listen to the moral voices of children in a deeply engaged manner, and not trivialize them. In Ethics in Practice 16-1, for instance, this meant sitting with William to listen to his fears rather than only rewarding the behaviour we wanted.

In a more extreme situation, for Robbie in Ethics in Practice 16-6, engagement meant ensuring that Robbie was able to continue to express his psychological as well as his physical pain. In fact, after expressing my dismay over the possibility of losing him in my life, by which I aimed to emphasize his moral significance, Robbie told me that my relationship with him helped him to talk about all his pain and lighten the meaninglessness he felt in his life.

The promotion of authentic listening is particularly important for fostering a deepened awareness of the moral lives of children among the significant adults in their world. Parents are commonly moved by their children's expressed wishes, especially when these are articulated with a demonstration of the richness of their moral awareness. In Ethics in Practice 16-3, in which six-year-old Gloria's parents wanted to end her life-support, we were able to engage her in a dialogue through which she was able to explicitly express that she enjoyed many aspects of her life. Although she was frustrated by her dependence on technology, she clearly indicated that it was better to be alive in this manner than to not be alive at all.

In Ethics in Practice 16-5, David had demonstrated that he was highly capable of assessing his chronic pain in an ongoing manner and determining which pain-management strategies would be most effective in different circumstances. He was able to make important decisions and assume significant responsibility for his care. However, he was so distraught over his parents' fighting that he was unable to speak with them about how this aggravated his pain (and for Robbie in Ethics in Practice 19-6, this gave rise to suicidal feelings). Children in such situations can benefit from advocacy that facilitates the revealing of their masked sentiments. For example, when I arranged a family conference to help David express his feelings, he said that he felt safe in knowing that I would be there as an adult who would help ensure that he was heard. David's parents were very upset with themselves after hearing their child's despair. They promised him that they would do everything they could to stop fighting.

In Ethics in Practice 16-2 and 16-4, the cases of Benjamin and Marianne each involve situations in which some of the adults in the children's lives were withholding significant information from them. Although keeping such secrets may be intended to protect children from emotional pain, they in fact distance the children from the significant moral matters at hand. This impedes the children's ability to understand what is happening, as well as their ability to express how this matters to them morally. In such situations, I have found that parents themselves appear morally distressed about such secrets. Commonly, parents demonstrate a form of relief once the secret is broken (because they believe that on some level it is wrong to not tell the truth), and a deeper intimacy between the parents and the child is fostered. It is also important to recognize that parents commonly strive to protect their children from harm, which can give rise to a profound sense of burden when they acquire emotionally painful information about their children's lives.

The promotion of authentic listening is also important for enhancing health professionals' awareness of children's moral worlds. In caring for children like William in Ethics in Practice 16-1, this can involve discussing how the use of normative terms such as "good boy" can significantly limit the range of feelings that children will openly express while privately experiencing fear, pain, and distress.

Summary

Much has been written regarding ethical issues surrounding treatment decisions for children. This literature has predominantly been focused on that which adults are most suited to decide on behalf of children and the normative standards that should be employed for such decisions. In this chapter, I strive to give voice to the silent agents that are the objects of these decisions: morally aware youthful subjects living their own moral experiences.

For Reflection

1. How does this chapter affect your understanding of the role of parents?

2. Identify a situation from your practice where a child's moral agency was under-recognized.

3. How would you approach a child differently after reading this chapter?

Endnotes

1. Portions of these narratives have been modified in an attempt to preserve the anonymity of the persons involved. For example, all of the names presented are pseudonyms.

2. This discussion is exclusively limited to the context of *treatment* decisions. Children's consent to participate in *research* also raises a number of challenging questions (Baylis and Downie 2003; Carnevale et al. 2008; Ross 2006), but these are beyond the scope of this chapter.

3. Although the family is generally viewed as the most suitable unit for creating the moral milieu conducive for fostering the healthy development of children, it is also recognized that, on occasion,

some families can neglect or abuse children. In such cases, there is some acceptance of state interference in family life.

4. See *B.(R.) v. Children's Aid Society of Metropolitan Toronto* (1995) 1 S.C.R. 315 and *A.C. v. Manitoba (Director of Child and Family Services)* (2009).

5. This resembles Freedman's (1999) central argument in his study of adult children of incompetent parents.

6. Decision-making capacity should be judged on the basis of an ability to understand relevant information, think and choose with some degree of independence, and assess the potential for benefit and harm, as well as the achievement of a fairly stable set of values (Harrison et al. 1997). Decisional sophistication among adolescents has been further discussed by Weir and Peters (1997).

7. This view can be traced to a fundamental ethos of individualism in modern Western societies, wherein each human ought to become an independent or autonomous agent capable of judging morally significant matters through a developed faculty of rational discernment (Carnevale 1999).

8. This highlights a fundamental tension whereby cognitive "maturity" is presumed as a necessary condition for moral agency. Moral development is related to the development of general skills of rational reasoning (Kohlberg 1981; Piaget 1932/1965). This presumption is valid for an adult-centred conception of moral agency. However, I argue for a recognition of children's moral agency, regardless of their level of cognitive development.

9. Kohlberg subsequently put forth a reformulated theory that attempted to address criticisms of his earlier work (Kohlberg, Levine, and Hewer 1983). This was regarded as complex and unclear, such that his earlier work persisted as his most influential (Shweder, Mahapatra, and Miller 1987).

10. Although I am employing the metaphor of voice in this discussion, drawing on Gilligan's (1982) acclaimed work, "listening" to the moral experiences of children should not be limited to attending to their *verbal* expressions. Children commonly express outrage and protest or comfort and acceptance through various modes of *bodily* and verbal expression (Carnevale 1997; 1998). Also, see Kagan and Lamb (1987) for a discussion of the relation of culture to moral development in children.

11. In regard to my discussion of moral responsibility, I am deeply indebted to Carl Elliott (1996) for his philosophical analysis of responsibility in mentally ill offenders.

12. According to Aristotle, the type of *ignorance* that can make an action involuntary refers to an ignorance of the particular circumstances of an action (e.g., injuring someone in response to a suspected yet false threat, an ignorance-based involuntary injury). *Compulsion* refers to an act where the drive resides outside the person. This essentially refers to acts committed out of necessity or duress, wherein many would agree that they could not really have done otherwise under those particular circumstances.

13. This is further related to the clinical care of children in Schultz and Carnevale (1996).

14. This acknowledges the importance of (1) retaining some form of the best-interests standard for a preliminary discernment of which treatment options might be best for a child, and (2) continuing to recognize the significance of parents as surrogate decision makers because the common intimacy of their relationship predisposes them (more than most other adults) to think in terms of the child's interests. However, a corresponding recognition of the moral views of children problematizes objections or exclusions they experience toward treatment decisions made by their parents. This fosters a greater consideration of the child's voice as well as enriches the parents' understanding of the benefits and harms attributed to various treatments by better recognizing that certain courses of action are *morally* distressing for the child. It is noteworthy that in the context of *research,* it is widely held that a child's expression of dissent should be respected (Ross 2006; Tri-Council 2010). "Children can be seriously harmed by having something done to them without their knowledge or understanding" (Baylis, Downie, and Kenny 1999, 8).

References

A.C. v. Manitoba (Director of Child and Family Services). 2009. SCC 30, [2009] 2 S.C.R. 181, Supreme Court of Canada.

Alderson, P., Sutcliffe, K., and Curtis, K. 2006. Children's competence to consent to medical treatment. *Hastings Center Report, 36* (6), 25–34.

American Academy of Pediatrics (AAP). 1994. Guidelines on forgoing life-sustaining medical treatment. *Pediatrics, 93* (3), 532–536.

American Academy of Pediatrics (AAP). 1995. Informed consent, parental permission, and assent in pediatric practice. *Pediatrics, 95* (2), 314–317.

Aristotle. 350 BCE/1985. *Nichomachean ethics.* D. Ross (Trans.). Oxford: Oxford University Press.

Attig, T. 1996. Beyond pain: The existential suffering of children. *Journal of Palliative Care, 12* (3), 20–23.

Baylis, F. and Downie, J. 2003. The limits of altruism and arbitrary age limits. *American Journal of Bioethics, 3* (4), 19–21.

Baylis, F., Downie, J., and Kenny, M. 1999. Children and decision making in health research. *IRB: A Review of Human Subjects Research, 21* (4), 5–10.

Bluebond-Langner, M. 1978. *The private worlds of dying children.* Princeton: Princeton University Press.

B.(R.) v. Children's Aid Society of Metropolitan Toronto. 1995. 1 S.C.R. 315.

Brinchmann, B.S., Forde, R., and Nortvedt, P. 2002. What matters to the parents? A qualitative study of parents' experiences with life-and-death decisions concerning their premature infants. *Nursing Ethics, 9* (4), 388–404.

Canadian Charter of Rights and Freedoms, Canada Act 1982 (U.K.), c. 11.

Canadian Pediatric Society (CPS). 2004. Treatment decisions regarding infants, children and adolescents. *Pediatrics and Child Health, 9,* 99–103.

Carnevale, F.A. 1997. The experience of critically ill children: Narratives of unmaking. *Intensive and Critical Care Nursing, 13,* 49–52.

Carnevale, F.A. 1998. "Striving to recapture our previous life"—The experience of families of critically ill children. *Dynamics—Official Journal of the Canadian Association of Critical Care Nurses, 9* (4), 16–22.

Carnevale, F.A. 1999. Toward a cultural conception of the self. *Journal of Psychosocial Nursing and Mental Health Services, 37* (8), 26–31.

Carnevale, F.A. 2002. Moral binds and conflicts of interests: Ethical considerations for innovative therapies. *Pediatric Intensive Care Nursing, 3* (2), 4–6.

Carnevale, F.A. 2003. The injured family. In P.A. Moloney-Harmon and S.J. Czerwinski (Eds.), *Nursing care of the pediatric trauma patient* (pp. 107–117). Philadelphia: W.B. Saunders.

Carnevale, F.A. 2005a. Ethical care of the critically ill child: A conception of a "thick" bioethics. *Nursing Ethics, 12* (3), 239–252.

Carnevale, F.A. 2005b. Families are not visitors: Rethinking our relationships in the ICU. *Australian Critical Care, 18* (2), 48–49.

Carnevale, F.A., Alexander, E., Davis, M., Rennick, J.E., and Troini, R. 2006. Daily living with distress and enrichment: The moral experience of families with ventilator assisted children at home. *Pediatrics, 117* (1), e48–60.

Carnevale, F.A., Canoui, P., Cremer, R., Farrell, C., Doussau, A., Seguin, M-J., Hubert, P., Leclerc, F., and Lacroix, J. 2007. Parental involvement in treatment decisions regarding their critically ill child: A comparative study of France and Quebec. *Pediatric Critical Care Medicine, 8* (4), 337–342.

Carnevale, F.A., Macdonald, M.E., Bluebond-Langner, M., and McKeever, P. 2008. Using participant observation in pediatric health care settings: Intellectual demands and ethical solutions. *Journal of Child Health Care, 12* (1), 18–32.

Carnevale, F.A. and Rafman, S. 1998. *Socio-moral transformations in childhood trauma.* Proceedings of the XXII International Congress of Pediatrics, Amsterdam, August, 407.

Coles, R. 1986. *The moral life of children.* New York: Atlantic Monthly Press.

Elliott, C. 1996. *The rules of insanity: Moral responsibility and the mentally ill offender.* Albany: State University of New York Press.

Erikson, E.H. 1950. *Childhood and society.* New York: W.W. Norton.

Freedman, B.1999. *Duty and healing: Foundations of a Jewish bioethic.* New York: Routledge.

Gilligan, C. 1982. *In a different voice: Psychological theory and woman's development.* Cambridge, MA: Harvard University Press.

Harrison, C., Kenny, N.P., Sidarous, M., and Rowell, M. 1997. Bioethics for clinicians: Involving children in medical decisions. *Canadian Medical Association Journal, 156* (6), 825–828.

Kagan, J. and Lamb, S. (Eds.). 1987. *The emergence of morality in young children.* Chicago: University of Chicago Press.

Kenny, K., Downie, J., and Harrison, C. 2008. Respectful involvement of children in medical decision-making. In P. Singer (Ed.), *The Cambridge textbook of bioethics* (pp. 121–126). Cambridge: Cambridge University Press.

Kohlberg, L. 1981. *The philosophy of moral development.* San Francisco: Harper and Row.

Kohlberg, L., Levine, C., and Hewer, A. 1983. *Moral stages: A current formulation and a response to critics.* New York: Karger.

Levinson, D.J. 1978. *The seasons of a man's life.* New York: Alfred A. Knopf.

McPherson, G. 2007. *Children's participation in chronic illness decision-making: An interpretive description.* Unpublished doctoral dissertation, University of British Columbia, Vancouver, British Columbia.

Melton, G.B. 1999. Parents and children: Legal reform to facilitate children's participation. *American Psychologist, 54* (11), 935–944.

Nelson, H.L. and Nelson, J.L. 1995. *The patient in the family: An ethics of medicine and families.* New York: Routledge.

Piaget, J. 1932/1965. *The moral judgment of the child*. New York: The Free Press.

Rogers, C. 1951. *Client-centered therapy*. Boston: Houghton Mifflin.

Ross, L.F. 1998. *Children, families and health care decision making*. Oxford, UK: Oxford University Press (Clarendon Press).

Ross, L.F. 2006. *Children in medical research: Access versus protection*. Oxford, UK: Oxford University Press (Clarendon Press).

Scheper-Hughes, N. and Sargent, C. 1998. Introduction: The cultural politics of childhood. In N. Scheper-Hughes and C. Sargent (Eds.), *Small wars: The cultural politics of childhood* (pp. 1–33). Berkeley: University of California Press.

Schneider, M.D., Bersoff, D.N., and Podolsky, S.R. 1989. Brief for *amici curiae* American Psychological Association, National Association of Social Workers, and the American Jewish Committee in *Ohio v. Akron Center for Reproductive Health* and *Hidgson v. Minnesota*. Washington, DC: Jenner and Block.

Schultz, D.S. and Carnevale, F.A. 1996. Engagement and suffering in responsible caregiving: On overcoming maleficence in health care. *Theoretical Medicine, 17* (3), 189–207.

Shweder, R.A., Mahapatra, M., and Miller, J.G. 1987. Culture and moral development. In J. Kagan and S. Lamb (Eds.), *The emergence of morality in young children* (pp. 1–83). Chicago: University of Chicago Press.

Sourkes, B.M. 1995. *Armfuls of time: The psychological experience of the child with a life-threatening illness*. Pittsburgh: University of Pittsburgh Press.

Tri-Council: Canadian Institutes of Health Research, Natural Sciences and Engineering Research Council of Canada, and Social Sciences and Humanities Research Council of Canada. 2010. *Tri-Council policy statement: Ethical conduct for research involving humans*.

Weir, R.F. and Peters, C. 1997. Affirming the decisions adolescents make about life and death. *Hastings Center Report, 27* (6), 29–40.

Wright, P.W.G. 1988. Babyhood: The social construction of infant care as a medical problem in England in the years around 1900. In M. Lock and D. Gordon (Eds.), *Biomedicine examined* (pp. 299–329). Dordrecht: Kluwer Academic Press.

Yalom, I.D. 1980. *Existential psychotherapy*. New York: Basic Books.

CHAPTER 17

Ethics and End-of-Life Decisions

Janet L. Storch, Rosalie Starzomski, and Patricia Rodney

. . . [T]he issue is not one of life or death. The issue is which kind of death, an agonized or peaceful one. Shall we meet death in personal integrity or in personal disintegration? Shall there be a moral or demoralized end to mortal life? (Fletcher 1954, 208)

Fletcher's questions about death are as important today as they were in 1954 as we continue to develop ways to provide ethical end-of-life care in the twenty-first century. In our studies in the area of nursing ethics, we learned that caring for people at the end of life was one of the most ethically problematic issues for nurses (see Chapter 1). Nurses told us many deeply troubling stories about their inability to provide good ethical care for patients at the end of life (Rodney et al. 2002a; 2006; Storch et al. 2002; Varcoe et al. 2004; Varcoe et al. in review). They often spoke about their distress in not being able to effect a good death for their patients because sometimes physicians did not take actions they believed were necessary to assist the individuals to have a good death. They indicated their sense of being morally compromised (i.e., experiencing moral distress). In the end, we found that a great deal of nurses' moral distress arose from their disagreement with others (physicians, family members, other health care team members) about end-of-life care. We wondered why, after all these years of clearly identifying ethical issues, concerns, and potential guidelines for end-of-life care, this agony was still ongoing in practice.

In this chapter, we do not intend to provide an extensive overview of end-of-life issues since many others have already provided important informative and analytical work in this area.[1,2] Rather, we intend to build on the writings of others and our own research, observations, and experiences around end of life situations. Together, we (the three editors of this book) have been engaged in providing ethics consultation, chairing ethics committees, conducting research, focusing on education (academic teaching as well as professional and community education), responding to guidelines and policies, and helping to develop public policy about end-of-life care for many years. We have shared our reactions, responses, and stories with each other, often consulting each other. It is these experiences and reflections—and, of course, our reading of expert literature from a variety of sources—that inform our approach in this chapter.

In what follows, we will address several areas from the wide range of potential topics, providing examples from our research and experience related to (1) the meaning of a good death, (2) good care at the end of life, including "living wills" or advance treatment directives, (3) relief of pain and discomfort, (4) information and truthfulness, and (5) fostering family and friendship support. We also offer some updates and our preliminary thoughts about euthanasia and assisted suicide: a re-emerging ethical-legal issue in Canada in this decade. We begin and end with a moral imperative for nurses to provide leadership to enhance the quality of end-of-life decision making for all. We hope to provide readers with updates and to stimulate insights into their own important roles in end-of-life care and decision-making.

A MORAL IMPERATIVE FOR NURSES

Despite over five decades of research and policy work aimed at improving care at the end of life, it is still the case that far too many patients and their families face uncertainty, pain, and suffering at this time (Carstairs 2005; 2010; see also Chapter 13).

The technological imperative, where if something *can* be done to preserve life, it *should* be done, contributes to the moral distress of patients/clients, families, physicians, other care providers, and nurses. Families often feel uncertain and want to trust health professionals to make good judgments for their loved ones. Nurses frequently feel caught between the family and friends and the physician's need to preserve a patient's life. Often what nurses witness during their steady 8- to 12-hour periods of caring for a dying patient (or weeks of daily and twice daily visits to the homes of those who are dying) gives them a growing conviction that the person is wanting and waiting to die. When the nurse's voice is not heard to convey that understanding to the physician, or when nurses are not included in end-of-life discussions and decisions, they experience a sense of *moral distress* (Corley 1995, 2002; Hamric and Blackwell 2007; Rodney et al. 2002b; Storch et al. 2002; see also Chapter 9).

Many aspects of end-of-life care and decision making fall squarely within the realm of nursing practice on an individual and collective level. As we have indicated above, our research shows that these areas of practice continue to raise very troubling moral issues for nurses and for their colleagues in other professions. Nurses must act on this knowledge of their difficulties to improve their own education in end-of-life care. This will allow them to be better able to provide culturally sensitive end-of-life care, and to do so with confidence and competence. In learning to listen to, advocate for, and support people who are dying, nurses will then be able to fulfill the mandate of care in a way that respects different views of a *good death*. They will also be able to provide leadership within nursing and across other health care professions in a crucial arena of practice.

Nurse leaders for a number of years have called upon nurses to be the "catalysts for improving end-of-life care." For example, Scanlon (1996) challenged nurses to act upon their concerns that adequate and timely disclosure be given to persons who are dying. Carol Taylor (1995) urged nurses to take a leading role in bringing clinicians as well as patients and families together to negotiate end-of-life decision making, particularly when conflict is beginning to be apparent and when the patients' prognoses are poor. And more recently, on the basis of a research study she completed with dyads of patients and family members, Robinson (2011) has argued for a *relational* approach to end-of-life dialogue with patients and their families such that we attend to the engagement of people in relationships rather than just focusing on information to present (see also Chapters 5, 7, and 8 for discussions of relational ethics). Stadjuhar (2011) and her research team have signaled that an urgent need also exists for all those with *life-limiting* conditions, such as chronic obstructive pulmonary disease, end stage renal disease, and heart disease, to have access to end-of-life care comparable to those receiving palliative care due to cancer. Nurses can and should be pivotal forces in shaping such initiatives.

The Meaning of a "Good Death"

In his seminal research, palliative care physician Dr. David Kuhl (2002) sought to answer the question, What does it mean to have a *good death*? In this chapter, we draw from his research findings. We first acknowledge that because the term "euthanasia" in its simplest form also means "an easy and painless death" (De Wolf et al. 1997), open discussions about a *good death* have often been avoided because there can be confusion and anxiety about this controversial topic. The matter of euthanasia as "a painless killing, especially to end a painful and incurable disease, or mercy killing" (De Wolf et al. 1997) will be discussed briefly later in this chapter. At this juncture, our focus is on the meaning of a *good death,* which is different from the meanings embodied in contemporary discussions of euthanasia.

According to Kuhl (2002), patients' perceptions of a *good death* include the relief of pain; being close to loved ones and being in good relationship with them; having the support of family and friends; feeling free to talk openly about death and about care; reflecting upon their lives and having those reflections valued by others; having trusting relationships with professional caregivers; and finding meaning in their lives and deaths. Each individual holds his or her own particular meaning of a good death, and it is important to seek to understand that meaning. Not all individuals want technologies that will prolong their lives. Yet discussions about end-of-life decisions and narratives of individual struggles too often feature language about fighting, conquering, and battling terminal illness. Such language may valorize patients' resistance in ways that imply that those who make other choices are falling short of what they ought to do. Sensitivity to the choices individuals make to fight—to "rage against the dying of the light" (Thomas 1969)—or *not* to fight, is critical. Nurses can be active in understanding the importance of this choice and in facilitating communication of it to patients and families. Such manifest understanding and good communication are evident in Ethics in Practice 17-1 where a good death experience of a nursing colleague is recounted.

ETHICS IN PRACTICE 17-1

Living While Dying: A Good Death

Sharon[3] first learned about a potential life-threatening problem when her physician informed her during an office visit that biopsy tissue showed signs of melanoma. A referral to an oncologist led to the recommendation that surgery be performed as quickly as possible. In preparation for her unanticipated absence from the workplace for a matter of weeks, she elected to ask for a meeting of the nursing staff to tell them directly of her lab results, to ask for their support, and to confirm that she wanted channels of communication to be honest and open with respect to her condition. Surgical findings meant that further treatment was required, involving more extensive time away from work. Through-out the months she was away, one nursing colleague had been selected by Sharon as the point of contact for staff in order to update them on her condition. She wanted all information to be available in order to give her colleagues an opportunity to help her with the moral and/or physical support she needed or might need. Telling her RN colleagues about her experiences meant that she could trust their responses and their care.

During the weeks that stretched to a year, Sharon had many treatments, made many choices involving both traditional care and alternative therapies, and relied upon her family, her friends, members of her church, and her colleagues to support her will to live. At first her main discomfort was excessive fatigue from the treatments, but, as interferon therapy was replaced by chemotherapy, she experienced pain, nau-sea, and weakness. Home care nursing staff and her colleagues came to support her and to encourage her. All efforts were made to keep her as the key decision maker regard-ing her care, including making decisions about her pain control and management. To that end, she kept detailed notes in her jour-nal, often referring back to previous entries to help keep track of medications and labo-ratory results.

Her family was very important to her, and her grandchildren gave her particular joy. Sharon and her closest friend (her husband) planned that their children and grandchildren would come home on a more regular basis. Meanwhile, Sharon, her family, and her friends sought all advice possible about any potential for cure or hope for a remis-sion. They also sought good information about her care.

The time came when cancerous tumours had so thoroughly invaded her body that she had to succumb to further surgery. That sur-gical intervention took her to hospital for a matter of weeks. But when it was clear that nothing further could or should be done, her family brought her home where home care nurses, her nursing colleagues, her friends, and her family cared for her for several weeks. The day after Christmas Day it was clear that this would be her final day, and, surrounded by family and friends, she died in the evening. Her nursing colleagues gave her body its final care, and her family elected to have her rest in peace with them at home until the morning.

As exemplified in the case above, a good death is possible; however, for many peo-ple it is difficult to plan in the face of potentially "futile" medical treatments. The con-cept of futility, and the issues surrounding it, are fraught with complex problems that are important for nurses to understand. We present in what follows a brief background on medical futility and some of the challenges with the use of this term as we strive to ensure that each patient has the opportunity for as good a death as possible.

Medical Futility (or Inappropriate Care)

Toward the end of the 1980s, a combination of enhanced life-sustaining technologies, an entrenched belief in patients' rights, and growing concerns about ethical resource alloca-tion in health care led to academic discussions/debates and practice policies about medi-cal futility. Medical futility was defined as, "a medical treatment that is seen to be non-beneficial because it is believed to offer no reasonable hope of recovery or improvement of the patient's condition" (Canadian Nurses Association 2001, 1). Schneiderman, Jecker, and Jonsen (1990) believed futility had two distinct components—physiological effect and benefit from the patient's perspective. Schneiderman et al. considered that some treatments could be futile because they did not produce a desired physiological effect or the anticipated goal of treatment. However, it can be argued that this determination is difficult to apply because the outcome data with which to determine the potential physiological effect is not usually available and leads to a question about what percentage of success would be considered adequate to consider a treatment beneficial. Even with outcome data, each case must be evaluated in terms of the potential benefits *as seen through the eyes of the patient*. The patient must be the one, when presented with the information about the benefits and burdens of treatment, to make a choice based on his or her own individual interpretation of well being.

For the above reasons, as well as agreement by many other authors that the use of futility places end-of-life care in the category of decisions based on economic goals (e.g., utility), the term *inappropriate care* was considered as preferable. Thus, it became the term invoked in discussions about a "way to set some reasonable boundaries to health care" that would be beneficial to the welfare of the patient and reasonable for society" (Callahan 1991, 30-31). There was a growing sentiment among administrators and policy-makers that it would be possible to collect some good evidence about medical conditions and human responses to treatment at the end of life, as well as evidence related to socio-economic indicators. Such evidence, they believed, could lead to clearer decision making about medical futility or inappropriate care. Varcoe and Rodney (2003) have suggested that the problem identified as *inappropriate care* could be considered as a problem of unnecessary suffering resulting from dehumanizing practices (11).

As Callahan (1991) points out,

> It turns out that there are facts and there are facts. . . . Values, it soon became evident, can influence not only what facts are identified as facts, but also which ones are thought worth having and which are worth dismissing. (30)

Since the anticipation of outcomes in beneficial patient care involves an inter-play of physical well-being and improved overall well-being, information about both facts and values is involved. In considering the matter of medical futility, Taylor (1995) suggests four classifications of futility:

1. not futile: beneficial to both physical and overall well-being;
2. futile: non-beneficial to both physical and overall well-being;
3. futile from the patient's perspective: medically indicated but not valued by the patient; and
4. futile from the clinician's perspective: valued by the patient but not medically indicated (301).

Clearly, these classifications have objective and subjective, quantitative and qualitative dimensions. Only some judgments, therefore, could rest with physicians and other health professionals, while a good many rest with the patient or family. Given that physicians may feel morally compromised by feeling obliged to provide treatment they believe will not benefit the person, the problem of who has priority in decision making is very real for all involved. Taylor (1995) presents a strong case for her recommendation

. . . that nurses play a leading role . . . by identifying patients, families and health care teams at risk of experiencing conflict about futile care, and then initiating dialogue that may prevent or resolve conflict. The focus in negotiation should be on everyone working together to obtain the best possible outcome for a particular patient, not on any person or group asserting their primacy of authority. (303)

The difficulties of embarking upon such negotiation were recognized by professional bodies at the national level in Canada, leading to the *Joint Statement on Preventing and Resolving Conflicts Involving Health Care Providers and Persons Receiving Care* in 1999. Shortly thereafter, the Canadian Nurses Association issued a paper in their *Ethics in Practice* series to guide nurses in addressing the matter of futility (Canadian Nurses Association 2001). While futility as a topic is not addressed as much in recent ethics literature as it used to be (primarily because of the problems described above) difficulties with end-of-life decision making have not decreased. Many of the discussions in the area of futility and inappropriate care involve tension between patient autonomy and professional autonomy—that is, the tension between what patients and/or families may want in regard to their treatment and what health care professionals believe they can offer based on their professional judgment. As Robinson's (2011) recent research suggests, more dialogue and a focus on relational ethics are essential in helping to resolve these conflicts.

Do-Not-Resuscitate (DNR) Orders

One of the most dramatic ways in which decisions about medical futility are exercised is in documenting a "do-not-resuscitate" (DNR) decision as a physician's order, and in executing that order. Some organizations use the terms "do not attempt resuscitation," or "allow natural death" (Venneman et al. 2008). However, for the purposes of our discussion, we will use the term DNR. While it should be recognized that DNR orders represent only one of the many decisions an individual might make to decline technological prolongation of life, the majority of these types of decisions are difficult for caregivers and for families. Nurses, in particular, continue to experience the morally traumatic effects of the dilemmas involved in the application of DNR policy.

In many instances, nurses have had to deal with verbal physician orders only, including a physician's directives calling for a "slow code." Physicians' reticence to commit a DNR order to paper has centered on their (legitimate) concerns about being pressured into DNR decisions before they have an opportunity to adequately assess the individual and his or her wishes. This reticence may also be due to the physicians' own misinformation, misunderstanding, or fear of legal liability. In a study of ethical conflicts of physicians and nurses in clinical care (Gaudine et al. 2011), one physician spoke about the difficulties for families in making a decision about cardio-pulmonary resuscitation (CPR) because it depends upon how one asks the question. In observing junior residents and others asking families about CPR, this physician stated: "But what I think is brutally unfair is to ask the patient's family [if] they want resuscitation treatment. They don't have the knowledge to make that decision" (12). The importance of clarifying roles and responsibilities in CPR and DNR decision making is critical (Keatings and Smith 2010; Kuhl 1998; Kuhl and Wilensky 1999). Patients and their families need to be well informed about the potential for CPR to make a difference for their health and life or not

(Puopolo et al. 1997). Examination of various hospital policies about DNR suggests that variation continues to exist in who is allowed to make the DNR decision, what patients and families are told, whether health professionals are obligated to provide active life-sustaining treatments, and what the role of nurses might be in such decisions and actions.

Merely by being present with patients in hospital on a more constant basis than other health professionals, nurses are frequently in attendance when a cardiac arrest occurs. Nurses ". . . often find themselves initiating or withholding cardiopulmonary resuscitation (CPR) in situations characterized by verbal orders, euphemistic documentation and poor communication, and when consultation with patients about their CPR choices often do not take place" (Schultz 1997, 227). The need for attention to sound policies supported by administrative structures, as well as continued education about DNR policies and processes, is critical to successful decision making about, and implementation of, "do-not-resuscitate" orders. Included in this education is the importance of removing the widespread conflation of DNR with "no treatment"—a mistaken assumption that often hinders effective discussion and decision making about DNR (see also Chapter 13).

Limited information about non-treatment is also common with regard to other life-preserving technologies such as renal dialysis, mechanical ventilation, and delivering food and fluids by artificial means. This is a serious oversight in the provision of full information to patients and may also represent a reluctance to entertain the idea of a natural death, often referred to as a good death when good care is provided at the end of life.

GOOD CARE AT THE END OF LIFE

The story of Sharon's final days in Ethics in Practice 17-1 was unique to Sharon, as each life and death is unique. Others may not have the type of family, friends, or colleagues who are able to offer the level or kind of support Sharon received. Others may not have the will or ability to be as open and honest as Sharon was with those most significant to her. Respect is due to those who choose to be more private about their terminal condition and the choices they wish to make to deal with it. At the same time, nurses and other caregivers need to be aware that traditions surrounding "death talk" keep some people prisoners to custom, when what they may need most is openness and the support of their fellow human beings. With sensitivity to these individual needs, and awareness of the effect of societal constraints on actions, all caregivers need to engage with people at the end of their life. Such engagement allows caregivers to create situations for the dying that represent who they are and how they wish to spend their final days. All this should occur with careful attention to family wishes (Sahlberg-Blom, Ternestedt, and Johansson 2000). What might that kind of care be like?

Over time, based upon interviews with people who were dying, researchers have been consistent in identifying the wishes of those individuals. People want to have adequate pain and symptom management. They do not want to have their dying prolonged, to lose a sense of control, or to be a burden to others. They want to strengthen their relationships with loved ones (Davies et al. 1995; Fry and Johnstone 2008; Kuhl 2002;). To that end, preparing a living will or an advance directive affords people an opportunity to think about their lives and the meaning of their lives, and to be engaged with family and friends (Godkin 2002). Thus, advance directives are not as much about dying as they are about living while one is entering one's final years and days. This suggests that advance directives really are "living wills"—that is, directions about planning for and living one's final days well.

Living Wills and Advance Directives

The format of the "living will" documents, now commonly called advance directives, varies somewhat but most agree that the advance directive is "a written document containing a person's wishes about life-sustaining treatment" that "extend[s] the autonomy of competent patients to future situations in which the patient is incompetent" (Singer 1994, 111; see also Storch, Rodney, and Starzomski 2009, 467). Advance directives include an *instruction* directive, which "allows the person to specify which life-sustaining treatments he or she would not wish in various situations" as well as a *proxy* directive, which "allows individuals to identify a substitute decision maker should they ever be rendered incompetent" (Keatings and Smith 2010, 240). This can be as simple as a letter or as complex as a many-page form. Most forms include several direct situational categories of treatment decisions and/or some accompanying guidance to assist the individual to consider his or her wishes regarding treatment or no-treatment options.

After the individual is guided through the various interventions that can be taken to sustain life, the directives are often categorized under different levels of intensity. These levels can vary from "full acute care" (including critical care) to "palliative interventions only." For example, some long-term care facilities have used a form that includes four levels of care: comfort care (palliation); limited care, which includes comfort care; surgical care, which includes limited care; and intensive care, which includes surgical care. These advance directives, which include provision for a proxy to represent the wishes of the individual if the person is unable to do so, should fulfill the need health professionals, families, and friends have for guidance at a time of personal anguish and allow the individual's wishes to be respected. Unfortunately, advance directives are not always followed.

Many experts involved in the area of advance directives are now stressing the importance of telling others and giving others, who might be speaking for them, a copy of the advance directive. Some health regions are suggesting that a form be kept to indicate when the client has spoken to his or her physician or nurse, and who else has been informed. Informal caregivers, as well as health care providers, are also encouraged to keep records of advance directive actions taken, changes made, and contacts described. One example is the Interior Health Authority in B.C.'s Advance Care Planning Tracking Record, designed to be used by the health care team. Recording spaces include date, topic of conversation, with whom, location of detailed documentation (e.g., progress notes), action taken, and signature of health care provider.

Problems with Advance Directives

Despite the prevalence of talk about advance directives over the past three to four decades, we have found that in any group assembled to discuss advance directives only a handful of people will indicate that they have actually developed a directive. Researchers have found the use of advance directives to be less than predicted or desired (Blondeau et al. 2000; Tulsky et al. 2008; Zronek, Daly, and Lee 1999). Why is implementation of this idea so elusive? What stops individuals from completing an advance directive? What limits health professionals in responding to advance directives? The subcommittee of the Standing Senate Committee on Social Affairs, Science and Technology, chaired by Carstairs and Beaudoin (2000), urged that advance directives "should not be viewed as purely legal documents" (12). Regardless of whether too much or too little detail is provided in an advance directive, there will always be challenges in interpretation of its contents and difficulties specifying in advance a person's wishes with regard to every possible medical situation. Instead, an advance directive should be *only part* of the communication and planning to help people prepare for death. If the people the dying person cares most about have been engaged in this communication, problems of interpretation are less likely to arise and "[the] passage to death is eased, the level of comfort rises, and the burden of care is lightened for the substitute decision-maker" (Report of the Special Senate Subcommittee 2000, 13).

An integral feature of an advance directive is ensuring that a person is named as a substitute or surrogate decision maker and that this person is made aware of the wishes and values of the person for whom he or she will be acting (see also Moorhouse, Yeo, and Rodney 2010). This is essential, as with a written advance directive, not every scenario can be considered and often the substitute decision maker is called upon to consider what the person would want in a particular situation when there may be no documentation to provide direction.

Public Resistance

Some resistance to advance directives resides within patients, families, and the general public. We are a death-denying society, or, at least, we are in denial that a situation requiring an advance directive will ever happen to us. Our societal mind-set is about living, with an assumption that we can leave death decisions until later because we will be among the 10 percent of Canadians who die a sudden and clear death. For some, who realize they may not die suddenly, their denial is likely due to their inability to personally face death. For others, the mental and emotional work of preparing an advance directive is too difficult to have to think through or is not considered a priority. Others may have difficulty trusting that the directives will be honoured. Some are unsure if they will be able to change the advance directive once made, and they fear making a lasting commitment. Many forms and guides for completion of an advance directive are complex and confusing. This means that individuals have to block off time to accomplish the task, and for many people time is a rare commodity. Some provinces also require legal certification in certain cases for the advance directive to be valid.

Health Professionals' Reluctance

A surprising number of health professionals are only vaguely aware of advance directives and may fail to see the relevance or worth of such directives. Often a barrier to health professionals' engagement with advance directives is their lack of knowledge and their reluctance to engage in "death talk" (Godkin 2002; Rodney and Howlett 2003; Tulsky et al. 2008). Given that past practices discouraged physicians from conveying bad news to patients for fear of upsetting them and interfering in their recovery, it is not surprising that they might withhold information or be reluctant to engage in discussion of death with patients. Often those who do share the "bad news" are poorly prepared for the task and do not give themselves sufficient time to stay with the patient; such situations can lead to upset patients and distressed health care professionals. The mistaken assumption that withholding information is safer may then be reinforced, leading to further avoidance of end-of-life discussions. In Ethics in Practice 17-3 we provide one nurse's illustration of the type of difficulty health professionals have in telling a patient about his impending death.

In summary, good care at the end of life includes attention to understanding what the patient (the person) wants, documenting the patient's wishes, and encouraging patients to share those wishes with family and friends. In the study by Gaudine et al. (2011), both physicians and nurses shared concerns about nine main thematic issues including ". . . others not respecting a patient's wishes; patient not receiving quality end-of-life care; and patient and/or family not having informed consent of full disclosure" (11). And, as we indicated at the outset of this chapter, in her study, Robinson (2011) points out that we ought to understand advance care planning as a relational process in which we should understand and support the relationships involved, not just provide information.

RELIEF OF PAIN AND DISCOMFORT

Although nurses may well intend to provide relief of pain and discomfort at the end of life, there is good evidence that their efforts often fall short of that goal. White, Coyne, and Patel (2001), in a study of the adequacy of nurses' preparation for end-of-life care, found that the highest ranked areas for additional education identified by nurses included pain control techniques and comfort care interventions. A fear of providing too much relief for pain through analgesics (particularly narcotics) seems pervasive in nursing for a number of reasons, including fear of creating an addiction, fear of prematurely ending a life, lack of understanding about pain relief through analgesia, poor pain assessment, and a belief that suffering serves an important purpose (Hunter 2000). Most of these fears and biases are both unfounded and misguided, and these motives of caregivers must be carefully discerned and corrected, with priority given to patients' needs and desires (see also, Stajduhar 2011).

Furthermore, culturally sensitive care demands that differing views about the role of suffering and the acceptability of opioid analgesics be considered and respected. Tensions may be heightened when nurses must deal with particular family members' values and beliefs about pain relief, as illustrated in Ethics in Practice 17-2.

ETHICS IN PRACTICE 17-2

Family Resistance to Pain Control

And it was a horrible time for all the staff because this woman was terminal and she was in a lot of pain. And we had to play with that fine line between [having] the patient pain-free and keeping her awake so that her son could still see her. He did not want his mother to be unconscious or to not be able to respond to him; as far as he was concerned that was killing her. So we would have to justify all of the treatments that we were able to give her. And try as we might, by discussing with the husband, the other son, physicians, even managers . . . we could not get this young gentleman to change his mind, and we had horrible fears of coming into her room in the middle of the night and finding her dead and having to resuscitate her (Storch et al. 2000).

I Challenges in Pain and Symptom Control

In addition to pain control through medication, a better understanding of alternative and complementary therapies is also important. Different individuals and communities may have their own particular pain-relieving methods that they associate with their own cultural traditions. For example, Aboriginal elders may use prayer, or burn sage, sweet grass, or cedar (Fisher, Ross, and MacLean 2000). Pain might be decreased through massage, hydrotherapy, music therapy, and other means (White, Coyne, and Patel 2001). Moreover, sometimes the most distressing symptoms may not involve pain—for example, nausea, vomiting, breathlessness, hiccups, edema, dry mouth, pruritus, anorexia, fatigue, vertigo, insomnia, and many other physical conditions (Ferris et al. 2002). Alleviating these symptoms often takes nursing empathy and creativity, as well as the input of members of the entire health care team. In Ethics in Practice 17-2 we also raise the need for better family assessment and support.

Kuhl (2002) reminds us that pain in life and in dying extends beyond physical pain. He suggests that the dying may experience unnecessary suffering because of the poor communication between caregivers and patients. He describes this as *iatrogenic suffering* because it is pain and suffering inflicted upon another person unintentionally but as a result of the way physicians and other health professionals speak to patients. Kuhl also underscores the fact that pain is comprised of psychological and spiritual features as well as physical. He maintains that too often physicians and nurses minimize the extent of pain an individual feels and neglect to provide the information and the support needed by those facing the end of their lives. Salas and Cameron (2010) provide a further illustration of suffering. In an interpretive study of palliative home care in Canada, they analyzed how nurses engage with "whatever is going on in the patient's home" (653). Ruth, a very ill patient, is visited by Sarah, the home care nurse, and Ruth is found to be in serious need of care. Although Sarah knows that other patients are waiting for her, she is entirely immersed in her final act of care for Ruth. That care involves changing her diaper and washing her following severe diarrhoea. The researcher observing this action states:

> Ruth's home holds Sarah up and does not let her go. The stench is everywhere. Ruth is silent, mortified. Yet, there is something in Sarah's actions that make this moment a little less unbearable, something in this nursing act that turns this horrific moment into a more liveable human experience (660).

INFORMATION AND TRUTHFULNESS

Throughout his book, Kuhl (2002) emphasizes the importance of caregivers being honest with patients to facilitate the patients' control of their final days. Yet such truthfulness continues to be the exception in end-of-life care. Kristman-Scott (2000) provides an historical analysis of the "movement toward greater disclosure of health information to patients" (47) over the past half-century. She notes that the cycle of pretense may rob an individual of power and control over what remains of his or her final days.[4]

ETHICS IN PRACTICE 17-3

Lack of Truthful Disclosure of Impending Death

The condition of a 55-year-old man, who had undergone a bone marrow transplant 50 days prior, began to deteriorate rapidly on Friday that week. His wife questioned the physician in charge of his care about this setback. The physician assured her that her husband would be going home soon. On Saturday, her husband's condition worsened and late that night a medical resident visited the room. The resident told the patient's wife and sister that before they left the hospital he wanted clear direction about what should be done if the patient's condition deteriorated further. When the wife questioned the meaning of this request, the resident said, "Didn't they tell you?" He then proceeded to state that the transplant had not worked. In tears, the wife conveyed this information to her husband by saying, "Sweetheart, it is time to let go." His whispered, laboured response to her was, "Why would I want to let go?" following which she told him the transplant had not worked. His shuddering body expressed his grief and (perhaps) betrayal. In retrospect, it seemed clear that the nurses knew, and were trying different ways to help the family find out that their loved one's condition was terminal. This seemed to be information they understood they were not allowed to give.

Reflecting on this sad death, it seemed clear that many people on, or visiting the hospital unit, knew for some days that this man's transplant had not worked and he that was dying. The nursing care he received after the event described in Ethics in Practice 17-3 was of the highest quality. The 16 medications he had been receiving prior to that time were reduced to six by Sunday morning, and only pain relief and comfort measures were given. The nurse told the family (who had by then converged in the room) that the room was theirs to use, and that she would be in and out steadily but did not need anyone to leave or to move for her—she would work around the family. She checked that family members were nourished in body and soul, until the patient died at 5 p.m. on Sunday night.

What this man and his family most needed when it was clear that his life was ending was clear communication that this was so, and assistance to make connections within, to self, to others, to nature, and to transcendence (Mount 2010). It is not only the patient who needs these connections. In the case cited above, the young adult children suffered unremitting grief from not having been allowed this final connection to their dad. Carstairs (2010) states that: "We know that each death in Canada affects the immediate well-being of, on average, five other people" (12). Those who continue to live following a loved one's death can experience poor health due to a poor death experience.

Kristman-White (2000) traces the belief of serious danger in disclosing a prognosis of terminal illness to patients back to the teachings of Hippocratic medicine. According to this tradition, patients will "take a turn for the worse" if they are told the truth. The halting efforts to change medical views on this dictum, based upon the principle of nonmaleficence, have led to only modest changes in practice. Early studies by Glaser and Strauss (1965) and Kubler-Ross (1969) exposed the myth of harm (as opposed to benefit) in revealing a fatal prognosis. Even decades later, the practice of non-disclosure prevails in many settings. Struggles with levels of disclosure continue to exist, especially when family and/or the health care team is in conflict. More recently, it has been suggested that anxiety may prevent physicians from discussing the eminence of a person's death. The lack of open discussion with the patient and the family often precludes nurses from knowing what the physician has in mind and this, in turn, limits nurses ability to better support the patient, family, and physician. In Ethics in Practice 17-3 the harm that lack of honest communication can cause is illustrated.

It is equally important that information not be forced upon patients. Individual's cultural values vary with respect to truth-telling about serious and incurable illness, and this can be highly problematic for the health care team. Sometimes, too, there may be gaps between generations within communities; younger members of the community may consider it important that seniors be told about a fatal prognosis while older members may continue to believe that information about serious illness should not be shared with the individual who is dying (Fisher et al. 2000).

More difficult for patients and nurses is that physicians often believe that they tell patients the truth, even when the information given is considerably modified. This occurs, for example, when patients are given information about their treatments but blurred information about their prognoses, rendering a flexible meaning to the truth. To be fair, such vagueness—at least in the way patients understand what has been told to them—may occur for at least two additional reasons. Physicians may try to tell the truth about the person's condition in a sensitive and careful way that in fact has the effect of obscuring the message, or patients may not be able to comprehend the bad news at the first telling.

In 1984, Jameton raised yet another problem. He stated that, for nurses, sharing difficult news with people who are dying is not simply a matter of *what* to tell. Concomitant questions are *who* is to do the telling, and who *will* tell if those entrusted to tell do not make it their responsibility to do so. Unfortunately, some 26 years later, assurance that people will receive a full disclosure of their terminal condition is not yet universal (Krisman-Scott 2000; Starzomski 2009), although significant progress has been made (Yeo and Khan 2010).

FOSTERING FAMILY AND FRIEND SUPPORT

Just as birth should be an event supported by family and friends, so should death be (Chambers-Evans 2002; Kuhl 2002). It is a time of "people needing people" to assist them in a significant life passage. Thus, for example, the writers of a protocol for decision making at one major urban hospital emphasized that end-of-life decisions require collaboration among the patient, family, family physician, and health professionals to fulfill an imperative to give appropriate and compassionate care (Rodney et al. 1999). These writers also spoke to culturally sensitive end-of-life care that acknowledges diverse value systems within and between diverse cultures and ethnic communities. Urging that stereotyping be avoided, this directive includes the need for health professionals to recognize that "patients from other cultures and/or ethnic groups may defer to the wishes of their family to avoid conflict and to fulfill their duty to their family. Decisions may be made as a unit, rather than by the patient" and "families may decline to give permission to limit aggressive care, since this might be seen as a sign of disrespect for the patient" (Rodney et al. 1999, 30; see also Chapter 13).

While most advance directives focus on allowing medical interventions (or not), other aspects of care are also critical to an individual's final days of life, as illustrated in Ethics in Practice 17-4.

ETHICS IN PRACTICE 17-4

Saying Good-bye: Who Is in Control?

A 45-year-old actor with a wide network of admirers and a close group of friends was diagnosed with cancer at too late a stage to respond to treatment. He subsequently died within only a few months of his diagnosis. He had left some fairly clear messages about his treatment wishes but had not left directives about who he wished to see before he died. Because he became confused and semi-comatose much sooner than expected, decisions about who was allowed to see him during wakeful periods were taken over by someone who did not seem to appreciate who his closest friends were nor sympathize with those who needed to see him to say goodbye.

Those who are dying need to make clear what is important to them in their final days. Since they may not be able to anticipate how soon they may become incapable of being the decision-maker, nurses can assist patients in thinking ahead, and making notes about what the dying person wishes to do and whom they wish to see. If they are alert to their needs for final connection, and the needs of their friends, the well-being of those grieving their loss can also be recognized and addressed.

Researchers emphasize the importance of attending to cultural and personal meaning and support. For instance, in a study of ways in which patients participate in end-of-life decision making, Sahlberg-Blom, Ternestedt, and Johansson (2000) found that patients' participation in care planning could be classified according to four main variations in participation with respect to decision making: self-determination, co-determination, delegation, and nonparticipation. These authors suggest that their findings support the notion that people's dying and death are a reflection of the way they have lived.

LISTENING, REFLECTING, AND DEVELOPING TRUST

Kuhl (2002) found that most people who are at the end of life need to know that someone is listening to them. Byock (2003) emphasizes that a core value for end-of-life care is community. She maintains that as a community we have certain commitments to each other, including keeping company with those who are suffering and dying so that they will not be alone and not be abandoned. She speaks of this type of obligation as a covenantal value involving trust and connection. Among our responsibilities to the dying is the enhancement of their quality of life and the life of the community by bearing witness and promoting opportunity. In bearing witness, we promise to listen to their stories and to remember the stories of their passing. In promoting opportunity, we remember that "some people change in ways that are valuable and important to them and their families during the time they are dying. . . . [In] reviewing their lives, sharing bad news, reconciling (when needed) and exploring existential and spiritual aspects of life, some people value assistance" (Byock 2003, S41). This may be the greatest gift that nurses and other caregivers can give to the dying. Attentive listening and reflecting back to an individual what we are hearing are powerful ways to assist another to understand him or herself and others in new ways. It is in *hearing oneself talk,* and knowing what has been heard, that clarification occurs. And since attentive listening builds relationships, trust can develop between nurse and patient.

NURSES AND PALLIATIVE CARE

In a CBC Radio interview on November 29, 2010, Balfour Mount, founder of palliative care in Canada, stated that the goal of palliative care is exclusively to enhance the quality of life of a person who is dying. He also noted that these are the sickest people with the most complex needs; this was the reason palliative care became a specialty in the United Kingdom in 1987. Responding to a challenge that the connotation of palliative care means "giving up," he stated that dying is *part of the human voyage* and that dying is charged with special potential for the person and his or her significant others. They will carry that legacy of care. Mount stated that "As we die, we become healed."

Carstairs (2010), a Canadian senator and advocate for palliative care over a 15-year period, provides a definition for palliative care that accords with Mount's concept. She states that palliative care in its broadest sense,

> . . . is used to refer to whole-person health care that aims to relieve suffering and improve the quality of living and dying. It is multi-disciplinary. It includes all settings of care, such as the home, the community, the residential hospice, and the hospital. It is care that starts at diagnosis of a life-threatening condition, carries through until death and continues on into bereavement care. (6)

Carstairs believes it should be the right of every Canadian to have access to palliative care (7). She also drew attention to the reality that sudden death occurs for only 10 percent of Canadians: 90 percent will die from either a terminal illness, organ failure, or frailty and will likely need palliative care. She outlined a vision for palliative care to include developing a culture of care, building capacity, support for caregivers, integration of services, and greater leadership in palliative care (16). Carstairs' vision is that this care should be available to patients and their family members regardless of whether or not they are in a designated palliative care unit since palliative care principles need to be part of practice in all areas of nursing. Stadjuhar (2011) supports this view with a modified definition of palliative care, which she and her team describe as "an approach to care focused on improving the quality of life of persons with life-limiting conditions, and their families. It is provided in all health care settings." (10-11)[5] Many believe that if such palliative care services were available to all people, requests to legalize assisted suicide and euthanasia would diminish. While the three of us who have authored this chapter support that belief, we also believe it is important to better understand such requests.

ASSISTED SUICIDE AND EUTHANASIA IN CANADA

While a variety of definitions are provided for euthanasia and assisted suicide, widely used Canadian definitions are provided by Dickens, Boyle, and Ganzini (2008). "Euthanasia is defined as a deliberate act undertaken by one person with the intention of ending the life of another person to relieve that person's suffering"; whereas assisted suicide "has been defined as intentionally killing oneself with the assistance of another who deliberately provides the knowledge, means, or both" (72).

Most researchers, legal experts, and philosophers write and speak about assisted suicide and euthanasia in somewhat apologetic terms, knowing that for many, these are troubling, emotionally laden, and spiritually conflicting matters. This was the context in which the Select Committee of the Parliament of Quebec released a consultation document on "Dying with Dignity" in May 2010. In introducing what the committee described as a delicate subject, they drew attention to the legal cases of Nancy B. and Sue Rodriguez (see Endnote 2) as raising questions that need to be addressed. In addition to recognizing the intense debates on euthanasia and assisted suicide, they coin a term, *therapeutic obstinacy,* that they define as "use of aggressive treatment to prolong the life of a patient in the terminal stages of an illness, with no real hope of improving his or her condition" (Select Committee 2010, 10).

The Quebec Select Committee provides other definitions to refine the discussion about euthanasia and assisted suicide as they review the law (the Criminal Code of Canada, the Civil Code of Quebec, and Canadian and Quebec Charters of Rights) providing case examples to complement this discussion. Based on international comparisons, questions are raised for public reflection about what could be acceptable in addressing compassionate, ethical end-of-life care.

Several years earlier, Downie (2004), a leading legal-ethical expert in Canada, published her treatise for decriminalizing euthanasia and assisted suicide. Downie argued for clarification and reform of Canadian law and practices, noting that the "absence of a clear legislative or judicial statement on withholding and withdrawing potentially life-sustaining treatment and providing for potentially life-shortening palliative care" (3) was causing a number of harms to people at the end of life. These harms included receiving unwanted treatment, variations in treatment across the country, not receiving adequate pain control, experiencing the practice of defensive medicine, requiring people to press their case before the courts of law; and having law made on a case-by-case basis with inconsistencies and confusion as a result (3–4). After carefully dissecting the criminal law as well as other provincial legislation, and international experiences in relation to euthanasia, she provided recommendations of how laws should be understood and reformed with respect to withdrawing medical treatment, assisted suicide, and euthanasia.

Many others have entered into these debates for or against euthanasia and assisted suicide (see for example, Moreno 1995 and Jeffrey 2009), and, as noted at the outset of this chapter, more books of readings contain stories and arguments for and against these practices as well. So too have nurses been engaged in these discussions. One prime example is recorded in an article by Quaghebeur et al. (2009) in which the authors conducted a thorough review of argument-based ethics literature complete with a detailed table of their findings. Overall, they found "a lack of consensus among nurses on euthanasia in general, and on their involvement in particular" (483). These authors suggested that nurses need to focus their attention on this debate, and they outlined four specific areas including better analysis, sound dialogue, position papers and codes of ethics from professional nursing organizations, and participation of nurses in the public debates (483). A second example is presented by Begley (2008) who defended a known legal case of voluntary active euthanasia by a physician, constructing her defense from the perspective of virtue ethics. Her aim in doing so was to encourage critical reflection by nurses and other colleagues on euthanasia and assisted suicide. Begley's paper was published in the journal *Nursing Ethics* where the editors, invited others to comment and respond, and a rebuttal by the author was included. This type of dialogue is needed to help nurses critically reflect on situations of this sort in advance, as urged in Chapter 1 of this book.

A challenge for nurses entering into dialogue about euthanasia and assisted suicide will be to set aside prejudices of the past, clarify their personal and professional values, and be open to contextual considerations. An important goal of such dialogue is to advocate for refining laws and guidelines in ways that are clearly understood and that are ethical.

NURSES LEADING AND INFLUENCING CHANGE IN END-OF-LIFE CARE

Nurses need to consider ways in which they can lead and influence change in regard to end-of-life care. It is critical that palliative care be available to everyone in need of it; nurses have a pivotal role in ensuring that this happens. Mount (2010) provides reasons why palliative care is a specialty, and there is a pressing need to make that specialized, complex care a reality for *all*. For example, we know that in some parts of Canada the philosophy of hospice care in the community is well entrenched, and health services are provided to make a "good death" possible. But, despite numerous calls for greater access to palliative care across Canada (Canadian Hospice Palliative Care Association 2002; Commission on the Future of Health Care in Canada 2002; National Health Forum 1997; Ferris et al. 2002; Report of the Special Senate Subcommittee 1995; Report of the Special Senate Subcommittee Report 2000), many Canadians do not have access to such care as they enter their final months and days. In fact, at this time for instance, only a small majority are admitted to hospice, while thousands die waiting (to get into hospice or other programs of palliative care) in crowded hospital wards or alone at home. The absence of end-of-life care attuned to the needs of the dying creates a moral imperative for nurses to become more sensitized to the dying and more capable of doing their part to foster and provide care that leads to a good death (Canadian Nurses Association 2008; McCarthy, Donnelly, Dooley et al. 2010).[6] This is particularly important given the changing culture of health care organizations (with and without walls) where such care might be considered a frill rather than an evidence-informed practice.

All health professionals who work with patients at the end of life must see it as their role to ask patients about their wishes, listen to their responses, and urge them to document those wishes and communicate them to their family members or substitute decision-makers. When patients are unable to carry out this task without assistance, nurses and physicians should enable this work in whatever way they can. To ensure such assistance can be given, all health professionals need education about advance directives and about discovering an individual's wishes, transmitting those wishes to others, and respecting those wishes (Blondeau et al. 2000; Justin and Johnson 1989; Robinson 2011; Storch 1998).

Trusting relationships are critical to ensuring that individuals' wishes are understood, that they receive their desired type of assistance in managing their discomfort, and that they receive full information to meet their needs. Moral imperatives for nurses underscore the need for nurses to enhance their education in end-of-life care and to be the catalysts to improve end-of-life care. In order to succeed in carrying out these moral imperatives, nurses must show leadership at the micro, meso, and macro levels of the health care system and be involved in ethical decision making at all these levels (see Chapters 4, 9, 13, and 18).

At the *micro level,* nurses have a responsibility to provide compassionate, competent, and ethical end-of-life care. They must provide education about end-of-life care in a manner that individuals and their families can understand (Canadian Nurses Association 2008). Nurses have a unique role to play in encouraging people to

> . . . express their goals and desires related to end-of-life care (for example preferred location of death, choices about organ donation, and whether or not they would like life-sustaining treatments such as cardiopulmonary resuscitation, artificial nutrition and hydration, dialysis and mechanical ventilation). The plan of care should include current and future treatment options, as well as the right to refuse treatment (Canadian Nurses Association 2008, 11; see also, Price 2003).

If nurses are to assist people to make good ethical decisions, then they need to understand and emphasize the importance of interdisciplinary team communication and collaboration and continue to strive for better collaborative methods of delivering end-of-life care.

At the *meso level,* all nurses must advocate for programs that provide access to end-of-life care. Nurses can help shape the programs, guidelines, and policies that provide direction for this care by participating in local working groups, ethics committees, and program evaluation committees. In Chapter 18 of this book we explore how nurses can enact their leadership in organizations and in policy work.

When developing curricula, nurse educators must ensure that undergraduate and graduate nursing programs, as well as continuing education programs, include content about end-of-life and palliative care. Nurse researchers have a role to play in establishing programs of research aimed at ensuring that quality end-of-life care can be identified and provided to ensure optimal outcomes for those requiring it. End-of-life situations are not limited to elderly people or to people with cancer. Nurses need to understand better the needs of all persons who require end-of-life care and to determine the most effective ways of delivering that care. Nurse researchers such as Kelli Stajduhar (2011) and her team in British Columbia are doing just that as they advance the palliative approach to care in areas outside of the realm of cancer care where palliative care has been most visible (see endnote 5).

At the *macro level* of the system, we need a collaborative approach to care as we work together with members of the public and governments to improve end-of-life care for all citizens. Nurses have the knowledge and skill to assist in the development of health care and public policy (including legislation that pertains to health care consent and advance directives) that enhances the access people have to the type of end-of-life care they require when and where they need it. In the creation and dissemination of health care and public policy, emphasis should be placed on the need to encourage more open, public discussion about resource allocation for end-of-life care to ensure that all societal voices are heard, values respected, and the best decisions are made about the just allocation of health care resources.

Summary

In this chapter, several topics have been explored based upon the authors' research, experience, and the findings of others. The meaning of a "good death" was discussed with a detailed case situation provided to illustrate the many elements comprising a good death. Care at the end of life, along with attention to advance directives (living wills) was explored with an analysis of public and health professional constraints in developing such directives. Pain and symptom relief, through specialized care (palliative care) was shown to be improved, and situations were described that *may* add to a dying individual's pain. The importance of providing truthful and fulsome information was highlighted by a particular case showing the negative impacts of withholding information. At the same time, sensitivity to how much information individuals and families may want was underscored. Supporting those dying, their families, and their friends was emphasized with examples of different ways those individuals can be supported.

Although much has been done in the last number of years to ensure that end-of-life care services and programs are available to all who need them, there are still challenges to be met. Leadership by nurses and other interdisciplinary health care team members, along with the ideas, support, and commitment of all citizens, will ensure that end-of-life care will receive the attention required. We need to move beyond rhetoric to a place where there is true collaboration and consultation among members of our communities as we strive to open moral space for continued societal ethical discourse about the provision of optimal end-of-life care.

For Reflection

1. Consider situations you might describe as continuations of futile care at the end of life. Does the concept of "futility" assist or impede good decision making in end-of-life care? Does a change of terminology, for example, "inappropriate care" make a difference toward enhancing better decision making?

2. In your experience with DNR orders, what types of guidelines are most helpful to you and other nurses in sound implementation of such policies?

3. What are the predominant factors, in your experience, that have prevented greater attention to advance directives? What role do you see for advance practice nurses in creating a better environment for discovering, recording, and transmitting patients' wishes about their end-of-life care?

4. What role might nurses take in fostering better communication amongst health professionals, families, and individuals in end-of-life care?

5.   In your role, what do you think you can do to enhance end-of-life care in your setting and in your community?

Endnotes

1.   Since the beginning of bioethics, matters of death and dying have received significant attention (Dugdale 2010). Almost all major books of readings on bioethics or health ethics (Canadian and American) have focused on conceptual ethical problems, such as determination of death, neurological determination of death, brain death, persistent vegetative state, euthanasia or mercy killing, prolongation of life, death and dignity, assisted suicide, cessation of treatment, and resuscitative interventions. More recently there is renewed emphasis on advance treatment directives, substitute decision making, and quality of end-of-life care. The books of readings referred to include those by Baylis et al. (2004); Beauchamp and Walters (1978 or 1982); Gorovitz et al. (1976), Kluge (1999), Singer and Viens (2008); and Yeo et al. (2010).

2.   In addition, a number of Canadian legal cases have made more visible the conceptual and practical ethical concerns at the end of life. Examples of cases that focused on self-determination are the cases of Nancy B. and Sue Rodriquez, cases of substitute decision making are Golubchuk and Tyrell Dueck, and a case of mercy killing is the case of Tracy Latimer. The reader would do well to become acquainted with these legal cases. Information about the cases of *Nancy B. (N) v. Hotel Dieu de Quebec, Rodriguez v. British Columbia (Attorney General), and R. v. Latimer* are summarized in Baylis et al. (2004), and discussed in Moorhouse, Yeo, and Rodney (2010). The case of Tyrell Dueck (a 13-year-old boy) is noted briefly in Moorhouse et al.2010, and the case of *Golubchuk v. Salvation Army Grace General Hospital et al.* 2008 is available through the Court of Queen's Bench of Manitoba.

3.   This Ethics in Practice 17-1 account is written as a tribute to Sharon Nield. At the time of her diagnosis, Sharon was director of nursing policy at the Canadian Nurses Association, where she had previously served as a nursing policy consultant since 1990. In the latter position, she was the CNA person responsible for ethics. Sharon was instrumental in developing the ethics program at CNA to maximize ethics education following the publication of the 1997 Code of Ethics, and she was instrumental in preparing for the 2002 Code of Ethics revision. Under her guidance, the *Everyday Ethics* booklet to serve as companion to the 1997 Code of Ethics was developed, and five of a series of "Ethics in Practice" papers were commissioned. She was instrumental in facilitating breakfast or noon-hour sessions for nurses involved and interested in ethics who were attending the Canadian Bioethics Society Annual Conferences and the Canadian Nurses Association Biennial Conferences.

4.   For a thoughtful analysis of disclosure as a concept, including how disclosure should be approached, see d'Agincourt-Canning and Johnston (2008).

5.   For example, in 2011, Dr. Stajduhar and a colleague were awarded a four-year infrastructure team grant from the Michael Smith Foundation for Health Research in British Columbia to address the question, "How and in which contexts can a palliative approach better meet the needs of patients with a life-limiting illness and their family members and guide the development of innovations in health care delivery systems to better support nursing practice and the health system?" Through a bulletin posted on their website, they invite other nurses to participate in answering their research questions. Visit www.ipanel.ca. iPANEL stands for "Initiative for a Palliative Approach in Nursing Evidence and Leadership."

6.   Working with the Irish Hospice Foundation, McCarthy (2010) and her colleagues in Ireland have prepared a series of eight study sessions suitable for a noon-hour discussion for nurses and other health professionals. The sessions include topics germane to nurses and other health professionals

involved in end-of-life care. Topics such as "The Ethics of Breaking Bad News," "The Ethics of Managing Pain," "The Ethics of Life-Prolonging Treatments (LPTs)," and "The Ethics of Confidentiality" are included. These study sessions are complete with cases for discussion and they are accessible from http://www. hospicefriendlyhospitals.net/ethics.

References

Baylis, F., Downie, J., Hoffmaster, B., and Sherwin, S. (Eds.), 2004. *Health care ethics in Canada* (2nd ed.). Toronto: Thomson Nelson.

Beauchamp, T.L. and Walters, L. (Eds.). 1978, 1982. *Contemporary issues in bioethics* (2nd ed.). Belmont, CA: Wadsworth Publishing Co.

Begley, A.M. 2008. Guilty but good: Defending voluntary active euthanasia from a virtue perspective. *Nursing Ethics, 15* (4), 434–445.

Blondeau, D., Lavoie, M., Valois, P., Keyserlingk, E.W., Hebert, M., and Martineau, I. 2000. The attitude of Canadian nurses towards advance directives. *Nursing Ethics, 7* (5), 399–411.

Byock, I. 2003. Rediscovering community at the core of the human condition and social covenant. In B. Jennings, T. Ryndes, C. D'Onofrio, and M.A. Baily (Eds.), "Access to Hospice Care: Expanding Boundaries, Overcoming Barriers." *Hastings Center Report,* Special Supplement (S40–S41). New York: The Hastings Center.

Callahan, D. 1991. Medical futility, medical necessity: The problem-without-a-name. *Hastings Center Report, 21* (4), 30–35.

Canadian Healthcare Association, Canadian Medical Association, Canadian Nurses Association, and the Catholic Hospital Association. 1999. *Joint Statement on preventing and resolving ethical conflicts involving health care providers and persons receiving care.* Ottawa: Authors.

Canadian Hospice Palliative Care Association. 2002. *Canadian strategy for palliative and end-of-life-care.* Available online: http://www.chpca.net/canadian_strategy_for_palliative_and_eol_care

Canadian Nurses Association. 2001. *Futility presents many challenges for nurses.* Ethics in Practice series paper. Ottawa: Author.

Canadian Nurses Association. 2008. *Providing nursing care at the end of life. Position Statement.* Ottawa: Author.

Carstairs, S. 2005. *Still not there: Quality end of life care: A progress report.* Ottawa: The Senate of Canada.

Carstairs, S. 2010. *Raising the bar: A roadmap for the future of palliative care in Canada.* Ottawa: The Senate of Canada.

Chambers-Evans, J. 2002. The family as window onto the world of the patient: Revising our approach to involving patients and families in the decision-making process. *Canadian Journal of Nursing Research, 34* (3), 15–32.

Commission on the Future of Health Care in Canada. 2002. *Building on values: The future of health care in Canada.* Ottawa: Commission on the Future of Health Care in Canada.

Corley, M.C. 1995. Moral distress for critical care nurses. *American Journal of Critical Care, 4* (4), 280–285.

Corley, M.C. 2002. Nurse moral distress: A proposed theory and research agenda. *Nursing Ethics, 9* (6), 636–650.

d'Agincourt-Canning, L., and Johnston, C. 2008. Disclosure. In P.A. Singer and A.M. Viens (Eds.), *The Cambridge textbook of bioethics* (pp. 24–30). Cambridge: Cambridge University Press.

Davies, B., Brown, P., Reimer, J., and Martens, N. 1995. *Fading away: The experience of transition in families with terminal illness.* New York: Baywood Publishing Company, Incorporated.

De Wolf, G.D., Gregg, R.J., Harris, B.P., and Scargill, M.H. 1997. *Gage Canadian Dictionary.* Toronto: Gage Educational Publishing Company.

Dickens, B.M., Boyle, J.M., and Ganzini, L. 2008. Euthanasia and assisted suicide. In P.A. Singer and A.M. Viens (Eds.), *The Cambridge textbook of bioethics* (pp. 72–76). Cambridge: Cambridge University Press.

Downie, J. 2004. *Dying justice: A case for decriminalizing euthanasia and assisted suicide in Canada.* Toronto: University of Toronto Press.

Dugdale, L. 2010. The art of dying well. *Hastings Center Report, 40* (6), 22–24.

Ferris, F.D., Balfour, H.M., Bowen, K., Farley, J., Hardwick, M., Lamontagne, C., Lundy, M., Syme, A., and West, P.J. 2002. *A model to guide hospice palliative care: Based on national principles and norms of practice.* Toronto: Canadian Hospice Palliative Care Association.

Fisher, R., Ross, M.M., and MacLean, M.J. 2000. *A guide to end-of-life care.* Ottawa: University of Ottawa.

Fletcher, J. 1954. *Morals and medicine.* Princeton, NJ: Princeton University Press.

Fry, S.T. and Johnstone, M.J. 2008. *International Council of Nurses ethics in nursing practice: A guide to ethical decision making* (3rd ed.). Oxford: Blackwell Publishing.

Gaudine, A., LeFort, S.M., Lamb, M., and Thorne, L. 2011. Clinical ethical conflicts of nurses and physicians. *Nursing Ethics, 18* (1), 9–19.

Glaser, B.G. and Strauss, A.L. 1965. *Awareness of dying.* Chicago: Aldine Publishing Co.

Godkin, M.D. 2002. *Apprehending death: The older adult's experience of preparing and advance directive.* Unpublished doctoral dissertation. University of Alberta, Edmonton.

Gorovitz, S., Jameton, A.E., Macklin, R., O'Connor, J.M., Perrin, E.V., St. Clair, B., and Sherwin, S. 1976. *Moral problems in medicine.* Englewood Cliffs, NJ: Prentice Hall, Inc.

Hamric, A.B. and Blackhall, L.J. 2007. Nurse-physician perspectives on the care of dying patients in intensive care units: Collaboration, moral distress, and ethical climate. *Critical Care Medicine, 35* (2), 422–429.

Hunter, S. 2000. Determination of moral negligence in the context of the undermedication of pain by nurses. *Nursing Ethics, 7* (5), 380–391.

Jameton, A. 1984. *Nursing practice: The ethical issues.* Englewood Cliffs, NJ: Prentice Hall.

Jeffrey, D. 2009. *Against physician assisted suicide: A palliative care perspective.* New York: Radcliffe Publishing.

Justin, R.G. and Johnson, R.A. 1989. Recording end-of-life directives on hospital admission. *Nursing Management, 20* (3), 65–68.

Keatings, M. and Smith O. 2010. *Ethical & legal issues in Canadian nursing* (3rd ed.). Toronto: Elsevier.

Kluge, E-H. W. (Ed.). 1999. *Readings in biomedical ethics: A Canadian focus.* Scarborough, ON: Prentice Hall Canada Inc.

Krisman-Scott, M.A. 2000. An historical analysis of disclosure of terminal status. *Journal of Nursing Scholarship,* First Quarter, 47–52.

Kubler-Ross, E. 1969. *On death and dying.* New York: Macmillan.

Kuhl, D. 1998. *Hospital bioethics committee: DNR Task Force.* Vancouver: St. Paul's Hospital.

Kuhl, D. 2002. *What dying people want: Practical wisdom for the end of life.* Toronto: Doubleday Canada.

Kuhl, D. and Wilensky, P. 1999. Decision-making at the end of life: A model using an ethical grid and principles of group process. *Journal of Palliative Medicine, 2* (1), 75–86.

Law Reform Commission of Canada. 1981. *Criteria for the determination of death.* Ottawa: Author.

Law Reform Commission of Canada. 1982. *Euthanasia, aiding suicide and cessation of treatment.* Working Paper 28. Ottawa: Author.

McCarthy, J., Donnelly, M., Dooley, D., Campbell, L., and Smith, D. 2010. *An ethical framework for end of life care. Modules 1–8.* Dublin: Irish Hospice Foundation.

Moorhouse, A., Yeo, M., and Rodney, P. (2010). "Autonomy." In M. Yeo, A. Moorhouse, P. Kahn, and Rodney, P. (Eds.), *Concepts and cases in nursing ethics* (3rd ed.; 143–205). Peterborough, ON: Broadview Press.

Moreno, J. (Ed.). 1995. *Arguing euthanasia.* Toronto: Simon and Schuster.

Mount, B. 2010. CBC Radio interview conducted by Michael Enright, November 29.

National Health Forum. 1997. *Canada health action: Building on the legacy.* Final report of the National Health Forum. (Volumes 1 and 2). Ottawa: Minister of Public Works and Government Services.

Price, C. 2003. Resources for planning palliative and end of life care for patients with kidney disease. *Nephrology Nursing Journal, 30* (6), 649–664.

Puopolo, A.L., Kennard, M.J., Mallatratt, L., Follen, M.A., Desbiens, N.A., Conners, A.F., Califf, R., Walzer, J., Soukup, J., Davis, R.B., and Phillips, R.S. 1997. Preferences for cardiopulmonary resuscitation. *Journal of Nursing Scholarship, 29* (3), 229–235.

Quaghebeur, T., Dierckx de Casterle, B., and Gastmans, C. 2009. Nursing and euthanasia: A review of argument-based ethics literature. *Nursing Ethics, 16* (4), 466–486.

Regan, T. (Ed.). 1980. *Matters of life and death: New introductory essays in moral philosophy.* New York: Random House.

Standing Committee on Social Affairs, Science and Technology. 2000. *Report of the Special Senate Subcommittee to update Of Life and Death.* Chaired by S. Carstairs and G.A. Beaudoin. Ottawa: Supply and Services.

Report of the Special Senate Committee on Euthanasia and Assisted Suicide. 1995. *Of life and death.* Ottawa: Supply and Services.

Robinson, C.A. 2011. Advance care planning: Re-visioning our ethical approach. *Canadian Journal of Nursing Research, 43* (2).18–37.

Rodney, P., Dodek, P., Thompson, T., Kuhl, D., Calam, B., Chung, M., Jolliffe, C., and Nicholson, R. 1999. *Constructing bioethics policy through stakeholder participation and collaboration: Development of the St. Paul's hospital "do not resuscitate" protocol.* Unpublished manuscript. Vancouver: St. Paul's Hospital.

Rodney, P. and Howlett, J. 2003. *Elderly patients with cardiac disease: Quality of life, end of life, and ethics.* (Paper in unpublished Canadian Cardiovascular Society Consensus Document on the Elderly and Cardiac Disease.)

Rodney, P.A., Thompson, T., Calam, B., Chung, M., Frost, L., Jolliffe, C., Murphy, K., McKenzie, L., Mulcahy, M., Dodek, P., Young, D., Mackinnon, M., Kuhl, D., and Budz, B. 2002a. *Constructing bioethics policy through consensus building and community participation: An evaluation of the St. Paul's Hospital DNR Protocol.* Unpublished research report sent to Providence Health Care and the Associated Medical Services Incorporated (Bioethics Division).

Rodney, P., Varcoe, C., Storch, J.L., McPherson, G., Mahoney, K., Brown, H., Pauly, B., Hartrick, G., and Starzomski, R. 2002b. Navigating towards a moral horizon: A multisite qualitative study of ethical practice in nursing. *Canadian Journal of Nursing Research, 34* (3), 75–102. Reprinted in *Canadian Journal of Nursing Research, 41* (1), 292–319.

Rodney, P., Doane, G.H., Storch, J., and Varcoe, C. 2006. Toward a safer moral climate. *Canadian Nurse, 102* (8), 24–27.

Sahlberg-Blom, E., Ternestedt, B.M., and Johansson, J.E. 2000. Patient participation in decision-making at the end of life as seen by a close relative. *Nursing Ethics, 7* (4), 296–313.

Salas, A.S. and Cameron, B.L. 2010. Ethical openings in palliative home care practice. *Nursing Ethics, 17* (5), 655–665.

Scanlon, C. 1996. Nurses as catalysts for improving end-of-life care. *Center for Ethics and Human Rights Communique.* Washington, DC: American Nurses Association, *5* (1), 1–2.

Schneiderman, L., Jecker, N., and Jonsen, A. 1990. Medical futility: Its meanings and ethical implications. *Annals of Internal Medicine, 11 2*(12), 949–954.

Schultz, L. 1997. Not for resuscitation: Two decades of challenge for nursing ethics and practice. *Nursing Ethics, 4* (3), 227–238.

Select Committee of the Parliament of Quebec. 2010. *Dying with dignity: A consultation document.* Quebec City, QC: National Assembly.

Singer, P.A. 1994. Advance directives in palliative care. *Journal of Palliative Care, 10* (3), 111–116.

Singer, P.A. and Viens, A.M. (Eds.). 2008. *The Cambridge textbook of bioethics.* Cambridge: Cambridge University Press.

Stajduhar, K.I. 2011. Chronic illness, palliative care, and the problematic nature of dying. *Canadian Journal of Nursing Research, 43* (3), 7–15.

Starzomski, R. 2009. Truth-telling at the end of life. *Canadian Association of Nephrology Nurses and Technicians Journal, 19* (2) 36–37.

Storch, J. 1998. Advancing our thinking about advance directives: Ethics at the end of life. In E. Banister (Ed.) *Focus on research: Mary Richmond lecture series* (pp. 73–91). Victoria: University of Victoria School of Nursing.

Storch, J., Rodney, P., Hartick, G., Varcoe, C., and Starzomski, R. 2000. *The ethics of practice: Context and curricular implications for nursing.* Victoria: University of Victoria.

Storch, J.L., Rodney, P., and Starzomski, R. 2009. Ethics and health care in Canada. In B.S. Bolaria and H.D. Dickinson (Eds.), *Health, illness and health care in Canada* (pp. 409–444). Toronto: Nelson Thomson Learning.

Storch, J.L., Rodney, P., Pauly, B., Brown, H., and Starzomski, R. 2002. Listening to nurses' moral voices: Building a quality health care environment. *Canadian Journal of Nursing Leadership, 15* (4), 7–16.

Taylor, C. 1995. Medical futility and nursing. *Journal of Nursing Scholarship, 27* (4), 301–306.

Thomas, D. 1969. Do not go gentle into that good night. In C.M. Coffin (Ed.), *The major poets: English and American* (2nd ed.; p. 553). New York: Harcourt Brace Jovanovich.

Tulsky, J.A., Emanuel, L.L., Martin, D.K., and Singer, P.A. 2008. Advance care planning. In P.A. Singer and A.M. Viens (Eds.). *The Cambridge textbook of bioethics* (pp. 65–71). Cambridge: Cambridge University Press.

Varcoe, C. and Rodney, P. 2003. Trends and new thinking. In G. Doane (Ed.), *Rethinking ethics education in nursing* (pp. 40–59). Unpublished manuscript. University of Victoria School of Nursing, Victoria, B.C.

Varcoe, C., Hartrick, G., Pauly, B., Rodney, P., Storch, J.L., Mahoney, K., McPherson, G., Brown, H., and Starzomski, R. 2004. Ethical practice in nursing—Working the in-betweens. *Journal of Advanced Nursing, 45* (3), 316–325.

Varcoe, C., Pauly, P., Storch, J., Schick Makaroff, K., and Newton, L. In review. Nurses perceptions and responses to morally distressing situations.

Venneman, S., Narnor-Harris, P., Perish, M., and Hamilton, M. 2008. Allow natural death versus do not resuscitate: Three words that can change a life. *Journal of Medical Ethics, 34,* 2–6.

White, K.R., Coyne, P.J., and Patel, U.B. 2001. Are nurses adequately prepared for end of life care? *Journal of Nursing Scholarship,* Second Quarter, 147–151.

Yeo, M. and Khan, P. 2010. Truthfulness. In M. Yeo, A. Moorhouse, P. Khan, and P. Rodney (Eds.), *Concepts and cases in nursing ethics* (3rd ed.; 207–220). Peterborough, ON: Broadview Press.

Yeo, M., Moorhouse, A., Khan, P., and Rodney, P. (Eds.). 2010. *Concepts and cases in nursing ethics* (3rd ed.). Peterborough, ON: Broadview Press.

Zronek, S., Daly, B., and Lee, H. 1999. Elderly patients' understanding of advance directives. *Journal of Nursing Administration's Healthcare Law, Ethics and Regulation, 1* (2), 23–28.

CHAPTER 18

A Further Landscape: Ethics in Health Care Organizations and Health/Health Care Policy[1]

Patricia Rodney, MaryLou Harrigan, Bashir Jiwani, Michael Burgess, and J. Craig Phillips

Nursing sees its professional mandate as solidly grounded within a set of values and ethical principles such as social justice, spirituality, cultural safety, but has considerable difficulty figuring out how these ideas might fit within the knowledge production and application arena in health care. (Thorne 2009, 150)

Throughout this book we have pointed to the importance of ethical action at individual, organizational, and larger societal levels to address the difficulty that Dr. Sally Thorne has articulated above. It is our premise that to actualize ethical practice requires that nurses and other health care professionals maintain the *integrity* of their practice at each level, *advocate* for resources at each level, and address the *interactivity* of action at each level[2] (Pellegrino 1979; Yeo et al. 2010; see also Exhibit 18-1).

EXHIBIT 18-1

Ethical Practice at All Levels

Ethical practice at the *micro* level involves decisions and policy about the allocation of resources (money, time, expertise) that primarily affect *individuals*. *Meso*-level practice involves decisions and policy *within* an institution or communities. *Macro*-level practice involves decisions and policy involving broader public policy issues and includes the allocation of resources *to* an institution or community—for example, decisions made by federal, provincial, and territorial governments about funding and priorities.

Micro, meso, and macro practice take place at *progressively higher levels of generality*. Decisions at a higher level of generality constrain decision making at a lower level of generality. For example, government macro allocation decisions about how much money will go to health as against other sectors establish limits that constrain allocation decisions *within* health spending. In turn, decisions at this level, such as how much money will go to hospitals as against community health, health promotion, and other programs, set limits on and constrain decision making at a lower level, such as *within* a hospital or a neighbourhood health centre. Eventually, we reach the micro level, at which decision makers allocate to or among individuals a resource that is limited in supply as a *consequence* of meso and macro allocations made at higher levels of generality. (Adapted from Yeo et al. 2010, 307–314)

As we indicated in Chapter 4, much of the original focus in bioethics was at the individual (micro) level. Yet we simultaneously need a firm grounding in organizational (meso) and societal (macro) influences on ethical practice, and we need to develop strategies that start to address these other two levels. *In other words, by recognizing the interactivity of ethical practice at each level we can work on policy and political action to advocate for all levels while still maintaining the integrity of our practice at each level.* For example, in addressing inadequate pain relief for home care clients who are recovering postoperatively we could ensure that we use best practices for pain management with our individual clients and their families, advocate for better discharge planning processes between hospital and home care organizations, and engage with our health regions and nursing associations to address the need for better home care support services provincially and nationally (see also Chapter 19). It is this challenge of extending our ethical expertise to meso and macro levels that we explicitly take up in this chapter. Acting with expertise at *all* levels is, we are convinced, the key to influencing knowledge production and application to benefit health and health care. While we are certainly not claiming to have the final word on ethical practice at organizational and societal levels, we do believe that what we offer in this chapter will be of use to our colleagues in nursing and other health care professions, health care ethics, and other fields such as policy analysis.

We start by laying out some of the powerful (and often unconscious) ideological influences operating in today's Western societies. We then follow by discussing how health care organizations might support ethical practice despite some of the negative influences of ideologies. This will lead us to begin to articulate how we might influence health and health care policy to actualize ethical practice at individual, organizational, and larger societal levels.

THE CONTEXT: THE MALAISE OF MODERNITY

The major forces of modernity significantly affect all areas of society, especially the health care system. Modernity, as a conceptual construction, has arisen over the past century or more as a complex nexus with many images—the unprecedented amalgam of new practices and institutional forms and new ways of living (Taylor 2001, 1). Recognition of the nature of the influences of modernity is paramount to understanding the challenges for contemporary health care and the implications for the ethics of organizations and policy development. Of course, modernity co-exists with postmodernity—the former based on a foundationalist philosophy of science where we look for "truths" and grand narratives of progress, and the latter questioning such certainty by pointing out that constructions of meaning and human power dynamics are inextricably interwoven in what we think we know and do (Crotty 1998).[3] In this chapter we are, in fact, offering a postmodern critique of some of the influences of modernity, and we are also using postmodern scholarship to open up possibilities for ethical action at all levels.

Over the past couple of decades, Canadian philosopher Charles Taylor's work has highlighted the disengaged instrumental and individual mode of life central to modernity, which he claims has resulted in a pervasive sense of malaise.[4] He argues that contemporary society has dissolved traditional communities and their ways of living with nature, resulting in fragmentation of identities so that those bound up in it lose their common purpose and communities are divided. The change both removes meaning from life and "threatens public freedom, that is, the institutions and practices of self-government" (Taylor 1989, 500). Thus, the negative consequences are two-fold: the individual experiences change that devalues heroism or higher purposes of life and the societal change causes disengagement and dissolution of traditional communities, marginalizing deeply entrenched values so as to replace community life with a series of mobile, changing, revocable associations (Taylor 1989, 500–502; see also Taylor 1991; 1994; 2004). In such a disengaged world, where each looks after him or herself, those who are seen as less worthy, or are "othered" (Canales 2010) because of attributes such as age, language fluency, physical ability, sexual orientation, and so forth, fare badly. *Two principal kinds of institutions in our society—the market and bureaucracy—reflect further aspects of the malaise: powerful steering mechanisms operate in impersonal ways, reducing moral responsibility for decisions that are made.* Together they give rise to decisions that are, "in a sense, in their aggregate form decided by nobody" (Taylor 1994, 175). Such features of modernity are problematic for ethical practice in Western society, and are especially incompatible with the cultural, feminist, and relational ethical perspectives we advocated for in Chapters 5 and 13—for instance, Aboriginal perspectives that emphasize interconnectedness between people and the land and transgenerational meaning (Ermine 2007).

MacIntyre, another fierce critic of modernity, attacks the failure of modernity (1984, 36–50) by painting an image of "catastrophe," all the more destructive because many are not even aware of it. He argues that the unifying frameworks necessary for coherent moral discourse have been lost so that human beings, regarded as atomistic individuals, cannot see themselves as having in common a meaning and purpose underpinning a shared conception of the ethical good. Notions of utility and of rights, he argues, are disconnected fictions because one cannot argue from individual desires to an interest in the good of others or to inviolable rights for all. Enlightenment liberalism cannot therefore construct a coherent ethics able to influence institutions so that they are conducive to care and a regard for shared human excellence. Lacking any way of giving substance to that goal, institutions can threaten to corrupt and demoralize practitioners by subordinating the pursuit of *the Good* to that of exchangeable or marketable *goods*. He claims that societal practices become dominated by bureaucracies and the marketplace, and that major forces for deprofessionalism, including commercialism and commodification of services, arise (MacIntyre 1984, 193–195).

Together, Taylor and MacIntyre provide serious critiques of what has been generally seen as "progress" in our society.[5] While we would also note that there have concurrently been significant areas of positive progress (e.g., in our philosophical commitment to human rights), the impact of the malaise of modernity on health and health care has been profound. Indeed, the challenges Taylor and MacIntyre portray are evident in many of the chapters of this text, particularly Chapters 9 through 11 and Chapters 19 through 21. Modernity is imbued with a strong ideology[6] of *liberal individualism*—an ideology that sees people as isolated, rational individuals who are "able" to choose what they need. Liberal individualism is largely blind to the contextual meanings and power dynamics that postmodern analyses would illuminate (Anderson et al. 2009; Browne 2001). And liberal individualism is closely tied to *globalization,* where monies too often flow around the world in a way that most benefits corporate elites (Saul 2005; 2008). In the meanwhile, there are widening inequities globally in the access to resources for the social determinants of health (such as income, food security, education, and child care) within and between countries (Coburn 2010; World Health Organization 2008a).[7] And there are widening inequities in access to health care within and between countries. This is certainly true in Canada, and is evident in most of the chapters of this text.

In 2002, the Commission on the Future of Health Care in Canada issued a groundbreaking report, *Building on Values: The Future of Health Care in Canada* (also known as the *Romanow Report*), which chronicled the results of continuing changes in health care services delivery combined with cost-cutting measures. The toll on those recipients of health care who are made most vulnerable in our society—including older adults, Aboriginal people, people living in rural and remote locations, and those with mental health problems—were noted as especially pronounced. And the impact on health care providers (at every level) working within the system has been significant (see also Chapters 10 and 11). The report noted that, while problems "differ for different health care providers, the malaise is widespread . . ." (Commission on the Future of Health Care in Canada 2002, 91). There are certainly areas of strength we can and should look to for hope and inspiration (Rachlis 2004)—such as the proliferation of interdisciplinary clinics to help people with chronic illnesses—but such areas of strength are somewhat isolated.

At the time this chapter is being written, despite a seemingly endless cascade of health care "reforms" across Canadian provinces (and notwithstanding areas of positive progress), the malaise of modernity has been growing worse, particularly in terms of cost constraints and their compounding impacts on health and health care delivery (Austin 2011; Coburn 2010; Health Council of Canada 2008; Rodney and Varcoe in press; Storch 2010). While the espoused intent of the health care reforms occurring in Canada and other Western countries is to improve the quality, accessibility, and sustainability of health care, the implementation of the reforms is fuelled by a powerful corporate ideology that views actions to save money in health care or other social services as inherently justifiable (Moorhouse and Rodney 2010; Myrick 2004; Rankin and Campbell 2006; Rodney and Varcoe in press; Stein 2001). *As the language of the "cult of efficiency" (Stein 2001) infiltrates the public institution of health care, health care professionals are expected to work under the ethos of efficiency as an end in itself and adopt it as a value more important than others.* When efficiency is elevated to an end in itself rather than a values-based means, Stein claims that it obscures the impact on individuals and it obscures questions of value and accountability.[8]

Further, an emphasis on efficiency can co-opt managers who may attempt to affect the actions of others by manipulation rather than by rational argument (Bakan 2004; MacIntyre 1984, 75–78).[9] Canadian historian John Ralston Saul observes that efficiency does not produce direction and that management is not leadership—it does not provide meaning, ideas, or purpose, but rather "works effectively as a function or servant of policy" (1999, 11). A focus on management at the expense of genuine effectiveness produces an increase in passivity and frustration among nurses, physicians, and other health providers who resent "being locked up in corporations." Saul argues that as mere functionaries, individuals cannot influence policy or choose directions of development, even when information is available from those who work in the system and appreciate its internal dynamics (1999, 14–15). Overall, what Taylor has called the malaise of modernity provides a challenging backdrop for ethical professional practice in health care organizations and ethical policy development (Kenny 2002; MacIntyre 1984; Saul 1999; Taylor 1989).

As a result, "some of the most pressing empirical and ethical questions facing us today are rooted in systemic inequities in access to resources for health and health care in Canada and around the globe" (Rodney 2011; see also Anderson et al. 2009; Austin 2003; 2004; Benatar and Brock 2011; Canadian Nurses Association 2009; World Health Organization 2008a; 2008b; Chapters 12, 19, 20, and 21). And, "as cost constraints proliferate in health-care delivery there are serious concomitant challenges to the moral agency of nurses and other health professionals" (Rodney 2011, 9; see also Austin 2011; Canadian Nurses Association and Registered Nurses Association of Ontario 2010; Pringle 2009; Rodney and Varcoe in press, as well as Chapters 9, 10, and 11). This leaves those of us working in nursing, ethics, and health care overall with organizational and policy challenges that are both practical and political. The challenges "are practical in the sense that we need to know more about how to make progress towards better ethical practice and policy, and political in the sense that we need to know more about how to foster stronger democratic dialogue within diverse care-delivery and policy structures" (Rodney 2011, 9). Yet most work in health care ethics "lacks a serious critical challenge to the organization of health practice and policy writ large" (Sherwin 2011, 77).

ETHICS IN HEALTH CARE ORGANIZATIONS

Given the challenges we have sketched out above, it is important to understand the ways in which the social processes of health care institutions affect health care practices and outcomes (Mishler 1981, 79). As Anderson, Blue, and Lau (1991) have stated, "the vocabularies of the larger social organization are reproduced in micro level interactions between [patients/families] and health professionals through a set of ideologies that structure health care delivery" (102). Thinking of ethics at the organizational level can help us to both unpack and strategize around these kinds of issues (see also Suhonen et al. 2011).

Organizations such as hospitals, long-term care facilities, community centres, and research institutes are characterized by hierarchy, a complex division of labour, administrative positions based on technical expertise and/or knowledge, collective outputs, reliance upon rules and policies, and multiple institutional/staff relationships (Buchanan 1996, 419–420). *Health care agencies are therefore entities that have responsibility and accountability that transcend the responsibility and accountability of individual health care providers.* These responsibilities and accountabilities simultaneously and reciprocally are shaped by and shape policy and law at local to global levels and are often codified in human rights documents.

Organizational Virtues

A relevant concept for our understanding of organizational ethics is that of the *common good*.[10] In MacIntyre's work, concepts of virtue, practice, tradition, and narrative units of moral experience create an ethical theory of the good (MacIntyre 1984; 1998; 1999). MacIntyre (1998) uses the example of a fishing crew to illustrate that the good of each member of the fishing crew cannot be characterized independently of the good common to all members of the crew. Thus, in his view, the space in which common goods are possible is the space of practices. The goods internal to the activity are relevant to answer questions about how the practices (i.e., ethical actions) in a community's life are to be ordered (MacIntyre 1998, 239–250).

MacIntyre builds his definition of virtue from three elements—from three acquired qualities. These elements are (1) necessary to achieve the good internal to practice; (2) necessary to sustain communities in which individuals can seek a "higher good" as the good of their own lives; and (3) necessary to sustain traditions that provide historical contexts. There is a complex relationship of virtues to practices and to institutions. The ability of a practice to retain its integrity will depend on the way in which the virtues can be and are exercised in sustaining institutions that are the social holders of the practice. "The integrity of a practice causally requires the exercise of the virtues by at least some of the individuals who embody it in their activities" (MacIntyre 1984, 195). The tension between the institutions (such as hospitals) and the practices (such as nursing and medicine) lies between the external goods and the internal goods: *MacIntyre argues that only through exercise of the virtues can the practice maintain its integrity.*

Health care organizations can be described as a collection of practices embedded in culture influenced by a mission and vision. By offering help, health care providers and the health care organization implicitly promise competence and good judgment in the interest of the person who seeks help. "This is their 'act of profession,' their commitment to the good of the patient" (Pellegrino 2004, 88). Health care organizations and the providers within them are all morally required to be faithful to this trust, and can therefore be thought of as members of *moral communities* (Aroskar 1995; see also Chapter 10 and Chapter 11). Discussing the relationship between hospitals and nursing practice, Day (2007) reflects that, "At best, the hospital supports and furthers the goods internal to nursing, such as attentiveness to the individual personhood of patients and protection of the vulnerable" (615); however, a hospital's commitment to efficiency and a hierarchal modernist focus can result in conflicts with goods internal to nursing and other health care providers. Indeed, MacIntrye warns that "Without virtues and a sense of tradition, practices cannot resist the corrupting power of institutions" (1984, 194).

Organizational Practices

Given the above, health care agencies have a role in the resolution *as well as* the creation of ethical problems in health care (Storch, Rodney, and Starzomski 2009). As we indicated at the outset of this chapter, attention to the ethics of organizations is a relatively new phenomenon, but is gaining increasing attention in a number of fields of applied ethics, including health care.[11] Our society has learned—often through painful experience—that organizations do not always operate in the best interests of the people they serve and/or the people they employ. In the aerospace industry, for example, the 1986 *Challenger* disaster (in which the space shuttle crashed immediately after takeoff) raised questions about the willingness of management to listen to the advice of their engineers (Boisjoly, Curtis, and Mellican 1991; Martin 1992/2005). In health care, the unexpected deaths of 12 infants who had undergone cardiac surgery in Winnipeg between March and December 1994 raised questions about the willingness of management to listen to the concerns of nurses practicing in the operating room (Sinclair 2000; Ceci 2004; see also Chapter 2). The nurses (and some anaesthetists) had repeatedly expressed concern about the unexpected complications that the infants were experiencing, but were left feeling not listened to, and even threatened. Associate Chief Judge Murray Sinclair's *Pediatric Cardiac Surgery Inquest Report* (2000) determined that the pediatric cardiac surgery program at the Winnipeg hospital involved was under-resourced, the competence of the sole pediatric cardiac surgeon was questionable, and the nurses and anaesthetists had been justified in taking their concerns to hospital management. Tragically, their concerns were not acknowledged until after many deaths had occurred.[12]

High-profile incidents such as the *Challenger* disaster and the infant cardiac surgery deaths in Winnipeg—and multiple everyday problems such as short-staffing—make it clear that we need to pay attention to the ethics of organizations, not just those of professionals/providers. In Exhibit 18-2 below we summarize the scope of what ought to be attended to in organizational ethics.

EXHIBIT 18-2

Organizational Ethics

The scope and character of organizational ethics includes (but are not limited to)

1. theories of organizational ethics (for instance, the organization as moral agent);
2. issues and concepts that are particularly relevant for organizations (for instance, conflict of interest, allocation of resources);
3. the use of professional guidelines or explicit statements of responsibilities for

individuals at all levels the organization (for instance, codes of ethics and job descriptions);

4. virtues that contribute to organizational ethics (for instance, promise keeping, prudence, and trustworthiness); and
5. structures and processes that contribute to organizational ethics (for instance, mission and value statements, policies and procedures, and ethics committees). (Adapted from Boyle et al. 2001, 17–18)[13]

In a sense, what we aim to do in organizational ethics is to change the *cultural ethos* (Jameton 1990; Liaschenko 1993) of the organization so that it better serves the diverse but legitimate interests of the people it serves as well as the people it employs. Within health care, we have much more work to do to figure out *how* to achieve this change.[14] Action at the organizational level is important, but it is not enough. Liaschenko (1993) reminds us that cultural ethos is "a complex term that includes both explicit and implicit ideals of conduct, ideology, and social and political structure and organization" (71). In other words, the push to launch the *Challenger* on schedule and the push to have an active pediatric cardiac surgery program in Winnipeg were embedded in influences that went beyond organizational walls.

Resource Allocation

Resource allocation is a key area where organizational ethics are highly visible and highly salient. And resource challenges were, at least in part, implicated in the *Challenger* and

Winnipeg pediatric cardiac surgery tragedies. Not surprisingly, then, while the initial focus of ethics committees from their inception in the late 1970s was on difficult decision making at the micro level, ethics committees are increasingly grappling with meso-level decisions about the allocation of resources (Storch, Rodney, and Starzomski 2009).[15] In Ethics in Practice 18-1 we illustrate by returning to a practice example from earlier in this text.

ETHICS IN PRACTICE 18-1

An Illustration of Resource Challenges

In Chapter 13 we presented the story of Mr. Johansen, an older gentleman who was on an acute medical ward after suffering a terminal stroke and whose mental status was deteriorating because of an undiagnosed urinary tract infection (adapted from Rodney 1997). His daughter was distraught at his deterioration, and, until a clinical nurse specialist and on-call physician intervened, was apparently being largely ignored by nursing and medical staff. In Chapter 13 we then illustrated how the application of an ethical decision-making model at the individual level could help us to address his situation, the situation of his daughter, and the moral integrity of the health care providers. However, if palliative care and home care expertise were not available, if the clinical nurse specialist and spiritual care liaison were not able to free up time to spend with Mr. Johansen's daughter, and if the nursing staff on the medical ward had such excessive workloads that they could not attend staff meetings, it would be difficult to implement the ethical care we recommended for Mr. Johansen.

How can decisions about the allocation of these kinds of resources be made ethically? This poses a huge challenge for health care agencies and health care regions—a challenge that is, fortunately, gaining more explicit ethical reflection from nursing, ethics, and other health care arenas.

Health care organizations face diverse economic, social, political, and legal pressures from different public groups (e.g., patients versus taxpayers). The public expects careful stewardship, with fair and efficient use of resources, while patients (such as Mr. Johansen) expect that their interests will be served (Commission on the Future of Health Care in Canada 2002; Health Council of Canada 2008). Health care administrators and regional health authorities wield significant power as intermediate and mediating figures (Yeo, Williams, and Hooper 1998). Practically speaking, the tone that health care leaders set will influence decision making and the "good" of health care. They are in important—albeit difficult—positions to ameliorate the effects of the malaise of modernity on their organizations (as we explored in Chapters 10 and 11).

From an ethical stance, meso-level resource allocation decisions should proceed with fair *processes* as well as fair *outcomes*. Thus, ethical decision-making frameworks can be beneficial for resource allocation decisions as well as patient-focused decisions. Some work is starting to be done to provide ethical direction for health care providers and administrators involved in resource allocation at the meso level. Norman Daniels, who has been writing about justice in health care for over two decades now (see also Chapter 4 and Chapter 5), and a number of colleagues have been working on a fair and accountable approach for meso-level resource allocation (see Daniels and Sabin 1997; 2008; Martin, Ableson, and Singer 2002). In Appendix C we have made available Michael McDonald's Ethical Framework for Making Allocation Decisions, which is a promising resource at the meso level. Nonetheless, *actualizing* ethical practice at all levels with advocacy, integrity, and interactivity requires attention to policy work and democratic political processes, which we turn to next in this chapter.

ETHICS IN HEALTH/HEALTH CARE POLICY

Health care organizations are imbued with policy, and health is closely linked to public policy, which is inclusive of health, social, and educational realms (Clarke 2010; see also Chapter 20).[16] The integration of ethics into health care policy development and decision making is becoming increasing important in the current health care environment. Relative to the attention paid to case-resolution, health care ethics has, until fairly recently, tended to underplay issues related to development of health policy and health care delivery (Fox 1990; Fox and Swazey 2008; see also Chapter 5). We are increasingly realizing that all levels of health policy have a significant moral dimension (Baylis, Kenny, and Sherwin 2008; Churchill 2002; Giacomini, Kenny, and DeJean 2009; Malone 1999). *Thus, the interface of ethics and health policy at meso and macro levels is important, both in terms of generating policies to address ethical issues and in critiquing existing policies in terms of their ethical implications* (Sherwin 2003; Storch, Rodney, and Starzomski 2009).

Public policy in health care is a primary avenue through which leadership expresses itself, grounding policy in clear and consistent values (Mason, Leavitt, and Chaffee 2007). Every level of health care leadership needs to address basic questions that involve "fundamental conceptual issues that require reflection and in-depth analysis," and recognize the interplay among the various levels—local, provincial, and federal—of health care policy-making (Kenny et al. 2000, 143). Moreover, at the macro level, further consideration needs to be given to implementation of human rights–based approaches and their potential influence on organizational policy. The inclusion of human rights–based approaches to ethical issues can offer additional legal guidance to more adequately inform policy-maker decisions that are respectful of human dignity and of human rights for all persons. The application of human rights–based approaches when combined with epidemiological evidence can facilitate resource allocation where health care resource needs are highest.[17]

Illustration: Aging Issues

A multidimensional process, policy development is embedded within social contexts and institutional traditions (Howlett and Ramesh 1995). The significance of these contexts and traditions comes to light when exploring aging issues, as our discussion of Mr. Johansen so far has indicated. Aging of the population is currently one of the most discussed topics in Canada. On the one hand, this is seen as a dramatic success story, with a growing percentage of people living into later life. On the other hand, there are concerns related to this "social and demographic phenomenon" (Turcotte and Schellenberg 2007, 7), with required services to support the physical, mental, and social well-being of these older adults (see also Callahan 2011, Dodds 2005, and Suhonen et al. 2010).

In what ways do present-day societal views influence the attitudes of health care professionals toward care of seniors and, ultimately, public policy? Butler coined the term "ageism" in 1968, contending that old age is equated by society as powerlessness, as a result of disease, disability, or uselessness (1989, 138). Ageism is, unfortunately, one of the features of the malaise of modernity, even though it constitutes a human right violation. Ageism and stereotypes are the root of many myths and misunderstandings about older adults, and lead to significant consequences: services may be limited for rehabilitation and health promotion in the older population; older adults can be segregated from mainstream society (Tabloski 2010, 3); and health care research may overlook issues particular to older adults (Zulman et al 2011). Ageism—as unacceptable as any other prejudice—often leads to older adults being treated with a lack of dignity and respect (British Medical Association 2009, 8). In Ethics in Practice 18-1 ageism was likely at least partly behind the problems that Mr. Johansen was experiencing. At the extreme, we find elder abuse (Harrigan 2010; Varcoe and Einboden 2010). Indeed, a 2010 report of the chief public health officer of Canada emphasizes that a significant issue for the well-being of seniors is the potential for physical, psychological, and financial abuse or neglect. The report acknowledges that it is difficult to determine the extent of this problem since the data are limited and very likely under-reported; *however, research estimates that between 4 percent and 10 percent of Canadian seniors experience some form of abuse or neglect* (Chief Public Health Officer of Canada 2010).

The literature emphasizes that abuse of older adults is a complex social, legal, and ethical issue, with multiple dimensions. In an international review of the literature, Lysne (2010) concluded that the prevalence rate of elder abuse of persons with dementia is considerably higher than the prevalence rate for elder abuse in general (16). O'Connor and Donnelly (2009), exploring reasons why persons with dementia are at risk for abuse, identify that they are more vulnerable due to increasing dependency on others, deteriorating social networks, and cognitive difficulties that affect their ability to take action and seek support (107). Another perspective relates to how they are valued. The personhood literature (Jaworska 1999; O'Connor and Purves 2009; Sabat 2005) proposes that older adults with dementia are undervalued as people (Kitwood 1997). Kitwood described a paradigm of dementia including a "malignant social psychology" that depersonalized persons with dementia by labelling, infantilization, and banishment. Current Australian research provides an illustration, indicating that prevailing attitudes to older people who require assistance with managing their assets allow some people to think that it is acceptable to "help yourself" to their assets even though this can significantly harm the older person (Tilse, Wilson, and Setterland 2009, 138). What all the previous literature points to is the absence of effective public policy (health as well as social and educational) to protect seniors.

Policy Gaps

The absence of effective public policy for older adults is a gap. It is, of course, not the only gap. *Indeed, what gets noticed as deserving of ethical reflection and policy work is itself a challenge worthy of more attention.* For instance, family violence is strikingly absent as an issue in ethics literature (Varcoe 2004; Varcoe and Einboden 2010), as is the widespread prejudice experienced by gay, lesbian, bisexual, transsexual, and gender questioning people (McCarthy 2006).

Further to the policy gaps in ethics-related work, Post (2000) contends, "We live in a culture that is, at least in large segments, dominated by heightened expectations of rationalism and economic productivity, so clarity of mind and productivity inevitably influence our sense of the worth of a human life" (5). In our malaise of modernity, this culture focuses on the rational and economic views of health policy as a "product." Malone (1999) asks what kinds of ethics and policies emerge from such a conceptualization of policymaking, and her response is that the major deficiency in the product-market metaphor rests in the moral dimension. The market appears to have no concept that corresponds to policy's moral mandate to appreciate problems from the perspective of those affected (20). Even if the *product* is in place, the *process* can undermine the policy intent. In an example from another population too often marginalized by society, Aboriginal anthropologist Caroline Tait (2008) gives a disturbing account of the experiences of impoverished First Nations and Métis women struggling with substance abuse and other mental health problems (and their front-line service providers) in a small community. An effective, nationally funded treatment program in the community was piloted and then unexpectedly discontinued. Not only was the policy that led to the program violated, but the trust of the community in health care was significantly eroded by the process. And, of course, the effect on the health and well-being of all members of the community was likely significant.

Policy Progress

The literature we have cited thus far points to serious challenges related to human rights, social welfare, justice, economics, and related policy needs. Fortunately, we are beginning to see proactive policy work make a difference in some areas. Policy concerns about the increasing proportions of older adults with dementia, for instance, have fostered an emphasis on policy initiatives to support later life planning, assessment of capacity, and substitute decision making (Tilse, Wilson, and Setterland 2009, 134). Leadership for policy development that supports community and societal change to reduce ageism and promote positive and valued roles for older people is a cornerstone to moving forward.

While ethical policy analysis is relatively new territory in health care generally, it is even newer when specifically applied to *health technology assessment* (HTA). Health technology assessment is an important emerging area in health care policy, and addresses technology in the technical treatment sense as well as in terms of systems of care delivery. In a recent European document on HTA, the authors define it as

> a multidisciplinary process that summarizes information about the medical, social, economic and ethical issues related to the use of a health technology in s systematic, transparent, unbiased, robust manner. Its aim is to inform the formulation of safe[,] effective health policies that are patient focused and seek to achieve best value. (European Network for Health Technology Assessment [EUnetHTA] 2008, 3)

Within the EUnetHTA document it is also made clear that "analysing ethical aspects should be conducted and developed through the entire HTA organization, and not as an add-on to selected HTA projects" (102; see also Rogers 2004 and Ten Have 2004). Various theories and models are available for ethical analysis of health technology assessment and other ethical policy analyses (EUnetHTA; Giacomini, Kenny, and DeJean, 2009). The process steps for HTA recommended by the EUnetHTA include (1) defining the focus of the overall assessment; (2) identification of all stakeholders; (3) answering a core set of questions; (4) presentation of the ethical analysis and evidence; (5) judging the transferability of the ethical analysis; and (6) reflection on concomitant legal and societal evaluation (117–121). Reflecting on Ethics in Practice 18-1, an ethical process of HTA at regional, provincial, and national levels could help us to better understand and address how to balance acute medical interventions with patients' quality of life; how to make palliative care and home care expertise more available; how to create better access to specialists such as the clinical nurse specialist, spiritual care liaison, and gerontologist; how to institute programs of support for grieving families; and how to more appropriately match registered nurse staffing with patient care requirements.

Trust is foundational to success in all the ethical policy work we have pointed to above, and at all levels—from micro through to macro. And that trust is best achieved by a *relational* approach to ethics and policy.[18] Baylis, Kenny, and Sherwin (2008) claim that we need a relational ethical approach to policy so that we can better attend to the vulnerability of subpopulations lacking in social and economic power so as to promote the public interest and the common good. We agree. Engaging relationally means attending to the postmodern meanings and power dynamics that infuse every layer of action within our health care organizations, and having the voices of patients, families, communities and health care providers—including nurses—better heard in policy arenas. Peggy Chinn (2009) puts our task this way:

> The most basic challenge, I believe, is to continue to make the voice of nursing stronger, louder, better understood, and heard (even among our own colleagues). . . . Our primary motive should be, and must be, a conviction that what we offer is exactly what the majority of people need the most from healthcare, regardless of where on the globe they reside. (281)

Addressing this challenge necessitates that we foster sound democratic policy processes.

DEMOCRATIC POLICY PROCESSES[19]

Democratic engagement is foundational to any ethical policy work, especially from a relational stance. Democratic engagement is also consistent with the principles of HTA we sketched out above, Reflecting on the examples we have just cited, this means that the elderly and Aboriginal people as well as their families, communities, and health care providers ought to be substantively engaged throughout policy design, implementation, and evaluation.

Galarneau (2002) emphasizes the importance of community in democratic justice-based deliberations, explaining that "because conflicts of meaning and value within and between communities are inevitable, we will need political processes that ensure effective community voice, deliberation, and decision making" (38).Who should be included in deliberations about justice and other ethical values? Political theorist Iris Marion Young's (1999) test for inclusion is relevant here:

If a public debate usually refers to a social segment in the third person, if that social segment rarely if ever appears as a group to whom deliberators appeal, and if there are few signs that public participants in deliberation believe themselves accountable to that social segment, among others, then that social segment has almost certainly been excluded from deliberations. (157)[20]

Until a strategy is in place, an infrastructure is developed, and the broader public sphere is effective, policy leaders should employ a short-term public involvement strategy. In particular, policy leaders should determine ways of linking their decisions to moments of public engagement. These could involve the creation of "minipublics"[21] (Fung and Wright 2003) to address specific issues such as managing patient flow through a system or even regional budget redesign. Or it could include much more humble approaches such as meaningfully open board meetings, structured conversations with community groups, focus groups, engaging community health councils (Gibson, Martin, and Singer 2005) and the like. Careful attention should be paid to ensure dialogue in these forums meet deliberative standards such that all those involved, but especially vulnerable subpopulations, are effectively heard. In other words, the *process* of the policy creation should match the intended ethical product.

As part of this strategy, policy leaders should also help the communities they serve to think about the values immanent in the system and engage in deliberative dialogue around value tensions where they exist. This should include dialogue around how these values are honoured in the context of the Canadian health system, and where they are not honoured (see Exhibit 18-3).

EXHIBIT 18-3

Procedural Standards for Democratic Policy Processes

The following key procedural standards are foundational for democratic policy processes for engaging the public or participants in a deliberation:

- Participants should have confidence in their ability to influence the decision process such that they feel it worthwhile to continue in the process.
- The public should have access to the types of complex decisions that need to be and are regularly made.
- The public should be supported in developing an understanding of the relevant information needed to make such decisions.
- Participants should expect to have their perspectives meaningfully engaged.
- To the extent that these ideal characteristics of the public sphere are realized in a

given minipublic, these minipublics should be empowered with the authority to make decisions.[22]

- The process should treat different voices with respect, such that the reasons of all should be heard, understood, and responded to in it.
- There should be opportunity to review and revise past decisions.
- There should be room for all types of reasons to be engaged, including presumed "dogmatic" perspectives that holders are likely not going to change.
- The approach should always be to seek solutions that respect a broad range of value perspectives.
- The conditions for fair moral compromise should be pursued.
- Where fundamental disagreements (deep conflicts) persist, these differences

should be handled with mutual respect and the goal should be to identify these and continue to meaningfully engage, even if time-sensitive decisions must be made.

- There should be room to question the assumptions behind decisions and the conceptual framework against which decisions are being made, to challenge prevailing discourses. Changing the

agenda and revising the questions should be possible.

- There should be intentional consideration of what forms of expression are acceptable and room for different types of communication should be ensured.
- Policy leaders should address the reasons delivered by public engagement and respond to these in the decisions that they make. (Adapted from Jiwani 2008)

Overall, democratic engagement in health and health care policy work can help to mitigate some of the damages caused by our malaise of modernity. Such work is, fortunately, growing. For example, based on Aboriginal anthropologist Caroline Tait's (2008) research with impoverished First Nations and Métis women struggling with substance abuse and other mental health problems (cited earlier in this chapter), she and Aboriginal elder Bill Mussell led a national project sponsored by the Mental Health Commission of Canada. For two years they listened to Aboriginal peoples and mental health care providers across Canada in order to create ethical guidelines for mental health policy. The insights generated by that work have led to ongoing policy follow up.

FURTHER REFLECTIONS: ECOLOGICAL AND POLITICAL

Promoting virtuous organizational practices and democratic policy processes requires that we reflect on broader ecological and political issues. Organizations exist within a nexus of complex structural, geographic, biological, social, and political environments. For this reason, an organization "can be considered an ecosystem, and its study an ecology. . . ." (Boyle et al. 2001, 7). As Marck explored in Chapter 11, we need to better understand some of these relationships in order to foster the ethical practice of nurses and other health care providers. In the Winnipeg example we cited earlier in this chapter, the relative geographical isolation of Winnipeg in the middle of the Canadian prairies meant that there were not as many specialized medical resources for the pediatric cardiac surgery program as there might have been in a city like Toronto. And the unique specialization and geographic isolation of the operating room meant that it was not easy for the nurses and anaesthetists to have their concerns about standards of practice heard.

We ought to be concerned about how complex structural, geographic, biological, social, and political environments affect the ethical dimensions of health care delivery and work in health/health care policy. This wider view is especially important in reflecting on the concept of justice (Powers ad Faden 2006).

Writing from the field of ethics and geography, David Smith (2000) warns of "a fundamental and deeply geographical distinction in morality" (9), indicating that we are more likely to have sympathy for "close and familiar persons" (9) than for "distant and different others" (9; see also Anderson et al. 2009 and Chapters 11 and 21).[23] Our discussion earlier in this chapter of the malaise of modernity and the challenges faced by groups such as the elderly and Aboriginal peoples would suggest that our concern for the latter two groups are not well developed, or at least not well acted upon. In other words, the individual orientation of much health care shapes the ethical issues to be those about identifiable individuals and not populations; about familiar case or management problems and not the political-social-economic context that shapes them. We believe that the remedies include the organizational and policy work we have articulated in this chapter. And we believe that one additional remedy is a critical human rights discourse and analysis of human rights–based approaches to health care—such as those proposed for the management of HIV disease globally (UNAIDS, 2008a; 2008b)—in order to clarify contextual challenges inherent in many ethical issues locally and globally. *Overall, it is our conviction that ethicists, policy-makers, and health care providers need to better explore the interface of ethics at all levels with policy, human rights law, and democratic political engagement.*

Politics can be seen as distinct from ethics in that politics is the realm of public affairs where decisions are made about the terms of association of individuals living together in a polity. Amidst this is the idea of democracy—itself a contested notion with many different interpretations. Politics is understood as the domain of questions about decisions that are to govern groups of people living together in community. On this approach, for political decisions (such as system-level decisions in the Canadian health care context) to be justified, they will need to be *ethically* justified, which means they will have to be based on a reasonable understanding of the context of health care delivery (facts)[24] and a well-considered understanding of what matters most in the situation (values).

On the view offered here, the central idea of the democratic ideal is that decisions that determine the terms of a collective's association are legitimate to the extent that those affected are able to influence them, either directly or through some mediated mechanism. In our discussion of democratic policy processes earlier in this chapter we started to point to *how* such democratic engagement can be facilitated.[25] In terms of health policy, the questions about how society organizes itself and the guidelines that direct this organization are political issues, in that they are about the decisions that will govern people living in the same political community. For these political issues to be legitimate is for them to be transparent to those whom they impact and to be open for influence by those impacted.

Summary

On the basis of his experiences in national policy work over two decades ago, Daniels (1996) noted that "the gap between [the justice] principle and guidance in institutional design is quite wide and . . . we do not yet know how to fill it" (108). His conclusion was that "we must pay much more attention to problems of fair process and to refinements of democratic theory" (112). This is still true. We would add that paying attention to problems of fair process and democratic theory means engaging in political action. As we have indicated above, political action should foster respect for *all* individuals so that they can have meaningful participation in decisions that will affect the community that they live and/or work in (Mann 1994; McGowan 1998). This requires promoting a constructive dialogue that embraces diverse viewpoints-—processes that are at the heart of democracy (Chinn 2008; Mouffe 1993). This is past/future terrain. Almost three thousand years ago, Aristotle (1985/320 BC) is reported to have spoken on politics immediately after he spoke on ethics. He saw these two disciplines as continuous and interdependent. We have lost this insight in our "modern" times, and it is time to retrieve it. The contemporary political philosopher Mark Kingwell (2000) claims that we need to rethink citizenship for ethics to be actualized through politics:

> What we don't have, but desperately need, is a global politics to balance and give meaning to these troubling universal realities. . . . At its best, a best we have yet to realize, citizenship functions as a complex structure for realizing our deeply social nature, even as it acknowledges and copes with the terrible vulnerability of humans, the myriad fragilities and risks of our existence on the mortal plane. (3–5)

We are, indeed, diverse people experiencing diverse realities, but sharing existential vulnerabilities. Throughout this book we have made the case that health care ethics therefore needs to draw on diverse sources of wisdom—sources that we hope will continue to evolve and flourish.

For Reflection

1. List some of the challenges to health care that you believe have arisen from the malaise of modernity. What strengths do you also see that have emerged over the past 10 years or so?

2. What positive virtues do you see in the health care organization(s) you are involved with? What virtues would you like to promote?

3. In what ways can a health care organization demonstrate its commitment to organizational ethics?

4. What ethical values do you believe should drive policy work related to new reproductive technologies? (See also Chapter 23)

5. How might we be able to promote better public dialogue around genetics and identity? (See also Chapter 24)

6. How might nursing and other health care professions use political theorizing to complement ethical theorizing?

Endnotes

1. This chapter includes content that was originally presented in McPherson, G., Rodney, P., Storch, J., Pauly, B., McDonald, M., and Burgess, M. 2004. Working within the landscape: Applications in health care ethics. In J. Storch, P. Rodney, and R. Starzomski (Eds.), *Toward a moral horizon: Nursing ethics for leadership and practice* (pp. 98–125). Toronto: Pearson-Prentice Hall. Content from that 2004 chapter is now contained and expanded in Chapters 13 and 18 in this revised edition.

2. Rodney is indebted to Dr. Michael McDonald, Founding Director of the W. Maurice Young Centre for Applied Ethics at the University of British Columbia, for his articulation of these relationships between levels.

3. In Chapter 3 of this book Johnson and Pesut offer a thoughtful analysis of how modernity and post-modernity have influenced nursing's uptake of knowledge, theory, and philosophy. Further, Chapter 7

by Bergum and Chapter 8 by Doane and Varcoe on relational ethics are both based on a postmodern reading of nursing ethics per se.

4. By disengaged and instrumental, we take Taylor to mean isolated and individualistic, with an over-emphasis on reason and (a narrow view of) productivity.

5. Another postmodern theorist, Giddens (1990), paints a dramatic third contemporary metaphor of modernity—the juggernaut—"a runaway engine of colossal power." He depicts this powerful run-away engine as one which, "collectively as human beings, we can drive to some extent but which also threatens to rush out of our control" (1990, 139). The path of the juggernaut is steady at times; at other times, it is erratic and crushes those who resist it. Giddens contends that the ride is not com-pletely unpleasant or unrewarding; it also may be exhilarating and charged with hopeful anticipa-tion; however, out of control, the journey of the runaway engine is uncertain. The path and the pace of the journey cannot be regulated; the terrain is fraught with risks and feelings of ambivalence. Within this image, four dialectically related frameworks of experience intersect in significant ways: estrangement and familiarity; intimacy and impersonality; expertise and reappropriation; and abstract systems and day-to-day knowledgeability. Thus, the imagery of the juggernaut of modernity is not an engine with integrated machinery, but rather one that includes tensions and contradictory influ-ences (Giddens 1990, 139).

6. An ideology is a taken for granted societal belief. It is not in itself good or bad, but an ideology goes unchallenged too often because it is taken for granted (Thomas 2003).

7. See also Chapter 20 by MacDonald and Chapter 21 by Pauly in this book.

8. An anonymous reviewer of this chapter has raised two further interesting points to consider here. The reviewer wonders if efficiency, when raised to an end instead of a means, obscures the impact on individuals or whether it directly impacts individuals and their practice. The reviewer also won-ders if efficiency as an end instead of a means obscures questions of accountability, or whether it obscures evaluation and dialogue regarding value and accountability.

9. The moral positions of managers in our current health care system are fraught with challenges, and are likely significant sources of moral distress for managers as well as other health care providers. However, this is an area that has not been well enough researched. See Chapter 9 in this text as well as Gaudine and Beaton (2002), Harrigan (2005), and Mitton et al. (2011).

10. A related theory here is *communitarianism.* Bellah et al. (1991) explain that "communitarians believe that more substantive ethical identities and a more active participation in a democratic polity are necessary for the functioning of any decent society" (6). However, they also caution that the term communitarianism "runs the risk of being misunderstood" (6).

11. An early foundational paper here is Reiser (1994).

12. This is *not* to say that specialized medical resources ought not to be located in cities such as Winnipeg, which serve a number of isolated communities. Across Canada, there are serious regional (especially rural) inequities in access to health care (Commission on the Future of Health Care in Canada 2002).

13. Note that in Canada addressing the ethics of health care organizations also requires addressing the ethics of the health care regions they are usually clustered in. See Yeo, Williams, and Hooper (1998).

14. See Chapter 10 for a discussion of action research indicating how leaders and health care providers at all levels of the organizational hierarchy can pull together to improve the moral climate of their health care organizations.

15. See also Chapters 4, 5, and 21 for discussions of the principle of justice.

16. Delineating the various categories of policy can be challenging. Clarke (2010) offers some useful distinctions. She identifies *public policy* as the larger category that is inclusive of (1) *health policy* (health goals and health care principles); (2) *social policy* (e.g., poverty and crime); and

(3) *educational policy* (funding, academic quality, and student affairs). She sees these three subsets as interrelated with each other as well as *institutional* policy (e.g., mission, quality assurance, and health human resources), *nursing* policy (e.g., practice guidelines), and *organizational* policy (e.g., nursing association position statements) (69–70).

17. Such work falls in the category of *policy-oriented jurisprudence* (Weissner and Willard 1999; 2001). According to Weissner and Willard, policy-oriented jurisprudence addresses value categories such as power, enlightenment, wealth, well-being, skill, affection, respect, and rectitude (responsibility for conduct). Procedural principles include delimiting the problem and clarifying goals; identifying conflicting claims; looking at past trends in decisions; projecting of future trends; and identifying alternatives and recommendations for the global common interest.

18. See Chapters 5, 7, 8, and 13 for discussions of relational ethics.

19. Parts of the following sections are adapted from Jiwani (2008).

20. For a comprehensive resource on the thinking of political theorists such as Iris Marion Young, Nancy Fraser, Amy Gutmann, Charles Taylor, and many others, see Farrelly (2004).

21. This is a term of art that is attributed to Goodin and Dryzek (2006).

22. This analysis addresses both "the public" and "participants" in engagements, reflecting processes as diverse as voting and representative democracy through more active forms of direct democracy and engagement. Burgess and colleagues (Burgess 2004; Longstaff and Burgess 2010) now describe "the public" as being "constructed" in their deliberative engagements through choosing demographic and other proxies for diversity across the population for particular issues. The critical literature is full of reflections on how the participants in events can function to replace rather than represent the wider public, perhaps intentionally on the part of some organizers, sponsors and analysts. Alternatively, some critics claim that the broad construal of the public is irrelevant or an abstraction, and that engagement of stakeholders is more important. In some ways, this is a debate between wide surveys of the public's "top of the head" responses against informed, deliberative groups structured to represent diversity. Wide surveys are clearly less reflective of the wider public for their level of information and deliberation. *Such are the kinds of complexities in public participation that need to be addressed in future ethical policy work at all levels.*

23. For an interesting application of moral geography, see Valentine (2003).

24. "Facts" ought to be studied from diverse epistemological positions—from quantitative through to qualitative and critical (Avis and Freshwater 2006; Goldenberg 2006; Holmes, Perron, and O'Byrne 2006; Upshur 2005; Yeo 1994).

25. For more specific insights into principles and methods for democratic dialogue, see Chambers (2003) and Dryzek (2000).

References

Anderson, J.M., Blue, C., and Lau, A. 1991. Women's perspectives on chronic illness: Ethnicity, ideology and restructuring life. *Social Science and Medicine, 33* (2), 101–113.

Anderson, J.M., Rodney, P., Reimer-Kirkham, S., Browne, A.J., Khan, K.B., and Lynam, M.J. 2009. Inequities in health and healthcare viewed through the ethical lens of critical social justice: Contextual knowledge for the global priorities ahead. *Advances in Nursing Science, 32* (4), 282–294.

Aristotle. 1985. *Nicomachean ethics.* (T. Irwin, Trans.) Indianapolis, IL: Hackett. (Original work published c. 320 B.C.)

Aroskar, M.A. 1995. Envisioning nursing as a moral community. *Nursing Outlook, 43* (3), 134–138.

Austin, W. 2003. Using the human rights paradigm in health ethics: The problem and the possibilities. In V. Tschudin (Ed.), *Approaches to ethics: Nursing beyond boundaries* (pp. 105–114). Edinburgh: Butterworth Heinmann. (Reprinted from *Nursing Ethics* 2001; *8* (13), 183–195).

Austin, W. 2004. Global health challenges, human rights, and nursing ethics. In J. Storch, P. Rodney, and R. Starzomski (Eds.), *Toward a moral horizon: Nursing ethics for leadership and practice* (pp. 339–356). Toronto: Pearson Prentice Hall.

Austin, W.J. 2011. The incommensurability of nursing as a practice and the customer service model: An evolutionary threat to the discipline. *Nursing Philosophy, 12,* 158–166.

Avis, M. and Freshwater, D. 2006. Evidence for practice, epistemology, and critical reflection. *Nursing Philosophy, 7* (4), 216–224.

Bakan, J. 2004. *The corporation: The pathological pursuit of profit and power.* Toronto, ON: Penguin Group.

Baylis, F., Kenny, N.P., and Sherwin, S. 2008. A relational account of public health ethics. *Public Health Ethics, 1* (3), 196–209.

Bellah, R.N., Madsen, R., Sullivan, W.M., Swidler, A., and Tipton, S.M. 2001. *The good society.* New York: Vintage Books.

Benatar, S. and Brock, G. 2011. *Global health and global health ethics.* Cambridge: Cambridge University Press.

Boisjoly, R.P., Curtis, E.F., and Mellican, E. 1991. Roger Boisjoly and the Challenger disaster: Ethical dimensions. In D.C. Poff and W.J. Waluchow (Eds.), *Business ethics in Canada* (2nd ed.; pp. 178–192). Scarborough, ON: Prentice-Hall.

Boyle, P.J., DuBose, E.R., Ellingson, S.J., Guinn, D.E., and McCurdy, D.B. 2001. *Organizational ethics in health care: Principles, cases, and practical solutions.* San Francisco: Jossey-Bass.

British Medical Association. 2009. *The ethics of caring for older people* (2nd ed.). Chichester, West Sussex, UK: John Wiley & Sons Ltd.

Browne, A.J. 2001. The influence of liberal political ideology on nursing science. *Nursing Inquiry, 8,* 118–129.

Buchanan, A. 1996. Toward a theory of the ethics of bureaucratic organizations. *Business Ethics Quarterly, 6* (4), 419–440.

Burgess, M.M. 2004. Public consultation in ethics: An experiment in representative ethics. *Journal of Bioethical Inquiry, 1* (1), 4–13.

Butler, R.N. 1989. Dispelling ageism: The cross cutting intervention. *Annals of American Academy of Political and Social Science, 503,* 138–147.

Callahan, D. 2011 End-of-life care: A philosophical or management problem? *Journal of Law, Medicine and Ethics,* (Summer), 114–120.

Canadian Nurses Association. 2009. *Position statement: Determinants of health.* Ottawa: Author.

Canadian Nurses Association and Registered Nurses Association of Ontario. 2010. *Nurse fatigue and patient safety: Research report.* Ottawa, ON: Canadian Nurses Association.

Canales, M.K. 2010. Othering: Difference understood?? A 10-year analysis and critique of the nursing literature. *Advances in Nursing Science, 33* (1), 15–34.

Ceci, C. 2004. Gender, power, nursing: A case analysis. *Nursing Inquiry, 11* (2), 72–81.

Chambers, S. 2003. Deliberative democratic theory. *Annual Review of Political Science, 6*, 307–326.

Chief Public Health Officer of Canada. 2010. *The chief public health officer's report on the state of public health in Canada 2010.* Available at http://www.phac-aspc.gc.ca/cphorsphc-respcacsp/2010/fr-rc/cphorsphc-respcacsp-06-eng.php.

Chinn, P.L. 2008. *Peace and power: Creative leadership for building community* (7th ed.) Boston: Jones and Bartlett.

Chinn, P.L. 2009. Healthy people beyond 2010. *Advances in Nursing Science, 32* (4), 281.

Churchill, L.R. 2002. What ethics can contribute to health policy. In M. Danis, C. Clancy, and L.R. Churchill (Eds.), *Ethical dimensions of health policy* (pp. 51–64). New York: Oxford University Press.

Coburn, D. 2010. Health and health care: A political economy perspective. In T. Bryant, D. Raphael, and M. Rioux (Eds.), *Staying alive: Critical perspectives on health, illness, and health care* (2nd ed.; pp. 65–91). Toronto, ON: Canadian Scholars' Press.

Commission on the Future of Health Care in Canada. 2002. *Building on values: The future of health care in Canada.* Ottawa, ON: Authors.

Crotty, M. 1998. *The foundations of social research: Meaning and perspective in the research process.* London: Sage.

Daniels, N. 1996. Wide reflective equilibrium in practice. In L.W. Sumner and J. Boyle (Eds.), *Philosophical perspectives on bioethics* (pp. 96–114). Toronto: University of Toronto Press.

Daniels, N. and Sabin, J. 1997. Limits to health care: Fair procedures, democratic deliberation, and the legitimacy problem for insurers. *Philosophy and Public Affairs, 26* (4), 303–350.

Daniels, N. and Sabin, J.E. 2008. Accountability for reasonableness: An update. *British Medical Journal, 337* (a1850).

Day, L. 2007. Courage as a virtue necessary to good nursing practice. *American Journal of Critical Care, 16* (6), 613–616.

Dodds, S. 2005. Gender, ageing, and injustice: Social and political contexts of bioethics. *Journal of Medical Ethics, 31*, 295–298.

Dryzek, J.S. 2000. *Deliberative democracy and beyond.* Oxford: Oxford University Press.

Ermine, W. 2007. The ethical space of engagement. *Indigenous Law Journal, 6* (1), 193–203.

European Network for Health Technology Assessment [EUnetHTA]. 2008. *Core model for diagnostic technologies: Work package 4: The HTA core model: FinOHTA.* Finland: Finnish Office for HTA.

Farrelly, C. (Ed.). 2004. *Contemporary political theory: A reader.* London: Sage Publications.

Fox, R.C. 1990. The evolution of American bioethics: A sociological perspective. In G. Weisz (Ed.), *Social science perspectives on medical ethics* (pp. 201–217). Philadelphia: University of Pennsylvania Press.

Fox, R.C. and Swazey, J.P. 2008. *Observing bioethics.* Oxford: Oxford University Press.

Fung, A., and Wright, E. 2003. *Deepening democracy: Institutional innovations in empowered participatory governance.* New York: Verso.

Galarneau, C.A. 2002. Health care as a community good: Many dimensions, many communities, many views of justice. *Hastings Centre Report, 32* (5), 33–40.

Giacomini, M., Kenny, N., and DeJean, D. 2009. Ethics frameworks in Canadian health policies: Foundation, scaffolding, or window dressing? *Health Policy, 89*, 58–71.

Gibson, J., Martin, D., and Singer, P. 2005. Evidence, economics and ethics: Resource allocation in health service organizations. *Health Quarterly, 8* (2), 50–59.

Giddens, A. 1990. *The consequences of modernity.* Stanford, CA: Stanford University Press.

Goldenberg, M.J. 2006. On evidence and evidence-based medicine: Lessons from the philosophy of science. *Social Science and Medicine, 62*, 2621–2632.

Goodin, R.E. and Dryzek, J.S. 2006. Deliberative impacts: The macro-political uptake of mini-publics. *Politics & Society, 34* (2), 219–244.

Hacking, I. 1995. *Rewriting the soul: Multiple personalities and the science of memory.* Princeton, NJ: Princeton University Press.

Harrigan, M.L. 2005. *Leadership challenges in Canadian health care: Exploring exemplary professionalism under the malaise of modernity.* Unpublished doctoral dissertation, Simon Fraser University, Burnaby, B.C.

Harrigan, M.L. 2010. *Older adult abuse and dementia: A literature review.* Toronto, ON: Alzheimer Society of Canada. Available at http://www.alzheimer.ca/docs/Care/Alzheimer_Society_of_Canada_Elder_Abuse_Prevention_Literature_Review_ENG.pdf.

Health Council of Canada. 2008. Rekindling reform: Health care renewal 2003–2008. Toronto, ON: Authors.

Holmes, D., Perron, A., and O'Byrne, P. 2006. Evidence, virulence, and the disappearance of nursing knowledge: A critique of the evidence-based dogma. *Worldviews on Evidence-Based Nursing, 3* (3), 95–102.

Howlett, M. and Ramesh, M. 1995. *Studying public policy: Policy cycles and policy subsystems.* Toronto, ON: Oxford University Press.

Jameton, A. 1990. Culture, morality, and ethics: Twirling the spindle. *Critical Care Nursing Clinics of North America, 2* (3), 443–451.

Jaworska, A. 1999. Respecting the margins of agency: Alzheimer's patients and the capacity to value. *Philosophy and Public Affairs, 28* (2), 105–138.

Jiwani, B. 2008. *Ethically justified system-level decisions in health care: Toward a decision support workbook for healthcare leaders.* Unpublished doctoral dissertation, University of Alberta Public Health Sciences, Edmonton, Alberta, Canada.

Kenny, N.P. 2002. *What good is health care? Reflections on the Canadian experience.* Ottawa, ON: CHA Press.

Kenny, N.P., Downie, J., Ells, C., and MacDonald, C. 2000. Organizational ethics Canadian style. *HealthCare Ethics Committee Forum, 12* (2), 141–148.

Kingwell, M. 2000. *The world we want: Virtue, vice, and the good citizen.* Toronto: Penguin.

Kitwood, T. 1997. *Dementia reconsidered: The person comes first.* Buckingham, UK: Open University Press.

Kitwood, T. 2007. The dialectus of dementia: With particular reference to Alzheimer's disease. In C. Baldwin and A. Capstick (Eds.), *Tom Kitwood on dementia: A reader and critical commentary* (pp. 34–51). Maidenhead, UK: Open University Press.

Liaschenko, J. 1993. Feminist ethics and cultural ethos: Revisiting a nursing debate. *Advances in Nursing Science, 15* (4), 71–81.

Longstaff, H. and Burgess, M.M. 2010. Recruiting for representation in public deliberation on the ethics of biobanks. *Public Understanding of Science, 19* (2), 212–224.

Lysne, L. 2010. *Elder care, elder abuse and neglect: An international literature review.* Ottawa, ON: Division of Aging and Seniors, Public Health Agency of Canada.

MacIntyre, A. 1984. *After virtue: A study in moral theory* (2nd ed.). Notre Dame, IN: University of Notre Dame Press.

MacIntyre, A. 1998. Politics, philosophy and the common good. In K. Knight (Ed.), *The MacIntyre reader* (pp. 235–252). Notre Dame, IN: University of Notre Dame Press.

MacIntyre, A. 1999. *Dependent rational animals: Why human beings need the virtues.* Chicago and LaSalle, IL: Open Court.

Malone, R.E. 1999. Policy as product: Morality and metaphor in health policy discourse. *Hastings Center Report, 29* (3), 16–22.

Mann, P.S. 1994. *Micro-politics: Agency in a postfeminist era.* Minneapolis: University of Minnesota Press.

Martin, M.W. 1992/2005. Whistleblowing: Professionalism, personal life, and shared responsibility for safety in engineering. In D.C. Poff (Ed.), *Business ethics in Canada* (4th ed.; 223–234). Toronto: Pearson Prentice Hall. (Reprinted from *Business & Professional Ethics Journal, 11* (2) (1992); 21–40.)

Martin, D., Abelson, J., and Singer, P. 2002. Participation in health care priority-setting: Through the eyes of the participants. *Journal of Health Services Research & Policy, 7* (4), 222–229.

Mason, D.J., Leavitt, J.K., and Chaffee, M.W. 2007. Policy and politics: A framework for action. In D.J. Mason, J.K. Leavitt, and M.W. Chaffee (Eds.), *Policy and politics in nursing and health care* (5th ed.; pp. 1–20). St. Louis, MO: Saunders Elsevier.

McCarthy, J. 2006. A pluralist view of nursing ethics. *Nursing Philosophy, 7* (3), 157–164.

McGowan, J. 1998. *Hannah Arendt: An introduction.* Minneapolis: University of Minnesota Press.

Milley, P. 2002. Imagining good organizations: Moral orders or moral communities? *Educational Management and Administration, 30* (1), 47–64.

Mishler, E.G. 1981. Social contexts of health care. In E.G. Mishler, L. Amara Singham, S.T. Hauser, R. Liem, S.D. Osherson, and N.E. Waxler (Eds.), *Social contexts of health, illness and patient care.* Cambridge, UK: Cambridge University Press.

Mitton, C., Peacock, S., Storch, J., Smith, N., and Cornelissen, E. 2011. Moral distress among health system managers: Exploratory research in two British Columbia health authorities. *Health Care Anal, 19,* 107–121.

Moorhouse, A. and Rodney, P. 2010. Contemporary Canadian challenges in nursing ethics. In M. Yeo, A. Moorhouse, P. Khan, and P. Rodney (Eds.), *Concepts and cases in nursing ethics,* (3rd ed.; pp. 73–101). Peterborough, ON: Broadview Press.

Mouffe, C. 1993. *The return of the political.* London: Verso.

Myrick, F. 2004. Pedagogical integrity in the knowledge economy. *Nursing Philosophy, 5,* 23–29.

O'Connor, D. and Donnelly, M. 2009. Confronting the challenges of assessing capacity: Dementia in the context of abuse. In D. O'Connor and B. Purves (Eds.), *Decision-making, personhood and dementia: Exploring the interface* (pp. 106–118). London, UK: Jessica Kingsley Publishers.

O'Connor, D. and Purves, B. (Eds.). 2009. *Decision-making, personhood and dementia: Exploring the interface* (pp. 11–21). London, UK: Jessica Kingsley Publishers.

Pauly, B. 2004. Shifting the balance in the funding and delivery of health care in Canada. In J.L. Storch, P. Rodney, and R. Starzomski (Eds.), *Toward a moral horizon: Nursing ethics for leadership and practice* (pp. 181–208). Toronto, ON: Pearson Education.

Pellegrino, E.D. 1979. Toward a reconstruction of medical morality: The primacy of the act of profession and the fact of illness. *Journal of Medicine and Philosophy, 4* (1), 32–56.

Pellegrino, E.D. 2004. Prevention of medical error: Where professional and organizational ethics meet. In V.A. Sharpe (Ed.), *Accountability: Patient safety and policy reform* (pp. 83–98). Washington, DC: Georgetown University Press.

Post, S.G. 2000. *The moral challenge of Alzheimer disease: Ethical issues from diagnosis to dying* (2nd ed.). Baltimore and London: The Johns Hopkins University Press.

Powers, M. and Faden, R. 2006. *Social justice: The moral foundations of public health and health policy.* Oxford: Oxford University Press.

Pringle, D. 2009. Alert—Return of 1990s healthcare reform. *Nursing Leadership, 22* (3), 14–15.

Rachlis, M. 2004. *Prescription for excellence: How innovation is saving Canada's health care system.* Toronto: HarperPerennial Canada.

Rankin, J.M., and Campbell, M.L. 2006. *Managing to nurse: Inside Canada's health care reform.* Toronto: University of Toronto Press.

Reiser, S.J. 1994. The ethical life of health care organizations. *Hastings Center Report, 24* (6), 28–35.

Rodney, P.A. 1997. *Towards connectedness and trust: Nurses' enactment of their moral agency within an organizational context.* Unpublished doctoral dissertation, University of British Columbia, Vancouver, B.C.

Rodney, P. 2011. Nursing inquiry to address pressing empirical and ethical questions. *Canadian Journal of Nursing Research, 43* (2), 7–10.

Rodney, P., and Varcoe, C. in press. Constrained agency: The social structure of nurses' work. In F. Baylis, J. Downie, B. Hoffmaster, and S. Sherwin (Eds.), *Health care ethics in Canada* (3rd ed.). Toronto: Nelson. (Revision of Varcoe, C. and Rodney, P. 2009. Constrained agency: the social structure of nurses' work. In B.S. Bolaria and H.D. Dickinson [Eds.], *Health, illness, and health care in Canada* [4th ed.; pp. 122–151]. Toronto: Nelson Education.)

Rogers, W.A. 2004. Evidence based medicine and justice: A framework for looking at the impact of EBM upon vulnerable or disadvantaged groups. *Journal of Medical Ethics, 30,* 141–145.

Sabat, S. 2005. Capacity for decision-making in Alzheimer's disease: Selfhood, positioning and semiotic people. *Australian and New Zealand Journal of Psychiatry, 19* (11–12), 1030–1035.

Saul, J.R. 1999. Health care at the end of the twentieth century: Confusing symptoms for systems. In M.A. Somerville (Ed.), *Do we care? Renewing Canada's commitment to health: Proceedings of the first directions for Canadian health care conference* (pp. 3–20). Montreal, PQ: McGill-Queen's University Press.

Saul, J.R. 2005. *The collapse of globalism and the reinvention of the world.* Toronto: Penguin Canada.

Saul, J.R. 2008. *A fair country: Telling truths about Canada.* Toronto: Viking Canada.

Sherwin, S. 2003. The importance of ontology for feminist policy-making in the realm of reproductive technology. *Canadian Journal of Philosophy, 26,* (Supplementary volume Feminist Moral Philosophy), 273–295.

Sherwin, S. 2011. Looking backwards, looking forward: Hopes for bioethics' next twenty-five years. *Bioethics, 25* (2), 75–82.

Sinclair, M. 2000. *Pediatric cardiac surgery inquest report.* Winnipeg, MB: Manitoba Chief Medical Examiner.

Smith, D.M. 2000. *Moral geographies: Ethics in a world of difference.* Edinburgh: Edinburgh University Press.

Stein, J.G. 2001. *The cult of efficiency.* Toronto, ON: House of Anansi Press.

Storch, J.L. 2010. Canadian healthcare system. In M. McIntyre and C. McDonald (Eds.), *Realities of Canadian nursing: Professional, practice, and power issues* (3rd ed.; pp. 34–55). Philadelphia: Wolters Kluwer Health.

Storch, J., Rodney, P., and Starzomski, S. 2009. Ethics in health care in Canada. In B.S. Bolaria and H. Dickinson (Eds.), *Health, illness, and health care in Canada* (4th ed.; pp. 458–490). Toronto: Nelson Education.

Suhonen, R., Stolt, M., Launis, V., and Leino-Kilpi, H. 2010. Research on ethics in nursing care for older people: A literature review. *Nursing Ethics, 17* (3), 337–352.

Suhonen, R., Stolt, M., Virtanen, H., and Leino-Kilpi, H. 2011. Organizational ethics: A literature review. *Nursing Ethics, 18* (3), 285–303.

Tabloski, P.A. 2010. *Clinical handbook for gerontological nursing* (2nd ed.). Upper Saddle River, NJ: Pearson Prentice Hall.

Tait, C.L. 2008. Ethical programming: Towards a community-centred approach to mental health and addiction programming in Aboriginal communities. *Pimatisiwin: A Journal of Aboriginal and Indigenous Community Health, 6* (1), 29–60.

Taylor, C. 1989. *The sources of self.* Cambridge, MA: Harvard University Press.

Taylor, C. 1991. *The malaise of modernity.* Toronto: House of Anansi Press.

Taylor, C. 1994. Philosophical reflections on caring practices. In S.S. Phillips and P. Benner (Eds.), *The crisis of care: Affirming and restoring caring practices in the helping professions.* Washington, DC: Georgetown University Press.

Taylor, C. 2001. *Contemporary sociological theory: On social imaginary.* Available at http://www.nyu. edu/classes/calhoun/Theory/Taylor-on-si.htm.

Taylor, C. 2004. *Modern social imaginaries.* Durham, NC: Duke University Press.

Ten Have, H. 2004. Ethical perspectives on health technology assessment. *International Journal of Technology Assessment in Health Care, 20* (1), 71–76.

Thorne, S. 2009. Ideas and action in a terrain of complexity. *Nursing Philosophy, 10,* 149–151.

Tilse, C., Wilson, J., and Setterland, D. 2009. Personhood, financial decision-making and dementia. In D. O'Connor and B. Purves (Eds.), *Decision-making, personhood and dementia: Exploring the interface* (pp. 133–143). London, UK: Jessica Kingsley Publishers.

Turcotte, M. and Schellenberg, G. 2007. *A portrait of seniors in Canada: 2006.* Ottawa, ON: Statistics Canada, Social and Aboriginal Statistics Division.

UNAIDS. 2008a. *Policy Brief: Criminalization of HIV transmission.* Geneva: Author.

UNAIDS. 2008b. *Report on the global HIV/AIDS epidemic 2008.* Geneva: Author.

Upshur, R.E.G. 2005. Looking for rules in a world of exceptions: Reflections on evidence-based practice. *Perspectives in Biology and Medicine, 48* (4), 477–489.

Valentine, G. 2003. Geography and ethics: In pursuit of social justice—ethics and emotions in geographies of health and disability research. *Progress in Human Geography, 27* (3), 375–380.

Varcoe, C. 2004. Widening the scope of ethical theory, practice, and policy: Violence against women as an illustration. In J. Storch, P. Rodney, and R. Starzomski (Eds.), *Toward a moral horizon: Nursing ethics for leadership and practice* (pp. 414–432). Toronto: Pearson-Prentice Hall.

Varcoe, C. and Einboden, R. 2010. Family violence and ethics. In J. Humphreys and J.C. Campbell (Eds.), *Family violence and nursing practice* (2nd ed., pp. 381–410). New York: Springer.

Veatch, R.M. 2003. *The basics of bioethics* (2nd ed.). Upper Saddle River, NJ: Prentice Hall.

Weissner, S. and Willard, A.R. 2001. Policy-oriented jurisprudence. *German Yearbook of International Law, 44,* 96–112.

Weissner, S. and Willard, A.R. 1999. Policy-oriented jurisprudence and human rights abuses in internal conflict: Toward a world public order of human dignity. *American Journal of International Law, 93* (316), 325–334.

World Health Organization. 2008a. *Closing the gap in a generation: Health equity through action on the social determinants of health.* (Final Report of the Commission on Social Determinants of Health). Geneva: Authors.

World Health Organization. 2008b. *World Health Report 2008: Primary health care: Now more than ever.* Geneva: Authors.

Yeo, M. 1994. Interpretive bioethics. *Health and Canadian Society, 2* (1), 85–108.

Yeo, M., Rodney, P., Moorhouse, A., and Khan, P. 2010. Justice. In M. Yeo, A. Moorhouse, P. Khan, and P. Rodney (Eds.), *Concepts and cases in nursing ethics* (3rd ed.; pp. 293–316). Peterborough, ON: Broadview Press.

Yeo, M., Williams, J.R., and Hooper, W. 1998. Ethics and regional health boards. In L. Groarke (Ed.), *The ethics of the new economy* (pp. 125–141). Waterloo, ON: Wilfrid Laurier University Press.

Young, I.M. 1999. Justice, inclusion and deliberative democracy. In S. Macedo (Ed.), *Deliberative politics: Essays on democracy and disagreement*. New York: Oxford University Press.

Zulman, D.M., Sussman, J.B., Chen, X., Cigolle, C.T., Blaum, C.S., and Hayward, R.A. 2011. Examining the evidence: A systematic review of the inclusion and analysis of older adults in randomized controlled trials. *Journal of General Internal Medicine, 26* (7), 783–790.

PART 3

Broadening the View of Health Care Ethics/Nursing Ethics

CHAPTER 19

Home Health Care: Ethics, Politics, and Policy[1]

Elizabeth Peter

Ethics tries to find out whether certain things are really right or good, and whether some ways to live are really better than others. I see the task of fully normative reflection as intrinsically comparative; in other words, when we ask ourselves what can be said for some way of life, we are asking whether it is better or worse than some other way we know or imagine. (Walker 1998, 13)

Many nursing services and other health services that were previously provided in institutional settings are now being offered in the homes of Canadians. Over the past decade, there has been a 51 percent increase in the number of home care recipients in Canada (CHCA 2008a). This change in setting is the result of health system restructuring and health policy shifts. Technological advances have also allowed for more medical treatments and assistive and monitoring devices to be offered in the home including "high-tech" interventions that involve chemotherapy, intravenous therapy, and dialysis. Today, home care offers "an array of services for people of all ages, provided in the home and community setting, that encompasses health promotion teaching, curative intervention, end-of-life care, rehabilitation, support and maintenance, social adaptation and integration and support for the informal (family) caregiver" (CHCA 2008a, viii). The demand for home care services is expected to rise as more patients are discharged from hospital earlier and sicker and as older persons expect to live independently in their homes and communities as long as possible (Williams et al. 2010).

Currently, however, Canadians are not entitled to home care services under the Canada Health Act (CHA) (CHA 1985). There exists tremendous variation among provinces and territories with respect to the access and availability of covered home care services. Some provinces provide extensive coverage for home nursing care, while

384

others strictly limit nursing services to a fixed dollar or hourly amount. Wide variations also exist with respect to the provision of supportive services such as homemaking and access to assisted living facilities. Therefore, no "floor," or basic set, of services is available to all Canadians (CHCA 2008a). As a result, many people are without adequate resources and must rely on family members, when they are available, to provide care that is often extensive and highly sophisticated. As the population ages, with many seniors living with chronic conditions, the sustainability of our health system is threatened if more resources are not provided to the home care sector. The demand will not be met (CHCA 2008b).

Health restructuring has also eroded the role of home care nurses, along with the associated autonomy of this role. Traditionally, home care nurses have embraced the importance of home and family as foundational to practice. Home care nurses have held a deep commitment to holistic and family-centred care that encompasses health promotion and disease prevention. As guests in the homes of their patients, home care nurses have valued collaborative relationships with patients and have striven to adapt to a never-ending variety of patient-controlled environments. Home care nurses have had the privilege of coming to know their patients and families as they actually live their lives. Fiscal restraints, however, have constrained home care nurses' capacity to provide care holistically and have led to role conflict and confusion because the range of care activities deemed necessary by nurses is often not considered worthy of remuneration (Bjornsdottir 2009; CHNAC 2003; Stajduhar et al. 2010). Constraints are not only experienced by nurses who provide direct care, but are also experienced by home care case managers as economics play an increasingly influential role in care provision. Organizational priorities often take precedence over professional judgment in this era of cost containment (Ceci 2006).

This lack of available resources, and the transfer of responsibility for care from the state to the family, are of great ethical importance, having major implications for patients and their families, health care organizations, health care professionals, and governments. In this chapter, I argue that this lack of resources is the result of shifting services to the home outside of the protection of the Canada Health Act. This shift has been made possible by a political ideology that is neo-liberal in nature. I address some of the implications of current home care policy, particularly those that concern the well-being of patients, families, and home care workers and those that have an impact upon nurse-patient-family relationships. I then offer recommendations that challenge neo-liberal values and beliefs that can inform the work of both nurses directly providing care and those who are in leadership roles. While there are numerous community health nursing roles, including occupational health nurses, public health nurses, parish nurses, primary care nurses, outpost nurses, mental health nurses, and home health nurses (CHNAC 2009), in this chapter, I will focus on home care nursing in order to provide a rich analysis of the kind of ethical issues that a community nurse may face.

THE POLITICAL CONTEXT: NEO-LIBERALISM

Prior to the CHA, two federal acts—the Hospital Insurance and Diagnostic Services Act (1957) and the Medical Care Act (1968)—governed hospital and medical care insurance in such a way that all Canadians were entitled to medically necessary hospital and insurance programs. The passage of the CHA in 1984 replaced these acts but retained the basic principles underlying the existing national health insurance program and also eliminated extra-billing. The CHA contains five well-known requirements that the provinces and territories must meet to qualify for full federal funding, including public administration, comprehensiveness, universality, portability, and accessibility. These, however, apply to insured health care services only, that is, medically necessary hospital services, physician services, and surgical dental services provided in a hospital. They do not apply to extended health care services, that is, aspects of long-term residential care and the health aspects of home care (CHCA 2008b). Consequently, as home care becomes more prevalent, the CHA is becoming increasingly incapable of protecting the health care needs of Canadians. Today's health care involves more than the one privileged place (the hospital) and more than the one privileged provider (the physician), resulting in many health care services falling outside of the scope of the CHA (Coyte 2002). In fact, there are close to one million Canadians receiving home care services today (CHCA 2008a).

The rise of neo-liberalism underlies these health care reforms that have left many without coverage, including those who require home care services. Within **neo-liberalism**, or the "New Public Management," as a political and social philosophy, the following are emphasized:

1. The reduction of public/state responsibility for health through the shift of responsibility to individuals and families.
2. The use of the market as the best allocator of health and social resources.
3. The requirement of individuals to take responsibility for their own health and health improvements, including the need for self-care and the care provided for family members during long-term illnesses.
4. The idea that society is composed of competitive and economically focused autonomous individuals.
5. The belief that health promotion is about individually driven behavioural changes as opposed to an understanding that involves the ability of all citizens to access the social determinants of health (Bjornsdottir 2009; Coburn 2000; Navarro 2009).

With markets functioning as resource allocators, the lack of state intervention in the form of welfare and income redistribution can be justified from a neo-liberal perspective. Furthermore, the autonomous, economically motivated individual has little to no responsibility for the well-being of others. In this political culture, individuals are framed in terms of their rights and freedoms (Rose 1998). Others merely function as competition to material goods (Coburn 2000).

Neo-liberalism promotes a view of justice such that persons receive a fair distribution of goods according to free-market exchanges. Market inequalities are seen as "just" because what one puts into the market one gets out. Inequalities from this viewpoint, therefore, can be justified because it is presumed that individuals are equally equipped to compete for resources. Adherents of neo-liberal ideologies view public and social expenditures, like health care, as a source of inefficiency and waste. In the end, free-market forces and private profits are substituted for the collective public good (Navarro 2009; Williams et al. 2001).

At the heart of neo-liberalism are two core ideals that threaten the values fundamental to the CHA and to Canadian identity and that are contrary to the stated values of home care nurses. The first is the belief that the free market is a just allocator of resources, such that each person fairly receives his or her share of resources by virtue of market exchanges. In contrast, the CHA is based largely on the belief that justice is served when each person receives his or her share of resources according to need, a central principle informing Canadian identity. As the Commission on the Future of Health Care in Canada (2002) states, "Canadians view medicare as a moral enterprise, not a business venture" (xx). The Canadian Community Health Nursing Standards of Practice also do not support a market sense of justice. Instead, community nurses believe in advancing social justice by facilitating universal and equitable access to conditions for health and to health services. They recognize that socio-political issues may underlie individual and community problems (CHNAC 2008).

Social justice can be viewed as an opposing perspective to market justice (Beauchamp 1999). Matters of social justice "concern whether the background conditions of people's actions are fair, whether it is fair that whole categories of persons have vastly wider opportunities than others, how among the opportunities that some people have is the ability, through the way institutions operate, to dominate or exploit others, or benefit from their domination and exploitation" (Young 2011, 38). Beauchamp (1999) further argues that unless collective burdens are assumed, the environment, heredity, or social structures will prevent all persons from receiving health protection and a minimum income. Market justice is not appropriate for the distribution of health-related resources because factors such as disability, gender, age, and poverty impede people's abilities to access formal health care services and the determinants of health. The disparities that exist between members of one social group and another because of factors such as race, class, sexual orientation, and sex must be addressed to achieve justice (CNA 2006; Drevdahl et al. 2001).

The neo-liberal emphasis upon the self-interested and autonomous individual is individualistic, not collectivist, in nature. Outside of immediate family and friends, others are viewed as competitors for scarce resources and are blamed and punished for their problems rather than helped. This individualistic market orientation elevates the level of social fragmentation and lowers the level of social cohesion and trust and heightens the sense of relative deprivation in a society. It also contributes to income inequalities, higher rates of violence and racism, less community involvement, more chronic anxiety, and a lowered health status of citizens (Coburn 2000; Lynch 2000; Wilkinson and Pickett 2007). This individualistic orientation is antithetical to the core values of equity, fairness, and solidarity that are central to a Canadian understanding of citizenship (Commission on the Future of Health Care in Canada 2002). It is also antithetical to the home care nurse's core belief in connecting with and caring for individuals, families, and communities (CHNAC 2008).

ETHICAL IMPLICATIONS: THE EVERYDAY LIVES OF CLIENTS, FAMILIES, AND HOME CARE NURSES

Many researchers have identified issues in home care that have arisen as a result of health reform (Bee, Barnes, and Luker 2008; Exley and Allen 2007; Peter et al. 2007; Stajduhar et al. 2010). These issues have not always been explicitly conceptualized as ethical in nature, but they are of ethical importance particularly on an everyday level because they affect the health and well-being of care recipients and caregivers alike. In the following discussion, I will draw upon these issues to describe the ethical implications of neo-liberal health reforms.

ETHICS IN PRACTICE 19-1

Self-Care and Family Care

I have been a case manager for a Community Care Access Centre in Ontario (CCAC) for the past five years. Before that I worked in the ICU at a teaching hospital. I used to think that I had seen pretty much everything in terms of ethical problems, but I was really wrong. The community is very different and there are things that I just can't seem to resolve. There are cases that bother me so much that I believe that I can't work here much longer. When I was in the ICU, although sometimes beds were an issue, we still always seemed to be able to have enough to go around. Here in the community I find that there are never enough resources for everyone. Sometimes we have clients who are so sick that we need to help them get admitted into hospital. The problem is they are generally discharged just a few days later. Some of these people just can't take care of themselves or don't have family around. I feel terrible that we can't provide them with all of the care they need because we only can give each person so many hours.

One client, I'll call him Joe, was one I have really tried to help. He was diagnosed with schizophrenia and Type 2 diabetes and had few supports available to him. He came from Kenya eight years ago with his family when he was 15 years old but started to get sick a few years later. After a short hospitalization last spring, we did our best to address his medical, psychiatric, and social needs the best we could, but services available are so limited and fragmented. Joe needed many things that we found difficult to find for him, such as job training and a sense of belonging. His mother called the other day to tell us he is not doing well again and she is having difficulty coping not only with his symptoms, but also financially because she has needed to take off time from work to care for him.

In Ethics in Practice 19-1, a nurse describes many of the consequences of neo-liberal health policies. Expenditures for home care services have not met the increased demand for them; instead family must take up the slack (Duncan and Reutter 2006). Thus, many sick and disabled people must rely on themselves or their families and friends, if available, to provide care. The moral distress of this home care nurse is evident as she describes the experience of wanting to provide care, but of being incapable of doing so because the resources are simply not available. On the one hand, the nurse is attempting to help Joe attain the highest level of health possible for him, consistent with the expectation within the CNA (2008) Code of Ethics, but cannot achieve her goal given the lack of services to help promote Joe's health. She is also concerned that Joe's mother is having difficulty coping with the demands of caregiving, which include not only physical and emotional demands, but also financial ones. The latter reflects the declining involvement of the state in providing services and also the need for better integration of services.

As this nurse suggests, others must be there to provide care when covered professional home care services are not available or are limited. High-income Canadians may be able to purchase their own professional services, but for most Canadians the onus falls on them to provide care for their loved ones. It is estimated that over the last year, 25 percent of Canadians cared for either a family member or a friend with a serious health condition, many taking time off from work, using personal savings, and experiencing emotional difficulties and a decline in their own health (Duxbury, Higgins, and Schroeder 2009). Low-income Canadians may be particularly affected because they often do not have extended health care benefits to cover the cost of pharmaceuticals and additional home care services, and many may not have the kinds of homes that are suitable for caregiving. As Anderson (2001) suggests, home care policy is dependent upon a particular notion of home that reflects the privileged middle class who are more likely to have the resources necessary to provide care.

The transfer of caregiving responsibilities from the state to the family also represents the state's reliance on the social positioning of women and the assumption that women will be available to care for others in the home, as the example of Joe's mother illustrates. It is expected that women will provide this care in the home for their sick, dying, or disabled family members (MacKinnon 2009) because caring for the home and the family has been the expected focus of many women's lives to the extent that "the house is identified as a place that is 'female' and caring as 'female' work" (Bowlby, Gregory, and McKie 1997, 346). Indeed, in Canada, the greatest burden of both informal and formal care does fall upon women (CHCA 2008a; Duxbury, Higgins, and Schroeder 2009) The level of care provision can be extraordinary, encompassing both personal and high-tech care. It can include assistance with activities of daily living (e.g., bathing, eating, cooking, laundry, cleaning, and transportation) and also the provision and management of medications, injections, IVs, catheterizations, dialysis, tube feeding, and respiratory care). These informal caregivers are often responsible for 24-hour care with little available public support and often with inadequate training for the responsibilities they are expected to assume (Duxbury, Higgins, and Schroeder 2009).

Addressing the underlying social injustices in Ethics in Practice 19-1 most likely has the best potential to make the greatest difference for Joe and his mother. Referring them to any available community service that would take into account their socio-economic status, along with the fact that they are immigrants living with a persistent mental illness, could be helpful. Challenging the underlying service deficits in home care at a policy level is also a possible action that could be undertaken within the context of participation within a professional organization.

In Ethics in Practice 19-2 the neoliberal values of cost-savings and efficiency under-lying the health care system are also shown to have an impact on the working conditions of home care workers.

ETHICS IN PRACTICE 19-2

Working Conditions

I used to be a physician in Brazil, but I haven't been able to pass my exams here in Canada. My husband, who used to be a teacher, is unemployed so I need to work as many hours as I can as a home support worker. Most of the people I take care of are very happy to see me, but I find the work heavy and there is a lot of travel around the city on the bus. Sometimes people talk to me like I don't know any-thing, but I need this work for my family to live.

The home support worker in Ethics in Practice 19-2, like the majority of formal home care workers in Canada, is an unregulated health provider. These home health aides, at-tendants, and support workers are mainly women, many of whom are drawn from immi-grant and visible minority populations. Although many community workers enjoy the autonomy and varied work environments that providing home care can offer, they gener-ally work alone without the assistance and team support normally available in institutional settings. The requirement of round-the-clock services poses risks for all workers, but par-ticularly for personal and home support workers who often rely on public transportation. While employers are required to comply with health and safety regulations, many of these rest on the premise that employers can exert control over the workplace. Employers, how-ever, do not have this power when work is conducted off site, such as in private homes. Conditions in patients' homes can be highly variable and can fluctuate over time. It is not unusual for workers to face unsanitary conditions, harassment, abuse, and exposure to illegal activities and domestic violence. Along with concerns regarding safety, home care work is poorly paid, is of low status, and must be completed within highly constrained amounts of time (CHCA 2008a; Liaschenko and Peter 2002; Wojtak 2002).

The poor employment opportunities for the home care worker and her husband in Ethics in Practice 19-2 may also reflect the lack of community supports offered to them as they attempt to adapt in a highly competitive society that expects autonomy. Biases related to foreign credentials and language may make them less capable of competing with others. Consequently, poorly paid home care work may be one of few options available to them. Ultimately, this economic arrangement, along with the unpaid work of family, permits the health care system to continue to function in an efficient, but exploitative manner.

Nurses, particularly in leadership positions in home care provider agencies, can help address these working conditions by attending to workload, travel arrangements, sched-uling, and potential discrimination/safety concerns in homes. Providing a forum for workers to bring their suggestions for an improved working environment could also be helpful. Drawing attention to some of these concerns when budgeting and seeking fur-ther funding could also be important.

ETHICS IN PRACTICE 19-3

Nurse–Patient–Family Relationships

Over the years, my role as a home care nurse has changed dramatically. I used to provide a lot of hands-on care, but now I mainly teach clients how to provide the care themselves. The other day, I taught a 91-year-old woman how to provide a complicated dressing for her husband and how to watch for signs of deterioration in his condition. I know she wasn't comfortable doing this and has difficulty given her own health problems. They would also benefit from help with fundamental things, like housekeeping and groceries. Although I think she is managing, I find myself worrying about them as soon as I leave.

The nurse in Ethics in Practice 19-3 describes the responsibilities of home care nurses as clients in the community become increasingly complex, often living with a number of chronic illnesses. The introduction of additional "high-tech" care has also changed the relationship among the nurse, client, and family. The nurse teaches the client and family how to do it themselves and then takes calls to trouble-shoot and problem solve. The client and family become more self-sufficient and the nurse's role becomes less hands-on, which for some may be desirable, but for others, such as the couple in the example, may be an enormous burden. The relationship eventually takes place at a greater distance, the nurse acting as more of a resource than a direct caregiver. This type of relationship may or may not fully support the well-being of all involved depending on the resources of the client and family. In other words, the individual situations of clients and families must be taken into account. In our current system, however, these parameters cannot always be followed. In keeping with neo-liberal trends, clients and their families must often take responsibility for their own care, even when they do not have sufficient personal and other resources to do so.

In fact, many of the responsibilities of family caregivers are those that, until recently, would normally only have been held by regulated, formal caregivers. Families often assume the responsibilities and attain the skills of nurses but are not given the remuneration or the regulated working conditions and protections of formal providers. As nurses have enacted the role of physician extender, or the "Hamburger Helper" of medicine, when medical responsibilities have become inconvenient, too expensive, or otherwise unappealing to perform (Sandelowski 1999), so too have families become the "Hamburger Helper" of nursing. Because this transfer of responsibility is occurring in homes, it can easily be hidden and justified as merely an extension of "usual" family responsibility. Caregivers are profoundly affected by this work, to the extent that they experience increased morbidity and mortality (Duxbury, Higgins, and Schroeder 2009).

A Canadian study by Ward-Griffin and McKeever (2000) examined the relationships between community nurses and family members caring for frail elders that described well the impact of the neo-liberal health reforms of the 1990s on nursing relationships. Four types of nurse–family–caregiver relationships were identified: (1) nurse–helper, (2) worker–worker, (3) manager–worker, and (4) nurse–patient. The latter two were most frequent. The nurse–helper relationship was the least common relationship found.

In this type of relationship nurses provided and co-ordinated most of the care, while family caregivers assumed a supportive role to nurses. Because of the cost of providing this type of care, nurses quickly moved to the second form of relationship—the worker–worker relationship. Care work was transferred to family caregivers, with nurses teaching them technical skills. These caregivers learned to assume much responsibility with little authority. Some family caregivers reported feeling afraid and unqualified to assume this level of responsibility much like the elderly woman in Ethics in Practice 19-3. In time, these relationships moved to the manager–worker type, at the point that family caregivers had taken on virtually all of the care. At this stage, nurses no longer provided actual caregiving, but focused on the monitoring of family caregivers' coping skills and competence. Many family caregivers resisted this type of support, wanting assistance with actual caregiving instead. The final type of relationship, the nurse–patient relationship, occurred as frequently as the previous one. With this type of relationship, many caregivers, because of pre-existing health problems and the heavy demands of caregiving, became the nurse's patient too. The authors concluded that these family caregiver–nurse relationships were not partnerships, but were exploitative in character. The work of caring was transferred to family caregivers who were left socially isolated and without adequate resources to provide care.

Through their research, Ward-Griffin and McKeever (2000) illustrate how the policies of health reform shaped the everyday lives of clients, families, and home care nurses. Over 10 years later, home care recipients and their caregivers often continue to be without the necessary resources to receive and provide care in such a way that the quality of care is maintained (CHCA 2008a). Every aspect of the work of home care nurses has been impacted, the well-being of all involved being threatened. This situation compromises the ability of nurses to enact one of nursing's most fundamental ethical values—the requirement to promote the health and well-being of persons (CNA 2008). Nurses can advocate for further services, including respite care, whenever possible to support clients like those in Ethics in Practice 19-3. Strategies must also be sought to make changes in Canadian home care policy such that care recipients are protected and nurses can practise ethically.

RECOMMENDATIONS

Home care policy, like other forms of policy, is based on the values of the politically dominant group. Consequently, policy has a moral dimension in that it results in those with power making decisions being involved in how others not involved in the decision making will be treated (Giacomini and Kenny 2005; Malone 1999). Reflecting the interests of the most powerful, current Canadian home care policy upholds values and beliefs consistent with market justice and individualism (Peter et al. 2007; Purkis, Ceci, and Bjornsdottir 2008). As such, home care policy constructs a neo-liberal notion of citizenship. This dominant vision of reality can be resisted, however. In recent years, a number of Canadian authors have offered alternative views.

Kenny (2002) presents the values of solidarity, equity, compassion, efficiency, and civility to supplant the market metaphor. She views health care not as a private commodity, but as a public and social good that must be distributed based on a communitarian sense of justice that embraces shared risk and collective responsibility.

The Romanow Report (Commission on the Future of Health Care in Canada 2002) also explicitly put forward alternatives to a market view of justice, offering the values of equity, fairness, and solidarity to challenge the view that health care is a business venture. Specifically, the authors of the report proposed that home care be targeted for additional funding in order to provide a foundation for a national home care strategy, and that the Canada Health Act be revised to include coverage for home mental health case management and intervention services, post-acute home care, and palliative home care. In addition, the authors recommended that informal caregivers be given ongoing support through direct remuneration, tax breaks, job protection, caregiver leave, and respite. Yet the authors fell short in leaving the provision of care for people with chronic illnesses and physical disabilities outside the focus of the report's priority areas. A danger exists that these individuals will become further marginalized and viewed as problems in the system.

In nursing, Rodney et al. (2002), Varcoe et al. (2004), and Varcoe and Rodney (2009) have described in rich detail how the underlying ideologies of corporatism and scarcity have had a constraining influence on nurses' moral agency. They offer examples of how nurses have resisted these ideologies in a variety of ways, including through the negotiation of better care, relationship building among workers and clients, and rule bending. They suggest strategies of further resistance that involve tactics that go beyond the efforts of individuals, such as the restructuring of nurses' work in ways that align it with the goals of health and the common good instead of the goals of corporatism. They also recommend unmasking current ideologies in such a way that values can be laid bare so that nurses can become more conscious and deliberate about the values they are enacting in their practice.

Innovative and politically savvy nurse reformers may realize some of these goals. More likely, however, change will be made possible through the everyday activities of nurses who adopt these strategies. We must guard against the common tendency in nursing of either viewing nurses as powerless or of viewing power as somehow separate from the usual activities of nurses (Lunardi, Peter, and Gastaldo 2002; Purkis 2001). With respect to home care nursing, Purkis (2001) suggests that the practice of home care nursing be re-conceptualized as a political practice that addresses and acknowledges the legitimacy of nurses' knowledge of the difficulties that they and their clients are experiencing. With this knowledge, nurses have the potential to resist managerial demands for efficiency by refusing to enact practices that exclude clients from the home care services they require. In my own previous work (Peter 2002), I have also examined the politics of home care by exploring how early twentieth-century home care/private duty nurses exercised power. Despite the emphasis in nursing upon duty and obedience to physicians at that time, nurses also plainly expressed their capacity to influence their clients through education, role modelling, and the re-ordering of homes. These nurses also later played a significant role in the rise of hospitalization, as private duty nursing came to be viewed as a waste of nursing skill and money. Thus, nurses were not powerless. Their values left a mark not only on individual clients and families, but also on the health care system as a whole. Today our values also have influence. Therefore, purposefully explicating them may foster a much-needed awareness that can move us collectively forward to a more humane and ethical health care system.

In a previous publication where this author and others analyzed home care policies across Canada (Peter et al. 2007), a preliminary ethical framework that could be used to examine and develop home care policy and could direct practice was developed that included the dimensions of relational autonomy, care, and social justice. Social justice is of particular importance because it can counter the predominance of market justice inherent in neo-liberalism.

Social justice is required to promote a belief in collectivism over individualism that can challenge neo-liberalism. Nurses who are in the position to develop policy can examine critically those policy dimensions that idealize the autonomy of home care recipients.

Striving for social justice often requires collective action to reduce the effects of factors such as age, disability, and poverty. Promoting awareness and action regarding human rights, homelessness, poverty, unemployment, stigma, and so on are ways of working toward social justice. Young (2006; 2011) recommends forward-looking strategies using the social connections among us. Because many of the issues underlying the problems that are inherent in home care policies and delivery have structural roots, it is difficult for individuals alone to make significant change. Nurses have the benefit of belonging to organized nursing groups that have the potential to make social change (Peter 2011). It is important that codes of ethics in nursing, such as the CNA Code of Ethics (2008), provide a vision of social justice that nurses can use as an ideal. While making social change is exceedingly difficult small steps forward are important.

Opportunities exist for nurses to become vocal with respect to issues of social justice. Writing letters to local Members of Legislative Assemblies or Members of Parliament and participating in activities of professional organizations in nursing are realistic ways to have influence. Nursing faculty through nursing curricula can also foster an understanding of social justice in future nurses. Students can become sensitized in the classroom and in clinical practice to the health concerns of marginalized groups and to the need not only to equitably distribute health care services, but also the determinants of health. The CNA's (2008) Code of Ethics for Registered Nurses can provide assistance in this manner, with its stance that nurses must endeavour to promote social justice through a variety of actions including changing systems and societal structures, incorporating the principles of primary health care, changing unethical policies, recognizing the importance of the social determinants of health, preventing environmental change, advocating for vulnerable and disadvantaged groups and advocating for access to the full continuum of health care services for all.

Summary

In this chapter, I have described the current state of home care in Canada, revealing inadequacies and inequities in our system that privileges hospital and physician services. The rise of home care has been made possible not only through advances in technology, but also by neo-liberal beliefs in market justice and individualism that have informed the development of home care policy. I have provided a number of recommendations based on social justice that have the potential to counter the market justice of neo-liberalism.

For Reflection

1. How has neo-liberalism affected your nursing practice?

2. What are the ethical dimensions of health policy? How can nurses challenge unethical policies?

3. Is an emphasis on social justice in nursing ethics compatible with the traditional ethical ideal of the caring nurse–client relationship? Why or why not?

4. With the current emphasis on acute care in home care provision, how can nurses ensure that the well-being of those with disabilities and chronic illnesses is protected?

Endnote

1. This work was supported through the funding of the Social Sciences and Humanities Research Council of Canada.

References

Anderson, J.M. 2001. The politics of home care: Where is "home"? *Canadian Journal of Nursing Research, 33* (2), 5–10.

Beauchamp, D. 1999. Public health as social justice. In D.E. Beauchamp and B. Steinbock (Eds.), *New ethics for the public's health* (pp. 101–109). New York: Oxford University Press.

Bee, P.E., Barnes, P., and Luker, K.A. 2008. A systematic review of informal caregivers' needs in providing home-based end-of-life care to people with cancer. *Journal of Clinical Nursing, 18*, 1379–1393.

Bjornsdottir, K. 2009. The ethics and politics of home care. *International Journal of Nursing Studies, 46*, 732–739.

Bowlby, S., Gregory, S., and McKie, L. 1997. "Doing home": Patriarchy, caring, and space. *Women's Studies International Forum, 20* (3), 343–350.

Canada Health Act. 1985. C.6, s.1.

Canadian Home Care Association (CHCA). 2008a. *Portraits of home care*. Ottawa: Author.

Canadian Home Care Association (CHCA). 2008b. *Home care: The next essential service*. Ottawa: Author.

Canadian Nurses Association (CNA). 2006. *Social justice . . . a means to an end, an end in itself.* Ottawa, ON: Author.

Canadian Nurses Association (CNA). 2008. *Code of ethics for registered nurses*. Ottawa: Authors.

Ceci, C. 2006. Impoverishment of practice: Analysis of effects of economic discourses in home care case management practice. *Canadian Journal of Nursing Leadership, 19* (1), 56–68.

Coburn, D. 2000. Income inequality, social cohesion and the health status of populations: The role of neo-liberalism. *Social Science and Medicine, 51*, 135–146.

Commission on the Future of Health Care in Canada. 2002. *Building on values: The future of health care in Canada*. Saskatoon: Commission on the Future of Health Care in Canada.

Community Health Nurses Association of Canada (CHNAC). 2003. *Understanding home health nursing: A discussion paper*. Available at www.communityhealthnursescanda.org.

Community Health Nurses Association of Canada (CHNAC). 2008. *Canadian community health nursing standards of practice*. Toronto: Author.

Community Health Nurses Association of Canada (CHNAC). 2009. *Definition of community health nursing practice across the lifespan*. Available at www.communityhealthnursescanda.org.

Coyte, P.C. 2002. Expanding the principle of comprehensiveness from hospital to home. Submission to the Standing Committee on Social Affairs, Science and Technology. Available at http://www.parl.gc.ca/Content/SEN/Committee/372/SOCI/rep/coyte1-e.pdf.

Drevdahl, D., Kneipp, S.M., Canales, M.K., and Dorcy, K.S. 2001. Reinvesting in social justice: A capital idea for public health nursing? *Advances in Nursing Science, 24* (2), 19–31.

Duncan, S. and Reutter, L. 2006. A critical policy analysis of an emerging agenda for home care in one Canadian province. *Home and Social Care in the Community, 14* (3), 242–253.

Duxbury, L., Higgins, C., and Schroeder, B. 2009. *Balancing paid work and caregiving responsibilities: A closer look at family caregivers in Canada*. Ottawa: Canadian Policy Research Networks.

Exley, C. and Allen D. 2007. A critical examination of home care: End-of-life care as an illustrative example. *Social Science and Medicine, 65* (11), 2317–2327.

Giacomini, M. and Kenny, N. 2005. Wanted: A new ethics field for health policy analysis. *Health Care Analysis, 13* (4), 247–260.

Kenny, N.P. 2002. *What good is health care? Reflections on the Canadian experience*. Ottawa: CHA Press.

Liaschenko, J. and Peter, E. 2002. The voice of home care workers in clinical ethics. *Healthcare Ethics Committee Forum, 14* (3), 217–223.

Lunardi, V.L., Peter, E., and Gastaldo, D. 2002. Are submissive nurses ethical? Reflecting on power anorexia. *Revista Brasileira de Enfermagem, 55* (2), 183–188.

Lynch, J. 2000. Income inequality and health: Expanding the debate. *Social Science & Medicine, 51*, 1001–1005.

MacKinnon, C.J. 2009. Applying feminist, multicultural, and social justice theory to diverse women who function as caregivers in end-of-life and palliative home care. *Palliative and Supportive Care, 7*, 501–512.

Malone, R.E. 1999. Policy as product: Mortality and metaphor in health policy discourse. *The Hastings Center Report, 29* (3), 16–22.

Navarro, V. 2009. What we mean by social determinants of health. *International Journal of Health Services, 39* (3), 423–441.

Peter, E. 2002. The history of nursing in the home: Revealing the significance of place in the expression of moral agency. *Nursing Inquiry, 9* (2), 65–72.

Peter, E., Spalding, K., Kenny, N., Conrad, P., McKeever, P., and Macfarlane, A. 2007. Neither seen nor heard: Children and home care policy in Canada. *Social Science & Medicine, 64*, 1624–1635.

Peter, E. 2011. Educating for social justice: The possibility of a socially connected model of moral agency. *Canadian Journal of Nursing Research, 44* (2).

Purkis, M.E. 2001. Managing home nursing care: Visibility, accountability and exclusion. *Nursing Inquiry, 8* (3), 141–150.

Purkis, M.E., Ceci, C., and Bjornsdottir, K. 2008. Patching up the holes: Analyzing the work of home care. *Canadian Journal of Public Health, 9* (Supplement 2), S27–S32.

Rodney, P., Varcoe, C., Storch, J.L., McPherson, G., Mahoney, K., Brown, H., Pauly, B., Hartrick, G., and Starzomski, R. 2002. Navigating towards a moral horizon: A multi-site qualitative study of ethical practice in nursing. *Canadian Journal of Nursing Research, 34* (3), 75–102.

Rose, N. 1998. *Inventing our selves: Psychology, power, and personhood.* London: Cambridge University Press.

Sandelowski, M. 1999. Venous envy: The post-world war II debate over IV nursing. *Advances in Nursing Science, 22* (1), 52–62.

Stajduhar, K.I., Funk, L., Roberts, D., McLeod, B., Coutier-Fisher, D., Wilkinson, C., and Purkis, M.E. 2010. Home care nurses' decisions about the need for and amount of service at the end of life. *Journal of Advanced Nursing, 67* (2), 276–286.

Varcoe, C. and Rodney, P. 2009. Constrained agency: The social structure of nurses' work. In B. Singh Bolaria and H.D. Dickinson (Eds.), *Health, illness, and health care in Canada* (pp. 122–150). Saskatoon: Nelson Thomson Learning.

Varcoe, C., Doane, G., Pauly, B., Rodney, P., Storch, J.L., Mahoney, K., McPherson, G., Brown, H., and Starzomski R. 2004. Ethical practice in nursing: Working the in-betweens. *Journal of Advanced Nursing, 45* (3), 316–25.

Walker, M.U. 1998. *Moral understandings: A feminist study in ethics.* New York: Routledge.

Ward-Griffin, C. and McKeever, P. 2000. Relationships between nurses and family caregivers: Partners in care? *Advances in Nursing Science, 22* (3), 89–103.

Wilkinson, R.G. and Pickett, K.E. 2007. The problems of relative deprivation. Why some societies do better than others. *Social Science & Medicine, 65* (9), 1965–1978.

Williams, A.P., Deber, R., Baranek, P., and Gildiner, A. 2001. From medicare to home care: Globalization, state retrenchment, and the profitization of Canada's health-care system. In P. Armstrong, H. Armstrong, and D. Coburn (Eds.), *Unhealthy times: Political economy perspectives on health and care* (pp. 7–30). New York: Oxford University Press.

Williams, A.P., Lum, J.A., Deber, R., Montgomery, R., Kuluski, K., Peckham, A., Watkins, J., Williams, A., Ying, A., and Zhu, L. 2010. Aging at home: Integrating community-based care for older persons. *Healthcare Papers, 10* (1), 8–21.

Wojtak, A. 2002. Practice-based ethics: A foundation for human resource planning in community healthcare. *Healthcare Management Forum, 15* (3), 67–72.

Young, I.M. 2006. Responsibility and global justice: A social connection model. *Social Philosophy & Policy Foundation, 23* (1), 102–130.

Young, I.M. 2011. *Responsibility for justice.* New York: Oxford University Press.

CHAPTER 20

Ethics of Public Health

Marjorie MacDonald

A public health ethics must begin with recognition of the values at the core of public health, not a modification of values used to guide other kinds of health care interactions. (Baylis, Kenny, and Sherwin 2008, 199)

Public health practitioners have long grappled with ethical issues in their practice but, until recently, there have been few relevant ethics frameworks that take into account the values base of public health (PH). Historically, those involved in both health care ethics and nursing ethics have failed to provide public health nurses with guidance geared to their unique ethical concerns. Usually, a rights-based deontological approach (Zahner 2000), or the health care ethics principles of autonomy, beneficence, non-maleficence, and justice (Beauchamp and Childress 1979) are invoked as the appropriate framework to support ethical public health nursing (PHN) practice (Chafey 1995; Vollman, Anderson, and McFarlane 2003). But, as I will demonstrate in this chapter, health care ethics provides neither an adequate theoretical foundation nor appropriate normative justification for PH ethics. Recent developments in nursing ethics, as influenced by feminist and relational ethics has broadened nursing ethics' focus to encompass *some* of PHN's ethical concerns; however, ethical issues in PHN may be more adequately addressed by emerging developments in PH ethics. What I will argue is needed are ethics frameworks for PHN that synthesize relevant aspects of nursing ethics, feminist ethics, and PH ethics.

Public health ethics is a relatively new field of applied ethics (Bayer et al. 2007; Baylis, Kenny, and Sherwin 2008; Dawson and Verweij 2007). Although a few writers some years ago proposed the need for an ethics of PH (Beauchamp 1976; Lappe 1986), the field of PH ethics has only been claimed and named as a distinct area of scholarship since the late 1990s and into the new millennium (Kass 2004). In fact, Kass says that the term "public health ethics" was rarely used prior to the year 2000.

In this chapter, I define PH and review the history and development of PH ethics, including its philosophical underpinnings. I then explore and critique emerging frameworks for PH ethics, the development of ethics in PHN, and the ethical issues in a current and significant PH issue—pandemic influenza planning. Finally, I conclude with a brief summary of the current status of PH ethics and speculation about the future of PH ethics.

WHAT IS PUBLIC HEALTH?

Nixon and colleagues (2005) discuss two historical streams in PH. One stream recounts an authoritarian and coercive history in which PH officials imposed severe restrictions on movement and association through quarantine measures during the epidemics of the

Middle Ages and later in Europe. While arguably necessary to contain the raging epidemics, these repressive actions were not always applied equitably. This history haunts PH to this day, particularly with the threat of new and re-emerging infectious disease epidemics that raise the spectre of loss of liberty, freedom, and rights of association (Petersen and Lupton 1996).

The second stream records a more positive history with PH engagement in progressive social movements, during which major PH advances were achieved such as improved water quality and sanitation, sewage treatment, maternal and child health services, improved working conditions and housing (Lalonde 1974; Rutty and Sullivan 2010; Szreter 1988; 2002). The result was a dramatic improvement in population health with increased life expectancy and reduced morbidity. In fact, we know that it is PH measures, rather than medical treatment and health care that have contributed most significantly to these improvements (Rutty and Sullivan). There has been a 30-year gain in life expectancy over the past century, 25 years of which can be attributed to PH measures (Canadian Public Health Association [CPHA] 2010a). Public health, including PHN, has had a long history of social justice and political action to improve population health (Beauchamp 1976; Buhler-Wilkerson 1993; Chafey 1995), although even this history is not untainted by discrimination, oppression, and coercion for some populations. To the extent that these concerns remain today, there are an abundance of ethical issues to confront in PH practice.

"Public health is a contested concept" (Verweij and Dawson 2007, 13) that has multiple meanings and is often misunderstood. Some understand PH to mean health care provided within the publicly funded health system. This misinterpretation occurs, in part, because PH operates under the radar; people are not aware of it until a crisis strikes and drastic PH measures need to be implemented. The health care system, on the other hand, is highly visible in our lives.

Definitions of PH include the following:

> [T]he science and art of preventing disease, prolonging life and promoting health through the organized efforts of society. (Acheson 1988)
>
> [W]hat we, as a society, do collectively to assure the conditions in which people can be healthy. (Institute of Medicine [IOM] 1988, 1)
>
> . . . [A]n organized activity of society to promote, protect, improve, and, when necessary, restore the health of individuals, specified groups, or the entire population. It is a combination of sciences, skills, and values that function through collective societal activities and involve programs, services, and institutions aimed at protecting and improving the health of all the people. (Last 2007, 306)

Common elements across all definitions include collective effort, societal responsibility, and attention to social and environmental health determinants. In all of them, the moral aim is to promote the health of the population as a social good that allows people to pursue other valued ends. More recently, as evidence of growing health inequities accumulates, a concern with vulnerable and marginalized populations has emerged.

Because PH aims to improve the health of whole communities, the strategies do not focus solely on individuals. Societally oriented interventions, by their very nature, are provided by local governing bodies such as state/provincial governments, municipalities, or regional health authorities. Providing safe water, ensuring a safe and accessible food supply, public sanitation, and taking action to control or prevent communicable diseases are just some of the PH interventions that require collective rather than individual action. The collective nature of these interventions often requires legislative authority and may infringe on the rights of individuals, thus raising distinctive ethical challenges.

WHO IS THE "PUBLIC" IN PUBLIC HEALTH?

Childress et al. (2002) identify three notions of *public* in PH: the numerical public, the political public, and the communal public. The numerical public is the target population that refers to an aggregate of individuals and is concerned with population health measurement. The political public refers to what is done collectively through public agencies and governments; it is the legislatively designated responsibility of governments to promote and protect health. Finally, the communal public includes all other forms of social and community action to promote health that extend beyond the practices of PH providers and agencies including non-governmental organizations, private groups and citizens, and other collectives. The Healthy Cities/Communities movement worldwide (Hancock 1997) is an example of PH action that involves a communal public.

Jennings (2007) provides a more evocative notion of public as "a community of individuals, intertwined through complicated institutional and cultural systems in (and through) which they act and carry out their lives" (36). He sees *public* as a normative concept "that provides an account of how that system should be structured and how our lives in common ought to be composed and lived" (36). Thus, the public is much more than an aggregate of individuals. It is a complex system comprising a network of interacting and interrelated elements. As a whole, it has properties that are not reflected in its individual components. A simplistic view of a population as an aggregate of atomistic elements is rejected. Instead, Jennings argues, drawing on Harre (1988), that an understanding of ethical conduct must encompass notions and concepts that "reflect the relational nature of the human self or actor and the contextual social nature of the actor's meaningful, symbolically mediated relationships with others" (37). As we shall see, these ideas about the meaning of *public* and the relational nature of persons undergird emerging perspectives in both PH and feminist ethics.

WHAT IS PUBLIC HEALTH ETHICS?

Gostin (2001) proposes three analytic perspectives on PH ethics; the ethics *of* public health, ethics *in* public health, and ethics *for* public health. Callaghan and Jennings (2002) added a fourth type they name *critical public health ethics*. Professional ethics, or the ethics *of* public health, relates to the mission of PH to protect and promote health and focuses on the virtues or professional character of PH practitioners who hold themselves accountable to standards or codes of ethics. The Public Health Leadership Society (2002) in the U.S. has developed a code of ethics to guide PH practitioners but there is no such code in Canada. In the ethics *of* PH questions include, to whom do PH professionals owe a duty of loyalty? Is it individual clients/patients or the community at large? How do professionals know what actions are morally acceptable? How would an ethical PH practitioner serve the community interest? (Gostin 2001).

Applied ethics, or ethics *in* PH, seeks to develop general principles that can be applied to practical situations to guide ethical practice. It is situation-specific in that it "seeks to identify morally appropriate decisions in concrete cases" (Gostin 2001, 125). However, the principles that should be applied to decision making in concrete PH situations are open to debate and many have been identified (Kenny, Melynchuk, and Asada 2006); there is no consensus on what these principles should be, which should have priority, or how trade-offs among them should be determined when there are conflicts. It is generally agreed that the principles of health care ethics (autonomy, beneficience, non-maleficence, and justice) are not always a good fit for the ethical issues that arise in PH (Kass 2001) because of their individualistic and clients-rights orientation, to the exclusion of the common good. The most common ethical theories that have been applied in PH derive from various strands of liberalism but there is an emerging view that liberalism does not provide an adequate moral foundation for PH (Callaghan 2003; Jennings 2007). Several authors have attempted to lay out a set of principles more relevant to the moral aims of PH (Baylis, Kenny, and Sherwin 2008; Upshur 2002).

Advocacy ethics, or ethics *for* PH, is a less theoretical approach and probably represents the most pervasive ethical orientation in practice. PH practitioners clearly see themselves as advocates. Advocacy ethics involves taking a stand for the goals, interventions, and reforms that are most likely to achieve the moral aims of PH. There is a strong orientation to social justice and equity primarily from a distributive justice and contractarian ethics perspective. Ethics for PH reflects a "populist ethic" (Gostin 2001) to serve the interests of populations, but in particular, the needs and interests of the marginalized and disadvantaged, and thus needs to account for more than distributive concerns (Rogers 2006; Young 1990). Gadow and Schroeder (1996) have described advocacy ethics applied specifically to community health nursing. One concern with advocacy ethics is that PH practitioners may be constrained by their positions within PH units or departments and thus their loyalties may be divided. Advocacy can be seen as "biting the hand that feeds you." Jennings (2003) suggests that advocacy ethics is limited in its ability to provide a critical perspective on taken-for-granted professional norms or orientations and that we need a perspective that is critical of powerful interests.

Critical PH ethics sheds light on issues that may be obscured from view by traditional ways of thinking or acting (Nixon 2006). Critical ethics is historically informed, practically oriented, and considers social values and trends in analyzing and understanding both the PH situation at hand and the moral problems it raises (Callaghan and Jennings 2002). PH problems are influenced by, among other things, "institutional arrangements and prevailing structures of cultural attitudes and social power" (172). This perspective calls for policies or interventions to be "genuinely public or civic endeavours" and suggests the need for "meaningful participation, open deliberation, and civic problem solving and capacity building" (172). This commitment to participation is a longstanding tradition within PH and is also consistent with a range of philosophical perspectives, including feminist and communitarian perspectives, and deliberative democracy.

Nixon (2006) goes further to suggest that a critical lens "prompts us to question the taken-for-granted and think about the ways in which power relations are represented in particular PH concerns. We need to uncover the assumptions underlying our positions and perspectives and interrogate these critically, asking "Why?" and "Whose interests are served?". Through a critical PH ethic, we are asked that we remember our social justice roots, recalling that "public health is social justice" (Beauchamp 1976). Jennings (2003) argues that development of critical ethics is the most important priority within the normative study of PH ethics. This analytic perspective is reminiscent of an older theoretical perspective on health promotion in nursing sometimes referred to as "critical social nursing" (Stevens 1989; Stevens and Hall 1992), "upstream nursing" (Butterfield 1990), or "emancipatory nursing" (Kendall 1992). Bringing together critical PH ethics and a critical perspective in nursing seems to be a promising avenue for the development of PHN ethics.

How Does Public Health Ethics Differ from Health Care Ethics?

The difference between health care ethics and PH ethics lies in the distinction between PH and health care. Health care and its ethics are focused on the needs, interests, and concerns of individual patients as they interact with and receive care from practitioners and the health care system for their illnesses. PH and its ethics, on the other hand, focus on the health of the population, made up of large numbers of people in the settings of their daily lives, particularly as they are affected by social and political structures and environmental conditions. Although concerned with the entire population, there is also a concern with equity in health and the health of those who are disadvantaged, oppressed, or marginalized.

Daniels (2006) says that the early bioethics focused on (1) the relationships between patients and physicians (or other health care providers) and between researchers and subjects and (2) the issues and challenges arising out of new medical technologies. The problem, according to Daniels, is that bioethics has largely ignored the broader institutional settings and policies that affect and mediate population health and has not addressed the context in which these relationships develop and play out in practice. He further suggests that the focus on "exotic technologies" has blinded bioethics to the broader determinants of health that are of primary concern in PH. This has led bioethics away from concerns with health inequities and issues of social justice. Others have also argued that bioethics has not typically demonstrated a concern with the social determinants of health (Baylis, Kenny, and Sherwin 2008; Pauly 2008).

Three features of PH create specific moral concerns (Dawson and Verweij 2007). First, in PH, the initiative comes from the professional not the patient. Classic PH strategies, like case finding and contact tracing, mean that the professional seeks out the patient and may have to use either persuasion or coercion to ensure essential care for protecting the public. In health care, patients voluntarily seek out professionals. Second, because interventions are aimed at populations, the benefits for any individual may be negligible—this is the classic "prevention paradox" (Rose 1985). Some interventions that will benefit the community as a whole may not benefit the individual in any significant way, or may even inflict harm. Third, PH interventions are potentially pervasive such that it is difficult for individuals to refuse participation. Examples include fluoridation of water, seat belt legislation, drinking and driving laws, and mandatory immunization. These distinct foci create very different demands for ethical analysis and each raises its own unique ethical challenges.

The overarching concern in health care for the individual patient is not comparable to the concern for the health of the population. Upshur (2002) points out that there is no clear analogy in PH to the fiduciary role of health care providers in terms of their therapeutic contract with the patient, which is legitimized by informed consent (Nixon et al. 2005). By contrast, the population focus of PH implies a contract with society at large that is legitimized in governmental policies and PH legislation.

In summary, it appears that there is a deep divide between the commitments of health care ethics and the values that inform PH ethics (Bayer and Fairchild 2004). "The core values and practices of PH, which often entail the subordination of the individual for the common good, seem to stand as a rebuke to the ideological impulses of bioethics" (474); therefore, the standards for guiding PH ethics cannot be derived from the assumptions of bioethics in which individualism is dominant and the principle of autonomy has pride of place. In later sections, I discuss perspectives on the philosophical basis of PH ethics, and discuss frameworks that have been proposed to guide ethical PH policy and practice.

What Is the History of Public Health Ethics?

Canada has lagged behind the U.S. and the U.K. in the development of a focus on PH ethics, although increasingly Canadian ethicists have recognized the need for a "robust, coherent and meaningful ethic for public health" (Kenny, Melynchuk, and Asada 2006, 402). Recent theoretical work by feminist ethicists in Canada position us to contribute meaningfully to the broader development of PH ethics (Baylis, Kenny, and Sherwin 2008; Kenny, Sherwin, and Baylis 2010).

Kass (2004) describes three stages of PH ethics development. In Stage I, during the 1970s and 1980s, health promotion and HIV/AIDS came on the scene to contribute foundational ideas for the later articulation of PH ethics. Stage II saw the development of frameworks for PH ethics, an emerging consensus that the field of PH ethics was distinct from that of health care ethics, and proposals for philosophical and political foundations as alternatives to the classical utilitarian and contractarian theories. Stage III is the future, which Kass suggests will focus on global and environmental justice and PH research ethics. I will add additional speculations about the future of PH ethics at the end of the chapter.

Stage I began with the emergence of health promotion as a new focus within PH. Because PH ethics had not been named as such, nor had its philosophical basis been proposed and debated, ethical analysis of health promotion drew primarily from liberal philosophy and bioethics that privileged the principle of autonomy (Bayer and Fairchild 2004). Challenges emerged to the legitimacy of state or professional interventions to change individual voluntary behaviour (e.g., diet, exercise, and smoking) because such interventions based on education and persuasion could stray dangerously close to coercion and thus violate individual autonomy. Even if coercion was not overtly involved, the ethics of persuading people to change their personal preferences, desires, and behaviours, particularly if there was no harm to others, was viewed as a violation of individual liberty and autonomy.

A number of authors, including ethicists and health promoters, weighed in on the ethics of health promotion (Faden and Faden 1978; McLeroy, Gottlieb, and Burdine 1987; Minkler 1978; Wickler 1978a; 1978b; 1987). Both the challenges and the ethical analyses were, however, based on an individually focused and uniquely American definition of health promotion that has been challenged by many authors (Hancock 1985; 1994; Labonte and Penfold 1981; MacDonald 2002; Pederson, Rootman, and O'Neil 1994) since the release of the Ottawa Charter on Health Promotion (World Health Organization 1986). Then, the emphasis shifted from individual behaviour change to social and community change to promote health with a focus on social determinants of heath and healthy public policy. This raised a different set of concerns that called on ethicists to grapple with the inherent paternalism of healthy public policy. In health care ethics, paternalism is a "dirty word" and PH has struggled to deal with this given that much PH policy is indeed paternalistic. Recent work in PH ethics has led to a reconceptualization, perhaps even reclaiming, of the notion of paternalism within the context of relational ethics drawing implicitly or explicitly on communitarian thinking (Beauchamp 1985; Gostin and Gostin 2009; Jennings 2009; Jones and Bayer 2007).

With the emergence of AIDS, many ethical issues became apparent and debates regarding policy responses were spawned. In addressing the moral challenges raised by HIV/AIDS, as with health promotion, health care ethicists were initially guided by the same principles and values that had shaped the development of their field (Bayer and Fairchild 2004). When AIDS arrived, PH already had a set of well-established practices related to screening, surveillance, reporting, and notification for infectious diseases that had proven effective in controlling epidemics (Burr 1999). HIV/AIDS, however, was understood to be very different from other infectious diseases; this led to a response that came to be known as "AIDS exceptionalism" (Bayer 1991; Smith and Whiteside 2010) defined as "departures from standard PH practice and prevention priorities in favour of alternative approaches to prevention that emphasize individual rights at the expense of public health protection" (Fisher, Kohut, and Fisher 2009, 45). In retrospect, Burr (1999) and others (Bayer 1991) questioned whether AIDS exceptionalism had its intended effects—to gain the cooperation of those affected and reduce the spread of the disease—or whether it contributed to a worsening of the problem. The contribution of HIV/AIDS to the development of PH ethics is a long and complicated story that cannot easily be summarized here. What is important is that HIV/AIDS raised many issues related to the dilemma of attending to individual human rights while protecting the health of the population.

In Stage II, from about the year 2000, PH ethics frameworks were proposed and theoretical work intensified to articulate an appropriate philosophical basis, including perspectives that went beyond the traditional liberal orientation. A journal dedicated solely to PH ethics was launched in 2008 (Dawson and Verweij 2008). A parallel track of development in feminist and nursing ethics, which drew on some of the same concepts and principles (e.g., relational autonomy and solidarity, social justice) was also developing. These ideas were applied to specific PH problems (e.g., harm reduction, violence against women) within a health care ethics context but without consideration as to how ethical analysis for these PH problems might help to articulate a broader PH ethics (Pauly 2008; Varcoe 2004).

It was in Stage II that PH ethics came into the limelight in Canada in the wake of SARS, which spurred efforts to renew the PH system and its infrastructure to be better prepared for the next PH crisis. SARS demonstrated that Canada was ill-prepared to deal with the ethical issues raised by serious epidemics (Singer et al. 2003). Some critics suggest, however, that the work on the ethics of pandemic planning in Canada has reflected a traditional bioethics perspective with a "too heavy reliance on an ethic of individual rights" (Baylis, Kenny, and Sherwin 2008, 196) and limited recognition that the burdens of a pandemic are most likely to affect disadvantaged groups. I will discuss the ethics of pandemic planning in more detail later in this chapter.

WHAT ARE THE PHILOSOPHICAL AND THEORETICAL UNDERPINNINGS OF PUBLIC HEALTH ETHICS?

We know that PH has long been tied to utilitarianism harkening back to Edwin Chadwick, the founder of the early PH movement in Britain, who was influenced by Bentham's utilitarianism (Nixon et al. 2005). PH activities are generally teleological or ends-oriented (Childress et al. 2002) with health outcomes the consequence of greatest concern. Quantitative models for priority setting in PH that include measures of health status like quality adjusted life years (QALYs) and disability adjusted life years (DALYs), and methods such as cost-effectiveness analysis and cost-benefit analysis, are grounded firmly in utilitarianism. Although the ethical issues associated with these have been widely debated (Anand and Hanson 2004; Brock 2004; 2007; Kamm 2004), these quantitative approaches have had a great appeal in the traditional, epidemiologically oriented fields of PH and policy analysis. Work in the ethics of communicable disease control and, more recently, pandemic planning has also been strongly reflective of utilitarian concerns, at least in Canada (Baylis, Kenny, and Sherwin 2008; Thompson et al. 2006).

Contractarianism and rights-based theories have also provided philosophical justification for PH actions, drawing on the work of John Rawls, grounded in the notions of freedom and equal moral worth of individuals and concerned about fundamental human, social, and political rights (Jennings 2003). Rawls' theory of justice (1971) is concerned with the rights of the least well off, and thus is congruent with PH considerations for the most disadvantaged in society. This perspective, however, has been criticized for the individualism inherent in its distributive justice focus, which is not adequately reflective of population health and not able to account for non-distributive concerns (Pauly 2008; Powers and Faden 2006; Young 1990).

Concerns with liberal individualism in contractarian ethics, and the limited conception of both human relationships and justice in utilitarianism, have led to communitarian formulations of the philosophical foundations for PH ethics (Jennings 2003). Communitarianism represents a disparate grouping of perspectives that share some common concepts and values. Such groupings include the Green Parties of Europe (Roberts and Reich 2002), feminists (Baylis, Kenny, and Sherwin 2008; Friedman 1992; Sherwin 2004), neo-Confucians (Zhang 2010), indigenous communities (Henry, Houston, and

Mooney 2004; Russell 2000), and the responsive communitarian movement in the U.S. (Etzioni 1998; 2003).

Communitarian theorists provide a critique of utilitarian and contractarian ethical theories as applied to PH (Beauchamp 1985; Bellah 1998; Callaghan 2003; Etzioni 2003; Jennings 2003; 2007; Selznick 1998). Jennings (2003) points out that social change has been a steady hallmark of PH. For this reason, he argued that liberalism, despite providing "a serious agenda for issues of public health ethics" (Jennings 2007, 31) is too narrow to provide either adequate normative justification or the kind of insights necessary to support the types of social change that PH aims to accomplish. A framework that goes beyond liberalism is necessary and he proposes *civic republicanism* as a theory able to provide an adequate moral foundation for PH. In the civic republican tradition, the common good refers to the welfare of the people taken together, the body politic, or commonwealth (Beauchamp 1985). But he also suggests that to engage fully in discussions of PH ethics and its applications, it is essential to understand the broader theoretical and ideological context within which PH controversies and conflicts occur (Jennings 2003).

Jennings (2003) provides a useful framework for tying together the various, and often competing strands of ethical and political theory, to help us sort through how seemingly disparate views are actually congruent in many respects. He categorizes two broad types of theory, ethical and political theory, and describes the interrelationships and connections between them. For example, he sees the political theories of liberal welfarism and democratic socialism as tied to utilitarianism; libertarian and egalitarian liberalism as tied to both utilitarianism and contractarianism; civic republicanism as tied to democratic communitarianism; and deliberative democracy as tied to both democratic communitarianism and contractarianism. Finally, elements of civic republicanism and cultural conservatism are tied to authoritarian communitarianism. (Note that neither democratic communitarianism nor civic republicanism bear any direct relationship to the philosophy and politics of the two major U.S. political parties.)

Jennings (2003) distinguishes two types of communitarianism: democratic and authoritarian, classified by others as relativist and universalist (Roberts and Reich 2002). Democratic communitarianism is the more left-leaning orientation with connections to Habermas' communicative ethics (Habermas 1990) and is strongly committed to social change, feminist theory, and philosophy, and has affinities with political theories of deliberative democracy (Fung 2005; Gutman and Thompson 2004) and civic republicanism (Beauchamp 1985; Jennings 2007; Nielsen 2011). Those using this theory see morality as contextual and defined by the community (Roberts and Reich 2002) but, at the same time, as needing to stand up to outside scrutiny. Authoritarian communitarianism has a greater affinity to a right-leaning political theory of cultural conservatism, religious traditions, and fundamentalism, where adherents tend to put forward a single view of the "good society" and the appropriate virtues of its citizens.

It is this cross-pollination of theoretical ideas between both liberal and conservative political theories and forms of communitarianism that have created some confusion among critics of communitarianism. Some feminist critiques of communitarianism (Friedman 1992; Stacey 1994), which do not appear to distinguish among the two types, primarily take aim at the authoritarian version with its emphasis on family values, and its sexual and cultural conservatism (Hauerwas 1977; Oakeshott 1991). Freidman's critique of communitarianism is based on the views of community put forward by Sandel (1982) and MacIntyre (1981) who present an idealized notion of community not well aligned with a feminist critique of the institutionalized oppression of women within families and communities. Etzioni (2003) responds to such critiques by arguing that communitarians clearly recognize that there are exploitive communities, just as there are exploitive individuals. He further argues that critics of communitarianism are making reference to an older, outdated understanding of community that is not compatible with current communitarianism. Moreover, Friedman's proposals for reorienting communitarianism to be more feminist in direction have also been proposed by communitarian theorists (Etzioni 2003; Selznick 1998). Nonetheless, feminists bring a useful critical perspective to communitarian thought.

Feminism, democratic communitarianism, communicative ethics (Habermas 1998), and civic republicanism share many of the same important concepts. Democratic communitarianism has benefitted from an infusion of critical and feminist theory as well as theories and critiques of deliberative democracy. Key concepts in democratic communitarianism that are shared with civic republicanism, deliberative democracy, critical PH ethics, feminist ethics, and relational ethics include the common good, relational autonomy, reciprocity, mutuality, (relational) solidarity, social justice, equity, participation, and inclusion (Baylis, Kenny, and Sherwin 2008; Callaghan 2003; Jennings 2003; Selznick 1998).

As mentioned previously, in a civic republican tradition, the common good refers to the welfare of the people taken together (Beauchamp 1985). The public holds interests in common often related to health, safety, security, and self-preservation from threats. This is congruent with the notion of the common good put forward by Baylis, Kenny, and Sherwin (2008) in their feminist relational framework for PH ethics. The common good is not an end in itself, but rather is created through the practices of citizenship (Jennings 2007); thus, it consists in having the social systems, institutions, and environments on which everyone depends available in a way that benefits all people (Velasquez et al. 1992). This understanding fits with the PH concern for the social and economic determinants of health and the need to address structural inequities through healthy public policy. It is also in keeping with the role of the PH system in supporting and maintaining the common good through collective action and cooperative efforts of the community.

In nursing ethics, Starzomski and Rodney (1997) proposed that nursing's professional responsibilities at the macro level focus on promoting the common good, particularly related to accessing health care services and the determinants of health; whereas, responsibilities to patients and families take place at the individual or micro level and relate more to the public interest than the common good. This understanding can bring nursing ethics and PH ethics into a more congruent and productive relationship than it has had in the past.

Different writers emphasize different concepts within the cluster of communitarian perspectives. Callaghan's (2003) understanding of communitarianism is organized around four key categories: (1) *Human nature*—human beings are social animals who exist within a network of other people and within social institutions and the culture of their society. This is consistent with the feminist notion of relational personhood and relational autonomy (Appleby and Kenny 2010; Baylis, Kenny, and Sherwin 2008).

(2) *The public and the private*—there can be no sharp distinction between the public and the private spheres of life and what counts as private is a societal decision. The feminist principle that "the personal is political" (Hanisch 1969) reflects a very similar notion. (3) *The welfare of the whole*—the welfare of society as a whole is the starting place for the communitarian, where welfare is understood in its broadest sense to encompass political institutions, traditions, practices and values, and cultural commitments of a society. Promoting human well-being and social justice, then, requires attention to the ways in which these institutions and traditions structure inequities. (4) *Human rights*—positive and negative rights are essential, both as a source of resistance to the power of governments and the community, and to establish the moral standing of individuals. At the same time, these rights are not unlimited and carry with them a balancing against responsibilities. When intervening for PH, the first question will be about what the intervention means for all of us together but there will also be a balancing with what it means for individuals. Democratic participation and inclusion is central to establishing an understanding of the common good; deliberative democracy is the mechanism by which this can occur. It has been defined as "a revolutionary political ideal that requires fundamental changes in political institutions, bases of collective decision making, and the distribution of resources" (Fung 2005).

In the liberal tradition, liberty is understood primarily as freedom from interference whereas communitarians understand liberty as freedom from domination and oppression. This idea is central to civic republicanism in which the harmful effects of domination and arbitrary power are the primary evil. This notion of freedom from arbitrary power and domination is also reflected in the work of feminist philosopher Iris Marion Young (2000; 2007) and her concern that liberal justice often ignores the claims of oppressed groups. The foregoing ideas bring together feminist, critical, and civic republican ideals into a communitarian vision of freedom as living life in the absence of oppression and domination. Although Young expresses caution about the pursuit of a common good because it can privilege those with the most power (Young 2000), when this notion of liberty is coupled with other communitarian concepts of mutuality, reciprocity, and solidarity, a framework of PH ethics can be created that both acknowledges and accounts for the challenges raised by liberalism about communitarian ideals.

What Kind of Frameworks Might Work for Public Health Ethics?

Over the past decade, a number of authors have developed more practical frameworks to guide ethical PH practice; many are nascent and not fully formed. Despite this development, there is nowhere near a consensus on the most appropriate frameworks for PH ethics and most authors agree that there is still a need for a framework (or frameworks) that can provide normative justification for PH activities (Wilson 2009). Kass (2001) argues that when analyzed within a traditional bioethics framework, PH actions are seen as allowable exceptions to ethical principles, if not quite a breach of ethics.

At this stage in the development of PH ethics, frameworks are primarily a collection of principles developed through ethical analysis rather than being empirically derived. Although principlism has come under criticism within health care ethics more broadly (Beauchamp 1995; Clouser and Gert 1990) and nursing ethics specifically (Rodney et al.

2004), the approach continues to retain appeal in practice as a robust and useful way of helping practitioners think about ethical issues (Upshur 2002). The challenge is that the few PH ethics frameworks that have been developed have not been widely debated by the PH community, and there have been only a few published applications. Thus, much work remains to be done.

In Exhibit 20-1, I present a range of PH ethics frameworks that vary considerably in their scope and focus, the principles and values they reflect, and the philosophical or theoretical perspectives from which they are derived. Nonetheless, there are some similarities. Although most of the framework authors do not explicitly identify the philosophical or theoretical underpinnings, it is not difficult to infer their origins. Utilitarianism is the most common ethical theory reflected in these frameworks because all have a consequentialist concern for population health as a moral aim. There are some frameworks containing specific principles that reflect a communitarian ethical perspective but only one (Baylis, Kenny, and Sherwin 2008) that could be categorized as primarily communitarian given that it draws heavily on communitarian and civic republican concepts and references key authors in these traditions; however, the authors themselves do not refer to their feminist relational framework as communitarian.

EXHIBIT 20-1

Public Health Ethics Frameworks

Authors	Purpose	Description	Underlying Philosophy or Theory	Critique
Upshur 2002 Principles for the Justification of Public Health Interventions	To provide a heuristic guide to public health (PH) decision making, for justifying PH decisions to reduce, control, or eliminate risks related primarily to environmental hazards and infectious diseases. It does not apply to health promotion, prevention, or screening. Focus is primarily on PH action in which individual liberties are curtailed to prevent harm.	This is a "stepwise" framework spelling out a logical ordering of steps through which analysis proceeds: 1. Harm principle—PH actions are justifiable to prevent harm to others, but not to prevent harm to oneself. 2. Least restrictive means—The full force of state authority should be reserved for exceptional circumstances. More coercive methods are only employed when less coercive methods have failed. 3. Reciprocity principle—Once PH action is warranted, the individual or community must be assisted in discharging their duties and be compensated for burdens imposed on them.	Utilitarian ethics Libertarian and egalitarian liberalism	Provides a practical, easy-to-use heuristic for practitioners. Limited to only some PH interventions. Does not consider community and relational aspects of public health practice. Reflects attempts

Authors	Purpose	Description	Underlying Philosophy or Theory	Critique
		4. Transparency principle—All stakeholders should be involved in decision making, with equal input, free of political interference or coercion.		to "bind" the harm principle in specific ways. Reflects a limited version of the trans-parency principle.
Public Health Leader-ship Society 2002 A Code of Ethics for Public Health	To clarify the dis-tinctive elements of public health and identify the ethical principles that follow from those elements. The focus of this code is on public health practice, specifically for institutions. Not designed to provide a means of untangling convo-luted ethical issues or resolving a particular dispute.	Comprises 12 principles with a set of 14 underlying values. 1. PH should address principally the fundamental causes of disease and requirements for health, aiming to prevent adverse health outcomes. 2. PH should achieve community health in a way that respects the rights of individuals in the community. 3. PH policies, programs, and priorities should be developed and evaluated through proc-esses that ensure an opportunity for input from the community. 4. PH should advocate and work for the empowerment of disen-franchised community members, ensuring basic resources and conditions for health are acces-sible to all. 5. PH should seek the informa-tion needed to implement effective policies and programs that protect and promote health. 6. PH institutions should provide communities with the information needed for decisions on policies/programs and should obtain the community's consent. 7. PH institutions should act in a timely manner on the information they have within the resources and the mandate given to them by the public.	Draws from utilitarian, deontologi-cal, and communi-tarian perspectives. Informed by theories of distributive justice and the social determinants of health. Duty as an ethical motivation is reflected in several prin-ciples and the concept of community is central; promoting the common good is implicit. Different principles reflect different theoretical orientations. The underly-ing values, not discussed here, make	What they call princi-ples are more like guidelines or "rules" for prac-tice. Provides specific guidance to PH institutions and practi-tioners and lays out the major commit-ments and orienta-tions of PH. No specific guidance about how to resolve ethical disputes or choose among alterna-tives. Second principle appears to privilege

Authors	Purpose	Description	Underlying Philosophy or Theory	Critique
		8. PH programs and policies should incorporate a variety of approaches that anticipate and respect diverse values, beliefs, and cultures in the community. 9. PH programs and policies should be implemented in a way that enhances the physical/social environment. 10. PH institutions should protect confidentiality of information that can harm an individual/community. Exceptions must be justified on the basis of the high likelihood of significant harm. 11. PH institutions should ensure the professional competence of their employees. 12. PH institutions and their employees should engage in collaborations and affiliations in ways that build the public's trust and the institution's effectiveness.	the communitarian aims more evident.	individual rights over community health, yet in the underlying values, this is not so.
Kass 2001 An Ethics Framework for Public Health	To provide an analytic tool to help PH professionals consider the ethical implications of proposed interventions, policy proposals, research initiatives, and programs. Intent is to help PH professionals recognize the multiple and varied moral issues in their work and consider means of responding. It is NOT a code of professional ethics.	Analytic tool and action guide organized into six steps to be considered in assessing the ethics of a given public health intervention. 1. What are the program goals? 2. How effective is the program in achieving stated goals? 3. What are the known or potential burdens? 4. Can burdens be minimized? Are there alternatives? 5. Is the program implemented fairly? 6. How can burdens and benefits be fairly balanced? Under each of these questions, more specific guidance is provided for making decisions.	Utilitarian and contractarian. Is consequentialist in its aim to improve health, decrease morbidity and mortality. Analysis of potential burdens relates to prevention of harms related to confidentiality, privacy, justice, liberty, and self-determination. In choosing	Provides a broad set of considerations in making ethical decisions but does not get into the specifics of how to make particular decisions. A body of literature describing applications of this framework is developing.

Authors	Purpose	Description	Underlying Philosophy or Theory	Critique
		among strategies, least restrictive means is prioritized. Draws on theories of distributive justice rooted in liberal egalitarianism. Procedural justice informs the balancing of burdens and benefits.		Focus on distributive versus social justice and beneficence is prioritized over justice and liberty/ autonomy.
Selgelid 2009 A Moderate Pluralist Approach to PH Policy and Ethics	To provide a principled means for striking a balance between the values of utility, liberty, and equality in cases of conflict. Rather than choosing among these independent values, because none would have absolute priority in all circumstances, we should seek creative ways of promoting all three values at the same time.	Drawing from frameworks identifying principles for making tradeoffs, the author proposes ways of striking a balance between principles that consider strategies, not as either acceptable or unacceptable, but as having degrees of acceptability using measures such as disability adjusted life years (DALYs). The principles are offered as a starting point are: 1. Liberty restriction is based on evidence of effectiveness in protecting/promoting health. 2. The least restrictive (liberty infringing) alternative should be used. 3. Extreme liberty infringing strategies should not be imposed unless consequences of not doing so are severe. 4. These strategies should be used equitably. 5. Liberty infringement should be minimally burdensome. 6. Those whose liberty is violated should be compensated (reciprocity).	Utilitarianism (utility), libertarianism (liberty), and egalitarianism (equality). Despite the argument that the approach is an integrated one that incorporates all three of the above ethical theories, the starting principles appear to give the highest priority to the value of liberty and the use of measures such as DALYs is utilitarian.	Creates a strong rationale for an integrated approach. Approaches for making tradeoffs have not yet been developed— author merely provides some plausible ideas about how this might be done. The notion that none of the values holds priority in all circumstances is

Authors	Purpose	Description	Underlying Philosophy or Theory	Critique
		7. Implementation of restrictions should involve due process (procedural justice). 8. Policy making should be democratic and transparent.		in line with "common-sense morality" in that there would likely be widespread agreement that none of these values are always "right" or "wrong."
Baylis, Kenny, and Sherwin, 2008 A Relational Account of Public Health Ethics	To provide a comprehensive framework that embraces the full spectrum of PH responsibilities based on a relational orientation that recognizes the need to pay attention to the vulnerability of subpopulations lacking in social and economic power. The aims are (1) to develop policies and programs aimed at a common interest in preventing illness, building physically and socially healthy communities, and eliminating health inequities; (2) promoting the public interest and the common good	Framework is based on the concepts of: 1. Relational personhood—Persons are thoroughly social who develop and are constituted through engagement and interaction with others. 2. Relational autonomy—Sees autonomy as a product of social relations, not an individual achievement. Choices depend on options available. We are not all equally situated in our opportunities for autonomy. 3. Social justice—Draws on Powers and Faden's (2006) theory of social justice, which is congruent with notions of relational justice. There are six distinct dimensions of well-being (one is health) that are interrelated. Each is a lens for evaluating the impact of patterns of social organization. 4. Relational solidarity—Goes beyond traditional notions of solidarity to acknowledge that a relational conception of solidarity already exists within PH and recognizes important differences	Implicitly reflects notions of Jenning's (2003) democratic communitarianism and draws on feminist relational theory and elements of civic republicanism but has consequentialist elements given explicit PH goals. Implies notions of deliberative democracy. Also draws on Powers and Faden's (2006) theory of social justice in PH, which in turn draws on Young's	Major strengths are its comprehensive focus and clear articulation of principles congruent with a communitarian perspective. Builds explicitly on moral aims of PH and the values inherent in its practices. Relational approach provides a framework for resolving polarized tensions in PH but a

Authors	Purpose	Description	Underlying Philosophy or Theory	Critique
	(i.e., our shared interests in survival, safety, and security).	among people. Does not devolve to an "us" and "them" mentality but considers "us all." Asks that we be cognizant of and responsive to the needs of those who are socially and economically disadvantaged among us.	(1990) critical theory of justice, which provides a critique of distributive justice.	weakness is that the implications are not spelled out and it requires greater elaboration for concrete application.

Most frameworks reflect elements of some form of both utilitarian and contractarian theories. One framework is really a professional code of ethics for PH (Public Health Leadership Society 2002), although it is aimed at both PH institutions and individual practitioners. A few of the frameworks incorporate more specific guidance for working through the ethical decision-making process and making tradeoffs or choosing among competing values and/or principles. Others provide only general guidance on the kinds of considerations that need to be taken into account.

Although within several frameworks some of the same values or principles are identified, there is a wide range of principles reflected. Yet there may be other important PH ethical principles that have not made their way into any framework (e.g., the precautionary principle) but which are being increasingly recognized as important to ethical decision making in PH (Chaudry 2008; Rosner and Markowitz 2002).

WHAT ABOUT ETHICS AND PUBLIC HEALTH NURSING?

Despite growth of the field of health care and nursing ethics over the past three decades, there has been little development in ethics for PHN. Few studies on ethics in PHN have been conducted or published in the peer-reviewed literature and only a small number of theoretical articles have been written. Early work by Mila Aroskar (1979; 1989) and Sara Fry (1983; 1985) and a later study by Oberle and Tenove (2000) identified that the moral concerns of PHNs might not be the same as those of most other nurses; that there is an ethical tension in PH nursing practice between promoting the health of a population versus the health of individuals; and that the professional codes of ethics in nursing might require PHNs to violate those codes while engaging in population-focused practice.

In a review of the ethics content of community health nursing textbooks, Zahner (2000) found that many had no ethics content at all and only 30 percent had separate chapters on ethics. The dominant ethical theory was a duty-based, deontological perspective. Surprisingly, given its prominence in PH more broadly, a utilitarian perspective was found in only 14 percent of the sample while human rights and distributive justice theories were the theoretical basis in 23 percent and 25 percent of the texts, respectively. None of the texts mentioned a communitarian ethical perspective nor did they discuss the distinction between PH and health care ethics. This is consistent with Kass' (2004) observation that very little appeared in the literature on PH ethics prior to the year 2000.

The definition of public health nursing provides important clues about the ethical challenges for PHNs. A PHN is a "community health nurse who synthesizes knowledge from public health science, primary health care (including the determinants of health), nursing science, and the theory and knowledge of the social sciences to promote, protect, and preserve the health of populations" (CHNAC 2003, 3). Although the focus is on population health, PHNs do some of their population-focused work with individuals. PHNs also recognize that individuals and communities are inextricably linked (Diekemper, Smith-Battle, and Drake 1999). This dual nature of the PHN role, with a concurrent focus on the care of individuals and the welfare of the population, creates unique ethical challenges for PHNs that are not experienced by nurses working in other areas of practice or by other types of PH professionals. Few other nurses, or PH workers, have the same type of intimate relationship with individuals while also working at the community level (CNA 2006).

Professional codes of ethics for nurses are important guides for practice because they reflect a professional consensus on matters of ethics; however, several authors have pointed out that, for some time, these codes did not reflect the nature of PHN practice, nor did they provide guidance for the unique ethical issues in PH nursing (Folmar et al. 1997; Fry 1983; 1985). Fortunately, the most recent version of the CNA Code of Ethics (2008) encompasses some of the concerns of PHNs and the language opens the possibility that ethical decisions might be different when the community or population is the primary concern. This is particularly evident in the code's values under the headings of Promoting Health and Well-being and Justice. However, handling a conflict between individual human rights and protecting the public's health is not specifically addressed and the answer to the conflict might be different for PHNs and nurses in hospital settings. In addition to the value statements and their accompanying ethical responsibilities, the Code of Ethics includes a set of ethical endeavours, which are broad aspects of social justice that relate to the need for social and system change to promote health equity. These are not considered to be part of nursing's *core* ethical responsibilities but are a part of ethical practice. I would argue, however, that these ethical endeavours actually do reflect PHN's core ethical responsibilities, even if they are not core responsibilities for the rest of nursing. Several statements under the heading Ethical Endeavours (CNA 2008, 20–21) are explicitly reflected in national community health nursing documents defining the roles, responsibilities, and competencies of PHNs (Community Health Nurses of Canada 2009; CPHA 2010b). Thus, the 2008 version of the CNA Code of Ethics represents a substantial step forward in reflecting the ethical responsibilities of PHNs, although there are still some gaps.

Clearly, the development of PHN ethics has lagged behind both PH ethics and nursing ethics. Recently, however, a feminist relational perspective on nursing ethics has begun to inform some areas of PHN practice such as tuberculosis care and treatment (Bender 2009), working with high-priority families (Browne et al. 2010), child protection clients (Marcellus 2004), and perinatal substance users (Marcellus 2005), all of whom might be considered vulnerable, oppressed, disadvantaged, or marginalized in some way. Drawing on the notions of relational practice (Hartrick Doane and Varcoe 2007), relational autonomy (Sherwin 2004), and relational ethics in nursing (Bergum 1994), the analysis of PHN practice with the population groups as described by the authors above reveals considerable congruence with a relational account of PH ethics (Baylis, Kenny, and Sherwin 2008; Kenny, Sherwin, and Baylis 2010), critical PH ethics (Callaghan and Jennings 2002; Nixon 2006), feminist ethics in PH (Rogers 2006), and a communitarian ethical perspective (Etzioni 2003; Friedman 1992; Jennings 2007; Selznick 1998).

Thus, one meeting place for nursing ethics and PH ethics may well be feminist relational ethics. What is necessary for advancement in the field is to draw on the work noted above to develop ethical frameworks or guidelines for PHNs in dealing with other major ethical challenges in PH, such as the issue discussed below related to pandemic ethics. For example, there is very limited guidance for PHNs in addressing issues related to pandemic ethics in the community, whereas case studies have been developed to assist hospital-based nurses in working through the ethical challenges of pandemics in institutional settings (National Collaborating Centre on Healthy Public Policy 2010).

PANDEMIC ETHICS

Pandemic planning is an important PH issue currently on the local, provincial, national, and international PH agenda. Selgelid (2009a) points out that the consequences of infectious diseases were unparalleled in the past and that epidemics have been among the most catastrophic events in history, yet have received little attention from bioethics (Selgelid 2005). I suggest that "pandethics" (Selgelid 2009b) provides a paradigm case of the classic ethical tension between individual liberty and the common good as well as issues that are new to current generations of practitioners and citizens because many have not experienced a serious epidemic. SARS and H1N1 have given us only a taste of what is likely to come. Pandethics requires a global perspective and intersectoral collaboration, bringing together the concerns of both the health care system and PH. It is thus a useful case for exploring a diverse range of ethical issues.

Communicable diseases threaten the health of populations and can constitute a global emergency. *Collateral damage* is one possible outcome, as was the case in the SARS epidemic in Toronto where severe restrictions on hospital admissions meant that many people did not receive needed treatment for life-threatening conditions (Singer et al. 2003) and there were considerable economic costs. Pandemics, and the fear they generate, have the potential to challenge our commitment to each other and the common good if not handled well because the measures required to control them are sometimes controversial, coercive, and liberty infringing. In addition, infectious diseases raise critical equity issues because the burden of illness is born inordinately by the poor and disadvantaged groups. For example, there is a much higher incidence of tuberculosis among First Nations and immigrant populations in Canada (Tapiéro and Lamarre 2003) and there was a disproportionate impact of the recent H1N1 pandemic in First Nations communities in Canada, the U.S., and New Zealand (Peters, Adams, and Waters 2010).

The success of PH has, in some ways, been its nemesis. The dramatic reduction and even elimination of some infectious diseases has lulled the public (and health care professionals) into a sense of complacency to the point of diminishing support for the PH measures (e.g., vaccination) that have prevented and controlled epidemics and drastically reduced the death toll. The World Health Organization (WHO) (2007) says that we can expect to experience three pandemics per century at intervals of 10 to 50 years and that a serious influenza pandemic in the near future is likely. Following a 2004 outbreak of the highly pathogenic H5N1 virus, the WHO (2005) stated that the world is moving closer to a serious pandemic. The recent H1N1 pandemic, which people initially thought might be the "big one," did not have the kind of economic and social impact that some expected. Although it is impossible to make accurate predictions about the seriousness of the next pandemic, PH officials warn that another influenza pandemic is inevitable with the potential for widespread morbidity and mortality, in addition to causing significant social and economic disruption (WHO). Thus, governments at all levels, businesses, health care, and other organizations have developed pandemic plans.

The WHO (2007) has produced a document on ethical considerations in developing a PH response to pandemic influenza, which has influenced the global development of pandemic plans. This was informed by the work of the Pandemic Influenza Working Group (PIWG) at the University of Toronto Joint Centre for Bioethics (a WHO Collaborating Centre), which produced the report "Stand on Guard for Thee" (PIWG 2005). This document has also informed the pandemic plans and ethical frameworks for some Canadian provinces (e.g., Ontario and Prince Edward Island) and other countries like New Zealand (National Ethics Advisory Committee 2007).

If pandemic ethics are not addressed in the planning phase, the response efforts to a pandemic could be seriously compromised (WHO 2007). In many pandemic plans, however, there is no discussion of the ethical underpinnings and the values intended to inform decision making have not been made public (PIWG 2005). The PIWG has argued that it is essential to discuss these issues openly in advance of a pandemic to ensure buy-in, legitimacy, and trust of the public. The urgency of the situation could result in ethical considerations being put aside if they are not considered in advance. Based on the SARS experience, researchers have found that ethical frameworks may reduce collateral damage and increase trust and solidarity among health care organizations (Thompson et al. 2006) and thus are essential elements of pandemic plans.

The four major ethical issues that have been identified in international and national pandemic plans are related to (1) allocating scarce resources for both prevention and treatment (e.g., vaccines, anti-virals, ventilators, and hospital beds); (2) obligations of health care workers to provide care in the face of risk to self and family and the reciprocal obligations of organizations to their workers; (3) implementing coercive restrictions and social distancing measures on individuals and groups (e.g., isolation, quarantine, restrictions on travel and movement, closure of public spaces, and limits on public gatherings); and (4) obligations of countries to one another in planning and response. Infectious agents do not honour national boundaries, so poor pandemic planning in one country can have serious global consequences. How each of these issues is dealt with will be determined by the underlying values of those responsible for developing and/or implementing the specific plans, or the public if an effective public engagement process has taken place.

The Canadian Pandemic Influenza Plan for the Health Sector (PHAC 2006) identifies two major goals; to minimize morbidity and mortality, and to minimize societal disruption. Similar goals are reflected in most of the provincial plans in Canada and in the plans of other countries. In addition, the Canadian plan identifies six underlying values: (1) to promote and protect the public's health; (2) to ensure equity and distributive justice; (3) to respect the inherent dignity of all persons; (4) to use the least restrictive means; (5) to optimize the risk/benefit ratio; and (6) transparency and accountability. Some of the same values are reflected in the ethical frameworks for the pandemic plans of other countries including the U.S. and New Zealand but both of these countries contain a more explicit focus on the common good.

A review of the pandemic ethical frameworks of the World Health Organization (2007), the Canadian Pandemic Influenza Working Group (PIWG) (2005), the Public Health Agency of Canada (PHAC) (2007), the United States (Kinlaw and Levine 2007), and New Zealand (National Ethics Advisory Committee 2007) reveals that there are not only many commonalities but also some distinct differences that reflect unique cultural, philosophical, and value systems among countries. For example, the values of equity, balancing liberty and collective interests, and reciprocity are shared across these ethical frameworks. Solidarity is a value in the WHO, Canadian, and New Zealand frameworks but not in the U.S. framework. The WHO and PHAC frameworks include the utilitarian values of utility and efficiency while the U.S. ethical framework explicitly rejects a classic utilitarian approach as "morally inadequate for pandemic influenza planning" (Kinlaw and Levine 2007, 6). The Canadian PIWG ethical framework includes four unique values not included in the other frameworks; privacy, trust, the duty to care, and stewardship. The duty to care in a pandemic may not always be explicit in professional codes of ethics although often it is implicit. Health care providers will need to weigh professional demands against competing obligations to themselves and their families, and in relation to limited resources, workplace conditions, and liability issues (PIWG 2005). Although New Zealand does not explicitly name the duty to care as a substantive value, it is encompassed in their value of reciprocity, which includes acting on social standing or special professional responsibilities.

Both the New Zealand and PIWG frameworks reflect the same procedural values. The U.S. framework shares responsibility/accountability, transparency, and inclusiveness with New Zealand and Canada. The notion of inclusiveness differs somewhat across groups. In the U.S., this means an acknowledgement of the historical abuse of vulnerable groups who may have strong distrust and suspicion of the health care system on the basis of past wrongs and the need to ensure attention to these groups in pandemic decision making. This value would be very useful to include in the Canadian frameworks given the history of colonialism, oppression, and discrimination of Aboriginal peoples in our country.

Both the U.S. and the WHO frameworks include the distinct procedural value of public engagement. This value is central to a communitarian ethical perspective drawing on civic republican and deliberative democratic political traditions. Public engagement is an important procedural value in some ethical frameworks. There have been some powerful demonstrations of the feasibility and efficacy of deliberative processes for engaging a diverse public in deciding on the values that should guide ethical decision making in a pandemic. These include the Minnesota Pandemic Ethics Project (Garrett et al. 2011) and the Public Engagement Project on Pandemic Influenza (PEPPI) (Keystone Centre for Science and Public Policy 2005; 2007), both of which used a deliberative democratic approach with broad public participation to develop frameworks for guiding rationing decisions in a pandemic. These reflect the principles of commitment to the common good, respect, and mutuality. When such deliberative processes are used, the public can come to consensus on how to deal with difficult ethical questions in an equitable and responsive way.

Unfortunately, few of the provincial pandemic influenza plans in Canada appear to have used any sort of deliberative public engagement process. The Stand on Guard for Thee framework (PIWG 2005) did utilize stakeholder consultation primarily at the organizational level, but this did not involve citizen engagement. Since the framework was released, however, the CanPREP research group at the University of Toronto Joint Centre on Bioethics (www.canprep.ca) has launched a research program exploring ethical issues in pandemics. One study is designed to engage the public to elucidate the normative basis of Stand on Guard for Thee and to solicit public perspectives on the four ethical challenges identified above for pandemic planning. The provinces would be well advised to undertake a similar public engagement process prior to the next major pandemic.

Clearly, the Stand on Guard for Thee framework has made a significant impact nationally and internationally on the development of pandemic ethics frameworks that cut across the acute care and PH sectors. It has not, however, gone without criticism. Other Canadian ethicists (Baylis, Kenny, and Sherwin 2008; Kenny, Melynchuk, and Asada 2006; Kenny, Sherwin, and Baylis 2010) have suggested there is "a too heavy reliance on an ethic of individual rights" (Baylis, Kenny, and Sherwin 2008, 196). In their view, there is an inordinate focus on the values and priorities of individuals, not just in the Stand on Guard for Thee framework (PIWG 2005) but in pandemic plans more generally including the Canadian plan (PHAC 2006). Kenny, Melynchuk, and Asada (2006) suggest that only three of the values in Stand on Guard for Thee focus on the common good—equity, trust, and solidarity. Baylis, Kenny, and Sherwin (2008) add reciprocity to the list with the caveat that persons likely to face a disproportionate burden include not just health workers and their families, but also the vulnerable and historically marginalized. They argue that the list of four ethical issues in Stand on Guard for Thee are narrowly focused on the individual, including duty to care, restricting liberties, and allocating scarce resources.

This individual focus in pandemic planning may not be so surprising given that many of the ethical issues that emerge in dealing with a pandemic will play out within the context of the health care system rather than solely in the community, except that New Zealand's plan stands as a beacon in its strong orientation to the common good. Although a health care ethics perspective is important, pandemic planning provides a unique opportunity to bring together the concerns and interests of both health care ethics and PH ethics with its explicit concerns about the most vulnerable populations and about the common good. This integration has not happened in the vast majority of provincial and national pandemic plans and ethical frameworks (where they exist) in Canada and will be important to encourage if we are to avoid many of the ethical challenges and resulting problems that emerge in pandemics.

Summary

So, where are we and were do we go from here? Despite its relative newness, PH ethics has come a long way with extensive theoretical and empirical work being conducted internationally as well as in Canada. Both the Canadian Institutes of Health Research—Institute of Population and Public Health (CIHR-IPPH) and the National Collaborating Centre for

Healthy Public Policy (NCCHPP) have been developing materials and resources to build capacity for public health ethics in Canada. For example, CIHR-IPPH sponsored a journal club in 2010 where a large group of people interested in PH ethics came together by teleconference to discuss relevant articles in the PH ethics literature and to hear presentations from key thought leaders and researchers (e.g., Françoise Baylis, Norman Daniels, Ross Upshur, James Wilson). This was followed up in 2011 with a Dialogue and Debate series that built on the earlier journal club and again brought in experts in the field to contribute to the dialogue (e.g., Angus Dawson, Daniel Wikler). The NCCHPP has been developing a range of resources to support PH ethics, including resources on deliberative democratic processes, case studies in pandemic ethics, background papers on important PH issues as well as philosophically oriented discussion documents (www.ncchpp.ca).

Developments in the philosophical underpinnings and frameworks to guide practice and decision making have been substantial but remain tentative, contradictory, and not always practically useful. Most frameworks remain grounded in a utilitarian or contractarian ethics perspective, with little development of communitarian frameworks. What work has been done from a communitarian perspective is more theoretical than practical. Thus, further development of communitarian frameworks to provide guidance to practitioners in making decisions in concrete situations would be very helpful.

PH nursing ethics has lagged behind developments in nursing, feminist, and PH ethics and requires some concerted work to bring it in line with these developments. In particular, frameworks are needed that build on the insights of feminist relational theory, nursing ethics, and PH ethics that are geared to the unique ethical challenges experienced by PHNs. To support this work, however, more research is necessary to clarify the nature of PHN's ethical challenges in working with communities and populations as distinct from those of nurses working in institutional settings with individuals. And, of course, attention to education for ethics in PHN as well as public health more broadly is important to ensure that there is capacity in the workforce to deal with the ethical challenges of public health.

A great deal more work in public engagement is necessary to inform the values underlying PH ethics, particularly for dealing with public health emergencies. The challenges that will arise in emergency situations will be difficult to address in fair and equitable ways if deliberation, dialogue, and priority setting is not done in advance. There will be no time to deal with these issues in the midst of an emergency and past experience suggests that vulnerable and marginalized populations will be most at risk in the wake of unfair decisions.

Overall, there are a wide range of important PH issues confronting us that demand ethical analysis as identified by Wickler and Brock (2007), including the following: defining societal versus individual responsibility for health; the relationship between health and human rights at the population level; priority setting in public health; cost-effectiveness analysis and its inability to take equity into consideration; the relationship between health and economic development; the ethics in emergency humanitarian interventions; environmental equity; population genetics; global aging; global health equity; the social determinants of population health; research ethics and social justice; the practice implications of a population perspective; and health system reform. For each of these, the authors identify key ethical questions but observe that ethical analysis related to most of these questions has been limited. More than a laundry list, these issues provide a useful agenda for further development in the field of PH ethics. With respect to each of them, however, it will be important for nurse ethicists to identify and define the ethical implications for PHN to advance the field of PHN ethics.

For Reflection

1. Are the ethics of public health more responsive to the ethical challenges of public health nursing than are nursing ethics? Why or why not?

2. Which of the ethical frameworks discussed in this chapter provide the most appropriate guide for the ethical challenges in your own population-focused practice? How might you apply this framework to ethical challenges in your practice?

3. What philosophical foundations for public health ethics resonate with you? In what ways?

4. Is there a place in nursing ethics for the "benevolent paternalism" inherent in most public health ethics frameworks?

5. How might you reconcile the individualist focus of most human rights approaches with the collectivist or population focus of public health ethics? Is it possible to reconcile a concern with individual human rights and population level or public health ethics?

Public Health Ethics Case Study Resources

Canadian Nurses Association (2006). Public health nursing practice and ethical challenges. This resource presents two case scenarios related to ethical challenges for public health nurses and provides guidelines and frameworks for working through these challenges. It also defines public health nursing and discusses some of the unique aspects of PHN that distinguishes this specialty and creates distinctive ethical issues. It is available at http://www.cna-aiic.ca/cna/documents/pdf/publications/Ethics_in_Practice_Jan_06_e.pdf

National Collaborating Centre for Healthy Public Policy (2010). *Case studies of ethics during a pandemic.* Montreal: Author.
This resource presents a collection of 11 cases that illustrate a wide range of pandemic and infectious disease control scenarios reflecting ethically complex situations that address professional roles and responsibilities. This resource is available at http://www.ncchpp.ca/127/Publications.ccnpps?id_article=320

University of North Carolina, Gillings School of Public Health. Public Health Ethics. This resource is a short course in public health ethics that discusses the basics of public health ethics and contains a variety of case scenarios related to challenging ethical situations in public health practice. It is available at http://oce.sph.unc.edu/phethics/

References

Acheson, D. 1988. *Public health in England.* London: HMSO.

Anderson, E.T. and McFarlane, J.M. 1996. *Community as partner: Theory and practice in nursing* (2nd ed.). Philadelphia: Lippincott.

Anand, S. and Hanson, K. 2004. Disability-adjusted life years: A critical review. In S. Anand, F. Peter, and A. Sen (Eds.), *Public health, ethics, and equity* (pp. 183–200). New York: Oxford University Press.

Appleby, B. and Kenny, N.P. 2010. Relational personhood, social justice and the common good: Catholic contributions toward a public health ethics. *Christian Bioethics, 16* (3), 296–313.

Aroskar, M.A. 1979. Ethical issues in community health nursing. *Nursing Clinics of North America, 14* (1), 35–44.

Aroskar, M.A. 1989. Community health nurses—Their most significant ethical decision-making problems. *Nursing Clinics of North America, 24* (4), 967–975.

Bayer, R. 1991. Public health policy and the AIDS epidemic: An end to HIV exceptionalism. *New England Journal of Medicine, 324* (21), 1500–1504.

Bayer, R. and Fairchild, A.L. 2004. The genesis of public health ethics. *Bioethics, 18* (6), 473–492.

Bayer, R., Gostin, L.O., Jennings, B., and Steinbock, B. 2007. *Public health ethics: Theory, policy, and practice*. New York: Oxford University Press.

Baylis, F., Kenny, N.P., and Sherwin, S. 2008. A relational account of public health ethics. *Public Health Ethics 1* (3), 196–209.

Beauchamp, D.E. 1976. Public health as social justice. *Inquiry, 13*, 1–14.

Beauchamp, D.E. 1985. Community—The neglected tradition of public health. *Hastings Centre Report, 15*, 28–36.

Beauchamp, T.L. and Childress, J.L. 1979. *Principles of biomedical ethics*. New York: Oxford University Press.

Beauchamp, T.L. 1995. Principlism and its alleged competitors. *Kennedy Institute of Ethics Journal, 5* (3), 181–198.

Bellah, R.N. 1998. Community properly understood: A defense of "democratic communitarianism." In A. Etzioni (Ed.), *The essential communitarian reader* (pp. 15–20). Lanham, MD: Rowman & Littlefield Publishers Inc.

Bender, A.C. 2009. *The welcome intrusion of TB nurses. An interpretive phenomenological study of relational work in public health nursing*. Unpublished doctoral dissertation, Lawrence S. Bloomberg Faculty of Nursing, University of Toronto, Toronto, ON.

Bergum, V. 1994. Knowledge for ethical care. *Nursing Ethics 1*, 71–79.

Brock, D.W. 2004. Ethical issues in the use of cost-effectiveness analysis for the prioritization of health care resources. In S. Anand, F. Peter, and A. Sen (Eds.), *Public health, ethics, and equity* (pp. 201–224). Oxford University Press.

Brock, D.W. 2007. Ethical issues in applying quantitative models for setting priorities in prevention. In A. Dawson and M. Verweij (Eds.), *Ethics, prevention, and public health* (pp. 111–128). New York: Oxford University Press.

Browne, A., Hartrick Doane, G., Reimer, J., MacLeod, M.L.P., and McLellan, E. 2010. Public health nursing practice with high priority families: The significance of contextualizing risk. *Nursing Inquiry, 17* (1) 27–38.

Buhler-Wilkerson, K. 1993. Bringing care to the people: Lillian Wald's legacy to public health nursing. *American Journal of Public Health, 83*, 1778–1776.

Burr, C. 1999. The AIDS exception: Privacy vs. public health. In D.E. Beauchamp and B. Steinbock (Eds.), *New ethics for the public's health* (pp. 211–224). New York: Oxford University Press.

Butterfield, P.G. 1990. Thinking upstream: Nurturing a conceptual understanding of the societal context of health behaviour. *Advances in Nursing Science, 12* (2), 1–8.

Callaghan, D. 2003. Individual good and common good: A communitarian approach to bioethics. *Perspectives in Biology and Medicine, 46* (4), 496–507.

Callaghan, D. and Jennings, B. 2002. Ethics and public health: Forging a strong relationship. *American Journal of Public Health, 92* (2), 169–176.

Canadian Nurses Association. 2002. *A code of ethics for registered nurses*. Ottawa: Author.

Canadian Nurses Association. 2006. Public health nursing practice and ethical challenges. *Ethics in practice for registered nurses, February*. Ottawa: Author.

Canadian Nurses Association. 2008. *A code of ethics for registered nurses*. Ottawa: Author.

Canadian Program of Research on Ethics in a Pandemic. *Program description*. Available at http://canprep.ca/index.php?option=com_content&task=view&id=40&Itemid=79.

Canadian Public Health Association. 2010a. *Celebrating a century of public health leadership: 12 great achievements.* Available at http://cpha100.ca/12-great-achievements.

Canadian Public Health Association. 2010b. *Public health–community health nursing practice in Canada: Roles and activities*. Ottawa: Author.

Chafey, K. 1995. Caring is not enough: Ethical paradigms for community-based care. *Nursing and Health Care: Perspectives on Community, 17* (1), 10–15.

Chaudry, R.V. 2008. The precautionary principle, public health and public health nursing. *Public Health Nursing 25*(2), 261–268.

Childress, J.E., Faden, R.R., Gaare, R.D., Gostin, L.O., Kahn, J., Bonnie, R.J., Kass, N.E., Mastroianni, A.C., Moreno, J.D. and Nieberg, P. 2002. Public health ethics: Mapping the terrain. *Journal of Law, Medicine & Ethics, 30*, 170–178.

Clouser, K. and Gert, B. 1990. A critique of principlism. *Journal of Medicine and Philosophy, 15*, 219–236.

Community Health Nurses Association of Canada. 2003. *Canadian community health nursing standards of practice*. Toronto: Author.

Community Health Nurses Association of Canada. 2009. *Public health nursing discipline specific competences. Version 1.0*. Toronto: Author.

Daniels, N. 2006. Equity and population health: Toward a broader bioethics agenda. *Hastings Centre Report, 36* (4), 22–35.

Dawson, A. and Verweij, M. 2007. Introduction: Ethics, prevention and public health. In A. Dawson and M. Verweij (Eds.), *Ethics, prevention, and public health* (pp. 1–12). New York: Oxford University Press.

Dawson, A. and Verweij, M. 2008. Public health ethics: A manifesto. *Public Health Ethics, 1* (1), 1–2.

Diekemper, M., Smith-Battle, L., and Drake, M.A. 1999. Bringing the population into focus: A natural development in community health nursing practice. Part 1. *Public Health Nursing, 16* (1), 3–9.

Etzioni, A. (Ed.) 1998. *The essential communitarian reader*. Lanham, MD: Rowman & Littlefield Publishers Inc.

Etzioni, A. 2003. Communitarianism. In K. Christensen and D. Levinson (Eds.), *Encyclopedia of community: From the village to the virtual world*, Volume 1, A–D, (pp. 224–228). Thousand Oaks: Sage Publications.

Faden, R. and Faden, A. 1978. The ethics of health education as public health policy. *Health Education and Behavior, 6* (2), 180–197.

Fisher, W.A., Kohut, T., and Fisher, J.D. 2009. AIDS exceptionalism: On the social psychology of HIV prevention research. *Social Issues and Policy Review, 3* (1), 45–77.

Folmar, J., Coughlin, S.S., Bessinger, R., and Sacknoff, D. 1997. Ethics in public health practice: A survey of public health nurses in Southern Louisiana. *Public Health Nursing, 14* (3), 156–160.

Friedman, M. 1992. Feminism and modern friendship: Dislocating the community. In E. Browning Cole and S.M. Coultrap-McQuin (Eds.), *Explorations in feminist ethics: Theory and practice*. Indiana: Indiana University Press.

Fry, S.T. 1983. Dilemma in community health ethics. *Nursing Outlook, 31* (3), 176–179.

Fry, S.T. 1985. Individual vs aggregate good: Ethical tension in nursing practice. *International Journal of Nursing Studies, 22* (4), 303–310.

Fung, A. 2005. Deliberation before the revolution: Toward an ethics of deliberative democracy in an unjust world. *Political Theory, 33* (2), 397–419.

Gadow, S. and Schroeder, C. 1996. An advocacy approach to ethics and community health. In E.T. Anderson and J.M. McFarlane (Eds.), *Community as partner: Theory and practice in nursing* (2nd ed.; pp. 123–137). Philadelphia: Lippincott.

Garrett, J.E., Vawter, D.G., Gervais, K.G., Prehn, A.W., DeBruin, D.A., Livingston, F., Morley, A.M., Liaschenko, J., and Lynfield, R. 2011. The Minnesota pandemic ethics project: Sequenced, robust public engagement processes. *Journal of Participatory Medicine, 3*. Available at http://www.jopm.org/evidence/research/2011/01/19/the-minnesota-pandemic-ethics-project-sequenced-robust-public-engagement-processes/.

Gostin, L.O. 2001. Public health, ethics and human rights: A tribute to the late Jonathan Mann. *Journal of Law, Medicine & Ethics, 29*, 121–130.

Gostin, L.O. and Gostin, K.G. 2009. A broader liberty: J.S. Mill, paternalism and the public's health. *Public Health, 123*, 214–221.

Gutman, A. and Thompson, D. 2004. *Why deliberative democracy?* Princeton, NJ: Princeton University Press.

Habermas, J. 1990. *Moral consciousness and communicative action*. Cambridge: MIT Press.

Habermas, J. 1998. *The inclusion of the other. Studies in political theory*. Cambridge: MIT Press.

Hancock, T. 1985. Beyond health care: From public health policy to healthy public policy. *Canadian Journal of Public Health, 76* (3, Suppl. 1), 9–11.

Hancock, T. 1994. Health promotion in Canada: Did we win the battle but lose the war? In A. Pederson, M. O'Neill, and I. Rootman (Eds.), *Health promotion in Canada: Provincial, national and international perspectives* (pp. 350–373). Toronto: WB Saunders.

Hancock, T. 1997. Healthy cities and communities: Past, present and future. *National Civic Review, 86* (1), 11–21.

Hanisch, C. 1969. *The personal is political.* Available at http://www.carolhanisch.org/CHwritings/PersonalisPol.pdf.

Hartrick Doane, G. and Varcoe, C. 2007. Relational practice and nursing obligations. *Advances in Nursing Science, 30* (3), 192–205.

Harré, R. 1998. *The singular self.* London: Sage Publications.

Hauerwas, S. 1977. *Truthfulness and tragedy.* South Bend, IN: University of Notre Dame Press.

Henry, B.R., Houston, S., and Mooney, G. 2004. Institutional racism in Australia. *Medical Journal of Australia, 180* (10), 517–520.

Institute of Medicine. 1998. *The future of public health.* Washington, DC: National Academy Press.

Jennings, B. 2003. Frameworks for ethics in public health. *Acta Bioethica, 9* (2), 165–176.

Jennings, B. 2007. Public health and civic republicanism: Toward an alternative framework for public health ethics. In A. Dawson and M. Verweij (Eds.), *Ethics, prevention and public health* (pp. 30–58). New York: Oxford University Press.

Jennings, B. 2009. Public health and liberty: Beyond the Millian paradigm. *Public Health Ethics, 2* (2), 123–134.

Jones, M.M. and Bayer, R. 2007. Paternalism and its discontents: Motorcycle helmet laws, libertarian values, and public health. *American Journal of Public Health, 97* (2), 208–217.

Kamm, F.M. 2004. Deciding whom to help, health adjusted life years and disabilities. In S. Anand, F. Peter, and A. Sen (Eds.), *Public health, ethics, and equity* (pp. 225–242). New York: Oxford University Press.

Kass, N.E. 2001. An ethics framework for public health. *American Journal of Public Health, 91* (11), 1776–1782.

Kass, N. 2004. Public health ethics: From foundations and frameworks to justice and global public health. *Journal of Law, Medicine & Ethics, 32,* 232–242.

Kendall, J. 1992. Fighting back: Promoting emancipatory nursing actions. *Advances in Nursing Science, 15* (2), 1–15.

Kenny, N.P., Melynchuk, R., and Asada, Y. 2006. The promise of public health: Ethical reflections. *Canadian Journal of Public Health, 97* (5), 402–404.

Kenny, N.P., Sherwin, S.B., and Baylis, F. 2010. Re-visioning public health ethics. *Canadian Journal of Public Health, 101* (1), 9–11.

Keystone Centre for Science and Public Policy. 2005. *Citizen voices on pandemic flu choices: A report of the public engagement pilot project on pandemic influenza.* Denver: Author.

Keystone Centre for Science and Public Policy. 2007. *The public engagement project on community control measures for pandemic influenza.* Denver: Author.

Kinlaw, K. and Levine, R. 2007. *Ethical guidelines in pandemic influenza. A report prepared for the ethics subcommittee of the advisory committee to the Director, Centres for Disease Control and Prevention.* Available at http://www.cdc.gov/od/science/integrity/phethics/panFlu_Ethic_Guidelines.pdf.

Labonte, R. and Penfold, S. 1981. Canadian perspectives in health promotion: A critique. *Health Education, 19* (3/4), 4–9.

Lalonde, M. 1974. *A new perspective on the health of Canadians.* Ottawa: Minister of Supply and Services Canada.

Lappe, M. 1986. Ethics and public health. In J.M. Last (Ed.), *Maxcy-Rosenau public health and preventive medicine* (12th ed.; pp. 1867–1877). Norwalk, CT: Appleton-Century Crofts.

Last, J.M. 2007. *A dictionary of public health* (p. 306). Oxford: Oxford University Press.

MacDonald, M. 2002. Health promotion: Historical, philosophical, and theoretical perspectives. In L.E. Young and V.E. Hayes (Eds.), *Transforming health promotion practice: Concepts, issues, and applications* (pp. 22–45). Philadelphia: FA Davis.

MacIntyre, A. 1981. *After virtue.* Notre Dame, IN: University of Notre Dame Press.

Mann, J. 1999. Medicine and public health, ethics and human rights. In D.E. Beauchamp and B. Steinbock (Eds.), *New ethics for the public's health* (pp. 83–93). New York: Oxford University Press.

Marcellus, L. 2004. Feminist ethics must inform practice: Interventions with perinatal substance users. *Health Care for Women International, 25*, 730–742.

Marcellus, L. 2005. The ethics of relation: Public health nurses and child protection clients. *Journal of Advanced Nursing, 51* (4), 414–420.

McLeroy, K., Gottlieb, N., and Burdine, J.N. 1987. The business of health promotion: Ethical issues and professional responsibilities. *Health Education Quarterly, 14* (1), 91–109.

Melynchuk, R. 2007. *Nova Scotia health system pandemic influenza plan. Reference 1: Ethical considerations and decision making framework.* Halifax: Nova Scotia Department of Health.

Minkler, M. 1978. Ethical issues in community organization. *Health Education and Behavior, 6* (2), 198–210.

National Ethics Advisory Committee. 2007. *Getting through together: Ethical values for a pandemic.* New Zealand: Author.

Nielsen, M.E.J. 2011. Republicanism as a paradigm for public health—some comments. *Public Health Ethics, 4 (*1), 40–52.

Nixon, S. 2006. Critical public health ethics and Canada's role in global public health. *Canadian Journal of Public Health, 97* (1), 32–34.

Nixon, S., Upshur, R., Robertson, A., Benatar, S.R., Thompon, A.K., and Daar, A.S. 2005. Public health ethics. In T.M. Bailey, T. Caulfield, and N.M. Ries (Eds.), *Public health law & policy in Canada* (pp. 39–58). Markam, ON: LexisNexis Butterworths.

Oakeshott, M. 1991. *Rationalism in politics and other essays.* Indianapolis: Liberty Press.

Oberle, K. and Tenove, K. 2000. Ethical issues in public health nursing. *Nursing Ethics, 7* (5), 435–438.

Pandemic Influenza Working Group. 2005. *Stand on guard for thee: Ethical considerations in preparedness planning for pandemic influenza.* Toronto: University of Toronto Joint Centre for Bioethics.

Pauly, B. 2008. Harm reduction through a social justice lens. *International Journal of Drug Policy, 19*, 4–10.

Peters, D., Adams, E., and Waters, S. 2010. *The impact of H1N1 on First Nations communities in BC.* Paper presented at Pacific Region Indigenous Doctors Conference, August 26, Whistler, British Columbia.

Petersen, A. and Lupton, D. 1996. *The new public health: Health and self in the age of risk.* London: Sage Publications.

Powers, M. and Faden, R. 2006. *Social justice: The moral foundations of public health and health policy.* New York: Oxford University Press.

Public Health Agency of Canada. 2006. *The Canadian pandemic influenza plan for the health sector.* Ottawa: Author. Available at http://www.phac-aspc.gc.ca/cpip-pclcpi/pdf-eng.php.

Public Health Leadership Society. 2002. *Principles of the ethical practice of public health.* Available at http://www.phls.org/home/section/3-26/.

Rawls, J. 1971. *A theory of justice.* Cambridge, MA: Harvard University Press.

Roberts, M.J. and Reich, M.R. 2002. Ethical analysis in public health. *Lancet, 259*, 1055–1059.

Rodney, P., Burgess, M., McPherson, G., and Brown, H. 2004. Our theoretical landscape: A brief history of health care ethics. In J.L. Storch, P. Rodney, and R. Starzomski (Eds.), *Toward a moral horizon: Nursing ethics for leadership and practice* (pp. 56–76). Toronto: Pearson Education Canada.

Rogers, W.A. 2006. Feminism and public health ethics. *Journal of Medical Ethics, 32*, 351–354.

Rose, G. 1985. Sick individuals and sick populations. *International Journal of Epidemiology, 14*, 32–38.

Rosner, D. and Markowitz, G. 2002. Industry challenges to the principle of prevention in public health: The precautionary principle in historical perspective. *Public Health Reports, 117*, 501–512.

Russell, D. 2000. *A people's dream: Aboriginal self-government in Canada.* Vancouver: UBC Press.

Rutty, C. and Sullivan, S.C. 2010. *This is public health: A Canadian history.* Ottawa: Author.

Sandel, M. 1982. *Liberalism and the limits of justice.* Cambridge: Cambridge University Press.

Selgelid, M.J. 2005. Ethics and infections disease. *Bioethics, 19* (3), 272–289.

Selgelid, M.J. 2009a. A moderate pluralist approach to public health policy and ethics. *Public Health Ethics, 2* (2), 195–205.

Selgelid, M.J. 2009b. Pandethics. *Public Health, 123*, 255–259.

Selznick, P. 1998. Social justice: A communitarian perspective. In A. Etzioni (Ed.), *The essential communitarian reader* (pp. 61–72). Lanham, MD: Rowman and Littlefield Publishers Inc.

Sherwin, S. 2004. A relational approach to autonomy in health care. In F. Baylis, J. Downie, B. Hoffmaster, and S. Sherwin (Eds.), *Health care ethics in Canada* (pp. 192–208). Toronto: Thompson Canada.

Singer, P.A., Benatar, S.R., Bernstein, M., Daar, A.S., Dickens, B.M., MacRae, S.K., Upshur, R.E.G., Wright, L., and Shaul, R.Z. 2003. Ethics and SARS: Lessons from Toronto. *British Medical Journal, 327*, 1342–1344.

Smith, J.H. and Whiteside, A. 2010. The history of AIDS exceptionalism. *Journal of the International AIDS Society, 13* (47). Available at http://www.jiasociety.org/content/13/1/47.

Stacey, J. 1994. The new family values crusaders. *Nation, 259* (4), 119–22.

Starzomski, R. and Rodney, P. 1997. Nursing inquiry for the common good. In S.E. Thorne and V.E. Hayes (Eds.), *Nursing praxis: Knowledge and action* (pp. 219–236). Thousand Oaks: Sage Publications.

Stevens, P.E. 1989. A critical social reconceptualization of environment in nursing: Implications for methodology. *Advances in Nursing Science, 11* (4), 56–68.

Stevens, P.E. and Hall, J. 1992. Applying critical theories to nursing in communities. *Public Health Nursing, 9* (1), 2–9.

Szreter, S. 2002. Rethinking McKeown: The relationship between public health and social change. *American Journal of Public Health, 92* (5), 722–725.

Tapiéro, B.F. and Lamarre, V. 2003. Tuberculosis in Canada: Global view and new challenges. *Pediatrics and Child Health, 8* (3), 139–140.

Thompson, A.K., Faith, K., Gibson, J.L., and Upshur, R.E.G. 2006. Pandemic influenza preparedness: An ethical framework to guide decision-making. *BMC Medical Ethics, 7*:12 Available at http://www.biomedcentral.com/1472-6939/7/12.

Upshur, R. 2002. Principles for the justification of public health intervention. *Canadian Journal of Public Health, 93* (2), 101–103.

Varcoe, C. 2004. Widening the scope of ethical theory, practice and policy: Violence against women as an illustration. In J.L. Storch, P. Rodney, and R. Starzomski (Eds.), *Toward a moral horizon: Nursing ethics for leadership and practice* (pp. 414–432). Toronto: Pearson Education Canada.

Velasquez, M., Andre, C., Shanks, T., and Meyer, M.J. 1992. *The common good.* Santa Clara, CA: Markkula Centre for Applied Ethics, Santa Clara University. Available at http://www.scu.edu/ethics/practicing/decision/commongood.html.

Verweij, M. and Dawson, A. 2007. The meaning of "public" in "public health." In A. Dawson and M. Verweij (Eds.), *Ethics, prevention, and public health* (pp. 13–29). New York: Oxford University Press.

Vollman, A.R., Anderson, E.T., and McFarlane, J.M. 2003.*Canadian community as partner.* Philadelphia: Lippincott Williams & Wilkins.

Wickler, D. 1978a. Persuasion and coercion for health: Ethical issues in government efforts to change lifestyles. *Millbank Memorial Fund Quarterly, 56* (3), 303–338.

Wickler, D. 1978b. Coercive measures in health promotion: Can they be justified? *Health Education and Behavior, 6* (2), 223–241.

Wickler, D. 1987. Who should be blamed for being sick? *Health Education and Behavior, 14* (1), 11–25.

Wickler, D. and Brock, D.W. 2007. Population-level bioethics: Mapping a new agenda. In A. Dawson and M. Verweij (Eds.), *Ethics, prevention and public health* (pp. 78–94). New York: Oxford University Press.

Wilson, J. 2009. Towards a normative framework for public health ethics and policy. *Public Health Ethics, 2* (2), 184–194.

World Health Organization. 1986. *The Ottawa charter for health promotion.* Ottawa: Canadian Public Health Association and Health and Welfare Canada.

World Health Organization. 2005. *Avian influenza: Assessing the pandemic threat.* Geneva: Author.

World Health Organization. 2007. *Ethical considerations in developing a public health response to pandemic influenza.* Geneva: Author.

Young, I.M. 1990. *Justice and the politics of difference.* Princeton, NJ: Princeton University Press.

Young, I.M. 2000. *Inclusion and democracy.* Oxford: Oxford University Press.

Young, I.M. 2007. *Global challenges: War, self-determination, and responsibility for justice.* Malden, MA: Polity Press.

Zahner, S.J. 2000. Ethics content in community health nursing textbooks. *Nurse Educator, 25* (4), 186–194.

Zhang, E. 2010. Community, the common good, and public health care—Confucianism and its relevance to contemporary China. *Public Health Ethics, 3* (3), 259–266.

CHAPTER 21

Challenging Health Inequities: Enacting Social Justice in Nursing Practice

Bernadette M. Pauly

Injustice anywhere is a threat to justice everywhere. We are caught in an inescapable network of mutuality, tied in a single garment of destiny. Whatever affects one directly, affects all indirectly. (Martin Luther King, Jr.)

As disparities in wealth and power increase, so have inequities in health, with differences in health being distributed along a social gradient both within and between countries (Commission on the Social Determinants of Health 2008). Reducing health inequities has been identified as an ethical imperative, key priority, and goal of health systems world-wide (Bryant et al. 2010; Commission on the Social Determinants of Health 2008; Graham 2004; Marmot 2005; 2007). Substantial health inequities have been identified in Canada with growing concerns related to poverty, housing, and food insecurity (Eggleton 2008; Eggleton and Segal 2009; Public Health Agency of Canada 2008).

Social conditions, where people live and work, play a critical role in determining the health of the population and those with least wealth and power are the most impacted (Commission on the Social Determinants of Health 2008). Income is a key determinant of health and has significant implications for housing and food security (Wilkinson and Pickett 2006). Housing is the nexus through which the other determinants of health operate and a home provides a place for the development of identity, relationships, and social inclusion (Despres 1991; Dunn et al. 2006; Dupuis and Thorns 1998; Padgett 2007; Shaw 2004). Lack of housing, poor nutrition, and inadequate income can exacerbate the harms of drug use, contribute to poor mental and physical health, social exclusion, and increase health care costs (Cheung and Hwang 2004; Corneil et al. 2006; Frankish, Hwang, and Quantz 2005; Hwang et al. 2009; Martens 2001; Patterson et al. 2007; Research Alliance for Canadian Homelessness Housing and Health 2010; Shannon et al. 2006; Werb et al. 2010). To add to this situation, people impacted by multiple social disadvantages often have the least access to health care. Such inequities in the health of the population and inequitable access to health care services are serious ethical concerns. They are morally relevant in that some groups are much worse off than others in the population (Powers and Fadden 2006; Whitehead and Dahlgren 2006).

My purpose in this chapter is to critically examine the structural conditions and marginalizing processes that contribute to health inequities and the implications for ethical nursing policy and practice. In particular, the relationship between structural conditions, overlapping systems of oppression (e.g., racism, classism, and sexism) and social positioning in the production of health inequities will be discussed using an intersectional framework. Intersectionality, as an overarching framework, specifically seeks to promote social justice (Hankivsky et al. 2010). Perspectives on social justice as theoretical underpinnings for ethical nursing practice will be explored. Finally, the role of registered nurses and potential strategies for enacting social justice in nursing practice that disrupts or dismantles systemic injustices will be discussed as means of promoting health equity.

HEALTH INEQUITIES

Access to the social determinants of health (e.g., housing, food, income, employment, education, social inclusion) are more important in determining the health of the population than access to traditional health care services (Commission on the Social Determinants of Health 2008; WHO 2003). In particular, it is the relative difference between the wealthy and poor in society that has the greatest impact on the health of a country (Wilkinson and Pickett 2010). As Wilkinson and Pickett point out, growing inequities in wealth impact the health of everyone in the population, even the wealthy. For example, fear, justified or not, can impact the way that people move through their neighbourhoods and conduct daily activities.

Vulnerability to poor health occurs along a social gradient with those experiencing extreme poverty and social disadvantage being the most negatively affected. Access to the resources for health (e.g., education, food, shelter, and so on) is impacted by social positioning, which is characterized by differences in power and prestige (Graham 2004; Marmot 2007). For example, health inequities are particularly profound among indigenous populations throughout the world following a legacy of historical abuses of power and colonization (Nettleton, Napolitano, and Stephens 2007; Stephens et al. 2005). In Canada, the health of Aboriginal people, including First Nations, Inuit, and Métis people, is poorer than that of the general population (Frohlich, Ross, and Richmond 2006; Kendall 2009; Loppie Reading and Wien 2009; MacMillan et al. 2008; Waldram, Herring, and Young 2006; Willows et al. 2009). In the United States, African American people have a health status much lower than the rest of the population. This is doubly concerning when we consider that Canada and the United States are some of the wealthiest countries in the world.

Health inequities are unfair or unjust differences in health outcomes or access to health care that are structurally produced, unnecessary, avoidable, and potentially remediable (Braveman 2004; 2006; Graham 2004; Starfield 2006; Whitehead 1992; Whitehead and Dahlgren 2006). Whitehead and Dahlgren identify three features that distinguish health inequities from inequalities (differences that are not necessarily morally relevant): (1) health inequities "concern systematic differences in health status between different socioeconomic groups" (2); (2) inequities are outcomes of social processes and are potentially remediable; (3) inequities are the consequence of "unjust social arrangements" or social structures that perpetuate these differences. Health inequities are rooted in social conditions that shape health (e.g., the social determinants of health) and the determinants of inequities that are deeply embedded in our societal fabric (such as racism, sexism, and classism) with differential impacts on individuals and groups in society relative to one's social position in society.

Social positioning, as reflected in intersections of age, gender, ethnicity, sexual orientation, class and so on impact access to resources for health over the life course (Graham 2004). As Graham observes, particular social locations determine the nature and degree to which resources for health enter and exit individual life course trajectories. For example, individuals living in poverty do not have access to the same resources for health and may be disproportionately impacted by income, housing, and food insecurity, which are essential for health. Further, such groups and individuals may have limited power and privilege due to social positioning.

Although individuals may ascribe to certain social locations, social locations are constructed and serve to position individuals in relation to marginalizing discourses of oppression and domination as well as resistance. Those who are not members of dominant groups may be pushed to the margins of society on the basis of perceived identities and associations (Hall 1999; Hall, Stevens, and Meleis 1994). Poverty, drug use, homelessness, mental illness, ethnic identities, involvement in the sex trade, and so on can serve to marginalize individuals and groups of people unfairly. Individuals may be assigned to categories such as "the homeless," "junkie," or "addict" and be stigmatized on the basis of perceived identities and associations. Illicit drug use is one of the most highly stigmatized conditions in which people are often marginalized as villains or sinners rather than as those who are subject of injustices (Lloyd 2010). In current policy and research, people affected by homelessness are often referred to as "the homeless" as if they were one homogenous group of people. Other times, "the homeless" refers to those who are living outside and may be associated with assumptions that everyone who is on the street is mentally ill, addicted, or involved in drug use. Such stereotypical notions of homelessness are problematic and fail to acknowledge the diversity of people impacted by social disadvantages and can lead to use of damaging labels such as "addict," "vagrant," and so on.

INTERSECTIONALITY: SOCIAL POSITIONING AND SYSTEMS OF OPPRESSION

An understanding of intersectionality as well as knowledge of complex adaptive systems holds potential for understanding the interaction between social position, structural conditions, and systems of oppression in the development of health inequities. Individuals are variously positioned within institutions and regimes of social inequality (Walby 2007; 2009). Intersectionality focuses on the social location of individuals in relation to multiple intersecting systems of oppression, in particular historical and political contexts (Hankivsky and Cormier 2009; Yuval-Davis 2006). Importantly, intersectionality does not privilege one social division or category over another. Gender, race, ethnicity, age, class, and sexual orientation are important categories and axes of difference to counter essentializing of groups. For example, "the homeless" as a point of reference for people without adequate housing obliterates differences in this experience in relation to axes of differences such as gender, age, ethnicity, sexual orientation, and so on. In reference to intersectionality, Yuval-Davis states, "the point is to analyse the differential ways in which different social divisions are concretely enmeshed and constructed by each other and how they relate to political and subjective constructions of identities" (2006, 205).

Further, intersectional analysis does not simply add one category to another (e.g., gender plus class) but rather focuses on understanding experiences at the location of intersecting axes of differences and the interplay of social relations of inequality (Hankivsky et al. 2010; McCall 2005).

Differences in gender, ethnicity, social class, socio-economic status, and sexual orientation are closely intertwined and implicated in systems of social inequality that shape health inequities (Weber and Fore 2007). Further, these regimes of inequality intersect with various economic, political, social, and historical features of the broader social context. For example, the legacy of colonization in which Aboriginal peoples were disposed and displaced from their land and social policies of assimilation (e.g., residential schools) have adversely impacted the health and well-being of generations of Aboriginal peoples with differences in health outcomes among groups (Loppie Reading and Wien 2009). According to Walby (2007), "Within each domain (economic, polity, violence and civil society), there are multiple sets of social relations (e.g., gender, class, ethnicity). Each institutionalized domain and each set of social relations are here conceptualized as systems, not parts of a system" (454). Thus, engaging a notion of complex adaptive systems in which various systems "can be overlapping and non-nested" (454), Walby argues that this revision of systems theory makes it possible to more fully consider multiple systems of social inequality and power imbalances enacted at multiple levels (micro, meso, and macro).

SYSTEMIC PROCESSES:NEO-LIBERALISM AND BIOMEDICINE

There are multiple regimes of social inequity that variously impact individuals in relation to social positioning. To illustrate more fully, neo-liberalism and the dominance of biomedicine will be examined here as examples of systemic processes that operate at multiple levels and exacerbate health inequities and inequities of access to health care.

Neo-liberalism and Health Inequities

Coburn (2000; 2004) has highlighted the association between increasing neo-liberalism, increased income and health inequities. Neo-liberalism refers to "the dominance of markets and the market model" (Coburn 2000, 138). According to Coburn there are three philosophical tenets that underpin neo-liberalism: (1) markets are the most efficient way to allocate resources; (2) assumption of autonomous individuals who are motivated chiefly by material or economic factors; (3) innovations will be achieved through competition (Coburn 2000). In capitalist economies dominated by various forms of neo-liberalism, there are increasing disparities in wealth that come to be accepted and consequent declines in the welfare state. Neo-liberal values have been associated with sharp declines in the provision and rates of social assistance that have contributed to growing rates of poverty as well as housing, income, and food insecurity (Bryant et al. 2010; Eggleton 2008; Eggleton and Segal 2009; Food Banks Canada 2009; Public Health Agency of Canada 2008; Wellesley Institute 2010).

Poverty, housing, and food insecurity are felt keenly throughout Canada among both indigenous and non-indigenous peoples (Bryant et al. 2010; Eggleton 2008; Eggleton and Segal 2009; Food Banks Canada 2009; Public Health Agency of Canada 2008; Wellesley Institute 2010). Inadequate housing in Canada has been the object of international criticism. During a 2007 visit to Canada, the U.N. special rapporteur on housing observed that

> Everywhere that I visited in Canada, I met people who are homeless and living in inadequate and insecure housing conditions. On this mission, I have heard of hundreds of people who have died as a direct result of Canada's nation-wide housing crisis. (Kothari 2007, 3)

Lack of adequate housing is associated with poor health and increased mortality (Cheung and Hwang 2004; Hwang 2000; Hwang et al. 2009; Nordentoft and Wandall-Holm 2003; Shaw 2004; Wellesley Institute 2010; Wright and Tompkins 2005). People who are homeless or inadequately housed are not only sicker but die prematurely, often 20 to 25 years earlier than the rest of the population. The combination of substance use, poverty, homelessness, and being female is particularly lethal. In one Vancouver study, Spittal et al. (2006) found that women who were homeless and using drugs were 50 times more likely to die prematurely than other women in the population.

Increasing housing insecurity is a consequence of a series of "dehousing" policies including privatization of the Canadian housing market, welfare reform, and deinstitutionalization as a consequence of neo-liberal policies that favour the free market (Eggleton and Segal 2009; Hulchanski 2009; Shapcott 2009). For example, the withdrawal of federal government funding for affordable housing and the reform of CMHC to a mortgage corporation in the 1990s has meant a loss of investment in social housing and the provision of housing controlled by market forces. Welfare reform and declining welfare rates have contributed to homelessness (Wallace, Klein, and Reitsma-Street 2006). Deinstitutionalization of those with mental illness without access to affordable housing or adequate services has contributed to increasing numbers of people on the streets in British Columbia. For Aboriginal communities impacted by colonization, the poor quality of on-reserve housing is a serious concern.

Housing and income insecurity are associated with increased food insecurity. In 2009, there were 884 food banks, 2900 affiliated agencies, and 790 000 individuals who used food banks (Food Banks Canada 2009). There was an 18 percent increase in food bank usage from 2008 to 2009, which is the largest increase on record. The profile of those who use food banks includes individuals, families, couples, and youth with the majority of people being on social assistance, pensions, or disability incomes. Food is often a flexible cost, unlike housing, which is fixed. While food banks struggle to respond to hunger, food insecurity persists because of a lack of secure access to food, fluctuating food supplies, and food that is often insufficient or of poor quality with consequences for poor health (Bocskei and Ostry 2010; Kirkpatrick and Tarasuk 2003; Tarasuk 2005).

In the current neo-liberal context, in which individual responsibility is highly valued, people who are poor, from diverse ethnic backgrounds, or using drugs are often blamed for their problems without recognition of the influence of systemic factors that have shaped opportunities and health of individuals and groups over the life course. For example, stigma and discrimination, although not always explicit, act as deterrents to accessing health care and can profoundly shape health care encounters (Browne and

Fiske 2001; Ensign and Planke 2002; Gelberg et al. 2004; Stajduhar et al. 2004; Wen, Hudak, and Hwang 2007). Perceived past or current status as a "drug user" has been associated with negative experiences in health care (Butters and Erickson 2003; Crockett and Gifford 2004). Aboriginal identity has been explicated as a source of racism that is often unacknowledged by health care providers but keenly felt by those who are the subjects of such behaviors (Browne 2005; 2007; Tang and Browne 2010). Stigma and discrimination not only act as barriers to accessing health care services but also contribute to further marginalization, feelings of low self-worth, and manifest in physical and mental health concerns (Bird, Bogart, and Delahanty 2004; Browne et al. 2002; Dinos et al. 2004; Krieger 1999; Wen and Hudak 2007; Zickmund et al. 2003).

Privileging of Biomedicine

Canada has a publicly funded health care system that ensures access to doctors and hospitals. However, costs of transportation, child care, and pharmaceutical costs may act as barriers to accessing health care services. In the U.S., there are 50.7 million people without health care insurance contributing to even greater inequities in access to health care (DeNavas-Walt, Proctor, and Smith 2010). Available health care services in Canada have been dominated by biomedicine, which has almost exclusively focused on the management and treatment of disease. Biomedicine has been concerned with the biological or genetic factors as the cause of disease, failing to consider broader social factors that shape the health of populations (Weber and Fore 2007). Health care services, with a dominant focus on biomedicine, have largely ignored the social determinants of health as fundamental causes of disease (Link and Phelan 1995). Further, biomedicine locates the source of the problem within the individual. As a result, individuals experiencing disease sequela associated with poor living conditions are viewed as being to blame or at fault for their situations that have been shaped by eroding social policies, gender bias, racial discrimination, and so on. These same forces often impact nursing practice as well as nurses' consequent power and ability to challenge biomedicine.

Health inequities are essentially the product of structural injustices that are potentially avoidable or remediable (Whitehead and Dahlgren 2006). While there has been growing evidence of health inequities, action on reducing health inequities has been limited (Bryant et al. 2010; Raphael 2003). This is due not merely to insufficient evidence or recognition of the importance of the social determinants of health but to the intersections of values, power, and political structures that shape policies and access to health and resources and the use of evidence (Pauly et al. under review; Varcoe et al. in press). Registered nurses, with specific commitments to social justice, have a role to play in challenging and dismantling systems of oppression. In the next section, theoretical perspectives on social justice will be discussed as an underpinning for ethical nursing practice to promote health equity.

PERSPECTIVES ON SOCIAL JUSTICE

Historically, public health nurses, such as Lillian Wald and Lavina Dock, focused their efforts on improving the conditions of those living in poverty, without adequate housing or access to basic resources for health (Drevdahl 2001). Lillian Wald, considered the founder of public health nursing, focused her work on redressing inequities in social policies that contributed to poor housing and employment conditions and advocated for reforms. Although codes of ethics embrace values in relation to the promotion of equity, underlying theoretical conceptions of social justice are often incoherent or inconsistent (Bekemeier and Butterfield 2005; Reimer Kirkham and Browne 2006). Further, enactment of social justice mandates as part of ethical nursing practice is often fraught with difficulties due to existing policy regimes, workloads, and other factors.

Of particular importance to reducing health inequities is an understanding of social rather than distributive justice. Within nursing, there has been critique of the limitations of distributive justice for addressing health inequities (Anderson et al. 2009; Drevdahl 2001; Pauly, MacKinnon, and Varcoe 2009; Reimer Kirkham and Browne 2006). Distributive justice is primarily concerned with the distribution or allocation of material resources but not the conditions that shape distribution (Young 1990). Current work to articulate social justice in nursing have emphasized feminist perspectives such as that of Iris Marion Young (Pauly 2008a; Pauly et al. 2009), relational justice (Doane and Varcoe 2005; Hartrick Doane and Varcoe 2005), and post-colonial perspectives (Anderson et al. 2009; Reimer Kirkham and Browne 2006) as part of a social justice lens in nursing. In this section, a brief overview of theoretical perspectives on social justice that have potential to further enhance work on reducing health inequities and social justice in nursing is provided. Specific attention is given to work in feminist and public health ethics.

Feminist Ethics

Work in feminist ethics and social justice provides a lens on health inequities that illuminates power, political structures, and social processes in the production of health inequities (Sherwin 2001; Young 1990). Iris Marion Young, in her critique of distributive justice, argued that the distributive justice paradigm tends to obscure the social structures and institutional contexts that shape distribution. She stated, "A large class of issues of social justice, and those that concern claims that inequalities are unjust in particular, concern evaluation of institutional relations and processes of society" (2). Young highlighted the importance of non-distributive goods including decision making, division of labour, culture, respect, and power that shape distributive patterns. Rather than beginning with distribution, Young argued that we begin with differences and the recognition that differences in age, gender, ethnicity, and social position act as constraints on individual choice and development of health inequities. The degree to which individuals can enact particular choices is constrained by the social circumstances and social positioning in which they are tightly bound (Sherwin 1998). People are not separate from, but rather are situated within historical, political, and social contexts and a complex array of social groups that determine the range of choices available to individuals (Sherwin 2002). For example, people may choose to sleep outside over sharing a room with three other strangers in an emergency shelter and being forced to leave their belongings or pets outside and unattended.

Young (1990) argues for full participation and inclusion of those affected by policies in the decision-making process both as a means to more equitable policy and also to enhance decision-making capacity and individual choice. Nancy Fraser (2007) in her articulation of a theory of justice brings together three key aspects: (1) who is represented in making policy; (2) the economic dimension of distribution; and (3) cultural dimension of who is recognized or counts in policy. All three dimensions are needed as a foundation for justice in a capitalist world. She differentiates between who is represented in policy making and who is recognized as suffering injustices, bringing to bear the importance of evidence, democracy, and intersecting vulnerabilities associated with social positioning in policy processes.

Public Health Ethics

Work in public health ethics has the potential to expand the development and application of social justice in redressing health inequities. Social justice is considered by some to be the foundation of public health (Beauchamp 1976; Powers and Fadden 2006). In an articulation of this claim, both distributive and non-distributive aspects of justice that impact health and the importance of attention to the health of the whole population and specific attention to the health of disadvantaged groups are highlighted. Powers and Faden state, "our claim is that justice is concerned with securing and maintaining the social conditions necessary for a sufficient level of well-being in all of its essential dimensions for everyone" (50). The focus is not on judging whether or not individuals have a certain level of well-being but rather the degree to which social systems and the social conditions allow for sufficiency or well-being. Baylis, Kenny, and Sherwin (2008) provide an account of relational justice that seeks to infuse social justice as described by Young and Powers and Faden with relational autonomy and relational solidarity. Relational autonomy recognizes that individual decision making is constrained by the social circumstances in which one lives (Sherwin 1998).

> A relational understanding of solidarity would not have us ignore important differences between people. A commitment to social justice requires us to recognize the special disadvantages that face members of social groups who are subject to systematic discrimination and reduced power. (Baylis et al. 2008, 204)

These authors go on to say that this endeavour is central to successful dismantling of systems of privilege and disadvantage that are located in social structures and public policies.

NURSING PRACTICE AND PROMOTION OF SOCIAL JUSTICE

Registered nurses have a professional ethical commitment to the promotion of health equity that is rooted in social justice (Canadian Nurses Association 2008). The current Canadian Nurses Association Code of Ethics states, "There are broad aspects of social justice that are associated with health and well-being and that ethical nursing practice addresses. These aspects relate to the need for change in systems and societal structures to create health equity for all" (20). Nurses are urged, through individual and collective actions, to contribute to reducing health inequities through action on primary health care, health promotion, social determinants of health, socio-economic and political factors, global health, environmental health, and universal health care. Specifically, the code encourages registered nurses to recognize that some groups in society are systemically disadvantaged, which impacts health and well-being, and urges nurses to work to address these disadvantages in health and inequitable access to health care. While codes of ethics for nurses often embrace such ideals and values related to health equity, enactment of ethical practice in relation to social structures and marginalizing processes may have limited uptake or be constrained in practice.

Social processes that shape inequities in health and access to health care are deeply embedded in social structures. Registered nurses can recognize and work to counter these processes in policy and practice. For example, nurses can examine their own social locations and be leaders in highlighting and discussing racialization and stereotypes associated with homelessness and drug use that contribute to discriminatory practices. All nurses, individually and collectively, from their positions in education, research, practice, and policy have the potential to enact social justice by raising and challenging social regimes that produce inequities. Nurses in policy, research, practice, and education are in key positions to assist in reframing policy problems through a socio-political lens and attention to evidence of the social, economic, and cultural roots of disadvantage that can contribute to equity-focused policies. Housing, food, income, and drug policy are key areas for future action that are needed to improve the health of the population (Bryant et al. 2010; Canadian Nurses Association in press; Pauly et al. 2007). These are important areas of action for professional nursing associations. For example, the Canadian Nurses Association has taken positions on the need for adequate housing as a determinant of health and on Insite (a supervised injection site) as an essential health care service for people who use drugs.

Involving people with direct experience of the situations at hand in decision-making processes can break down barriers (such as stigma), contribute to well-being and positive self-esteem, and improve the efficiency of services and client outcomes through development of programs that are in tune with the needs of people who use them. Principles of inclusion in policy development have emerged in discourses on disability and have been applied to the mental health consumer movement as well as in HIV/AIDS advocacy (UNAIDS 1999). These principles have also begun to inform discussions of substance use (Canadian HIV/AIDS Legal Network 2005) and homelessness (Owen 2009; Paasche et al. 2009). Increasingly, drug user groups (Friedman et al. 2007) and homeless persons have begun to self-organize to provide a voice for those who are often implicated but unheard in the policy process.

Registered nurses in public health with expertise in community development can facilitate and support the development of peer-based groups as means of supporting participation and fostering the inclusion of voices that are often overlooked in practice and policy. Community-based research (CBR) approaches such as photovoice methodology (Wang and Burris 1997; Wang et al. 2004) can be employed as participatory action research strategies that have social change as an explicit goal. CBR approaches to research seek to democratize knowledge, enhance participation, and reduce health inequities for disadvantaged communities by inclusion in the research process as a means of reducing power imbalances (Israel et al. 1998). However, working across differences in power is fraught with ethical issues that need to be considered (Wang and Redwood-Jones 2001).

Frequently, nurses in practice confront grave inequities associated with fundamental deficits in the social determinants of health. First, nurses should be aware of both the individual and cumulative impacts of intersecting policies (e.g., housing, income, and drug policy) that contribute to health inequities. In such situations, nurses have multiple and varied opportunities to influence the structural determinants of health in daily practice with individuals, groups, and communities (Pauly et al. 2009). For example, nurses in their practice can recognize and act on a need for housing post-discharge for individuals and advocate for innovations such as integrated discharge planning or primary health care services that promote access to the resources for health.

In practice, the adoption of equity-focused strategies such as *trauma-informed care, harm reduction,* and *cultural competency* are highly relevant to ethical nursing practice and the promotion of health equity. Trauma-informed care is an approach to nursing care that recognizes not only personal histories of trauma and abuse but also intergenerational and historical trauma (Elliott et al. 2005). Trauma-informed care for women is based on principles of respectful engagement, safety, focus on recovery, empowerment, and resilience. Trauma-informed care is culturally competent, relational, collaborative, maximizes choices, minimizes re-traumatization, and fosters participation in designing and evaluating services. Such principles are clearly aligned with nursing values and the promotion of social justice.

Adoption of a harm-reduction approach in practice can contribute to reducing health inequities through principles of respect and inclusion that can counter stigma and discrimination (Pauly 2008a; 2008b). Harm reduction aims to reduce the harms of an activity (such as drug use) without passing judgment on the activity. Harm reduction is both a philosophy and set of strategies that seek to prevent harms of substance use rather than eliminate substance use (International Harm Reduction Association 2010; Riley and O'Hare 2000). It is based on a pragmatic approach that acknowledges drug use as an enduring feature of human existence and advocates a compassionate response to inequities associated with drug use. There is a substantial evidence base for harm-reduction strategies (Canadian Nurses Association in press; Loxley et al. 2004; Marlatt and Witkiewitz 2010; Ritter and Cameron 2006). Harm reduction has the potential to shift moral norms toward more respectful and non-judgmental care for groups that are often highly stigmatized in society (Pauly 2008b). The principles of harm reduction are aligned with nursing values as described in the Code of Ethics and professional standards of practice (Lightfoot et al. 2009; Pauly et al. 2007). However, nurses are often caught between values and evidence for harm reduction and lack of organizational polices and public support for harm reduction. Clearly, professional and ethical standards of nursing practice that endorse values of respect and dignity, goals of health promotion and evidence-based practice are of critical importance in such situations.

Cultural competency and the creation of a culturally safe environment is a third strategy for nurses working with socially and economically disadvantaged populations. Cultural safety and related cultural competencies provide a conceptual framework for prompting nurses to reflect critically on issues of health and health care inequities, and nursing's role in mitigating health inequities (Anderson et al. 2010; Browne et al. 2009; Reimer-Kirkham et al. 2009). Recognizing one's own power and privilege relative to groups who have been marginalized and oppressed can assist one to better understand social locations and constraints on the decision making of others. Such understanding of the social context from which people make decisions can assist nurses in shaping nursing interventions that address the health needs of those impacted by social disadvantage. Cultural safety promotes awareness of assumptions and stereotypes that may be operating among individuals and systemically, a recognition of the way these stereotypes and assumptions may be operating in the delivery of care, and a shift in practice to convey respect and unconditional regard for patients. Thus, cultural safety fosters equity and social justice in nursing practice. Although cultural safety was developed to improve health care for indigenous peoples, it holds relevance for nurses in caring for people experiencing inequities and marginalization associated with homelessness and drug use (Lightfoot et al. 2009).

Summary

In this chapter, I have reviewed the ethical dimensions of health inequities associated with marginalization of those impacted by poverty, homelessness, and drug use. Health inequities are a product of social conditions and social processes. Addressing health inequities is central to the role of registered nurses and embedded in the CNA Code of Ethics. Registered nurses can enact their social justice mandate through recognition of the conditions that shape inequities, addressing the structural determinants of health, drawing on a wide range of evidence, and addressing power imbalances.

For Reflection

1. How do structural determinants of health and determinants of inequities operate in the production of health inequities?

2. What stereotypes and assumptions do you, as a nurse, bring to interactions with groups of people whom you perceive as different from yourself (e.g., in terms of ethnicity, socio-economic status, sexual orientation)?

3. How do these stereotypes impact nursing practice? What strategies can be implemented to resist such marginalizing practices?

4. How can nurses contribute to health inequity reduction in policy, practice, research, and education?

5. How can the Canadian Nurses Code of Ethics and Social Justice Gauge be used to support action to reduce health inequities?

References

Anderson, J., Rodney, P., Reimer-Kirkham, S., Browne, A.J., Khan, K.B., and Lynam, M.J. 2009. Inequities in health and healthcare viewed through the ethical lens of critical social justice. Contextual knowledge for the global priorities ahead. *Advances in Nursing Science, 32* (4), 282–294.

Anderson, J. M., Browne, A. J., Lynam, J. M., Reimer Kirkham, S., Rodney, P., and Varcoe, C. 2010. Uptake of critical knowledge in nursing practice: Lessons learned from a knowledge translation study. *Canadian Journal of Nursing Research, 42* (3).

Baylis, F., Kenny, N.P., and Sherwin, S. 2008. A relational account of public health ethics. *Public Health Ethics,* 1–14. doi: 10.1093/phe/phn025.

Beauchamp, D.E. 1976. Public health as social justice. [Invited paper]. *Inquiry, XIII,* 3–12.

Bekemeier, B. and Butterfield, P. 2005. Unreconciled inconsistencies: A critical review of the concept of social justice in 3 national nursing documents. *Advances in Nursing Science, 28* (2), 152–162.

Bird, S.T., Bogart, L., and Delahanty, D. 2004. Health-related correlates of perceived discrimination in HIV care. *AIDS Patient Care and STDs, 18* (1), 19–26.

Bocskei, E. and Ostry, A. 2010. Charitable food programs in Victoria, B.C. *Canadian Journal of Dietetic Practice and Research, 71* (1), 2–4.

Braveman, P. 2004. Defining equity in health. *Health Policy and Development, 2,* 180–185.

Braveman, P. (2006). Health disparities and health equity: Concepts and measurement. *Annual Review of Public Health, 27,* 167–194.

Browne, A. 2005. Discourses influencing nurses' perceptions of First Nations patients. *Canadian Journal of Nursing Research, 37* (4), 62–87.

Browne, A. 2007. Clinical encounters between nurses and First Nations women in a Western Canadian hospital. *Social Science & Medicine, 64* (10), 2165–2176.

Browne, A., Varcoe, C., Smye, V., Reimer Kirkham, S., Lynam, J., and Wong, S. 2009. Cultural safety and the challenges of translating critically oriented knowledge in practice. *Nursing Philosophy, 10,* 167–179.

Browne, A. J. and Fiske, J. 2001. First Nations women's encounters with mainstream health care services.. *Western Journal of Nursing Research, 23* (2), 126–147.

Browne, A.J., Johnson, J.L., Bottorf, J.L., Grewal, S., and Hilton, B.A. 2002. Recognizing discrimination in nursing practice. *Canadian Nurse, 98* (5), 24–27.

Bryant, T., Raphael, D., Schrecker, T., and Labonte, R. 2010. Canada: A land of missed opportunity for addressing the social determinants of health. *Health Policy.* doi: 10.1016/j.healthpol.2010.08.022.

Butters, J. and Erickson, P.G. 2003. Meeting the health care needs of female crack users: A Canadian example. *Women and Health, 37* (3), 1–17.

Canadian HIV/AIDS Legal Network. 2005. *Nothing about us without us: Great meaningful involvement of people who use illicit drugs: A public health, ethical, and human rights imperative.* Available at www.aidssida.cpha.ca.

Canadian Nurses Association. 2008. *Code of ethics for registered nurses.* Available at http://www.cna-nurses.ca/CNA/practice/ethics/code/default_e.aspx.

Canadian Nurses Association. in press. *Reducing the harms of illicit substance use: Implications for nursing policy, practice and research.* Ottawa, ON: Author.

Cheung, A.M. and Hwang, S.W. 2004. Risk of death among homeless women: A cohort study and review of the literature. *Canadian Medical Association Journal, 170* (8), 1243–1247.

Coburn, D. 2000. Income inequality, social cohesion and the health status of populations: The role of neo-liberalism. *Social Science & Medicine, 51*, 135–146.

Coburn, D. 2004. Beyond the income inequality hypothesis: Class, neo-liberalism, and health inequalities. *Social Science & Medicine, 58*, 41–56.

Commission on the Social Determinants of Health. 2008. *Closing the gap in a generation: Achieving health equity through action on the social determinants of health.* Geneva: World Health Organization.

Corneil, T., Kuyper, L., Shoveller, J., Hogg, R., Li, K., Spittal, P., and Wood, E. 2006. Unstable housing associated risk behavior, and increased risk for HIV infection among injection drug users. *Health Place, 12* (1), 79–85.

Crockett, B. and Gifford, S.M. 2004. "Eyes wide shut": Narratives of women living with hepatitis C in Australia. *Women and Health, 39* (4), 117–137.

DeNavas-Walt, C., Proctor, B., and Smith, J. 2010. Income, poverty, and health insurance in the United States: 2009. *Current Population Reports,* (pp. 60–238). Washington, DC: U.S. Census Bureau.

Despres, C. 1991. The meaning of home: Literature review and directions for further research and theoretical development. *Journal of Architectural and Planning Research, 8*, 96–115.

Dinos, S., Stevens, S., Serfaty, M., Weich, S., and King, M. 2004. Stigma: The feelings and experiences of 46 people with mental illness. *British Journal of Psychiatry, 184*, 176–181.

Doane, G. and Varcoe, C. 2005. Toward compassionate action: Pragmatism and the inseperability of theory/practice. *Advances in Nursing Science, 28* (1), 81–91.

Drevdahl, D. 2001. Reinvesting in social justice: A capital idea for public health nursing? *Advances in Nursing Science, 24* (2), 19–31.

Dunn, J., Hayes, M., Hulchanski, J.D., Hwang, S., and Potvin, L. 2006. Housing as a socio-economic determinant of health: Findings of a national needs, gaps and opportunities assessment. *Canadian Journal of Public Health, 97*, S11–S15.

Dupuis, A. and Thorns, D.C. 1998. Home, home ownership, and the search for ontological security. *The Sociological Review, 46* (1), 24–47.

Eggleton, A. 2008. *Poverty, housing and homelessness: Issues and options: First report of the subcommittee on cities of the standing senate committee on social affairs, science and technology* (pp. i–90). Ottawa: Government of Canada.

Eggleton, A. and Segal, H. 2009. In *from the margins: A call to action on poverty, housing and homelessness. Report of the subcommittee on cities.* Ottawa: Senate Canada.

Elliott, D., Bjelajac, P., Fallot, R., Markoff, L., and Reed, B. 2005. Trauma-informed or trauma-denied: Principles of implementation of trauma-informed services for women. *Journal of Community Psychology, 33* (4), 461–477.

Ensign, J. and Planke, A. 2002. Barriers and bridges to care: Voices of homeless female adolescent youth in Seattle, Washington, USA. *Journal of Advanced Nursing, 37* (2), 166–172.

Food Banks Canada. 2009. *Hunger count 2009: A comprehensive report on hunger and food bank use in Canada and recommendations for change.* Toronto: Author.

Frankish, C.J., Hwang, S.W., and Quantz, D. 2005. Homelessness and health in Canada: Research lessons and priorities. *Canadian Journal of Public Health, 96*, Suppl 2, S23–29.

Friedman, S.R., de Jong, W., Rossi, D., Touze, G., Rockwell, R., Des Jarlais, D.C., and Elovich, R. 2007. Harm reduction theory: Users' culture, micro-social indigenous harm reduction, and the self-organization and outside-organizing of users' groups. *International Journal of Drug Policy, 18* (2), 107–117.

Frohlich, K.L., Ross, N., and Richmond, C. 2006. Health disparities in Canada today: Some evidence and a theoretical framework. *Health Policy, 79*, 132–143.

Gelberg, L., Browner, C.H., Lejano, E., and Arangua, L. 2004. Access to women's health care: A qualitative study of barriers perceived by homeless women. *Women and Health, 40* (2), 87–100.

Graham, H. 2004. Social determinants and their unequal distribution: Clarifying policy understandings. *The Milbank Quarterly, 82* (1), 101–124.

Hall, J.M. 1999. Marginalization revisited: Critical, postmodern, and liberation perspectives. *Advances in Nursing Science, 22* (2), 88–10.

Hall, J.M., Stevens, P., and Meleis, A.I. 1994. Marginalization: A guiding concept for valuing diversity in nursing knowledge development. *Advances in Nursing Science, 16* (4), 23–41.

Hankivsky, O. and Cormier, R. 2009. *Intersectionality: Moving women's health research and policy forward.* Vancouver: Women's Health Research Network.

Hankivsky, O., Reid, C., Cormier, R., Varcoe, C., Clark, N., Benoit, C., and Brotman, S. 2010. Exploring the promises of intersectionality for advancing women's health research. *International Journal for Inequity in Health, 9* (5).

Hartrick Doane, G. and Varcoe, C. 2005. *Family nursing as relational inquiry: Developing health promoting practice.* Philadelphia: Lippincott, Williams and Wilkins.

Hulchanski, J.D. 2009. *Homelessness in Canada: Past, present, futures.* Paper presented at the Growing Home: Housing and Homelessness in Canada, University of Calgary.

Hwang, S. 2000. Mortality among men using homeless shelters in Toronto, Ontario. *Journal of the American Medical Association, 283* (16), 2152–2157.

Hwang, S., Wilkins, R., Tjepkema, M., O'Campo, P., and Dunn, J. 2009. Mortality among residents of shelters, rooming houses, and hotels in Canada: 11 year follow-up study. *British Medical Journal, 339.* doi: doi:10.1136/bmj.b4036.

International Harm Reduction Association. 2010. *What is harm reduction?* London. Available at http://www.ihra.net/files/2010/08/10/Briefing_What_is_HR_English.pdf.

Israel, B.A., Schulz, A.J., Parker, E.A., and Becker, A.B. 1998. Review of community-based research: Assessing partnership approaches to improve public health. *Annual Review of Public Health, 19*, 173–202.

Kendall, P. 2009. *Pathways to health and healing: 2nd report on the health and well-being of Aboriginal people in British Columbia.* Victoria, BC: Ministry of Healthy Living and Sport.

Kirkpatrick, S. and Tarasuk, V. 2003. The relationship between low income and household food expenditure patterns in Canada. *The Journal of Nutrition, 6* (6), 589–597.

Kothari, M. 2007. *United Nations special rapporteur on adequate housing, Miloon Kothari.* Ottawa: Main Ottawa Public Library.

Krieger, N. 1999. Embodying inequality: A review of concepts, measures, and methods for studying health consequences of discrimination. *International Journal of Health Services, 29* (2), 295.

Lightfoot, B., Panessa, C., Hayden, S., Thumath, M., Goldstone, I., and Pauly, B. 2009. Gaining insite: Harm reduction in nursing practice. *Canadian Nurse, 105* (4), 16–22.

Link, B. and Phelan, J. 1995. Social conditions as fundamental causes of diseases. *Journal of Health and Social Behavior, 35* (Extra issue), 80–94.

Lloyd, C. 2010. *Sinning and sinned against: The stigmatization of problem drug users.* London: U.K. Drug Policy Commission.

Loppie Reading, C. and Wien, F. 2009. *Health inequities and social determinants of Aboriginal peoples' health.* Prince George, BC: National Collaborating Centre for Aboriginal Health.

Loxley, W., Toumbourou, J., Stockwell, T.R., Haines, B., Scott, K., Godfrey, C., Waters, E., and. Patton, G. 2004. *The prevention of substance use, risk and harm in Australia: A review of the evidence.* Canberra: Australian Government Department of Health and Ageing.

MacMillan, H.L., Jamieson, E., Walsh, C.A., Wong, M.Y.Y., Faries, E.J., and McCue, H., MacMillan, A., Offord, D, and Technical Advisory Committee of the Chiefs of Ontario. 2008. First Nations women's mental health: Results from an Ontario survey. *Archives of Women's Mental Health, 11*, 109–115.

Marlatt, G.A. and Witkiewitz, K. 2010. Update on harm-reduction policy and intervention research. *Annual Review of Clinical Psychology, 6*, 20.21–20.16.

Marmot, M. 2005. Social determinants of health inequalities. *The Lancet, 365*, 1099.

Marmot, M. 2007. Achieving health equity: From root causes to fair outcomes. *Lancet, 370*, 1153–1163.

Martens, W. 2001. A review of physical and mental health in homeless persons. *Public Health Reviews, 29* (1), 13–33.

McCall, L. 2005. The complexity of intersectionality. *Journal of Women in Culture and Society, 30* (3), 1771–1800.

Nettleton, C., Napolitano, D.A., and Stephens, C. 2007. *An overview of current knowledge of the social determinants of indigenous health.* Geneva, Switzerland: World Health Organization Commission on the Social Determinants of Health.

Nordentoft, M. and Wandall-Holm, M. 2003. 10 year follow up study of mortality among users of hostels for homeless people in Copenhagen. *British Medical Journal, 327*, 1–4.

Owen, R. 2009. Participation of people experiencing homelessness: Sharing the power and working together. *The Magazine of FEANSTA: European Federation of National Organization Working with the Homeless, Autumn.*

Paasche, S., Williams, A., Laurberg, A.S., Sakamoto, I., Hall, J., Story, A., Jezek, R., and Le Floch, S. 2009. Participation of people experiencing homelessness: Sharing the power and working together. In R. Owen (Ed.), *Homeless in Europe.* Brussels: European Federation of National Organisations Working with the Homeless.

Padgett, D. 2007. There's no place like (a) home: Ontological security among persons with serious mental illness in the United States. *Social Science & Medicine, 64*, 1925–1936.

Patterson, M., Somers, J., MacIntosh, K., Shiell, A., and Frankish, C.J. 2007. *Housing and supports for adults with severe addictions and mental illness in British Columbia*. Vancouver: Centre for Applied Research in Mental Illness and Addiction.

Pauly, B. 2008a. Harm reduction through a social justice lens. [Commentary]. *International Journal of Drug Policy, 19*, 4–10.

Pauly, B. 2008b. Shifting moral values to enhance access to health care: Harm reduction as a context for ethical nursing practice. *International Journal of Drug Policy, 19*, 195–204.

Pauly, B., Goldstone, I., McCall, J., Gold, F., and Payne, S. 2007. The ethical, legal and social context of harm reduction. *Canadian Nurse, 103* (8), 19–23.

Pauly, B., MacKinnon, K., and Varcoe, C. 2009. Revisiting "Who gets care?" Health equity as an arena for nursing action. *Advances in Nursing Science, 32* (2), 118–127.

Pauly, B., Varcoe, C., MacPherson G., Laliberte, S., Reimer, J., Ponic, P., Hancock, T., and. Kenny, N. under review. *Conceptualizing an equity lens for public health: The contribution of health policy ethics*. Victoria, BC: University of Victoria.

Powers, M. and Fadden, R. 2006. *Social justice: The moral foundation of public health and health policy*. Toronto: Oxford University Press.

Public Health Agency of Canada. 2008. *The Chief Public Health Officer's report on the state of public health in Canada*. Ottawa: Health Canada.

Raphael, D. 2003. Barriers to addressing the societal determinants of health: Public health units and poverty in Ontario, Canada. *Health Promotion International, 18* (4), 397–405.

Reimer-Kirkham, S., Varcoe, C., Browne, A.J., Lynam, M.J., Khan, K.B., and McDonald, H. 2009. Critical inquiry and knowledge translation: Exploring compatibilities and tensions. *Nursing Philosophy, 10*, 152–166.

Reimer Kirkham, S. and Browne, A. 2006. Toward a critical theoretical interpretation of social justice discourses in nursing. *Advances in Nursing Science, 29* (4), 324–339.

Research Alliance for Canadian Homelessness Housing and Health. 2010. *Housing vulnerability and health: Canada's hidden emergency*. Toronto: Author.

Riley, D. and O'Hare, P. 2000. Harm reduction: History, definition and practice. In J. Inciardi and L. Harrison (Eds.), *Harm reduction: National and International Perspectives*. London: Sage.

Ritter, A. and Cameron, J. 2006. A review of the efficacy and effectiveness of harm reduction strategies for alcohol, tobacco and illicit drugs. *Drug and Alcohol Review, 25*, 611–624.

Shannon, K., Ishida, T., Lai, C., and Tyndall, M.W. 2006. The impact of unregulated single room occupancy hotels on the health status of illicit drug users in Vancouver. *International Journal of Drug Policy, 17* (2), 107–114.

Shapcott, M. 2009. Housing. In D. Raphael (Ed.), *Social determinants of health: Canadian perspectives* (pp. 201–215). Toronto: Canadian Scholar's Press Inc.

Shaw, M. 2004. Housing and public health. *Annual Review of Public Health, 25*, 297–418.

Sherwin, S. 1998. A relational approach to autonomy in health care. The Feminist Health Care Ethics Research Network, Susan Sherwin, Coordinator (Eds.), *The politics of women's health* (p. 19). Philadelphia: Temple University Press.

Sherwin, S. 2001. Moral perception and global visions. *Bioethics, 15* (3), 175.

Sherwin, S. 2002. The importance of ontology for feminist policy-making in the realm of reproductive technology. In S. Brennan (Ed.), *Feminist moral philosophy* (p. 273). Calgary: University of Calgary Press.

Spittal, P., Hogg, R., Li, K., Craib, M., Recsky, C., Johnston, J., Montaner, S., Schechter, M., and Wood, E. 2006. Drastic elevations in mortality among female injection drug users in a Canadian setting. *Aids Care, 18* (2), 101–108.

Stajduhar, K.I., Poffenroth, L., Wong, E., Archibald, C.P., Sutherland, D., and Rekart, M. 2004. Missed opportunities: Injection drug use and HIV/AIDS in Victoria, Canada. *International Journal of Drug Policy, 15* (3), 171–181.

Starfield, B. 2006. State of the art in research on equity in health. *Journal of Health Politics, Policy and Law, 31* (1), 11.

Stephens, C., Nettleton, C., Porter, J., Willis, R., and Clark, S. 2005. Indigenous peoples' health: Why are they behind everyone, everywhere? *The Lancet, 366* (9479), 10–13.

Tang, S. and Browne, A. 2010. 'Race' matters: Racilaization and egalitarian discourses involving Aboriginal people in the Canadian helath are context. *Ethnicity & Health, 13* (2), 109–127.

Tarasuk, V. 2005. Household food insecurity in Canada. *Topics in Clinical Nutrition, 20* (4), 299–312.

Varcoe, C., Pauly, B., MacPherson, G., and Laliberte, S. in press. Intersectionality, social justice and influencing policy. In O. Hankivsky (Ed.), *Health inequities in Canada*. Vancouver, BC: UBC Press.

Walby, S. 2007. Complexity theory, systems theory, and multiple intersecting social inequalities. *Philosophy of the Social Sciences, 37*, 449–470.

Walby, S. 2009. *Theorizing multiple social systems globalization and inequalities: Complexity and contested modernities*. London: Sage.

Waldram, J.B., Herring, A., and Young, T.K. 2006. *Aboriginal health in Canada: Historical, cultural and epidemiological perspectives* (2nd ed.). Toronto: University of Toronto Press.

Wallace, B., Klein, S., and Reitsma-Street, M. 2006. *Denied assistance: Closing the front door on welfare in BC*. Vancouver: Canadian Centre for Policy Alternatives & Vancouver Island Public Interest Research Group.

Wang, C., and Burris, M. 1997. Photovoice: Concept, methodology and use for participatory needs assessment. *Health Education and Behavior, 24* (3), 369–387.

Wang, C., Morrel-Samuels, S., Hutchinson, P., Bell, L., and Pestronk, R. 2004. Flint photovoice: Community building among youths, adults and policymakers. *American Journal of Public Health, 94* (6), 911–913.

Wang, C. and Redwood-Jones, Y. 2001. Photovoice ethics: Perspectives from flint photovoice. *Health Education and Behavior, 28* (5), 560–572.

Weber, L. and Fore, M. 2007. Race, ethnicity, and health: An intersectional approach. In H. Vera and J. Feagin (Eds.), *Handbooks of the sociology of racial and ethnic relations* (pp. 191–218). New York: Springer.

Wellesley Institute. 2010. *Precarious housing in Canada.* Toronto: Author.

Wen, C., Hudak, P., and Hwang, S. 2007. Homeless peoples' perceptions of welcomeness and unwelcomeness in health care encounters. *Journal of General Internal Medicine, 22*, 1011–1017.

Werb, D., Rowell, G., Kerr, T., Guyatt, G., Montaner, J., and Wood, E. 2010. *Effect of drug law enforcement on drug-related violence: Evidence from a scientific review* (pp. 1–25). Vancouver, BC: Urban Health Research Initiative of the British Columbia Centre for Excellence in HIV/AIDS.

Whitehead, M. 1992. The concepts and principles of equity and health. *International Journal of Health Services, 22* (3), 429.

Whitehead, M. and Dahlgren, G. 2006. Levelling up (part 1): A discussion paper on concepts and principles for tackling social inequities in health. *Studies on social and economic determinants of population health* (Vol. 2). Copenhagen: World Health Organization.

Wilkinson, R. and Marmot, M. (Eds.). 2003. *Social determinants of health: The solid facts* (2nd ed.). Copenhagen, Denmark: World Health Organization.

Wilkinson, R.G. and Pickett, K. 2006. Income inequality and population health: A review and explanation of the evidence. *Social Science & Medicine, 62*, 1768–1784.

Wilkinson, R.G. and Pickett, K. 2010. *The spirit level: Why equality is better for everyone.* Toronto: Penquin Books.

Willows, N.D., Veugelers, P., Raine, K., and Kuhle, S. 2009. Prevalence and sociodemographic risk factors related to household food security in Aboriginal peoples in Canada. *Public Health Nutrition, 12* (1150–1156).

Wright, N. and Tompkins, C. 2005. How can health care systems effectively deal with the major health care needs of homeless people? *Health Evidence Network Report.* Copenhagen: World Health Organization Regional Office for Europe.

Young, I.M. 1990. *Justice and the politics of difference.* Princeton, NJ: Princeton University Press.

Yuval-Davis, N. 2006. Intersectionality and feminist politics. *European Journal of Women's Studies, 13*, 193–208.

Zickmund, S., Ho, E., Masuda, M., Ippolito, L., and LaBrecque, D. 2003. They treated me like a leper. Stigmatization and the quality of life of patients with hepatitis C. *Journal of General Internal Medicine, 18*, 835.

CHAPTER 22

Opening Pandora's Box: The Ethical Challenges of Xenotransplantation: A Biotechnology Exemplar

Rosalie Starzomski

Men have become the tools of their tools. (Henry David Thoreau)

The twenty-first century is developing into the century of biotechnology, the application of science and engineering to the use of living organisms or their constituent parts with the intent to modify human health and the human environment. As the century unfolds, we find ourselves in the midst of a profound revolution in biotechnology—a revolution that is radically altering our view of who we are as human beings as well as our conceptions of health and health care (Dhanda 2002; O'Mathuna 2007; Rollin 2003; Susumu 2011). The seeds of this revolution were planted when Banting and Best first discovered insulin for the treatment of diabetes in Canada in 1921, thereby launching the field of biotechnology. In 2003, we marked 50 years since Watson and Crick solved the mysteries of DNA (Lemonick 2003), a period during which remarkable strides were made as a result of the historic discoveries in biotechnology. In the last few decades, the "biotech" industry has emerged as the cutting-edge industry of the new century. For instance, the identification of the human genome, and the breakthroughs that have arisen in the world of genetics, have resulted in significant changes regarding how we think about disease and disability (see also Chapter 24). In addition, we are faced with a myriad of new health care technologies emerging from research in areas such as human reproduction, cloning, regenerative medicine, xenotransplantation, and nanotechnology (Baylis 2001; Hovatta et al. 2010; Skloot 2010). The implications of this biotechnological reframing are vast. Today, developments are occurring at such a rapid rate that there is often insufficient discussion about the ethical and societal implications of the scientific advancements being made. Indeed, before the last half of the twentieth century, few people paid much attention to these implications.

Sometimes it appears that, as a society, we are prepared "to boldly go where no one has gone before" (as described in the science fiction television program *Star Trek*), often with minimal critique of the direction in which we are moving. However, whereas each episode of *Star Trek* provided opportunities for the show's writers and actors to examine the moral dimensions of a featured technological "wonder," as a society, we have not always reviewed the social and ethical consequences of biotechnological developments prior to their implementation (Midgely 2000; Latifah et al. 2011; O'Mathuna 2007; Rappert 2008; Susumu 2011). Consequently, the diffusion of biotechnology into the health care system continues to be haphazard at best.

My goal in this chapter is to review xenotransplantation as an exemplar of biotechnological development and to examine several of the ethical and societal challenges that are often pushed to the margins as we "boldly go where no one has gone before." Xenotransplantation, the transfer of living cells, tissues, or organs from one species to another for medical purposes, has arisen as one solution to increase the number of organs available for transplantation (Bloom et al. 1999; Brockbank et al. 2010; Einseidel and Ross 2002; Platt 1997). Many of the issues, concerns, and troublesome questions that emerge in the debate about whether to allow xenotransplantation to become part of the therapeutic armamentarium to treat end-stage organ failure are also evident in other domains of biotechnology development. In what follows, I offer some approaches to advancing the dialogue and debate about the ethical and societal concerns that are emerging as part of the discussion about biotechnology, particularly strategies to enhance nursing leadership in the area. I also illustrate what nurses need to know to assist people to make difficult choices and to be active and effective communicators in consultations with governments on public policy. Although my focus in this chapter will be primarily on reviewing developments in Canada, I briefly examine several international issues and challenges.

BIOTECHNOLOGY—PROMISES AND PITFALLS

Biotechnology changes come in many forms (e.g., the new developments in human genetics described in Chapter 24), and most share common features with respect to ethics. These include a rapid proliferation of the technology, corporate involvement in development and diffusion of the innovations, public pressure to make the biotechnology available, scientific progress with uncertain outcomes, and inadequate attention to societal values.

Even though there may be little question that, potentially, the capabilities and promises of biotechnology may be of benefit to society, there are concerns about the consequences of biotechnological innovation. For example, the worldwide public health crisis brought about by the outbreak of Severe Acute Respiratory Syndrome (SARS), the serious pandemic that occurred with the outbreak of H1N1 influenza, and the news that Bovine Spongiform Encephalopathy (BSE or Mad Cow Disease) was found in a few cows in Canada have fuelled fears about biotechnology and the crossover of viruses and other pathogens from animals and birds to humans (Health Canada 2003a; 2003b; Silva 2010). These developments have resulted in more emphasis being placed on the need for extensive societal discussion about the use of new technologies prior to their implementation.

Technological development and decisions about how to use new technology have largely been under the control of so-called "experts," including researchers, governments, vested interest groups, as well as corporations, and have been highly politicized. Today, there is widespread sentiment among a number of authors that societal input is required in the debate about the ethical issues that have surfaced in regard to biotechnology. Input from members of the public is required when making decisions about what type of research ought to be pursued, and also in the development of coherent public policy about the application of the innovations that emerge from the research. The call for public involvement about biotechnology policy and research comes from many sectors (Brunger and Cox 2000; Canadian Nurses Association 2006; Health Canada 2010) and for many years has been a theme in health care system reviews as well as in meetings to discuss biotechnology (Canadian Public Health Association 2001; Commission on the Future of Health Care in Canada 2002; National Forum on Health 1997; "Proceed with care" 1993; Sherwin 2000). Interestingly, although support exists for the idea that decisions about the research, use, and outcomes of biotechnology have major implications for society, input from members of the public has not always been sought. Further, in addition to the pivotal role members of the public could hold in determining the future direction for biotechnology, a substantial role is available for health care providers, such as nurses, not only to understand the ethical and societal concerns that surround the technology, but also to become involved in the ongoing debate about the manner in which to proceed with specific innovations.

Public and health care provider involvement in decision making about biotechnology is paramount in order to ensure that important societal values and expert knowledge are infused throughout the decision-making process. To illustrate how this can and should occur, I now turn to a discussion of the perplexing ethical and societal implications of biotechnology. Using xenotransplantation as an illustrative case, I first provide an Ethics in Practice narrative (Ethics in Practice 22-1) to contextualize the discussion. I then move on to review developments in the area and the benefits and concerns linked to the technology, especially as they apply to pathogen transmission and informed consent. Further, I elaborate on some of the challenges that arise in regard to corporate, research, and regulatory issues related to xenotransplantation. I conclude with a discussion about public participation in biotechnology policy development and provide an example of a comprehensive approach used when attempting to obtain citizen input into whether Canada should proceed with xenotransplantation.

XENOTRANSPLANTATION: AN ILLUSTRATION OF THE BENEFITS AND CHALLENGES OF BIOTECHNOLOGY

ETHICS IN PRACTICE 22-1

Advice about Xenotransplantation

Maria is an advanced practice nurse working within the transplant program in an urban quaternary care hospital. She, with other members of the transplant team, is responsible for the assessment, education, and support of potential kidney transplant recipients. One of her patients, Paul, is a 47-year-old married teacher and father of two adult children. Paul has been receiving hemodialysis for 10 years and has been on the transplant waiting list for over five years. Maria has met with Paul and his family several times and has developed a trusting relationship with them. Unfortunately, Paul has devel-

oped a number of complications from his chronic renal failure, including a severe peripheral neuropathy. He has exhausted all possibility of receiving an organ from a living donor, as the family members who have been tested are not compatible donors and no friends have come forward to offer him a kidney. In desperation, he put an advertisement on a social networking site where he asked people to respond if they could donate a kidney to him. Because of the number of unhelpful responses he received, he removed the request after a few months. He has been unsuccessful in obtaining an organ from a non-living donor, partly because he has a high level of panel-reactive antibodies, and with the waiting list growing, and the number of organs available for transplantation decreasing, Paul realizes he could be waiting for some time to receive a kidney transplant. Paul's only daughter is being married in several months and he does not believe he will survive to attend her wedding and walk her down the aisle. He is quite despondent and is feeling absolutely desperate about obtaining a transplant. He has even considered going to a developing country to buy a kidney on the black market, but cannot afford the cost. Recently, he has heard that xenotransplant human clinical trials are being conducted in some countries, and he wants to be a volunteer. Paul's wife does not support the idea as she is concerned about what could happen to him, and she is also worried about the transmission of viruses to her and her children if he follows through with his idea. Paul's good friend and neighbour also heard about the idea and believes that Paul is being irresponsible and putting his whole community at risk. Since Maria has been instrumental in helping Paul to make health care decisions in the past, he has approached her for advice about his idea. He also wants her to help him find a way to be a subject in a xenotransplant clinical trial in another country.

In this scenario, Maria is confronted with a variety of questions. How is she to advise Paul? How can she ensure that Paul has the information required to make an informed choice about xenotransplantation? What are the benefits and risks associated with xenotransplantation? What are her responsibilities as an advanced practice nurse in ensuring that patients and families in her care understand the risks, benefits, and implications of new technologies such as xenotransplantation? What are her responsibilities to the community regarding biotechnological innovations within the realm of her practice? In the sections that follow, I review several of the ethical and societal issues related to xenotransplantation emanating from Ethics in Practice 22-1. Further, by addressing the questions posed above, I will uncover ways in which Maria can demonstrate nursing leadership in the area of biotechnology.

Ethical and Societal Implications in the Development of Xenotransplantation

Organ, tissue, and cell transplantation have progressed from being impossible to becoming commonplace, with more than one million people worldwide benefiting from organ transplants alone in the last 55 years (Alexander 1962; Bailey 1990; Murray 1992; Canadian Organ Replacement Register [CORR] 2011; United Network for Organ Sharing [UNOS] 2011). With this success comes an increased demand for donor organs and a severe organ shortage, resulting in a growing number of individuals worldwide who die while waiting for suitable organs to become available (Canadian Blood Services—Organ Donation and Transplantation 2011; CORR 2011; Molzahn, Starzomski, and McCormick 2003; UNOS 2011).

Xenotransplantation has been proposed as one way to alleviate the shortage of organs, tissues, and cells available from non-living donors and to reduce the need for living humans to donate organs (a surgical process that is not without risk). Significant ethical and societal implications of biotechnology are reflected in the debates that have surfaced around xenotransplant technology—debates that raise fundamental questions about social justice, informed consent, our relationships with one another as humans, our relationships with other species, the roles of researchers and corporations, and the role of expert and public stakeholders in making decisions about biotechnology development and implementation (Canadian Public Health Association 2001; Daar and Phil 1997; Nuffield Council on Bioethics 1996).

The science of xenotransplantation has evolved over the past several decades, spurred on by major developments in genetics, and has transformed xenotransplantation from an area only being researched to one that may be clinically feasible (Health Canada 1997; 1999; Cozzi et al. 2009). Other potential solutions to ameliorate the organ short- age, such as the use of organs and tissues engineered from stem cells, may be options to increase the number of organs, tissues, and cells for transplantation, but the solution closest to clinical application for some conditions, such as the treatment of Type 1 diabe- tes with islet cells, will possibly be xenotransplantation (Cozzi et al. 2009; Schneider and Seebach 2010; Vanderpool 2009).

Most clinical developments in xenotransplantation have been in the area of cell transplantation, although there is growing emphasis on developing xenotransplant tech- nology for solid organ transplantation. The need for an appropriate ethical framework is paramount if this future clinical application is to be viable.

Although through xenotransplantation there is the potential to supply cells to treat such disorders as Parkinson's disease and diabetes, and to supply tissues such as skin and bone for transplant purposes (Canadian Public Health Association 2001; Council of Europe 2003), my emphasis in this chapter will be on the use of xenotransplantation in the field of solid organ transplantation. Further, while xenotransplantation can occur between animal species, I will be centering my review on transplantation of organs from animals to humans.

A major problem in the clinical application of xenotransplantation has been finding a suitable source animal from which to retrieve organs that will not be rejected by the human recipient (Cozzi et al. 2009; Platt 1997; Reemsta 1992). In the early days of xenotransplantation, the source animals were generally nonhuman primates. An example of such a case was that of newborn Baby Fae, one of the first humans to receive a xeno- graft. The case received much media attention in 1984 when Baby Fae received a heart transplant from a baboon to treat a condition often fatal in the first days of life called hypoplastic left heart syndrome—a condition in which her left atrium and ventricle were seriously underdeveloped. She died a few weeks post-transplant amid considerable con- troversy about the cause of her death since her heart did not show evidence of cellular rejection (McCormick 1985; National Institutes of Health 1985; Veatch 2000). Nonethe- less, in the midst of the analysis and disputes after her death, xenotransplantation trials in humans were stalled because of the concerns related to possible organ rejection.

Currently, nonhuman primates have largely been removed from consideration as source animals for xenotransplantation, partly because of the high risk of unknown infec- tions being transmitted from them to humans, as demonstrated by the HIV pandemic (Allan 1996; Cozzi et al. 2009). Major animal rights concerns exist regarding the use of nonhuman primates for research because of the close genetic link of these animals to humans (Singer 1992). Also, their long gestation period raises concern that insufficient numbers of animals would be bred to meet the need for organs (Allan 1996; Council of Europe 2003).

The current source animals of choice for xenotransplantation are transgenic pigs. Source animals, such as pigs, can be altered by genetic engineering to minimize rejection, thus optimizing organ function and providing potential advantages to the recipient. While some risks are reduced with the use of pigs as source animals because of their greater phylogenetic distance from humans, and the ability to breed them quickly in pathogen-free, closed environments, the risks associated with unknown infectious agents cannot be quantitatively assessed (Allan 1997; 1998; Cozzi et al. 2009; Fishman 1997). Because of the technological difficulties, few solid organ xenografts have been conducted worldwide. Most of the transplants done to date were for short-term bridging purposes—that is, while critically ill human recipients waited for human organs to become available (Council of Europe 2003; Schneider and Seebach 2010).

This situation is changing, however, as scientific developments in the area of xenotransplantation are accelerating. It is now possible to clone pigs, and scientists are altering genetic systems in order to reproduce litters of piglets with organs that the human immune system will not reject. Companies such as PPL Therapeutics, in addition to being the first in the world to clone piglets, have cloned pigs and "knocked out" the specific gene that has been implicated in transplant rejection, thereby moving the possibility of successful xenotransplantation closer to reality (Soulillou 2011). As a result of the speed at which the science is moving, many countries are involved in some way or another in attempting to develop an appropriate regulatory framework for xenotransplant human clinical trials and the therapeutic application of the technology, a topic I will take up later in this chapter.

Natural Law

Xenotransplantation, similar to other types of biotechnological innovation, is the focus of much controversy and debate, raising complex ethical, social, legal, and economic issues (Shapiro 2008; Sykes, d'Apice, and Sandrin 2003; Vanderpool 2009). The issues raised by xenotransplantation reflect the diversity of values, beliefs, and attitudes held by members of society about vital questions regarding who we are as humans and our role in the natural ecological order of our planet. Such questions are also important when discussing other forms of biotechnology such as genetics, regenerative medicine, and nanotechnology (Daar 2002; Scheufele et al. 2007).

Societal beliefs, attitudes, and values about the nature of xenotransplantation are quite diverse (Pearce, Thomas, and Clements 2006; Starzomski 1997; Tallacchini 2008). Some opponents of xenotransplantation suggest that the technology raises a problem of natural law because the intermixing of biological material from different species violates fundamental morality, impacting directly on who we are as humans (Canadian Public Health Association 2001; Veatch 2000). Some who support xenotransplantation propose that although the transplantation of organs from one species to another is cause for concern at first, it does not involve any more of a violation of natural law than does transplantation of an organ from one person to another, as long as the animal is treated with respect (Canadian Public Health Association 2001; Veatch 2000).

This diversity of societal opinion about the nature of xenotransplantation was clearly articulated by participants in a study conducted by the author several years ago, where 34 focus groups were held with consumers and health care providers to determine attitudes and beliefs about a number of ethical issues related to organ transplantation, including xenotransplantation (Starzomski 1997). One critical care nurse expressed her concern about xenotransplantation when she said,

> I'm a Christian, and I believe that death all along is natural; we are not immortal, and I see it as the final course of life, isn't it? And that's why, when you mentioned the pigs, I go no way! Because that is going to the mad scientist stage, and it's just beyond [imagination].

Providing a different view, an advanced practice nurse said,

> I would support it [xenotransplantation] as long as we are using, in real valued things, a lower-order animal like a pig (and I think there is still enough research done to know they already are lower-order animals) versus finding out later that they are actually smarter than we are, like the whales kind of thing. So, if there were some scientific assurances that that is the case then somehow I could bring myself to accept that.

> It sounds like a good idea, we eat them [animals] anyway, so we're not that sentimental about them. I wouldn't like to see them terribly exploited, but we exploit all over the place.

These opinions, generated by reflection on personal values, underscore several of the germane concerns related to xenotransplantation. In the next section, I will further explore many of the issues that have been raised in the discussion about biotechnology as I present a review of some of the benefits and concerns related to xenotransplantation.

Benefits and Challenges of Xenotransplantation

Although xenotransplantation has the potential to benefit many people, a number of societal and ethical concerns must be addressed if this technology is to move forward in a manner that optimizes its potential to benefit people while at the same time minimizing risk. In what follows, I will review the major benefits of xenotransplantation and discuss some of the potential problems that work against these benefits. Given the limited scope of this chapter, I will not address one of the concerns raised by xenotransplantation—that is, the rights of the animals who will be the donors if xenotransplantation becomes a reality (Canadian Public Health Association 2001; Singer 1992).

Potential Benefits of Xenotransplantation

Many potential benefits have been identified if xenotransplantation were to become a therapeutic treatment for end-stage organ failure. These include the following:

- The potential exists to eliminate the shortage of organs, tissues, and cells, as facilities would be established to produce pigs to serve as sources that would be available when required.

- In some jurisdictions where human organ donation has not been accepted because of ethical or ethnocultural concerns, xenotransplantation might provide an acceptable alternative.

- With ready access to organs, recipient selection criteria could be broadened, and the current ethical dilemmas surrounding transplant allocation would disappear as, theoretically, everyone who needed an organ would be transplanted.

- Xenografts could be conducted in an early, controlled fashion before the complications of diseases affected patients.

- Xenografts could offer advantages similar to those associated with the use of human living donor organs. For example, the transplant surgery could be pre-scheduled; pretreatment of recipients would be possible; the quality of the organs would be known; the organs would be out of the body for a limited period of time, thereby preventing rejection; and the effects of brain death on organ quality could be avoided.

- Finally, xenografts might not be susceptible to the human autoimmune diseases or viral infections that caused organ failure initially and which often limit the survival of organ transplants from human donors (Council of Europe 2003; Platt 1997; Shapiro, 2008; Sykes, d'Apice and Sandrin 2003, 195).

Through this review of the possible benefits of xenotransplantation I show that biotechnology has the *potential* to provide therapeutic advantages in health care delivery. Similarities to the benefits described above exist for other biotechnologies. For instance, successful gene therapy and cloning technology could make available treatments that are tailored to an individual's genetic profile, thus preventing further disease and disability.

Although xenotransplantation offers benefits, a number of scientific and ethical barriers exist that must be addressed to ensure that advances in biotechnology are developed in a manner that optimizes potential to benefit society and minimizes risk (Daar and Phil 1997; Shapiro 2008; Sykes, d'Apice, and Sandrin 2003). In the sections that follow, I will review some of the risks and concerns as they relate to xenotransplantation, recognizing that comparable challenges are evident in many other areas of biotechnology development.

Risk of Pathogen Transmission

One of the significant societal and ethical concerns involved in xenotransplantation is the worry about the risk of transmission of animal pathogens to humans and the subsequent consequences for society. As with all mammals, pigs have viruses that are active, latent, or represented only by a partial genetic sequence embedded in the pig genome. It is difficult to assign exact numbers to the risk, but many experts agree that it is possible that pig endogenous retroviruses (PERVs) could be transmitted to human xenograft recipients (Bach and Ivinson 2002; Fishman 1997; Muir and Griffin 2001; Schneider and Seebach 2008). The possibility has arisen that, under specific conditions, PERVs can infect human cells and be carried in tissue that is transplanted. Because PERVs could be transmitted to human xenograft recipients, it is further possible that such infections could be passed from recipients to other humans, and to society at large. Some authors have indicated that these fears are not unfounded by suggesting that technology in antibody screening for potential xenozoonoses is fraught with problems and is in need of further study (Bach and Ivinson 2002; Dillner 1996; Michaels et al. 1994; Muir and Griffin 2001). Although investigators disagree about the magnitude of the risk, few dismiss it and many agree that it is sufficient to merit serious concern (Dinsmore et al. 2000;

Fishman 1997; Gunzburg and Salmons 2000; Muir and Griffin 2001; Schneider and Seebach 2008).

Further complicating the issue of disease transmission is the reality that if researchers were aware of a particular virus or pathogen, they might be able to develop a test to determine if the pathogen was present. However, if it were a pathogen that had not yet been recognized, it would be impossible to determine if an animal were pathogen free (Sykes, d'Apice, and Sandrin 2003). This is a very serious concern as precedents exist for the survival, replication, and spread of animal viruses to humans with subsequent human-to-human transmission. For example, some scientists believe that HIV may have originated in monkeys before spreading to humans (Allan 1996). And some epidemiologists believe the Spanish flu, which killed close to 50 million people worldwide in the early part of the twentieth century, might have been triggered by swine flu. It is also thought that the influenza virus that struck people in Hong Kong in 1997 was spread from ducks to chickens to humans, killing 18 people. Experts indicate that if the outbreak had not been stopped in time, it would have caused a pandemic (Evanson 2000). Other situations linked to the jump of pathogens from animals to humans include the Ebola and Lassa fever outbreaks in Africa (Muir and Griffin 2001). Many gaps exist in our knowledge of the potential risks of disease transmission if xenotransplantation were to become a reality. Risks cannot be eliminated based on current evidence, and the uncertainty about the safety of xenotransplantation continues to be a significant obstacle to its implementation. Cloning and genetic modification techniques to address disease transmission are still in their early stages. Further scientific information may close the gap somewhat, but it will never be possible to say with absolute certainty that the risk is absent. Xenotransplantation falls into the category of experimental treatment where although the risk is perhaps low, and the benefits to humans substantial, the consequences for humanity could be catastrophic (Bach et al. 1998; Bach and Ivinson 2002; Fishman 1997; Fovargue and Ost 2010; Muir and Griffin 2001). As one consumer in my 1997 study said:

> You know at this point, I think [xenografting is] a good idea, but where will it lead? I'm not sure, and I don't think any of us know where DNA manipulation is going to lead. It could be really scary stuff, and we need the answers to the questions, I suppose, to think about it at this point. I worry about the transmission of disease. What will happen to our world if we get another bug like HIV?

Concerns about Informed Consent

The tension between individual and societal rights is part of the difficult ethical debate about xenotransplantation. While research subjects often accept risks arising from experimental treatment, believing them to be balanced by the potential benefits, one important distinction between xenotransplantation and other treatments is that xenotransplantation may put individuals other than the recipient at risk of contracting disease.

The concept of informed consent for individual patients is a central principle in Western health care delivery. When faced with health care decisions, the patient is informed of the various alternatives for treatment and the relative risks and benefits of each option. Given that the scientists and the clinicians in the area of xenotransplantation cannot answer all the questions about possible risks, a potential patient would be put in a very difficult situation if he or she were considering being a participant in a clinical trial (Bach and Ivinson 2002; Hughes 2007).

As evident in Ethics in Practice 22-1, the risk is not restricted to the individual who is receiving the xenotransplant, but is also of concern to close contacts, family members, and indeed the community at large. Xenotransplantation raises the problematic challenge of applying the principle of informed consent to an entire community since the community as a whole would be potentially exposed to the risk (Bach and Ivinson 2002; Fovargue and Ost 2010). The risk posed to the community by possible xenozoonoses after xenotransplantation requires that some form of "community consent" is necessary before solid organ animal-to-human xenotransplantation takes place. As the relevant community is global, and there are no existing agencies with the appropriate credentials sufficient to establish this consent, this presents obstacles to the implementation of xenotransplantation (Sparrow 2009).

In the situation in Ethics in Practice 22-1, Maria, the advanced practice nurse, will have to ensure that Paul has information about the risks of xenotransplantation and, as part of her responsibility, ensure that information is conveyed to Paul's family as well. To gain support in this work, Maria could access information about xenotransplantation, such as national standards and guidelines, and help to explain and interpret these to Paul and his family (Cozzi et al. 2009; Sykes, d'Apice, and Sandrin 2003). Even though Paul is not currently enrolled in a clinical trial, Maria might find it useful to review information available about the role of the nurse in research (as described in Chapter 14) to help her determine what she could and should convey to Paul and his family.

But what of the larger community? What is Maria's responsibility to it? Viruses, and other infectious agents, do not respect national borders. The 2003 cases of SARS and BSE have made that evident and, more recently, the 2009 worldwide H1N1 outbreak has made it clear that viruses know no geographic boundaries. Along with other health care providers and health care researchers, nurses in leadership roles have a responsibility to ensure that information about issues such as xenotransplantation, genetics, cloning, and regenerative medicine, that are within the realm of their practice, are discussed in the community. Further, it is essential that informed representatives of the public are given an opportunity to participate actively and meaningfully in the decisions about whether, and under what conditions, society is exposed to the risks associated with this and other biotechnological developments. If it is unethical to impose a health care risk on a patient, it is also unethical to expose the public to a risk without first considering societal opinion (Bach and Ivinson 2002). Strategies for nurses to become involved in the community at large in order to facilitate discussion about biotechnological advances will be discussed in more detail later in this chapter.

Corporate and Research Influences on Xenotransplantation

Xenotransplantation is big business, and it poses challenging problems from the perspective of business and corporate ethics as well as research ethics. The economic implications are considerable, and many pressures are brought to bear by stakeholders for whom these considerations are at the forefront (Bach and Ivinson 2002; Nicholson 1996). For example, the U.S. organ and tissue transplant market was thought to be worth 20 billion dollars by 2007, thus providing a huge potential market for biotechnology companies. Many companies have invested heavily in xenotransplantation and are eager to see their investment pay off ("Xenotransplant news" 2003).

When considering the diffusion of new biotechnologies, it is important to ask questions about who is likely to benefit from the various types of biotechnology and who is likely to suffer from them (Sherwin 2000). When considering biotechnology, wealth can be seen as a benefit and poverty a risk. It remains to be seen whether or not xenotransplantation and other technologies, such as gene therapies, will be accessible to the poor and disadvantaged. In the past, pharmaceutical and medical technologies have been readily available in the Western world but not accessible to the world's 50 poorest countries, which are inhabited by 75 percent of the world's population. Furthermore, issues regarding conflict of interest and research ethics have impacted on how companies choose to study new technologies and make them available globally (Baird 2003; Bodenheimer 2000; Neufeld et al. 2001).

Because many Western governments have been unwilling to sanction xenotransplant clinical trials, corporations and some investigators have moved to other countries, such as Mexico, to pursue research and human clinical trials. Clinical trials in Mexico, conducted under weak safety rules, opened the door for "international xenotourism," where desperate patients bypassed tight regulations in some developed countries by going to Mexico for treatment, an option discussed in Ethics in Practice 22-1 (Council of Europe 2003; Reuters Health 2002). Failure to implement international regulations, or loose interpretation of standards, has the potential to adversely affect already disadvantaged groups and populations, and possibly give rise to worldwide risks (Tallacchini 2008). Although some countries do not have the appropriate regulatory authorities to develop and maintain suitable guidelines to safeguard patients and their contacts, pressure from international bodies has sometimes influenced practice (BBC World 2002; Reuters Health 2002; Sykes and Cozzi 2006; Tallacchini 2008). For example, in Mexico, where clinical trials in children with Type 1 diabetes were conducted, and people from other countries came to Mexico for islet cell xenotransplants, the trials were shut down when it was found that international ethical standards were not upheld (Cook et al. 2011).

Moreover, it can be argued that in developing countries, biotechnology research is inappropriate when people are living without the basics of preventive care, maternal and child health services, and other fundamental health care needs (Veatch 2000). Further, xenotransplantation raises significant questions of international justice since there is the potential to place the lives of citizens of poor nations at risk to benefit the citizens of wealthy nations (Sparrow 2009). Although further discussion of these global issues is beyond my scope in this chapter, please see Chapter 4 for a more comprehensive discussion of the principle of justice.

Another challenging problem that falls within the corporate and research realm is the lack of access to data from international clinical trials of xenotransplantation. Usually, such data, and any adverse reactions resulting from treatment, are confidential, and may only be made public at the discretion of the sponsor, something that generally only happens if positive outcomes are observed.

Corporate and research issues and concerns must be part of the public debate about biotechnology, and there is a need for members of the public and health care providers to work together with corporations and investigators to ensure that they are able to meet their ethical and social responsibilities (Dhanda 2002). Shareholders, and society as a whole, must hold corporations and researchers accountable in future work related to xenotransplantation as well as innovations coming from areas such as stem cells, cloning, nanotechnology, and genetic research.

Regulatory Concerns

There are a variety of approaches used to regulate xenotransplantation research in different jurisdictions around the world. In Canada, xenotransplantation studies are currently being carried out using laboratory animals only. These pre-clinical or experimental trials do not involve human patients and are not regulated by Health Canada. Xenotransplants for humans are considered therapeutic products and can only be used in clinical trials if authorized by Health Canada. A request to conduct clinical trials could be submitted to Health Canada at any time (Health Canada 2006; 2010). For Health Canada, one of the principles guiding the identification and evaluation of risks related to xenotransplantation is the government of Canada's precautionary approach or principle. This is an approach used to manage threats of serious or irreversible harm when there is scientific uncertainty, recognizing that full scientific certainty will not be used as a reason to postpone decisions when faced with the threat of serious or irreversible harm (Government of Canada 2001).

In the United States, xenotransplant human clinical trials are approved and are tightly controlled. As a result, all experiments using animal tissues must be cleared through the Food and Drug Administration (FDA). In the past, the FDA has also banned xenotransplant recipients from donating blood because of the infection risk. As scientific knowledge about xenotransplantation increases, there is no consistency across the world about the status of xenotransplantation or how regulatory frameworks are developed and implemented. In January 1999, the Parliamentary Assembly of the Council of Europe called for a worldwide moratorium on xenotransplantation until the technology could be evaluated and guidelines could be established. However, countries worldwide implemented a wide range of decisions about xenotransplantation research and clinical trials, including outright bans, moratoriums, and more relaxed safety rules (Council of Europe 2003; Haddow et al. 2010). Authors such as Cozzi et al. (2009) and Vanderpool (2009) suggest that what is needed is a coordinated international effort by the World Health Organization aimed at harmonizing xenotransplantation protocols in accordance with the best available scientific data and with the highest ethical and regulatory standards, to ensure that clinical xenotransplantation trials are conducted with minimal risk to society. The Ethics Committee of the International Xenotransplant Association has suggested that trials on humans should only be performed with oversight from a governmental regulatory agency with guidelines similar to those developed in Western countries. The committee proposes that the trials should include information about the source animals as well as monitoring procedures for xenotransplant research subjects and, where deemed appropriate, their close contacts. In addition, the group suggests the development of a national repository for holding specimens from human subjects in countries in which clinical trials are conducted and, if a repository is not possible, then specimens should be properly obtained, tracked, analyzed, and stored. The committee goes on to recommend that in the absence of such oversight and monitoring, clinical xenotransplantation should not occur. The committee proposes that the International Xenotransplant Association take leadership in facilitating the development of universally accepted procedures, standards, and guidelines about xenotransplantation since many countries around the world are beginning xenotransplant programs. Like others involved in xenotransplantation, the committee raises the concern that without such co-operation, efforts of countries to minimize the potential risks may be jeopardized as possible recipients travel from countries with regulation to those without for the purpose of undergoing xenotransplantation. In addition, the committee also raises concern about xenotourism— the potential entry of individuals (or their close contacts) who have received a xenotransplant in a country without regulatory guidelines into other countries (Sykes, d'Apice, and Sandrin 2003, 201–202).

Schneider and Seebach (2010) reported that, over the past 15 years, there were a total of 29 human applications of xenotransplantation—mostly related to transplantation of xenogeneic cells. Of note, the procedures were performed in 12 different countries, nine of which had no national regulations on xenotransplantation. The authors proposed that this information should be used to inform national health authorities, health care staff, and the public, with the objective of encouraging internationally harmonized guidelines and regulation of xenotransplantation.

Although the issues discussed here are focused on xenotransplantation, they are also applicable to other biotechnologies such as cloning, gene therapy, and stem cell research, where similar regulations are required and are being discussed in many countries. Clearly, decisions about biotechnology require broad societal discussion and debate.

PUBLIC PARTICIPATION IN DECISIONS ABOUT XENOTRANSPLANTATION

I previously made the argument that members of the public are often overlooked as participants in the discussions about biotechnology. I also suggested that in order to ensure that the required values and perspectives are represented, multiple voices are needed in the debate about biotechnology, with a prominent position for members of the public. The idea of public and health care provider involvement in decision making is supported, but how can it happen in reality? Many people have been proponents of the public being more involved in decision making about technological diffusion into society and health care. A number of years ago, Winner (1993) proposed broad involvement in decision making about technology and pointed out that there was no moral community or public space in which technological issues were topics for deliberation and common action. Brunger and Cox (2000), in their discussion about genetics and ethics, suggested strategies for widening the space of public debate about technology, including providing the public with information about the production, distribution, and application of knowledge; legitimizing lay knowledge; attending to a multiplicity of voices; welcoming dissent as a sign that all voices are being heard; allowing the debate to be transparent in public; and promoting the accountability of government, industry, and science to the public (4). Other authors have proposed several conditions that must be met for meaningful public participation to occur in health care decision making, including assuring that consumers have adequate information; that there are a majority of consumers in the group; that there is a strong mandate from the community with formal and informal access to constituents; and that people selected to represent communities have strong personalities so that they will not be intimidated or dominated by the so-called experts within the group (Abelson et al. 2010; Blue et al. 1999; Charles and DeMaio 1993; Eyles 1993; Jennings 1991; Lenaghan 1999; Lomas and Veenstra 1995; O'Neill 1992; Starzomski 1997; 2002). What follows is a description of a public consultation process in which these strategies were evident in the discussion about whether Canada should proceed with xenotransplantation and, if so, under what conditions. This example stands as one of the most comprehensive processes undertaken in Canada to involve the public in the decision making about the implementation of a biotechnological development.

As part of efforts to hear the views and concerns of Canadians about xenotransplantation, Health Canada provided funding to the Canadian Public Health Association (CPHA) to strike a Public Advisory Group (PAG) to conduct an arm's-length public consultation. The PAG was given the task of reporting back to the federal Minister of Health with recommendations about whether Canada should proceed with xenotransplantation. Members of the PAG represented a diversity of perspectives, regions, and interests. The process they designed included several options for Canadians to voice their opinions, including a telephone survey of 1519 randomly selected adults; opportunities to submit letters, faxes, and e-mails to the CPHA office and website; a "have your say" questionnaire (which was located on the CPHA website and also mailed to 3700 organizations); and regional citizen forums (sometimes also called citizen juries) of between 15–23 demographically representative citizens held in six major cities across Canada. The forums were moderated by a professional facilitator and included opportunities for panellists to have discussions with experts and review resource material in the area of xenotransplantation. In addition, during each forum, prior to the private panellist's meeting, time was allocated for members of the general public to participate in the discussion (Canadian Public Health Association 2001; Einseidel and Ross 2002).

Before the two-and-a-half-day forums were held, the members of the citizen juries were asked to complete a questionnaire to determine their attitudes and beliefs about xenotransplantation. Many participants held a positive view, but after discussing the risks and concerns during the forums, the majority changed their thinking, concluding that Canada should not proceed with xenotransplantation at this time; 34 percent said no, 19 percent said no with qualifications, and 46 percent said yes with qualifications. It appeared from these results that the more Canadians learned about xenotransplantation, the more concerned they became. Although not absolutely opposed to xenotransplantation, the forum participants favoured a precautionary approach, expressing concerns about uncertain health risks, an insufficient level of scientific knowledge in the area of xenotransplantation, and inadequate regulations (Canadian Public Health Association 2001; Wharry 2002).

In contrast to the citizen jury experience, in the telephone survey of 1519 Canadian adults, 70 percent were not very, or not at all, knowledgeable about xenotransplantation and yet, of this number, 65 percent supported clinical trials. These findings must be interpreted cautiously and illustrate some of the problems that occur when public opinion polls (where participants have little data about the issues) are used to solicit information about complex areas such as xenotransplantation. In their final report, members of the PAG describe the results of the complete public consultation process (Canadian Public Health Association 2001). The report was delivered to the Minister of Health and subsequently released publicly in 2002. In the report, the CPHA did not close the door on xenotransplantation, but rather called for more research into potential risks, suggesting that those who wish to proceed with xenotransplantation need to determine the level of risk and demonstrate how the benefits of the procedure would outweigh those risks. In addition, among the recommendations, the CPHA suggested that pre-clinical research that did not involve humans, but which could provide more information about the viability of xenotransplantation, should occur. There was also a call for more stringent and transparent legislation and regulations covering all aspects of xenotransplant clinical trials. Further, it was recommended that Health Canada consider alternatives, such as disease prevention, the development of mechanical substitutes, and the pursuit of stem cell research to expand the human donor pool. Finally, in the report, it was suggested that efforts should continue to further the knowledge and public discussion of xenotransplantation and that the citizen forum model be considered for future consultations on complex and not widely understood policy issues.

The consultation process described here for xenotransplantation is a model for other areas where innovations in biotechnology are occurring. Regardless of the particular approach taken, if public consultation of this sort is to be effective, it is crucial that participants be well informed. All sides of the issue must be presented without attempts to steer the dialogue, allowing the public participants to arrive at their own conclusions. However, even with possible flaws (Wright 2002), the CPHA process to solicit public opinion about xenotransplantation stands as one of the only comprehensive experiments in Canada to engage the public in discussion about decisions regarding the diffusion of a new biotechnology into the health care system.

The practice of public consultation in biotechnology does not mean, however, that a few public representatives set policy. Such groups are not representative of the whole population and are not selected to represent the entire community (Bach and Ivinson 2002; Einseidel and Ross 2002; Ivinson and Bach 2002). In the example described above, the PAG report was presented to the federal Minister of Health to inform the decisions that must be made by policy-makers and the political representatives to whom citizens delegate such authority. The CPHA experience has provided valuable information about including the values of the public in decision making and engaging citizens in the debate about biotechnology development in Canada. On the Health Canada website, it is noted that xenotransplantation is currently not prohibited in Canada. However, as mentioned previously, the live cells, tissues, and organs from animal sources are considered to be therapeutic products. Thus, xenotransplants are subject to the requirements of the Food and Drugs Act, the Food and Drug Regulations, or the Medical Devices Regulations. To conduct a human clinical trial, a sponsoring company or research institute would have to apply to Health Canada for approval before proceeding. At the writing of this chapter, no human clinical trial involving xenotransplantation has yet been approved by Health Canada.

In summary, the public must be involved in all facets of societal development. In particular, in developing policy about biotechnology, it is clear that public values are essential in making ethical choices that will benefit the community. Good health care decisions are not possible until the public supplies the value framework to be used. Value systems drawn from cultural, religious, and philosophical ideological systems are central to planning health care directions and act as the guides and justifications for choosing the goals, priorities, and means that guide policy development (Abelson et al. 2010; Maxwell, Rosell, and Forest 2003; Veatch 1985; 1991).

In this section, I have made a case for public involvement in the decisions about biotechnology. In the following section, I discuss the implications for nurses in helping to open the moral space required for the discussion about the ethical and societal implications of biotechnology. As we have seen, the debate becomes all the more vital and complex with the introduction of ever more powerful biotechnologies that may offer potential benefits to individuals but that are counterbalanced by potential risks to society.

OPENING MORAL SPACE FOR DISCUSSION ABOUT BIOTECHNOLOGY: IMPLICATIONS FOR NURSES

In a rapidly changing world, we are inundated with material about biotechnology as well as information about the "good, the bad, and the ugly" of biotechnological innovations as we attempt to understand the vast amount of information that we are exposed to on a daily basis. Kingwell (2002) suggested that as conscientious citizens, we struggle to stay on top of what is happening in our technologically dominated and complex world and advised that we need to prepare ourselves for a "bumpy ride" as we try to determine where we are headed. Further, Saul (2001) pointed out that there are severe limitations to what we can understand in the face of constant technological change. He reminded us that

> In fact, with the explosion of technology over the last quarter-century, the percentage of what we understand versus what we know has probably slipped back to where it was a century ago (30).

As nurses, how do we sort through the information that is available, organize ourselves for the "bumpy ride," and ensure that we are prepared to deal with the societal and ethical implications of biotechnology? It is a difficult undertaking as the line between science and science fiction has become blurred, a plethora of information is available, and many conflicting points of view exist (Barnard 1997; 2002). We only have to review recent newspaper and magazine headlines to emerge with a sense of the complexity of the information provided for our perusal and the variety of perspectives and opinions that are presented to the public.

In this book, and elsewhere, there has been a call to expand social, environmental, and political thinking in nursing, a call for a focus on the common good, a term used to describe the well-being of the community at large based on shared goals and common purposes (Fry 1985; Rodney and Starzomski 1993; Starzomski and Rodney 1997; Stevens 1989; 1992). It is clear that nurses need to be involved in understanding and facilitating broad societal discussion of issues related to xenotransplantation as well as other emerging technologies as these raise profound changes in the human capacity to control diseases and human reproduction as well as to govern access to health information (Canadian Nurses Association 2002a; 2008).

The Canadian Nurses Association (CNA) has made claims about the importance of the involvement of nurses and the public in making policy decisions about biotechnology. Over time, in various position statements, documents, briefs, and the Codes of Ethics developed by the CNA, support is expressed for including nurses in discussions about technology at all levels of the health care system. The authors of these documents suggest that nurses must be involved in all aspects of technology use, including identifying the need for such use, developing and implementing technology, and evaluating the impact on client care. CNA policy statements, such as those related to technology, primary care, and leadership, all include some reference to supporting a nursing role in discussions about technology development and implementation (CNA 1992; 1995; 2002b, 2006; 2008). Further, CNA has shown national leadership in the area of biotechnology by ensuring that nurses are involved on committees and councils where decisions about biotechnology are made.

The scope of understanding about biotechnology can be overwhelming. It is neither practical nor possible for every nurse to keep abreast of all the ethical and societal developments; nor is it possible to speak out on every issue as the issues are numerous and priorities vary. However, nurses can act as expert navigators of biotechnology and become information brokers for their clients while ensuring that the core values of nursing are maintained. Further, there is a need for nursing leaders to examine the impact of biotechnological changes on nursing recruitment, nursing work design, and the nursing workforce. A solid understanding of nursing ethics can provide nurses with assistance to deal with the challenges related to biotechnology confronting them in health care settings and provide them with the ability to critically examine the issues and to devise solutions. In what follows, I suggest some strategies for continued nursing leadership in biotechnology at the micro, meso, and macro levels of the health care system. It is critical that nurses engage in this discussion with other health care providers and help to facilitate the involvement of members of the public. Many of the strategies that follow would be useful for Maria to consider (in Ethics in Practice 22-1) as she develops her plan about how to support Paul and his family.

Micro-Level Strategies

- Become educated about biotechnological developments and societal and ethical implications.

- Ensure that patients and families are informed about options, risks, and benefits when considering therapeutic biotechnological interventions.

- Help educate other nurses, health care providers, and members of the public.

- Ensure that ethical and societal issues about biotechnological developments are part of educational curricula, conferences, and symposia.

- Engage in advocacy to help patients and families have opportunities to express their views.

Meso-Level Strategies

- Participate in both clinical and research ethics committees where issues about biotechnology are being discussed.

- Conduct research examining the ethical and societal implications of biotechnology.

- Ensure that ethical and societal issues about biotechnological developments are part of hospital, community, regional health board, and health authority discussions.

- Work with provincial professional associations and groups to ensure that there is public dialogue about biotechnological concerns.

Macro-Level Strategies

- Participate in national committees, debates, and forums about health care and biotechnology.

- Use methods such as citizens' juries, consensus conferences, town hall meetings, and the Internet to engage the public and health care providers in debates about issues.

- Participate with professional associations to ensure that nurses are represented in the federal government and provincial/territorial legislatures where laws are being made that govern biotechnology.

There is no doubt that, in the future, decisions about biotechnology will continue to demand the involvement of consumers and all health care providers. These decisions will be complex and difficult, so that no one societal group or set of voices will be adequate to make the choices that are needed. Although, as a society, we may not always have the answers to questions related to choices about biotechnology, a collaborative effort will provide the best method to ensure that wise choices are made for future biotechnological developments.

Summary

Biotechnology raises major issues—issues of ethics, choice, trust, democracy, and globalization. Innovations in biotechnology come encumbered with intended and unintended social, political, and economic values. I have argued throughout this chapter that policies surrounding xenotransplantation, and other emerging biotechnological interventions, must be developed by those who consider the importance of balancing opportunity and risk. Further, I have advocated for an expansion in the debate about biotechnology that includes members of the public, nurses, and other health care providers in discussions about the societal and ethical issues facing us in the realm of biotechnology.

Public involvement in decisions about biotechnology is complex. There is no consensus on how to include the public in meaningful ways in the development of healthy public policy, although in this chapter I have presented several methods that I believe move us in the right direction. Clearly, we need to be sensitive to the contexts in which public participation is being asked to ensure that citizens are able to avail themselves of opportunities to be involved. This is an area where, definitely, "one size does not fit all" (Martin, Ableson, and Singer 2002).

Although the future of dialogue and debate on issues of biotechnology is by no means assured, there are promising signs. As discussed throughout this chapter, researchers and governmental and non-governmental organizations are turning more of their attention to the issues. The xenotransplantation public consultation process in Canada is one example of a move in that direction. There is still time to seek meaningful societal participation regarding many of the issues facing us in biotechnology in order to make the best possible choices about future technological opportunities that are coming our way.

By its very nature, science alone will not give us answers with absolute certainty and can only tell us about the likelihood of the benefits and dangers posed by biotechnology. As citizens, we will need to continue to review the science and to make decisions based on our value systems, as what we currently see is just the tip of iceberg. The future possibilities in biotechnology are beyond our imaginations and for many may seem like science fiction. Research in the areas of xenotransplantation, regenerative medicine, and nanotechnology may offer opportunities to address some of our health care concerns; but, in the future, the success of these approaches will depend not only on scientific development, but also careful consideration of the ethical and legal issues (Shapiro 2008).

Before us is a period of remarkable technological innovation. To our armamentarium of technological innovations we have added tools that have power over life and death. Will we use biotechnology to preserve our humanity and improve our quality of life, as exemplified in the optimistic future portrayed in *Star Trek*? Or will we choose a more pessimistic future such as that portrayed in Aldous Huxley's *Brave New World,* where humans have really become the tools of their tools. The manner in which we develop and use biotechnology today is a harbinger of what we can become as a society tomorrow (Atwood 2003; Starzomski 1994; 1997). We must use our tools wisely, keeping in mind that the wisdom we need for tomorrow comes from understanding the present and learning from the past. As T.S Elliot said, we shall not cease from exploration, and the end of all our exploring will be to arrive where we started and know the place for the first time.

For Reflection

1. Reflect on the situation described in Ethics in Practice 22-1. What actions do you think could support someone in Maria's position?

2. What are your personal views about xenotransplantation?

3. Think about your work setting and your role in your family and community. How can you facilitate discussion about the biotechnological innovations that affect you in those spheres of your life?

4. How can public input be obtained about biotechnology innovations like xenotransplantation, use of stem cells, cloning, and nanotechnology?

References

Abelson, J., Montesanti, S., Li, K., Gauvin, F., and Martin, E. 2010. *Effective strategies for interactive public engagement in the development of healthcare policies and programs.* Ottawa: Canadian Health Services Research Foundation.

Alexander, S. 1962. They decide who lives, who dies: Medical miracle puts a burden on a small committee. *Life,* November 9, 102–104, 106, 108, 110, 115, 117–118, 123–125.

Allan, J. 1996. Xenotransplantation at a crossroads: Prevention versus progress. *Nature Medicine, 2,* 18–21.

Allan, J. 1997. Silk purse or sow's ear. *Nature Medicine, 3,* 275–276.

Allan, J. 1998. Cross-species infection: No news is good news? *Nature Medicine, 4,* 644–645.

Atwood, M. 2003. *Oryx and crake.* Toronto: McClelland and Stewart.

Bach, F. and Ivinson, A. 2002. A shrewd and ethical approach to xenotransplantation. *Trends in Biotechnology, 20*(3), 129–131.

Bach, F., Fishman, J., Daniels, N., Proimos, J., Anderson, B., Carpenter, C., Forrow, L., Robson, S., and Fineberg, H. 1998. Uncertainty in xenotransplantation: Individual benefit versus collective risk. *Nature Medicine, 4* (2), 141–144.

Bailey, L. 1990. Organ transplantation: A paradigm of medical progress. *Hastings Center Report, 20* (1), 24–28.

Baird, P. 2003. Getting it right: Industry sponsorship and medical research. *Canadian Medical Association Journal, 168* (10), 1267–1269.

BBC World. 2002. *Cook Islands plans xenotransplant trials,* March 5.

Barnard, A. 1997. A critical review of the belief that technology is a neutral object and nurses are its master. *Journal of Advanced Nursing, 26,* 126–131.

Barnard, A. 2002. Philosophy of technology and nursing. *Nursing Philosophy, 3,* 15–26.

Baylis, F. 2001. The Canadian stem cell debate: Stuck in the '80s. *Journal of the Society of Obstetricians and Gynaecologists of Canada, 23* (3), 248–252.

Bloom, E., Moulton, A., McCoy, J., Chapman, L., and Patterson, A. 1999. Xenotransplantation: The potential and the challenges. *Critical Care Nurse, 19* (2), 76–82.

Blue, A., Keyserlingk, T., Rodney, P., and Starzomski, R. 1999. A critical review of North American health policy. In H. Coward and P. Ratanakul (Eds.), *An intercultural dialogue on health care ethics* (pp. 215–225). Waterloo, ON: Wilfred Laurier University Press.

Bodenheimer, T. 2000. Uneasy alliance—Clinical investigators and the pharmaceutical industry. *New England Journal of Medicine, 342* (20), 1539–1544.

Brockbank, K., Swaja, R., Wueste, D., and Sade, R. 2010. Resolving the shortage of organs for transplantation: Ethics, science, and technology. *The Journal of the South Carolina Medical Association, 106,* 209–212.

Brunger, F. and Cox, S. 2000. Ethics and genetics: The need for transparency. In F. Miller, L. Weir, R. Mykitiuk, P. Lee, S. Sherwin, and S. Tudiver (Eds.), *The gender of genetic futures: The Canadian biotechnology strategy, women and health* (pp. 27–31). Proceedings of the National Strategic Workshop, York University, Toronto, February 11–12, 2000. National Network on Environments and Women's Health Working Paper Series: York University. Available at http://www.cwhn.ca/groups/biotech/availdocs/workproc.htm.

Canadian Blood Services—Organ Donation and Transplantation. 2011. *Organ and tissue donation and transplantation.* Available at http://www.ccdt.ca/english/home.html.

Canadian Nurses Association. 1992. *The role of the nurse in the use of health care technology.* Ottawa: Author.

Canadian Nurses Association. 1995. *The role of the nurse in primary health care.* Ottawa: Author.

Canadian Nurses Association. 2002a. *Code of ethics for registered nurses.* Ottawa: Author.

Canadian Nurses Association. 2002b. *Position statement: Nursing leadership.* Ottawa: Author.

Canadian Nurses Association. 2006. *Toward 2020—Visions for nursing.* Ottawa: Author.

Canadian Nurses Association. 2008. *Code of ethics for registered nurses.* Ottawa: Author.

Canadian Organ Replacement Register. 2011. Available at http://secure.cihi.ca/cihiweb/dispPage. jsp?cw_page=statistics_results_source_corr_e&cw_topic=Canadian%20Organ%20Replacement%20Register%20(CORR).

Canadian Public Health Association. 2001. *Animal-to-human transplantation: Should Canada proceed? A public consultation on xenotransplantation.* Ottawa: Author.

Charles, C. and DeMaio, S. 1993. Lay participation in health care decision making: A conceptual framework. *Journal of Health Politics, Policy and Law, 18* (4), 883–904.

Commission on the Future of Health Care in Canada. 2002. *Building on values: The future of health care in Canada—Final report.* Ottawa: Government of Canada.

Cook, P., Kendall, G., Michael, M., and Brown, N. 2011. The textures of globalization: Biopolitics and the closure of xenotourism. *New Genetics and Society, 30* (1), 101–114.

Council of Europe. 2003. *Report on xenotransplantation.* Available at www.coe.int/T/E/Legal_Affairs/Legal_cooperation/Bioethics/Activities/XenotransplantationXENO(2003)1E_state_of_art_final_website.asp#TopOfPage.

Cozzi, E., Tallacchini, M., Flanagan, E., Pierson, R., Sykes, M., and Vanderpool, H. 2009. The International Xenotransplantation Association consensus statement on conditions for undertaking clinical trials of porcine islet products in type 1 diabetes—Chapter 1: Key ethical requirements and progress toward the definition of an international regulatory framework. *Xenotransplantation, 16*, 203–214.

Daar, A. 2002. Aspects of regenerative medicine today. *Proceedings of the International Congress on Ethics in Organ Transplantation,* Munich, Germany, December 10–13, 2002.

Daar, A. and Phil, D. 1997. Ethics of xenotransplantation: Animal issues, consent, and likely transformation of transplant ethics. *World Journal of Surgery, 21*, 975–982.

Dhanda, R. 2002. *Guiding Icarus: Merging bioethics with corporate interests.* Toronto: Wiley.

Dillner, L. 1996. Pig organs approved for human transplants. *British Medical Journal, 312* (7032), 657.

Dinsmore, J., Manhart, C., Raineri, R., Jacoby, D., and Moore, A. 2000. No evidence for infection of human cells with porcine endogenous retrovirus (PERV) after exposure to porcine fetal neuronal cells. *Transplantation, 70*, 1382–1389.

Einseidel, E. and Ross, H. 2002. Animal spare parts? A Canadian pubic consultation on xenotransplantation. *Science and Engineering Ethics, 8*, 579–591.

Evanson, B. 2000. What if there's a virus hiding in a pig organ? *National Post,* August 17, A16.

Eyles, J. 1993. *The role of the citizen in health care decision making*. McMaster University Centre for Health Economics and Policy Analysis. Policy Commentary C93-1.

Fishman, J. 1997. Xenosis and xenotransplantation: Addressing the infectious risks posed by an emerging technology. *Kidney International, 51* (58), S41–S45.

Fovargue, S. and Ost, S. 2010. When should precaution prevail? Interests in (public) health, the risk of harm and xenotransplantation. *Medical Law Review, 18*, 302–329.

Fry, S. 1985. Individual vs. aggregate good: Ethical tension in nursing practice. *International Journal of Nursing Studies, 22*, 303–310.

Government of Canada. 2001. *A Canadian perspective on the precautionary approach/principle*. Available at http://sd-cite.iisd.org/cgi-bin/koha/opac-detail.pl?biblionumber=24976.

Gunzburg, W. and Salmons, B. 2000. Xenotransplantation: Is the risk of viral infection as great as we thought? *Molecular Medicine Today, 6* (5), 199–208.

Haddow, G., Bruce, A., Calvert, J., Harmon, S., and Marsden, W. 2010. Not "human" enough to be human but not "animal" enough to be animal—The case of the HFEA, cybrids and xenotransplantation in the UK. *New Genetics and Society, 29* (1), 3–17.

Health Canada. 1997. *National forum on xenotransplantation—Clinical, ethical and regulatory issues*. Ottawa: Author.

Health Canada. 1999. *Proposed Canadian standard for xenotransplantation*. Ottawa: Author.

Health Canada. 2003a. *Summary of severe acute respiratory syndrome (SARS) cases: Canada and international*. Available at www.hc-sc.gc.ca/pphb-dgspsp/sars-sras/eu-ae/sars20030602_e.html.

Health Canada. 2003b. *Mad cow disease—Frequently asked questions*. Available at www.hc-sc.gc.ca/english/diseases/bse/faq.html.

Health Canada. 2006. *Science and research: Xenotransplantation*. Available at http://www.hc-sc.gc.ca/sr-sr/biotech/about-apropos/xeno-eng.php.

Health Canada. 2010. *Revised fact sheet on xenotransplantation*. Available at http://www. hc-sc.gc.ca/dhp-mps/brgtherap/activit/fs-fi/xeno_fact-fait-eng.php.

Holland, S., Lebacqz, K., and Zoloth, L. 2001. *The human embryonic stem cell debate: Science, ethics and public policy*. Cambridge, MA: MIT Press.

Hovatta, O., Stojkovic, M., Nogueira, M., and Varela-Nieto, I. 2010. European scientific, ethical, and legal issues on human stem cell research and regenerative medicine. *Stem Cells, 28*, 1005–1007.

Hughes, J. 2007. Justice and third party risk: The ethics of xenotransplantation. *Journal of Applied Philosophy, 24* (2), 151–168.

Ivinson, A. and Bach, F. 2002. The xenotransplantation question: Public consultation is an important part of the answer. *Canadian Medical Association Journal, 167* (1), 42–43.

Jennings, B. 1991. Possibilities of consensus: Toward democratic moral discourse. *Journal of Medicine and Philosophy, 16* (4), 447–463.

Kingwell, M. 2002. *Practical judgments: Essays in culture, politics and interpretation*. Toronto: University of Toronto Press.

Latifah A., Rezali, N., Samani, M., Hassan, Z., and Jusoff, K. 2011. Ethical issues on biotechnology in four mainstream newspapers. *World Applied Sciences Journal, 12* (11), 1939–1945.

Lemonick, M. 2003. The DNA revolution: A twist of fate. *Time, 161* (6), 31–40.

Lenaghan, J. 1999. Involving the public in rationing decisions. The experience of citizens' juries. *Health Policy, 49* (1–2), 45–61.

Lomas, J. and Veenstra, G. 1995. If you build it, who will come? Governments, consultation and biased publics. *Policy Options, 16* (9), 37–40.

Martin, D., Abelson, J., and Singer, P. 2002. Participation in health care priority-setting through the eyes of the participants. *Journal of Health Service Research Policy, 7* (4), 222–228.

Maxwell, J., Rosell, S., and Forest, P. 2003. Giving citizens a voice in healthcare policy in Canada. *British Medical Journal, 326*, 1031–1033.

McCormick, R. 1985. Was there any real hope for Baby Fae? *Hastings Center Report, 15*, 12–13.

Michaels, M., McMichael, J., Brasky, K., Kalter, S., Peters, R., Starzl, T., and Simmons R. 1994. Screening donors for xenotransplantation: The potential for xenozoonoses. *Transplantation, 57*, 1462–1465.

Midgely, M. 2000. Biotechnology and monstrosity: Why we should pay attention to the "yuk factor." *Hastings Centre Report, 30* (5), 7–15.

Molzahn, A., Starzomski, R., and McCormick, J. 2003. The supply of organs for transplantation: Issues and challenges. *Nephrology Nursing Journal, 30* (1), 17–28.

Muir, D. and Griffin, G. 2001. *Infection risks in xenotransplantation.* Prepared for U.K. Department of Health. Available at www.doh.gov.uk/pub/docs/doh/76035_doh_infection_risks.pdf.

Murray, J. 1992. Human organ transplantation: Background and consequences. *Science, 256*, 1411–1416.

National Forum on Health. 1997. *Canada health action: Building on the legacy* (Volumes 1 and 2). Ottawa: Author.

National Institutes of Health. 1985. *Report of the National Institutes of Health: The report of the NIH team investigating Baby Fae.* Washington, DC: Author.

Neufeld, V., MacLeod, S., Tugwell, P., Zakus, D., and Zarowsky, C. 2001. The rich–poor gap in global health research: Challenges for Canada. *Canadian Medical Association Journal, 164* (8), 1158–1159.

Nicholson, R. 1996. This little pig went to market. *Hastings Center Report, 26* (4), 3.

Nuffield Council on Bioethics. 1996. *Animal-to-human transplants: The ethics of xenotransplantation*: London: Nuffield Council on Bioethics.

O'Mathuna, D. 2007. Bioethics and biotechnology. *Cytotechnology, 53*, 113–119.

O'Neill, M. 1992. Community participation in Quebec's health system: A strategy to curtail community empowerment. *International Journal of Health Services, 22* (2), 287–301.

Pearce, C., Thomas, A., and Clements, D. 2006. The ethics of xenotransplantation: A survey of student attitudes. *Xenotransplantation, 13*, 253–257.

Platt, J. 1997. Xenotransplantation: A potential solution to the shortage of donor organs. *Transplantation Proceedings, 29*, 3324–3326.

Proceed with care. 1993. *Final report of the Royal Commission on New Reproductive Technologies.* Canada: Minister of Government Services.

Rappert, B. 2008. The benefits, risks, and threats of biotechnology. *Science and Public Policy, 35* (1), 37–43.

Reemtsma, K. 1992. Xenografts. *Transplantation Proceedings, 24* (5), 2225–2227.

Reuters Health. 2002. *Panel worried about "xenotourism" for animal organ transplants,* March 12.

Rodney, P. and Starzomski, R. 1993. Constraints on the moral agency of nurses. *The Canadian Nurse, 89* (9), 23–26.

Rollin, B. 2003. *The Frankenstein syndrome: Ethical and social issues in the genetic engineering of animals.* New York: Cambridge University Press.

Saul, J. 2001. *The unconscious civilization.* Toronto: Penguin.

Scheufele, D., Corley, E., Dunwoody, S., Tsung-Jen, S., Hillback, E., and Guston, D. 2007. Scientists worry about some risks more than the public. *Nature Nanotechnology, 2*, 732–734.

Schneider, M. and Seebach, J. 2008. Xenotransplantation literature update May–August, 2008. *Xenotransplantation, 15*, 344–351.

Schneider M. and Seebach J. 2010. Xenotransplantation literature update June–October 2010. *Xenotransplantation, 17*, 481–488.

Shapiro, R. 2008. Future issues in transplantation ethics: Ethical and legal controversies in xenotransplantation, stem cell, and cloning research. *Transplantation Reviews, 22*, 210–214.

Sherwin, S. 2000. Placing values at the center of biotechnology policy: The Canadian biotechnology strategy and women's health. Opening remarks. In F. Miller, L. Weir, R. Mykitiuk, P. Lee, S. Sherwin, and S. Tudiver (Eds.), *The gender of genetic futures: The Canadian biotechnology strategy, women and health* (pp. 1–8). Proceedings of the National Strategic Workshop, York University, Toronto, February 11–12, 2000. National Network on Environments and Women's Health Working Paper Series: York University. Available at http://www.cwhn.ca/groups/biotech/availdocs/workproc.htm.

Silva, D. 2010. H1N1 influenza: Global pandemic, global vulnerabilities. *Health Science Inquiries, 1* (1), 31–32.

Singer, P. 1992. Xenotransplantation and speciesism. *Transplantation Proceedings, 24* (2), 728–732.

Skloot, R. 2010. *The immortal life of Henrietta Lacks.* New York: Crown Publishing Company.

Soulillou, J.P. 2011. Xenotransplantation: Times are changing. *Current Opinion in Organ Transplantation, 16*, 188–189.

Sparrow, 2009. Xenotransplantation, consent and international justice. *Developing World Bioethics, 9* (3), 119–127.

Starzomski, R. 1994. Ethical issues in palliative care: The case of dialysis and organ transplantation. *Journal of Palliative Care, 10* (3), 27–33.

Starzomski, R. 1997. *Resource allocation for solid organ transplantation: Toward public and health care provider dialogue.* Unpublished doctoral dissertation, University of British Columbia, Vancouver.

Starzomski, R. 2002. Listening to multiple voices: Consumer involvement in health promotion. In L. Young and V. Hayes (Eds.), *Transforming health promotion practice: Concepts, issues and applications* (pp. 71–86). Philadelphia: F.A. Davis.

Starzomski, R. and Rodney, P. 1997. Nursing inquiry for the common good. In S. Thorne and V. Hayes (Eds.), *Nursing praxis: Knowledge and action* (pp. 219–236). Thousand Oaks: Sage Publications.

Stevens, P. 1989. A critical reconceptualization of environment in nursing: Implications for methodology. *Advances in Nursing Science, 114*, 56–68.

Stevens, P. 1992. Who gets care? Access to health care as an arena for nursing action. *Scholarly Inquiry for Nursing Practice, 6*, 185–200.

Susumu, S. 2011. The ethical issues of biotechnology: Religious culture and the value of life. *Current Sociology, 59* (2), 160–172.

Sykes, M., d'Apice, A., and Sandrin, M. 2003. Position paper of the Ethics Committee of the International Xenotransplantation Association. *Xenotransplantation, 10*, 194–2003.

Sykes, M. and Cozzi, E. 2006. Xenotransplantation of pig islets into Mexican children: Were the fundamental ethical requirements to proceed with such a study really met? *European Journal of Endocrinology, 154*, 921–922.

Tallacchini, M. 2008. Defining an appropriate ethical, social and regulatory framework for clinical xenotransplantation. *Current Opinion in Organ Transplantation, 13*, 159–164.

UNOS. 2011. Available at http://www.unos.org/.

Vanderpool, H. 2009. The International Xenotransplantation Association consensus statement on conditions for undertaking clinical trials of porcine islet products in type 1 diabetes—Chapter 7: Informed consent an xenotransplantation clinical trials. *Xenotransplantation, 16*, 255–262.

Veatch, R. 1985. Lay medical ethics. *Journal of Medicine & Philosophy, 10* (1), 1–5.

Veatch, R. 1991. Consensus of expertise: The role of consensus of experts in formulating public policy and estimating facts. *Journal of Medicine and Philosophy, 16* (4), 429–445.

Veatch, R. 2000. *Transplantation ethics.* Washington, DC: Georgetown University Press.

Wharry, S. 2002. Canadians not ready for animal-to-human transplants. *Canadian Medical Association Journal, 166* (4), 493.

Winner, L. 1993. Citizen virtues in a technological order. In E. Winkler and J. Coombs (Eds.), *Applied ethics—A reader* (pp. 46–69). Cambridge: Blackwell.

Wright, J. 2002. Alternative interpretations of the same data: Flaws in the process of consulting the Canadian public about xenotransplantation issues. *Canadian Medical Association Journal, 167* (1), 40–42.

Xenotransplant news. 2003. *Xenotransplantation, 10* (3), 191–193.

CHAPTER 23

Ethical Issues in Pregnancy and Reproduction

Chris Kaposy and Françoise Baylis

The woman's decision is not just about the fetus. It is about what she is and what she will become. (Boetzkes 1999, 122)

Through advances in science and technology, we have achieved an unprecedented level of control over our reproductive capacities. We can now safely and reliably end unwanted pregnancies. Using assisted human reproduction (AHR), we can medically circumvent various forms of infertility. We can assess the genetic characteristics of our potential children prior to birth using prenatal diagnostic techniques and, in the case of *in vitro* fertilization (IVF), we can do this prior to embryo transfer using pre-implantation genetic diagnosis (PGD). When AHR results in a multi-fetal pregnancy, we can selectively terminate one or more of the developing fetuses to reduce the pregnancy to twins or a singleton. In some cases, we can improve the health of a developing fetus through *in utero* interventions such as surgery to correct spina bifida, treatments to prevent the vertical transmission of HIV from an affected woman to her offspring, and vaccination of the pregnant woman to provide her newborn(s) with protective antibodies.

Nurses are involved in providing clinical care in all of these areas of reproductive health. As well, nurses may be involved in developing institutional policies and professional practice guidelines for reproductive care and research. This work can be ethically challenging for some nurses. For example, some nurses conscientiously object to participating in abortions chosen for social reasons. Some nurses have serious reservations about women who are not in a traditional heterosexual relationship accessing AHR services. Some nurses question policies and practices governing prenatal testing because of the frequency with which positive results (i.e., results confirming a fetal anomaly) lead to termination of pregnancy.

In this chapter, we examine ethical issues for nurses working in various capacities with a limited focus on induced abortion, AHR, and prenatal testing and screening. To be sure, there are a number of other important topics that could be addressed in this chapter—such as the ethics of elective caesarian section (Kukla et al. 2009), or research involving pregnant women (Baylis and Kaposy 2010; Lyerly, Little, and Faden 2008). Owing to space limitations, however, these and other relevant topics are not addressed.

Common themes in our discussion of induced abortion, AHR, and prenatal testing and screening are the importance of informed choice, and the wider social concerns brought about by technological advances in women's reproductive care (including issues of access, the status of women, and social attitudes toward disability).

INDUCED ABORTION

An induced abortion is the termination of a pregnancy through medical and/or surgical means. Early-term pregnancies can be terminated medically, through the administration of drugs such as Methotrexate and Misoprostol, which induce a miscarriage (Canadian Federation for Sexual Health 2008a). In Canada, however, most abortions are day-surgery procedures performed in the first or second trimester of pregnancy. In the first trimester of pregnancy, a surgical abortion usually involves the insertion of a vacuum aspirator device through the vagina into the uterus in order to suction out the embryo or fetus, placenta, and other products of conception (Canadian Federation for Sexual Health 2008b). Another technique, known as dilation and evacuation, can be used later in pregnancy (i.e., in the second trimester). With this technique, the cervix is opened with a dilator, and the uterus is emptied with the use of suction and surgical tools (Healthwise 2008). Abortions in the third trimester of pregnancy are rare in Canada (Abortion Rights Coalition of Canada 2005). When performed, late-term abortions usually involve a combination of surgical and medical techniques (Abortion Rights Coalition of Canada 2005).[1] Data from Statistics Canada for 2006 suggests that the rate of induced abortions in hospitals and clinics in Canada varies from a low of nearly 15 induced abortions per 100 live births in Saskatchewan to a high of nearly 40 abortions per 100 live births in the Yukon, with the national average at 25.7 for every 100 live births (Statistics Canada 2010).

In philosophical ethics, the abortion debate is dominated by two questions: (1) Do fetuses have a right to life, or a moral status that entitles them to protections against ending their lives? (2) Even if fetuses have a right to life, do they also have a right to occupy women's bodies when the pregnant women themselves do not want this? This second question is necessary because even if fetuses have a right to life, it might not follow that they also have a right to the intimate use of another's body for survival.

From the perspective of some, the exchange of argument and rebuttal in the ethics debate about abortion is unproductive (Kaposy 2010; Thomson 1995). The debate is irresolvable, and is therefore best dealt with as a matter of conscience. On this view, within liberal democracies (such as Canada) where freedom of conscience is an important protected value, the pro-choice position prevails when ethical arguments fail to show unequivocally that abortion is wrong. Consistent with the view that abortion is a matter of conscience is the view that freedom to access abortion care should be protected under constitutional provisions that protect freedom of conscience. This argument was advanced by Justice Bertha Wilson in the Canadian Supreme Court decision in 1988 that decriminalized abortion— *R. v. Morgentaler* (1988). A majority of the justices in this case argued that the law against abortion in effect at that time violated constitutional protections for security of the person (s. 7 of the Canadian *Charter of Rights and Freedoms*).[2] And, further rulings have clarified that only those who are born alive have legal rights, including the right to life (see *Winnipeg Child and Family Services [Northwest Area] v. G.[D.F.]* [1997]).[3]

Access to Abortion

Though abortion is not legally prohibited in Canada, limited resources, governmental policies, and the actions of health care workers (including nurses) create barriers to abortion

(Browne and Sullivan 2005; Peritz 2010). For example, only about 15 percent of all general hospitals in Canada provide abortions, and these hospitals are usually located in urban centres, making access difficult for women who live in rural or remote areas (Shaw 2006). Further, some provinces restrict public funding for abortion care in ways that create significant barriers for girls and women with limited financial means. Both New Brunswick and Prince Edward Island, for example, require physician approval confirming that an abortion is medically necessary (i.e., not chosen for social reasons) before the procedure will be paid for by the provincial health care system (Shaw 2006). New Brunswick specifically requires the approval of two physicians (Shaw 2006).[4]

In addition to structural barriers such as those set up by the governments of New Brunswick and Prince Edward Island, the actions of health care workers (unwittingly or intentionally) can also interfere with access to abortion. In the past 10 years, advocacy groups such as the Canadian Abortion Rights Action League (CARAL) and Canadians for Choice have conducted two thorough studies on access to abortion care in Canadian hospitals (Canadian Abortion Rights Action League 2003; Shaw 2006). These reports outline the various ways in which frontline health care staff—acting as self-designated gate-keepers to abortion—can foil a woman's efforts to terminate an unwanted pregnancy.

According to Canadians for Choice, if a hospital did not provide abortions, many staff members (including nurses) were unable or unwilling to provide helpful information about where to go for abortion care (Shaw 2006, 17–18). More surprisingly perhaps, if a hospital did provide abortion care, many frontline staff were unaware of this fact or were not forthcoming—"41% of hospitals that provide abortion services had staff members answer the phone who did not know if abortions were offered or where to transfer our researcher" (Shaw 2006, 42). When the call was transferred to nurses, in many cases these nurses either did not know or withheld information about the availability of abortion care at the hospital or in their geographic area (Shaw 2006, 17-18). Canadians for Choice report that

> Several times during this study, our researcher spoke with judgmental hospital staff members who insisted that no one in the area knew anything about abortion services. In one case, a nurse insisted that there were no doctors at the hospital who would be willing to talk to a pregnant woman about how to get a referral for an abortion. However, as discovered when our written questionnaire [sent to the hospital independently] was returned, the hospital from the experience mentioned above was actually one of the main providers in the province (Shaw 2006, 43–44).

Just as some nurses contribute to access problems, other nurses help improve access to abortion care. For example, Canadians for Choice commend the nurses on the Alberta Healthlink telehealth service for providing accurate and useful information about access to abortion care (Shaw 2006, 18).

Nurse educators also effectively address access problems when they inform nursing staff that they have no right in law or in ethics to deny women access to abortion care. Furthermore, nurses in leadership positions (e.g., nurses who are appointed to upper-level management positions and who serve on hospital boards or on the boards of regional health authorities) are sometimes effective advocates for their female patients in promoting access to good abortion care at their health care facilities.

From a broader perspective, reliable access to abortion care is only one component of good reproductive health care. Other components include access to reproductive counselling, to contraception (including emergency contraception), and to family planning services.

Conscientious Refusal

A nurse's right to refuse direct participation in an abortion on conscience grounds is recognized in law (Dickens and Cook 2000). However, conscientious refusal on the part of nurses is subject to limits by virtue of legal and ethical responsibilities. The justification for conscientious refusal diminishes in strength as the degree of a nurse's participation diminishes. For example, there is little ethical justification for a nurse's refusal to provide post-operative care to a woman who has terminated her pregnancy (Dickens and Cook 2000). Such a refusal could be construed as punitive in nature.

In general, conscientious refusal is justified to the extent that a health care worker's moral integrity is preserved by avoiding participation in a procedure deemed morally objectionable by that person. However, this justification runs up against a limit when a health care worker's patient will be harmed by a conscience-based refusal. Conscientious refusal does not enable a doctor or a nurse to force a woman to remain pregnant. Arguably, a conscience-based refusal of care can only be justified when the woman can be provided with other means for accessing an abortion (McLeod 2008). Consistent with this view, the Canadian Nurses Association's (CNA) Code of Ethics for Registered Nurses states that

> If nursing care is requested that is in conflict with the nurse's moral beliefs and values but in keeping with professional practice, the nurse provides safe, compassionate, competent and ethical care until alternative care arrangements are in place to meet the person's needs or desires. (Canadian Nurses Association 2008, 44).

Within the CNA Code of Ethics, it is recommended that nurses act proactively and notify prospective employers of practices and procedures in the workplace that they have moral objections to providing. If a nurse nonetheless finds herself or himself called upon to provide such care, the code states, "In all cases, the nurse remains until another nurse or health care provider is able to provide appropriate care to meet the person's needs" (Canadian Nurses Association 2008, 45).

From this it follows that while a physician who is asked to perform an abortion may refuse to provide this service on the ground of conscientious refusal,[5] a nurse who is expected to assist in providing an abortion is not always at liberty to refuse to participate. For example, a nurse working in obstetrics and gynaecology who is called upon to assist with a termination of pregnancy cannot respond to this request, in the moment, with a conscientious refusal. A nurse's conscience-based refusal to participate in abortion care would have to be dealt with as a policy matter regarding scheduling. The goal would be to ensure that there is always a nurse on shift able and willing to provide the requisite clinical care. This practice would be an effective way of respecting the moral views of nurses who object to participating in the termination of pregnancy, but it could also cause serious problems. Consider, for example, a situation where the number of nurses who do not want to assist in providing abortion care significantly exceeds the number who do, thereby constraining the range of practice for nurses who are willing to assist with termination of pregnancy, but who do not want this as a major part of their job description and workload.

In Ethics in Practice 23-1, we describe a nurse's refusal to participate in the care of a patient motivated by a concern other than religious or political beliefs. Regardless of the motivation, refusals may create difficult ethical dilemmas for those who must mediate them.

ETHICS IN PRACTICE 23-1

A Different Kind of Refusal to Providing Abortion Care

A hospital nurse with pro-choice convictions often assists with abortions. One day she is scheduled to participate in terminating the pregnancy of a teenage girl. While reading the patient's chart, the nurse realizes that she knows her—the teenager is the daughter of a close friend. The nurse appeals to her nurse-manager, asking to be re-assigned.

The nurse explains that the patient's mother is her friend and that she is likely unaware of the pregnancy or the planned termination. If the mother ever learned of the abortion and her role in assisting with this, the mother would consider this a personal betrayal of their friendship. The nurse doesn't want to deal with this potential conflict. The problem for the nurse manager is that there is no one she can re-assign to assist with the termination.

Objections to providing abortion care are often motivated by religious and political beliefs, but they need not be. This example may not be a refusal based on "conscience," but the implications are similar. The patient has an interest in accessing care, and the nurse has an interest in not participating in a procedure that will put her in a conflict situation. Unless another nurse can be assigned to participate in the abortion, satisfying one interest will prevent the realization of the other.

ASSISTED HUMAN REPRODUCTION

In North America, 8–12 percent of women are unable to conceive spontaneously (Fisher 2009) and recent data suggest that about half of these women will seek some type of medical care for their infertility (Boivin et al. 2007). These women may seek conventional fertility treatments such as surgical treatment for tubal disease, or they may be interested in AHR, which involves manipulation of the natural processes and materials of human reproduction in order to create a child (Baylis 2012; Mykitiuk and Nisker 2008). AHR techniques include artificial insemination (with or without donated sperm), *in vitro* fertilization (IVF) (with or without donor gametes, *in vitro* maturation of eggs, intra-cytoplasmic-sperm injection, egg freezing, or embryo freezing), PGD prior to embryo transfer, and contractual pregnancy.

Artificial insemination, arguably the earliest form of AHR, involves the placement of sperm in the female reproductive tract in an attempt to conceive a child. This infertility treatment is an option for women whose partners have a male infertility problem, for single women who do not have a male partner, and for women with a female partner.

IVF, arguably the most dramatic form of AHR, is an option for women with blocked fallopian tubes or endometriosis, or for couples with unexplained infertility. IVF often begins with ovulation induction, followed by egg retrieval. The eggs are exposed to sperm in a petri dish and resulting embryos are transferred to the uterus of the woman wishing to become pregnant. Embryos not transferred in the initial IVF cycle can be discarded or, if they are "healthy" embryos, they can be frozen for future reproductive use (by the woman or a third party). When the frozen embryos are no longer wanted for further attempts at pregnancy, they can be discarded or donated for research.

PGD involves the removal of one or two cells from a six- to ten-cell IVF embryo for genetic diagnosis and chromosomal tissue typing. Typically, the purpose of such testing is to avoid transferring embryos with genetic disease. PGD is an alternative to prenatal diagnosis (such as CVS or amniocentesis) and selective abortion for persons at risk of having a child with a genetic illness. Though PGD is typically used to select against embryos with undesired genetic characteristics, it can also be used to select embryos with desired genetic characteristics. Such examples are rare, but a couple with an older child suffering from leukemia might choose IVF followed by PGD to identify and selectively transfer an embryo that is a tissue match, so that stem cells could be harvested from the newborn's umbilical cord to treat the older sibling—a so-called "saviour sibling" (Sheldon and Wilkinson 2004). This procedure is ethically disquieting for those who believe that children are thereby treated instrumentally (i.e., as an object) (Habermas 2003).

Contractual pregnancy is a reproductive arrangement involving a woman who agrees to be inseminated or to accept an embryo transfer, and then to gestate a pregnancy with the intention of surrendering the live-born child to the person(s) who have contracted for the service and who intend to be the child's social parent(s). The child born of this arrangement may or may not be genetically related to the woman who bore the child, depending upon whose egg(s) were used to create the embryo(s). When a woman is inseminated and her own egg(s) are used, she is known as a genetic surrogate. When a woman accepts an embryo transfer where eggs from a third party are used (whether a donor or a woman contracting for services) she is known as a gestational surrogate.[6]

There are many ethical issues associated with AHR in the Canadian context. Among these issues are age restrictions on access to AHR (Goold 2005); payment for gamete providers (Baylis and McLeod 2007); and reproductive travel to get treatment(s) that are banned or difficult to access in Canada (Crozier and Baylis 2010; Whittaker 2010). Notwithstanding the importance of these discrete issues, we focus here on ethical issues in AHR that we deem most relevant for nursing care—issues of equitable access to fertility treatment, informed choice, and the commodification of reproductive tissues. For illustrative purposes we focus our discussion of these issues on IVF.

Access to IVF

For some, the availability of IVF enhances reproductive freedom by offering women and couples options for childbearing. For others, the availability of these technologies may actually constrain the freedom of women who use these technologies, or women who assist others in their use of these technologies. On this latter view, the patriarchal oppression of women is a potent force in the shaping of desires and one should ask why there is a market for IVF, given its great expense and attendant risks. One answer appears to be that IVF offers women, men, and couples a chance to have a "healthy" genetically related child. Underlying the strong desire to have one's "own" child, feminists see a pattern of children given value as limited-edition commodities, and women as lacking value unless they reproduce and raise children. Susan Sherwin argues that beneath the quest for biological parenthood is "a set of attitudes which views children as commodities whose value is derived from their possession of parental chromosomes [and where] . . . [w]omen are persuaded that their most important purpose in life is to bear and raise children" (Sherwin 1987, 537). These cultural values are oppressive, and as such IVF is seen as perpetuating oppressive social arrangements.

These criticisms notwithstanding, there is increasing demand for reproductive technologies and, in particular, increasing demand for IVF to be covered by provincial health insurance plans (see *Cameron v. Nova Scotia* 1999). At the time of writing, only two Canadian provinces pay for IVF. Ontario pays for three IVF cycles for women with bi-lateral blocked fallopian tubes (Nisker 2004). Quebec pays for three stimulated (or six natural) IVF cycles for all infertile women of childbearing age (Quebec 2010).

In Canada, the publicly funded provincial health insurance plans have long been under threat of privatization because of rising health care costs. For this reason, it seems both odd and offensive to some that a provincial government would finance IVF—a service desired by perhaps 5 percent of the population[7]—when there are health goods and services of potential benefit to the whole population that remain outside the medicare basket, such as pharmacare. Indeed, for many, the August 2010 Quebec decision to fund IVF had less to do with health care than pro-natalism—a desire to increase the birth rate (Wente 2010). This perspective is informed by the fact that no new funding was provided to prevent infertility, to address the lack of access to family practitioners, obstetricians, and midwives, or to provide less technologically intensive ways of addressing infertility (such as improved adoption processes) (Lippman 2010).

Informed Choice

Women and couples considering IVF must be able to make genuinely informed choices about fertility treatment. At minimum, this requires adequate disclosure of relevant information, including information about the nature of the procedure, the potential harms, the probability of success (in terms of healthy live births), and available alternatives. The Code of Ethics for Registered Nurses states that "Nurses, to the extent possible, provide persons in their care with the information they need to make informed decisions related to their health and well-being" (Canadian Nurses Association 2008, 11).

For example, when providing women and couples with information about the nature of IVF, it is important to explain (among other things) how many embryos will be transferred per cycle and the consequences of transferring more than one embryo (Van Voorhis and Ryan 2010). Globally, there is a move toward elective single embryo transfer in an effort to reduce the incidence of multiple births. Current practice in Canada, however, still involves the transfer of between two and four embryos per cycle depending upon such factors as the age of the woman, the cause of infertility, and the number of previous IVF attempts (Min, Hughes, and Young 2010). Women and couples must be informed of the risks of multi-fetal pregnancy for themselves and their offspring—for example, their babies may be born premature with low birth-weights and this may give rise to both short-term and long-term health problems (McGrath et al. 2010). They must be informed of the option of selective fetal reduction to reduce a multi-fetal pregnancy to twins or a singleton.

As regards the discussion of potential harms, women and couples should know that IVF is both physically and psychologically demanding. For example, women undergoing a stimulated IVF cycle may experience ovarian hyperstimulation syndrome (OHSS). At its most serious, "[l]ife-threatening complications of OHHS include renal failure, adult respiratory distress syndrome (ARDS), hemorrhage from ovarian rupture, and thromboembolism" (Practice Committee 2008, S189). In addition to the potential harms of OHSS, there are the potential harms of egg retrieval.[8] As well, women and couples may experience psychological harms, even after a successful pregnancy. These harms may include low self-esteem and doubts about one's competence as a parent and may require the care of a psychiatric clinical nurse specialist (McGrath et al. 2010).

For women considering IVF, these potential physical and psychological harms may seem worthwhile if the procedure enables them to conceive, gestate, and give birth to a healthy child. In Canada, data from 2008 show an overall pregnancy rate of 36.5 percent per cycle started, and a live birth rate of 29 percent per cycle started (Gunby 2008). Evidence regarding the efficacy of IVF specifically for unexplained infertility is mixed, however. A meta-analysis of four randomized studies comparing the success of IVF in cases of unexplained infertility with other reproductive strategies such as expectant management, ovarian stimulation alone, and intrauterine insemination was published in 2009 (Pandian et al. 2009). This review concluded that, "In vitro fertilisation (IVF) might result in more pregnancies than other options for unexplained infertility, but this is still uncertain and more research is needed on birth rates, adverse outcomes and costs" (Pandian et al. 2009). Those who are considering IVF for unexplained infertility should be informed of the uneven evidence concerning efficacy.

Finally, women and couples considering IVF should know what other options are available to them in pursuing their goal of becoming parents, including the option of adoption. In Ethics in Practice 23-2, we discuss the development of policies for accessing IVF. We show the difficulty in determining whether bias has influenced policy choices.

ETHICS IN PRACTICE 23-2

Age Restriction on Access to IVF: Good Policy or Ageist Bias?

A nurse working in a fertility clinic occasionally sees women in their late forties and early fifties who want to become parents using IVF. The nurse—who is herself in her fifties and a grandmother—believes that it is not right to help these women become pregnant and have children. She believes that motherhood at such an age is unnatural and is contrary to the best interests of the child.

The nurse uses her position on the clinic's policy committee to argue for a prohibition on fertility treatment in the clinic for women over 45 years of age. Another member of the committee argues that such a prohibition would be wrong because it would be a form of age discrimination.

The Commodification of Reproductive Material

Women and couples who use IVF sometimes have *in vitro* eggs and embryos they do not want for their own reproductive use. When this is the case, the options are to discard these reproductive materials, or donate them for (a) reproductive use by a third party, (b) improving or providing instruction in assisted human reproduction, or (c) research. This could be research aimed at (1) learning more about early embryonic development (e.g., to increase knowledge about congenital diseases and miscarriages); (2) developing or improving contraceptive techniques (and/or abortifacients); (3) developing or improving fertility treatments; (4) developing or improving early pre-implantation cell screening (e.g., pre-implantation genetic diagnosis); or (5) deriving human embryonic stem (hES) cell lines for future therapeutic interventions. In Canada, the purchase, sale, or exchange of gametes and embryos is legally prohibited (Assisted Human Reproduction Act 2004).

While some agree with prohibitions on the buying and selling of reproductive materials on the grounds that this contributes to the further commodification of reproductive tissues and labour, and potentially undermines voluntariness, others argue that it is unfair and exploitative of women to have them bear the potential harms of hormonal stimulation and surgical egg retrieval without appropriate financial compensation. In response, those who object to the commercialization of gametes and embryos maintain that while the providers of these materials are potentially capable of consenting to hormonal stimulation and egg extraction in exchange for money, for some women their precarious finances may place them in a weak bargaining position and at serious risk of exploitation (Baylis and McLeod 2007).

PRENATAL TESTING AND SCREENING

A wide range of prenatal tests and screens are available throughout pregnancy to obtain information about the developing fetus. These tests include ultrasound, maternal serum screening, amniocentesis, and chorionic villus sampling (CVS).

Ultrasound is an imaging technology usually performed at 18 to 20 weeks that can detect structural anomalies in the fetus, or physical markers that correlate with genetic anomalies. It is used to identify structural defects (such as spina bifida), congenital heart defects, gastrointestinal and kidney malformations, and cleft lip or palate (Ross 2008).

Maternal serum screening is a blood test taken from the pregnant woman between 15 and 20 weeks gestation that produces an odds ratio that the fetus has a chromosomal abnormality, such as Trisomy 21 (i.e., Down syndrome). If the blood test shows a high risk of chromosomal abnormality (typically a risk greater than 1 in 250), then the pregnant woman can opt for amniocentesis, which can give a definite diagnosis (Society of Obstetricians and Gynaecologists of Canada 2006). In an effort to improve the accuracy of prenatal screening, serum testing can be combined with prenatal ultrasound. The combination of tests (sometimes called "Integrated Prenatal Screening") produces a more reliable estimate of the risk of trisomies and neural tube defects (B.C. Prenatal Genetic Screening Program 2010).

Amniocentesis, usually done between 15 and 20 weeks, involves the extraction of amniotic fluid from the fetal amniotic sac using a needle. This fluid is then cultured and analyzed to see if there is a genetic disorder, a chromosomal anomaly, or a structural defect (Vorvick and Storck 2009). This test carries a 1 in 200 chance of causing a miscarriage (Society of Obstetricians and Gynaecologists of Canada 2006).

CVS involves the sampling of genetic material from the chorionic villi, which are part of the placenta and have the same genes and chromosomes as the fetus. This test, offered between 10 and 12 weeks gestation, is used to identify genetic disorders and chromosomal abnormalities. The risk of miscarriage with CVS is 1 in 100, which is considerably higher than the risk of miscarriage with amniocentesis. The benefit of CVS over amniocentesis is that CVS can be offered earlier in pregnancy, which is an important factor for those considering elective abortion (Vorvick and Storck 2008).

In addition to the above, there is research underway to develop prenatal tests for chromosomal abnormalities that would provide accurate diagnoses early in pregnancy, without the invasiveness of amniocentesis or CVS (Fan and Quake 2010; Lo et al. 2010). Such tests would require a maternal blood sample taken early in pregnancy—as with maternal serum screening—but unlike maternal serum screening the test would provide an accurate diagnosis and not just probabilistic information about a possible genetic abnormality. At present, there is research evidence showing that noninvasive prenatal diagnosis can be performed, and it may be just a matter of time until these tests are brought to market for clinical use (Greely 2011).

Access to Prenatal Testing and Screening

Prenatal surveillance technologies such as ultrasound and genetic testing are widely available in Canada and, for some, the normalized use of these technologies is problematic. For example, Susan Sherwin argues that the routine availability and use of prenatal testing and screening creates a crisis atmosphere around pregnancy that is harmful to women (Sherwin 2000). It sends a message that all pregnancies—even the healthiest, low-risk pregnancies—are crises waiting to happen, and must be carefully monitored. The medicalization of pregnancy takes gestation and childbirth out of the hands of women, and into the hands of health care professionals—symbolically alienating pregnant women from their own bodies. Sherwin argues as well that the options of midwifery care with minimal interventions, and home-birth for low-risk pregnancies, reverse this trend of medicalization (Sherwin 2000). Feminist ethicists are also concerned about the use of prenatal testing to identify and abort female fetuses because such use is an expression of misogyny, or reinforces patriarchal oppression (Bubeck 2002).

Prenatal testing and screening are also ethically contentious from the perspective of disability theorists who see this social practice as threatening to people living with disabilities. On the one hand, prenatal testing and screening allow women to make informed choices about their reproduction in deciding whether to continue a pregnancy when testing reveals that the fetus has a disabling condition. On the other hand, many are concerned about the implications of testing for, and eliminating, fetuses with disabling conditions. For instance, when prenatal testing reveals Down syndrome, women terminate their pregnancies at a high rate (around 90 percent) (Mansfield, Hopfer, and Marteau 1999). According to the "expressivist objection," genetic testing followed by the selective abortion of affected fetuses expresses a negative attitude toward those who are living with disabilities and thereby harms them (Buchanan 1996; Wendell 1996). The increase in, and normalization of, prenatal testing and selective abortion for disabilities is seen as a potential cause of discriminatory attitudes toward persons living with disabilities. It has also been suggested that the prevalence of prenatal testing and selective abortion could foster attitudes of intolerance toward women and couples who decide to continue pregnancies with affected fetuses (Parens and Asch 2000).

Furthermore, there is the fear that prenatal testing reinforces the tendency of the public to view people living with disabilities through the prism of one trait, rather than viewing them as fully complex human individuals with many traits (Asch and Wasserman 2005). This public view encourages women and couples to see their affected fetuses in a similar way, by assuming that the trait of having a disability is the only relevant factor determining whether a pregnancy ought to proceed (Asch and Wasserman 2005).

Some philosophers and ethicists contest the expressivist objection, arguing that the act of testing a fetus for disabling conditions can have many meanings that do not necessarily express a negative attitude toward disability (Kittay and Kittay 2000; Malek 2010; Nelson 2000). Others point to the fact that the historical emergence of prenatal testing coincides with the emergence of progressive legislation and policies that are favourable to people living with disabilities (Ross 2008). Examples are the Canadian Human Rights Commission's policies for employment accommodation for people living with disabilities (Canadian Human Rights Commission 2006) and the Americans with Disabilities Act passed in 1990. The argument here is that since progressive disability policy is a feature of societies that have introduced prenatal testing for disability, there is little reason to believe that prenatal testing reinforces discrimination. To further explore these issues, in Ethics in Practice 23-3 we illustrate the dilemma that arises in the process of gaining consent for prenatal testing and in the process of informing prospective parents about the results of a test diagnosing Down syndrome prenatally.

ETHICS IN PRACTICE 23-3

Prenatal Testing: A Personal Story

One of the authors (CK) has a son with Down syndrome.

When my wife had maternal serum screening, the test revealed a one in six chance that our son had a chromosomal abnormality. We were shocked by this—never having heard of such high odds resulting from a maternal serum screening test. The nurse who was responsible for counselling offered us amniocentesis, and explained that continuing the pregnancy and terminating the pregnancy were both options. We had the amniocentesis, and received a diagnosis of Trisomy 21, Down syndrome. The nurse gave us this information over the telephone once she had the lab results. At this time, she reminded us again of our options, and offered to give us information about Down syndrome and to put us into contact with members of the provincial Down syndrome society. We received a package of information and contacted the society. We decided to continue the pregnancy, and our son, Aaron, was born three months later. He is now a happy and healthy toddler.

Reflecting on the experience, I am aware of the fact that we could have faced this daunting set of decisions in virtual absence of any information about Down syndrome from our health care providers. We were given no information about Down syndrome when we were offered maternal serum screening. After amniocentesis, the nurse offered to give us information about Down syndrome, but we could have refused to find out anything about the lives of people living with Down syndrome.

Our nurse faced a dilemma when offering us information about Down syndrome. On the one hand, prospective parents should be informed about the disabilities for which they are testing. On the other hand, nurses should avoid directive counselling that could influence decision making about continuing or terminating a pregnancy.

Informed Choice

It is widely accepted that pregnant women and couples must make informed choices about prenatal testing or screening. However, ensuring that women and couples make informed choices is often challenging for health care providers. For example, the current guidelines in British Columbia for offering Integrated Prenatal Screening (maternal serum testing plus ultrasound measurement of the nuchal translucency) to pregnant women characterized as high risk are highly detailed and may invite confusion from health care workers and patients alike (B.C. Prenatal Genetic Screening Program 2010). There are six different eligibility categories in B.C. for Integrated Prenatal Screening, and a detailed understanding of the mathematics of risk may be required to explain the benefits of the integrated approach to patients. Furthermore, empirical evidence suggests that in Canada and elsewhere, health care providers regularly fail to achieve the elements of informed choice for prenatal testing. A recent article by Victoria Seavilleklein documents how "any of disclosure, understanding, voluntariness and consent can be challenged as inadequate in light of the empirical evidence of current practice" (Seavilleklein 2009, 70). Interactions with patients are often rushed, patients' understanding of testing procedures is often poor, and many health care providers offer prenatal testing in a way that virtually ensures the patient will agree to it.

Counselling about prenatal testing and screening may be provided by various health care professionals; physicians, genetic counsellors, midwives, or nurses. In these sensitive interactions, there is an ethical requirement to provide relevant information without attempting to influence a pregnant woman's decisions about undergoing prenatal testing, or about what to do with a positive diagnosis (i.e., a diagnosis confirming an anomaly). At the same time, disability rights advocates argue that accurate information about the disabilities for which tests are being done should be provided to pregnant women and couples prior to prenatal testing (Lindeman 2008). The standard of informed choice would require that women and couples be informed about the conditions for which they are being tested. Nurses and others who work in prenatal care must find a balance between ensuring they do not influence decision making, while also ensuring that pregnant women and their partners have adequate and accurate information to make informed decisions.

A positive prenatal diagnosis of a fetal genetic anomaly or impairment occasions a difficult choice between continuing the pregnancy or termination. Either of these options can be traumatic because each brings its own sense of loss. Those who opt to terminate lose a previously wanted pregnancy, whereas those who continue the pregnancy may experience a sense of loss that results from a change in their dreams and expectations about who their baby will be. Empirical research into the experiences of those given a positive prenatal diagnosis documents this sense of loss and the anguish felt by couples who must make "a series of nested and time-sensitive decisions" resulting from the diagnosis—for example, whether to terminate or continue the pregnancy; if terminating, what method to use; and what to tell friends and family about the pregnancy (Sandelowski and Barroso 2005, 310). These decision-points have been described as a "travesty" because the choices have been forced upon the pregnant women and their partners by the positive test result—a combination of choice and lack of choice—and all options have potentially devastating emotional consequences (Sandelowski and Barroso 2005).

These experiences have implications for nursing care. Nurses involved with counselling for prenatal testing and decision making after a positive diagnosis are in a position to facilitate coping strategies. Women and couples in this position develop narratives in order to cope with the difficult decisions they face—which may involve seeking additional information about disabilities, or about the fetus, or involve the control of information that may upset a decision that has already been made (Sandelowski and Barroso 2005). Sensitivity to the motives and details behind these coping strategies may allow nurses to assist women and couples in the construction of a healing narrative (Sandelowski 1994).

Summary

Nursing care in pregnancy and reproduction encompasses a variety of interventions including abortion, forms of assisted human reproduction such as IVF, and prenatal testing and screening. Nurses involved in providing these interventions will find that each raises unique ethical issues to which attention must be paid. However, there are some common threads. For instance, informed choice is an important ethical norm for nurse–patient interactions. More generally, our ability to control and harness the human powers of reproduction engages with wider societal concerns about the allocation of finite health care resources, the status of women, and our attitudes toward disability. A healthy and productive ethical discourse in the nursing profession and in society as a whole, requires that we focus our critical faculties on these issues with a view to providing women with high-quality reproductive health care.

For Reflection

1. Where do you stand on the issue of abortion? How would you justify your position? What makes you think you are right and others are wrong?

2. You have been scheduled to work a shift when you know that abortions are performed and that you will likely be asked to assist. You have serious moral objections to participating in termination of pregnancy and you were clear about this at the time that you were hired. Can you refuse to assist on the grounds of conscientious refusal?

3. Quebec recently decided to provide public funding for IVF for all infertile women of childbearing age. Should other provinces follow this lead and fund IVF? Why or why not?

4. An IVF patient asks you about her chances of getting pregnant following treatment. You could answer her question as asked, but you assume that what she really wants to know is what are her chances of having a healthy newborn (which are lower than her chances of getting pregnant). How should you answer her question?

5. Should prenatal testing be allowed for women and couples who want to select the sex of their child?

6. How should nurses who provide counselling for genetic testing deal with the difficulty of ensuring that they do not influence the decisions of the prospective parents, while also fulfilling the obligation to promote informed choice?

Endnotes

1. We do not address ethical issues specific to late-term abortion in this chapter (see Alward 2002).

2. For the pre-*Morgentaler* history of abortion law in Canada, see Brodie et al. 1992.

3. Since the *Morgentaler* ruling in 1988, there have been numerous legal challenges of abortion access barriers—for example, *Jane Doe 1* v. *Manitoba* (2004), and *Ontario (Attorney General)* v. *Dieleman* (1994).

4. At the time of writing, litigation against the government of New Brunswick's restrictions on abortion access is ongoing (Peritz 2010).

5. There are strong ethical arguments in support of the view that physician refusal is justifiable only when the physician refers the patient to another physician who can provide the service, or ensures that the patient is aware of other such physicians, and can likely access their services. Sanda Rodgers and Jocelyn Downie argue that this position is supported by the Canadian Medical Association's ethics policy on induced abortion and Code of Ethics (Rodgers and Downie 2006; 2007). Jeff Blackmer disagrees that these policies require a conscientiously objecting physician to provide a referral for abortion (Blackmer 2007). On this issue, see as well McLeod 2008.

6. For discussion of ethical issues arising from gestational contracts see Fry et al. 2011 and van Niekerk and van Zyl 1995.

7. As noted above, while 8–12 percent of women are unable to conceive spontaneously (Fisher 2009) only about half of these women will seek medical care for their infertility (Boivin et al. 2007).

8. Patients undergoing egg retrieval may be donors or they may be women planning to use IVF to get pregnant. The full scope of risks (emotional as well as physical) faced by female gamete donors, as well as the ethical duties of nurses dealing with these risks, will not be explored in this chapter. For a good discussion of the ethics of nursing care for female gamete donors, see Black 2010.

References

Abortion Rights Coalition of Canada. 2005. *Late term abortions (after 20 weeks)*. Available at http://www.arcc-cdac.ca/postionpapers/22-Late-term-Abortions.PDF.

Alward, P. 2002. Thomson, the right to life, and partial-birth abortion. *Journal of Medical Ethics, 28* (2), 99–101.

Asch, A. and Wasserman, D. 2005. Where is the sin in synecdoche? Prenatal testing and the parent-child relationship. In D. Wasserman, J. Bickenbach, and R. Wachbroit (Eds.), *Quality of life and human difference: Genetic testing, health care, and disability* (pp. 172–216). New York: Cambridge University Press.

Assisted Human Reproduction Act, S.C. 2004, c.2.

Baylis, F. 2012. Infertility. In R. Chadwick (Ed.), *Encyclopedia of applied ethics* (2nd ed.). San Diego: Elsevier Inc.

Baylis, F. and Kaposy, C. 2010. Wanted: Inclusive guidelines for research involving pregnant women. *Journal of Obstetrics and Gynaecology Canada, 32* (5), 473–476.

Baylis, F. and McLeod, C. 2007. The stem cell debate continues: The buying and selling of eggs for research. *Journal of Medical Ethics, 33*, 726–731.

BC Prenatal Genetic Screening Program. 2010. *BC prenatal genetic screening program update.* Available at http://www.perinatalservicesbc.ca/sites/bcrcp/files/spotlight/Pgsp_Newsletter.pdf.

Black, J.J. 2010. Egg donation: Issues and concerns. *MCN. The American Journal of Maternal Child Nursing, 35* (3), 132–137.

Blackmer, J. 2007. Clarification of the CMA's position concerning induced abortion. *Canadian Medical Association Journal, 176* (9), 1310.

Boetzkes, E. 1999. Equality, autonomy, and feminist bioethics. In A. Donchin and L.M. Purdy, (Eds.), *Embodying bioethics: Recent feminist advances.* New York: Rowman and Littlefield.

Boivin, J., Bunting, L., Collins, J.A., and Nygren, K. 2007. International estimates of infertility prevalence and treatment-seeking: Potential need and demand for infertility medical care. *Human Reproduction, 22*, 1506–1512.

Brodie, J., Gavigan, S.A.M., and Jenson, J. 1992. *The politics of abortion.* Toronto: Oxford University Press.

Browne, A. and Sullivan B. 2005. Abortion in Canada. *Cambridge Quarterly of Healthcare Ethics, 14*, 287–291.

Bubeck, D. 2002. Sex selection: The feminist response. In J. Burley and J. Harris (Eds.), *A companion to genethics.* Malden, MA: Blackwell Publishing.

Buchanan, A. 1996. Choosing who will be disabled: Genetic intervention and the morality of inclusion. *Social Philosophy and Policy, 13*, 18–46.

Cameron v. Nova Scotia (Attorney General). 1999. N.S.J. No. 297.

Canadian Abortion Rights Action League. 2003. *Protecting abortion rights in Canada.* Ottawa: Author.

Canadian Charter of Rights and Freedoms. 1982. Available at http://dsp-psd.pwgsc.gc.ca/Collection/CH37-4-3-2002E.pdf.

Canadian Federation for Sexual Health. 2008a. *Medical abortion.* Available at http://www.cfsh.ca/Your_Sexual_Health/Abortion/medical-abortion.aspx.

Canadian Federation for Sexual Health. 2008b. *Surgical abortion.* Available at http://www.cfsh.ca/Your_Sexual_Health/Abortion/surgical-abortion.aspx.

Canadian Human Rights Commission. 2006. *A place for all: A guide to creating an inclusive workplace.* Ottawa: Canadian Human Rights Commission. Available at http://www.chrc-ccdp.ca/pdf/publications/aplaceforall.pdf.

Canadian Nurses Association. 2008. *Code of ethics for registered nurses*. Ottawa: Author.

Crozier, G. and Baylis, F. 2010. The ethical physician encounters international medical travel. *Journal of Medical Ethics, 36*, 297–301.

Dickens, B.M. and Cook, R.J. 2000. The scope and limits of conscientious objection. *International Journal of Gynecology & Obstetrics, 71*, 71–77.

Fan, H.C. and Quake, S.R. 2010. In principle method for noninvasive determination of the fetal genome. *Nature Precedings,* doi:10.1038/npre.2010.5373.1.

Fisher, J. 2009. Infertility and assisted reproduction. In World Health Organization, *Mental health aspects of women's reproductive health: A global review of the literature* (pp. 128–146). Geneva: WHO Press.

Fry, S.T., Veatch, R.M., and Taylor, C. 2011. Genetics, birth, and the biologic revolution. In *Case studies in nursing ethics* (4th ed.). Mississauga, ON: Jones and Bartlett Learning.

Goold, I. 2005. Should older and postmenopausal women have access to assisted reproductive technology? *Monash Bioethics Review, 24* (1), 27–46.

Greely, H.T. 2011. Get ready for the flood of fetal gene screening. *Nature, 469*, 289–291.

Gunby, J. 2008. *Assisted reproductive technologies (ART) in Canada: 2008 results from the Canadian ART Register*. Available at http://www.cfas.ca/index.php?option=com_content&view=article&id=1085:cartr-2008&catid=1012:cartr.

Habermas, J. 2003. *The future of human nature*. Cambridge, UK: Polity Press.

Healthwise. 2008. *Dilation and evacuation (D&E) for abortion.* Available at http://www.webmd.com/a-to-z-guides/dilation-and-evacuation-de-for-abortion.

Jane Doe 1 v. *Manitoba*. 2004. M.J. No. 456 (Man. Q.B.).

Kaposy, C. 2010. Two stalemates in the philosophical debate about abortion and why they cannot be resolved using analogical arguments. *Bioethics* doi:10.1111/j.1467-8519.2010.01815.x.

Kittay, E.F. and Kittay L. 2000. On the expressivity and ethics of selective abortion for disability: Conversations with my son. In E. Parens and A. Asch (Eds.), *Prenatal testing and disability rights*. Washington: Georgetown University Press.

Kukla, R., Kuppermann, M., Little, M., Lyerly, A.D., Mitchell, L.M., Armstrong, E.M., and Harris, L. 2009. Finding autonomy in birth. *Bioethics, 23* (1), 1–8.

Lindeman, R. 2008. Take Down syndrome out of the abortion debate. *Canadian Medical Association Journal, 179* (10), 1088.

Lippman, A. May 25, 2010. *Saying "no" to the funding of assisted reproduction services in Québec.* Available at http://www.bionews.org.uk/page_61600.asp.

Lo, Y.M.D., Chan, K.C.A., Sun, H., Chen, E.Z., Jiang, P., Lun, F.M.F., Zheng, Y.W., Leung, T.Y., Lau, T.K., Cantor, C.R., and Chiu, R.W.K. 2010. Maternal plasma DNA sequencing reveals the genome-wide genetic and mutational profile of the fetus. *Science Translational Medicine, 2*, 61ra91.

Lyerly, A.D., Little, M.O., and Faden, R. 2008. The second wave: Toward responsible inclusion of pregnant women in research. *International Journal of Feminist Approaches Bioethics, 1*, 5–22.

Malek, J. 2010. Deciding against disability: Does the use of reproductive genetic technologies express disvalue for people with disabilities? *Journal of Medical Ethics, 36*, 217–221.

Mansfield, C., Hopfer, S., and Marteau, T.M. 1999. Termination rates after prenatal diagnosis of Down syndrome, spina bifida, anencephaly, and Turner and Klinefelter syndromes: A systematic literature review. *Prenatal Diagnosis, 19*, 808–812.

McGrath, J.M, Samra, H.A., Zukowsky, K., and Baker, B. 2010. Parenting after infertility: Issues for families and infants. *American Journal of Maternal/Child Nursing, 35* (3), 156–164.

McLeod, C. 2008. Referral in the wake of conscientious objection to abortion. *Hypatia, 23*, 30–47.

Min, J.K., Hughes, E., and Young, D. 2010. Elective single embryo transfer following in vitro fertilization. *Journal of Obstetrics and Gynecology Canada, 241*, 363–377.

Mykitiuk, R. and Nisker, J. 2008. Assisted reproduction. In P.A. Singer and A.M. Viens (Eds.), *The Cambridge textbook of bioethics* (pp. 112–120). New York: Cambridge University Press.

Nelson, J.L. 2000. The meaning of the act: Reflections on the expressive force of reproductive decision making and policies. In E. Parens and A. Asch (Eds.), *Prenatal testing and disability rights*. Washington: Georgetown University Press.

Nisker J. 2004. Anniversary of injustice: April fool's day, 1994. *Journal of Obstetrics and Gynaecology Canada, 26*, 321–322.

Ontario (Attorney General) v. *Dieleman*. 1994. O.J. No. 1864 (Ont. Ct. (Gen. Div.)).

Pandian, Z., Bhattacharya, S., Vale, L., and Templeton, A. 2009. In vitro fertilisation for unexplained subfertility (Review). *The Cochrane Library, 1*. Available at http://mrw.interscience.wiley.com/ cochrane/clsysrev/articles/CD003357/pdf_fs.html.

Parens, E. and Asch, A. 2000. The disability rights critique of prenatal genetic testing: Reflections and recommendations. In E. Parens and A. Asch (Eds.), *Prenatal testing and disability rights,* (pp. 3–43). Washington, DC: Georgetown University Press.

Peritz, I. 2010. Abortion access unequal across country. *The Globe and Mail,* June 18, 2010. Available at http://www.theglobeandmail.com/news/national/despite-being-legal-abortions-still-not-accessible-for-all-canadians/article1610254/?cmpid=rss1&utm_source=feedburner&utm_ medium=feed&utm_campaign=Feed%3A+TheGlobeAndMail-National+(The+Globe+and+Mail+-+National+News)&utm_content=Bloglines.

Practice Committee of the American Society for Reproductive Medicine. 2008. Ovarian hyper-stimulation syndrome. *Fertility and Sterility, 90 (Suppl 3),* 188–193.

Quebec. 2010. (August 5). *An Act respecting clinical and research activities relating to assisted procreation,* R.S.Q. c. A-5.01. Available at http://www.canlii.org/en/qc/laws/stat/rsq-c-a-5.01/latest/rsq-c-a-5.01.html; *Regulation respecting clinical activities related to assisted procreation,* R.R.Q., c. A-5.01, r.1.

R. v. Morgentaler. 1988. 1 S.C.R. 30.

Rodgers, S. and Downie, J. 2007. The authors respond. *Canadian Medical Association Journal, 176* (4), 494.

Rodgers, S. and Downie, J. 2006. Abortion: Ensuring access. *Canadian Medical Association Journal, 175* (1), 9.

Ross, L.F. 2008. Prenatal testing and newborn screening. In P.A. Singer and A.M. Viens (Eds.), *The Cambridge textbook of bioethics* (pp. 104–111). New York: Cambridge University Press.

Sandelowski, M. 1994. We are the stories we tell: Narrative knowing in nursing practice. *Journal of Holistic Nursing, 12*, 23–33.

Sandelowski, M. and Barroso, J. 2005. The travesty of choosing after positive prenatal diagnosis. *Journal of Obstetric, Gynecologic, and Neonatal Nursing, 34*, 307–318.

Seavilleklein, V. 2009. Challenging the rhetoric of choice in prenatal screening. *Bioethics, 23* (1), 68–77.

Shaw, J. 2006. *Reality check: A close look at accessing abortion services in Canadian hospitals.* Ottawa: Canadians for Choice.

Sheldon, S. and Wilkinson, S. 2004. Should selecting saviour siblings be banned? *Journal of Medical Ethics, 30*, 533–537.

Sherwin, S. 1987. Feminist ethics and in vitro fertilization. In T.A. Mappes and D. DeGrazia (Eds.), *Biomedical ethics* (6th ed.; pp. 536–540). Toronto: McGraw-Hill.

Sherwin, S. 2000. Normalizing reproductive technologies and the implications for autonomy. In R. Tong, G. Anderson, and A. Santos (Eds.), *Globalizing feminist bioethics* (pp. 96–113). Boulder, CO: Westview Press.

Society of Obstetricians and Gynaecologists of Canada. 2006. *Prenatal diagnosis.* Available at http://www.sogc.org/health/pdf/prenatal_e.pdf.

Statistics Canada. 2010. *Induced abortions per 100 live births.* Available at http://www40.statcan.ca/l01/cst01/health42a-eng.htm.

Thomson, J.J. 1995. Abortion. *Boston Review, 20* (3). Available at http://bostonreview.net/BR20.3/thomson.html.

van Niekerk, A. and van Zyl, L. 1995. The ethics of surrogacy: Women's reproductive labour. *Journal of Medical Ethics, 21*, 345–349.

Van Voorhis, B.J. and Ryan, G.L. 2010. Ethical obligation for restricting the number of embryos transferred to women: Combating the multiple-birth epidemic from in vitro fertilization. *Seminars in Reproductive Medicine, 28* (4), 287–294.

Vorvick, L.J. and Storck, S. 2008. Chorionic villus sampling. *Medline Plus Encyclopedia.* Available at http://www.nlm.nih.gov/medlineplus/ency/article/003406.htm.

Vorvick, L.J. and Storck, S. 2009. Amniocentesis. *Medline Plus Encyclopedia.* Available at http://www.nlm.nih.gov/medlineplus/ency/article/003921.htm.

Wendell, S. 1996. *The rejected body.* New York: Routledge.

Wente, M. 2010. In Quebec, infertility is now a disease. *Globe and Mail,* June 20, 2010 p. A15.

Whittaker, A. 2010. Challenges of medical travel to global regulation: A case study of reproductive travel in Asia. *Global Social Policy, 10* (3), 396–415.

Winnipeg Child and Family Services (Northwest Area) v. G.(D.F.). 1997. 3 S.C.R. 925.

CHAPTER 24

Genetics and Identity: Diagnosis, Management, and Prevention of Health Conditions

Susan M. Cox and Jehannine C. Austin

Genetics is an area that nursing must not ignore, or the profession "will find itself wholly unprepared" to deal with emerging health-care requirements (Gottlieb 1998, 4). Advances in human genetics are reshaping contemporary understandings of health and illness and transforming the practice of medicine and nursing. The first complete map of the human genome was completed a decade ago, and there is now a plethora of uses for genetic information in the prediction, diagnosis, treatment, management, and prevention of disease. The demand for genetic services is placing an increasing emphasis on the need to integrate genetics with the provision of primary health care (Guttmacher et al. 2001), and there is ongoing pressure from commercial interests to accelerate clinical utilization of predictive, diagnostic, and therapeutic interventions. Simultaneously, scientists, experts in population health, and policy analysts have long warned about the dangers of over-emphasizing genetics (Caulfield et al. 2001; Lewontin 2000) and now express concern that the potential of genomic science has been inflated (Evans et al. 2011).

Although a large number of conditions are caused entirely by genes, individually each of these conditions is rare. In fact, the vast bulk of common conditions that negatively affect human health (mental illness, arthritis, diabetes, cancer) are best described as complex or multifactorial disorders—that is, they arise as a result of genetic and environmental factors acting together. In this context, the simplistic message that "genes cause disease" overlooks other important socio-economic and environmental determinants of health (Baird 2002).

In this chapter, we focus on current applications of genetics in the area of human health. In the first section, we describe the Human Genome Project and some of its implications for the prediction, diagnosis, management, and treatment of health conditions. Though prenatal and other routinized forms of genetic testing raise many significant ethical issues, we focus on predictive testing because it creates a new subpopulation—that is, the "worried well" (Kenen 1996). In the second section, we explore the role of genetics in complex disorders, looking at the example of psychiatric illness (Peay and Austin 2011). In the third section, we identify practical challenges and opportunities for nurses and other health professionals seeking to assist patients, families, colleagues, and society in responding to recent advances in human genetics. In the final section, we offer some guidance for nurses and other health care professionals for integrating genetics into their practice.

Throughout the chapter, we introduce Ethics in Practice examples drawn from research, teaching, and clinical practice in which we have been engaged. The stories featured exemplify ethical practice issues identified by nurses, genetic counsellors, and other health professionals. Our perspectives are, however, that of a sociologist working within applied ethics (SMC) and a research-based genetic counsellor (JCA). We are especially interested in issues of genetics and identity and the value of listening to people's stories in order to identify enduring moral questions.

SOCIAL, FAMILIAL, AND ETHICAL IMPLICATIONS OF NEW GENETIC ADVANCES

The Human Genome Project

In 1990, the Human Genome Organization launched a multibillion dollar international effort to map and sequence the human genome.[1] Proponents of the Human Genome Project (HGP) promised that unlocking the secrets of the "book of life" would result in cures for common as well as rare diseases and that genome mapping would resolve long-standing puzzles of human development and cellular function (Kevles and Hood 1992). Critics argued that the HGP advanced an overly deterministic view of the relationship between genes, human health, and behaviour, and, moreover, that the project would siphon attention and resources away from other important health issues (Lippman 1992). Many also raised concerns about the consequences of an increasingly geneticized approach to health. These consequences include an overemphasis on individual risk, social stigmatization and discrimination, lack of respect for human diversity, commercialization and lack of regulation of genetic services, and eugenic applications of genetic knowledge and techniques[2] (Duster 1990; Hubbard and Wald 1993).

In recognition of these implications, the United States arm of the project established an Ethical, Legal, and Social Implications (ELSI) program to prospectively evaluate the various impacts of new genetic knowledge and techniques. In 1992, the Canadian Genome and Technology (CGAT) Program also included an ELSI program. Critics perceived these programs as a necessary and positive step, yet many remained concerned that the eugenic potential of the new genetics was not being taken seriously enough (Garver and Garver 1994).

History provides a potent reminder of the moral issues at stake. In Nazi Germany the campaign against all so-called "undesirable and useless" people included those with psychological illnesses and mental disabilities, schizophrenia, epilepsy, paralysis, Huntington disease and other neurological conditions, as well as those who were physically disabled, deaf, blind, elderly, or ill. The Nazis were, however, not alone in pursuing eugenic goals. Many U.S. states adopted mandatory sterilization programs. Nor did Canada escape unsullied. In 1933, British Columbia followed Alberta's lead in adopting legislation that sanctioned forced sterilization of the mentally ill and intellectually disabled. These programs remained in effect until the 1970s (McLaren 1990).

Although less overt, social processes like stigmatization continue to have a profound influence in shaping the lives of persons with physical and mental differences. Although much progress has been made, negative stereotypes still permeate popular culture, the practice of health care, and the policies guiding medical uses of genetic knowledge (Silvers 2001). As such, new genetic knowledge and techniques make it especially important to question predominant beliefs about health, illness, and disability; think critically about the social construction of "normality" and "abnormality"; and evaluate criteria used to define quality of life (Lippman 1992). Such issues arise in many practical settings—from assisting patients in decision making to evaluating the benefits and harms of new social policies on genetics and disability.

Now that a host of new diagnostic and other gene-based interventions are available, it is important to ask what this new knowledge and its application means for human health and well-being, as well as for social justice. How does possession of a computerized catalogue containing the biochemical "recipes" for life enhance detection and treatment of common as well as rare forms of disease? Do the predictive and diagnostic powers of genetics have the potential to contribute to new forms of discrimination (such as when persons who test positive for a gene that increases vulnerability to breast cancer are denied health insurance) and stigmatization (such as when persons diagnosed with Huntington disease experience a decline in self-esteem)? Will biobanking contribute to the development of personalized medicine? (See Exhibit 24-1). Answers to these questions are not straightforward. In fact, these issues have been of such concern that legislation to protect patients and families has been passed in the U.S. in the form of the Genetic Information Non-discrimination Act (GINA). Similar legislation is being developed in Canada but at present there are no legal regulations preventing genetic discrimination (Bombard et al. 2009).

Genome mapping has a dramatic impact in stepping up the pace of gene discovery and the range of available DNA-based tests. Genomic medicine is, perhaps, also qualitatively different in that there is an emphasis on the importance of understanding the interplay between genes and the environment in the causation of many common etiologically complex conditions. These are conditions such as heart disease, mental illnesses, cancer, diabetes, Alzheimer disease, and asthma (Guttmacher et al. 2001). This shift in thinking is ushering in a new medical paradigm—personalized (or genomic) medicine—in which therapeutic interventions will be tailored to each individual's genetic characteristics and disease (Feero, Guttmacher, and Collins 2010). This possibility opens up a Pandora's box of ethical challenges. Foremost at this historical juncture is the concern that, because the cost of whole genome sequencing has declined so rapidly, there will be increasing pressure for individuals to learn about their entire genome rather than specifically targeted differences related to a relevant health condition (Kohane et al. 2006). In fact, commercial entities have been exploiting these technological advances by offering consumers the opportunity to learn about their genetic risk for a wide variety of potential health conditions by simply submitting saliva to a direct to consumer (DTC) testing agency. Some believe this enhances accessibility while others question the quality and validity of the tests that these DTC testing companies are using (e.g., Khoury, Coates, and Evans 2010), and express concerns about how people will interpret the information they get without appropriate counselling. These are all significant health policy concerns and they continue to underscore the observation that medicine's growing ability to detect harmful genetic variations continues to outstrip the ability to offer treatment or cure for the resulting diseases.

Genetic Testing

The purpose of all genetic testing is to learn something about an individual's genotype (Clayton 2002).[3] Many genetic tests are now used in a wide range of clinical settings for many different purposes. Some genetic tests are applied broadly across many members of a population (e.g., newborn screening) while others are targeted more specifically to individuals (e.g., in the prediction and diagnosis of conditions like Huntington disease).[4] The decision to proceed with individual testing has typically been made within the context of the individual physician–patient or genetic counsellor–client relationship; at other times, decisions are made on a population basis. Increasingly, however, with the advent of direct to consumer marketing, this decision is made by consumers without consultation with a health care professional (McGuire and Burke 2010; Wade and Wilfond 2006).

Some types of genetic testing have been in use in Canada's health system for many years. A common example is newborn screening for phenylketonuria, a rare but treatable genetic metabolic disease that has been tested for since the 1960s. Another example is prenatal testing for detection of chromosomal anomalies such as trisomy 21 (Down syndrome). Pregnant women considered at "high risk" have been offered amniocentesis since the 1970s, as a routine part of prenatal care. Predictive or presymptomatic genetic testing for adult onset conditions is a more recent phenomenon. The first predictive test for an adult onset condition became available in the late 1980s, when scientists located genetic markers for Huntington disease (HD)[5] (Bloch et al. 1989). Since then, predictive and/or susceptibility tests have become available for many other adult onset conditions.

Early or presymptomatic detection of genetic variations that predispose at-risk individuals to particular conditions may lead to interventions that delay onset of disease or avert its most serious consequences. For instance, some women found to carry one of the variations strongly associated with hereditary breast and ovarian cancer may undergo prophylactic mastectomy and/or oophrectomy to reduce their chances of developing cancer (Hallowell et al. 1997). Alternately, the 1–2 percent of the population found to have a single-gene form of hyperlipidemia may, through diet and medication, avoid early heart disease (Baird 2002). There are, however, a great many cases in which there is no effective intervention available.

Even in the absence of effective treatment or cure, genetic testing and the provision of information about risk and disease susceptibility have emerged as new types of medical interventions in themselves. The paradigmatic example of this is Huntington disease. As psychologist Nancy Wexler (1990)—who is herself at risk for HD—pointed out at the outset, predictive genetic testing differs from other more routine forms of testing in several important ways.

First, predictive testing creates the novel situation in which some asymptomatic individuals learn, with a high degree of certainty, of impending illness while others learn they have escaped such a fate. This creates a new health status, that of the "worried well" (Kenen 1996). When there is no effective treatment available for the resulting disease, as is the case with HD, great care must be taken to ensure that there is adequate pre- and post-test counselling and support. Other dominantly transmitted genetic variations may demonstrate incomplete penetrance;[6] in these cases, genetic testing will not provide definitive information regarding whether the person will develop onset of the disease. For instance, women with BRCA1 mutations (associated with familial breast cancer) have an 80 to 85 percent lifetime risk of developing breast cancer, and so some women with BRCA1 mutations will not develop symptoms at all (Clayton 2002). However, those who do not have a mutation that is known to be pathogenic are not, however, free of risk. At the population level, the vast majority of breast cancer is not associated with BRCA variations.

The second aspect that distinguishes predictive genetic information from other types of medical information is that it does not "belong" to just one person. Given that we inherit DNA from both parents and share an average of 50 percent of the same genes as our siblings, predictive and/or susceptibility testing reveals information that is both individual and familial in orientation. The modification of risk that accompanies an informative test result may, therefore, have implications not only for the individual being tested but also for his or her family members. This can create ethical dilemmas for at-risk individuals, their families, and genetic service providers because there is an inherent tension between upholding the confidentiality of the person being tested and discerning where there may be a duty to warn other family members of potential harms related to an altered risk status. It is easy to imagine how genetic testing can have implications for family members beyond the tested individual by considering the situation in which one of a pair of identical twins wants predictive testing that the other does not.

Third, genetic information has an intimate connection with our individual (as well as collective) need to define ourselves in relation to others and, in so doing, to recognize both our similarity to, and difference from, others. Genetic information is, therefore, intertwined with ongoing existential processes of self-identity and perception—that is, one's sense of physical, intellectual, emotional, and spiritual "beingness" in the world. It is also deeply connected to our notions of uniqueness and personhood, agency, and self-determination (Brock 1994).

These aspects of genetic information (that is, predictive power, familial orientation, and existential quality) are central to understanding the social and ethical implications of hereditary risk and genetic testing for a range of adult onset conditions. The decision to undergo testing is highly personal, although it must be emphasized that many at-risk individuals feel responsible to other family members in making this decision (Burgess and Canning 2001; Cox 2003). For instance, some of the most common reasons given for testing for HD include relief of uncertainty; general planning for the future; specific planning in marital, reproductive, career, or financial areas; and the perceived responsibility to provide information to children (Bloch et al. 1989). Reasons for choosing not to be tested for HD include the burden of having knowledge of the increased risk of one's children, the absence of an effective cure, the potential loss of health insurance, financial or other genetic and discriminatory implications (Bombard et al. 2009), and the inability to "undo" the knowledge offered by predictive testing (Quaid and Morris 1993).

Whether or not genetic testing is employed, the implications of hereditary risk ripple through families, surfacing a welter of feelings about responsibilities to self and others (Burgess and Canning 2001). In Ethics in Practice 24-1, a nurse educator tells a story about a woman who has autosomal dominant polycystic kidney disease (ADPKD).[7] Through spending time at the woman's bedside, the nurse comes to understand that parental responsibility is often a significant source of moral distress for persons diagnosed with hereditary disease. The nurse in this example participated in a qualitative study on the social construction and clinical management of ADPKD (Cox and Starzomski 2004).[8]

ETHICS IN PRACTICE 24-1

Feeling Guilt-Ridden

There was one family that I spoke with and I remember how the woman was feeling quite guilt-ridden about knowing that one of her children was going to be experiencing what she was experiencing—having to come to the dialysis unit three times a week. It was very difficult for her. The whole issue around dialysis would have been easier for her to cope with if it was just her. But knowing that one of her children was actually in the process of realizing that their kidneys were starting to decline in function, I think it was becoming quite a difficult situation for her. We talked about it. This was a number of years ago, when I was working with her at the bedside and during the time when I was taking her off dialysis. I remember talking about her family and she went over the facts . . . her children all live back in Ontario. She didn't even have the opportunity to be close to them to support them because they were out of province. So I think there were a number of issues there for her, and you could see it was very painful for her. I mean her husband had passed away, she was in her late sixties, and it was so difficult. I think she had this huge feeling of responsibility on her shoulders.

As this example indicates, autosomal dominant[9] conditions (such as ADPKD and HD) impose a double burden. Patients must contend not only with their own symptoms and gradual loss of function, but also with the knowledge that their children may one day experience the same disease. Such knowledge may evoke profound feelings of responsibility, guilt, and shame (Cox and McKellin 1999).[10]

GENETICS AND COMPLEX DISORDERS: PSYCHIATRIC ILLNESS AS AN ILLUSTRATIVE EXAMPLE

Like most of the common health conditions (including diabetes, cancer, heart disease, asthma, arthritis), psychiatric disorders usually arise as a result of the combined effects of *both* genetic *and* environmental influences acting together (Thapar et al. 2007). Disorders that arise as a result of the combined effects of genes and environment are best conceptualized as "complex" or "multifactorial" disorders, rather than "genetic disorders" per se. Accordingly, although they certainly do aggregate, or "run in families," psychiatric disorders (and other common disorders like those listed above) are typically *not* inherited. Instead, it is a vulnerability to psychiatric disorders that is inherited. In the same way, the genetic variations that contribute to the development of psychiatric disorders are also best conceptualized as "vulnerability," "predisposition," or "susceptibility" genes rather than as genes that are "causative" of illness. As environmental influences contribute to the development of complex disorders, in general, genetic tests will not be able to predict with absolute certainty exactly who will and who will not develop them.

Although understanding cause of illness is important in many ways (as discussed in more detail below), historically, relatively little information about cause has been provided to individuals with psychiatric disorders and their family members. As a result, affected individuals and their family members generate explanations for the origins of illness that are based on their experiences. Often, these explanations involve roles for genes and environment, but the individual's understanding of the origin of illness is vague, uncertain, or inconsistent (Peay and Austin 2011). Interestingly, it seems that cognitively, people tend to understand genetic and environmental influences as quite separate entities, and developing a single, integrated causal explanation for illness that incorporates these two apparently disparate factors is difficult (Condit et al. 2009). Less frequently, individuals' existing causal explanations are certain and strongly held, but incorrect—for example, as illustrated in Ethics in Practice 24-2, some attribute their illness to "weak character" or "bad decisions" or "just genetics."

ETHICS IN PRACTICE 24-2

Schizophrenia and Genetics

I once talked with a woman who had been diagnosed with schizophrenia about the causes of her illness. At the time of our conversation she was an inpatient in a psychiatric ward, and was fighting with her psychiatrist about medications—she believed they wouldn't help, but he tried to persuade her to take them. She told me that she thought that "weak character and bad life decisions" caused her illness, and that she didn't need medications to get better, she just needed to try harder. I drew a family history based on information she gave me and showed her that both of her parents had experienced significant mental health problems themselves, and that it was very likely that she had inherited genetic vulnerability to mental illness from both of her parents. She broke down into tears as what she described as a huge weight of guilt lifted. Later, she told me that once she understood that the cause of her illness was in part genetic, then a biological treatment made more sense to her.

In the context of psychiatric disorders, correcting misunderstandings about the etiology of illness, or strengthening certainty in correct understanding, can have important implications for a person's sense of identity and management of illness. Specifically, with respect to identity, attributing illness to genetic factors alone can lead some individuals to adopt a fatalistic approach to their illness—that it was predetermined, and they have no power to influence their mental health. In these circumstances, facilitating an appreciation of the role of the environment may increase sense of control, hope for recovery, and ultimately self-esteem. Conversely, for individuals who attribute their illness to poor life decisions or weak character, facilitating an appreciation of the role of genetics in contributing to the development of their illness can mitigate self-blame.

With regard to issues related to management of illness, treatments make most sense to patients when they are congruent with their understanding of cause. For psychiatric disorders, the most efficacious treatment regimens involve invoking both psychotropic medications and psychosocial interventions. For individuals who attribute their psychiatric illness to poor life decisions (for example), a biological management strategy (taking psychotropic medications) is incongruent, and perhaps adherence will be problematic. Helping individuals to appreciate the role of genetic factors in contributing to development of illness may help them make sense of and buy in to the rationale for a biological treatment strategy. Helping those with no obvious family history to appreciate that genetics can still play an important role in illness causation rests on conveying the idea that having genetic vulnerability to psychiatric illness is not usually sufficient for an individual to experience illness. Environmental vulnerability factors are usually necessary for illness to manifest. Thus, even though no one else in the family may have appeared to be affected, it is likely that they had genetic vulnerability to psychiatric illness. (For nurses with interest in this area, see Peay and Austin 2011.)

PRACTICAL CHALLENGES AND OPPORTUNITIES FOR NURSING

The Canadian Nurses Association's Code of Ethics for Registered Nurses recognizes that genetic and other emergent technologies pose new challenges and opportunities for the ethical practice of nursing and medicine. A lack of basic knowledge about genetics and hereditary aspects of disease and disability is one challenge that nurses face. Other significant challenges include uncertainty about the most effective methods to convey complex information about genetic risk to patients and assist in promoting client-driven, ethically informed decision making (Jansen 2001). How can nurses begin to address these challenges and opportunities?

In assessing possible nursing roles in genetics, it is vital to distinguish between what is appropriate to expect of most nurses and what requires specific genetics training and education (see Exhibit 24-1). This means that there is both good and bad news in relation to nursing roles in genetics: The good news is that many of the skills that nurses should be prepared to use in relation to genetics, they are already using generally in day-to-day practice (e.g., empathy, clear communication). The bad news is that they may not realize how transferable these skills are to the domain of communication around genetics and (may) represent themselves as inadequate in these skills (Lashley 2000, 798).

A national survey conducted by the Health Canada Working Group on Public and Professional Educational Requirements Related to Genetic Testing of Late Onset Disease confirms that both nurses and physicians experience a lack of confidence with respect to competence in the provision of genetic services and, moreover, that this is often tied to a lack of specific knowledge about genetics (Bottorff et al. 2003).

In Ethics in Practice 24-3, a nephrology nurse reflects on her feelings of inadequacy when she imagines how she would respond if a patient asked about hereditary aspects of his or her condition.[11]

ETHICS IN PRACTICE 24-3

The Limits to Our Knowledge

We (nurses) would be of very little help to patients because we don't know much about hereditary aspects of disease. We don't know anything about genetic counselling so we would just be able to empathize. All we would be able to do is say "Oh" and "I know" and maybe send them back to their doctor. That is really all that we would be able to do. So other than just listening and trying to be supportive, we wouldn't be able to offer anything in particular, anything concrete if they were looking for that. We might talk about exercise, diet, those kinds of things. We can help them with lifestyle things but there is a limit to our knowledge, and certainly [to] our knowledge of genetic counselling! I remember in nursing school, 20 years ago, they would say "Huntington's is a genetic disease, so if you have it then chances are that your children will have it too." You know that's about as far as that went . . . [B]ut for us to delve into counselling about what that means for the child to grow up knowing their parent has Huntington's? Or maybe the grandparents died young, maybe nobody knew it was in the family, and now here it is, you have Huntington's at 43 *and* you've got two little kids?

The nurse in this example feels overwhelmed by the prospect of mastering a new and specialized area of knowledge. Although she is willing to empathize with patients' concerns and offer practical advice on lifestyle modifications, she is aware that she lacks basic knowledge about genetics. Recalling that her education about genetics was minimal, she recognizes that patients and families may need in-depth counselling to help them deal with the significant psychosocial and familial implications of hereditary risk. She also implies that because she is not equipped to offer this type of counselling, she has little to contribute to the delivery of genetic services. She may, however, be wrong in arriving at this conclusion.

Nurses already have many of the skills and abilities required to assist patients and families at risk for hereditary conditions. Nurses spend more hours interacting with patients than do most other health care providers. Further, nurses are often adept at deciphering complex medical information and communicating with patients in understandable language (Wright 2001). As such, nurses' "constant presence" (Weeks 1994)—whether at the bedside, in a community health clinic, or in the home—is an important contextual feature that must be factored into deliberations about how to integrate nursing with genetic services.

The nurse in Ethics in Practice 24-3 is an empathetic listener and clearly exercises moral sensitivity in imagining what it is like to grow up in a family affected by HD. She is aware of the limits of her own professional knowledge and recognizes that it might be appropriate to refer patients for specialized genetic counselling. Although there remains a need to provide nurses with specific genetics training and education, the skills and abilities she has already are important contributions to the delivery of genetic services.[12]

In Ethics in Practice 24-4, a social worker talks about her experiences in working with families with hereditary kidney disease. Like the nephrology nurse in Ethics in Practice 24-3, she acknowledges feelings of professional inadequacy in knowing how to respond to patients' fears.[13]

ETHICS IN PRACTICE 24-4

Being There

I don't know how to put this. Where some-times I feel at a little bit of a loss is with people who are having to deal with these major issues arising from genetic compo-nents of the disease and, you know, all the fears. Because the fears are real! Obviously you can't give false reassurance. But again it's like many other things in this job, you can't solve the problems, what you can do is be with the person as they're going through them and be as supportive as you can . . . I think social workers and many health care professionals feel inadequate in the face of the kinds of problems that patients have to deal with. You have to realize that you can't make it all better . . . But you can be there for people. I found again and again that you may think that you're doing nothing for a person, but you'll find later on that it's very important that you were there.

The social worker in this example does not want to offer false reassurance, nor does she want her clients to feel overwhelmed. She recognizes how important it is to be there *for* people, even if it is not possible to solve all of their problems. Providing accurate information and appropriate support is, in this sense, vital. As another social worker emphasized, families often operate on the basis of information that is out of date. Hence, their fears are sometimes based on unfounded concerns, and knowledgeable health care providers may be able to lay some worries to rest.

Nurses must not practise beyond their own level of competence, but when aspects of care demand the acquisition of new knowledge and skills, there is an ethical responsibility to seek out and employ such knowledge in their area of practice. Further, given that nurses have an ethical commitment to building trusting relations with patients and families, nurses also need to identify and respond to the range of issues that create moral distress for fami-lies affected by hereditary conditions (Canadian Nurses Association 2002).[14]

Nurses are well situated to play an important role in genetics within clinical and community, as well as research and educational, settings. Nurses can also do a lot to shift predominantly negative stereotypes of persons with physical and mental differences and to question the potentially eugenic uses of new genetic knowledge and techniques. Although there are many practical and theoretical challenges confronting nurses in these developing roles, there is also great potential for nurses to contribute to the humane and sensitive delivery of genetic services.

GENETIC COUNSELLING AND NURSES

As we saw above, one of the barriers to nurses engaging more fully with patients in issues around genetics relates to uncertainty about the most effective methods to convey complex information about genetic risk to patients and assist in promoting client-driven, ethically informed decision making (Jansen 2001). This is an area in which genetic counsellors excel, and in fact this constitutes the focus of their training. But, while there are specialist health care professionals—genetic counsellors—who exclusively engage in this activity, there are relatively few of them, and there is a need to develop a vision for how best to integrate genetic services within the existing health care system. Nurses are well positioned to play a key role in this endeavour, so in this section, we offer a genetic counselling perspective to provide a little insight for nurses as to how genetic counsellors approach these issues.

Genetic counselling as a specialist health care discipline is relatively new—master's-level training programs in genetic counselling have existed only since the 1970s, but there are several such programs in Canada as well as two organizations that offer professional certification for graduates. The term *genetic counselling* was first conceived of in the 1950s as "a kind of genetic social work without the eugenic connotations" (Reed 1955). In 2006, the largest professional organization for genetic counsellors, the National Society of Genetic Counsellors, defined genetic counselling as "a process of helping people understand and adapt to the medical, psychological and familial implications of genetic contributions to disease.

This process integrates the following:

- Interpretation of family and medical histories to assess the chance of disease occurrence or recurrence.

- Education about inheritance, testing, management, prevention, resources, and research.

- Counselling to promote informed choices and adaptation to the risk or condition" (Resta et al. 2006).

Fundamentally, whenever a "bad thing" happens (e.g., onset or diagnosis of a health condition), as human beings, we are driven to understand why, or what precipitated the negative event as we attempt to adjust to the new experience. Gaining this kind of understanding helps us make sense of the situation, allows us to gauge how much control we may have over future similar negative events and how we might manage the current situation, and ultimately helps us adapt (Godoy-Izquierdo et al. 2007). Our understanding of the cause also guides how we perceive strategies that are recommended for managing illness: treatment strategies make most sense when they are congruent with what we perceive to be the cause (Walter et al. 2004). Indeed, understanding the role of genetics in the development of a health condition can also affect an individual's sense of identity. Whereas one might anticipate that appreciation of the genetic etiology of a condition might result in a sense of "spoiled identity," it seems that if explored appropriately, this knowledge can actually contribute positively to the development of a revised sense of identity (Armstrong, Michie, and Marteau 1998). Genetic counselling aims to help with these issues.

It is important to explicitly address several common misconceptions about genetic counselling: first, it is not synonymous with genetic testing—the latter would always indicate genetic counselling, but genetic counselling does not necessitate genetic testing. Second, while genetic counselling is often traditionally associated with situations involving pregnancy and family planning, the definition above illustrates that the intervention can be applied meaningfully in a far broader range of circumstances than this. Last, genetic counselling is more than simply an educational intervention, rather it incorporates educational and supportive (counselling) aspects (McCarthy Veach et al. 2007), and embraces a stance whereby individual autonomy in decision making is promoted.

Not all nurses will be in roles where it is necessary or possible to engage in all of the components of genetic counselling described above, but all will undoubtedly encounter patients struggling to adapt, or to understand issues such as the cause of their condition and its implications for family members and the rationale for a particular treatment. These struggles may not be explicitly expressed, but almost all patients stand to potentially benefit from a discussion of these issues. It can be helpful for nurses to engage in an exploration of the patient's perception of cause of their condition, what that might mean for family members, and their feelings related to these issues. Often, for example, the explanations relating to cause of illness that individuals endorse evoke powerful emotions. Sometimes, these feelings are difficult to articulate, and helping patients identify them can facilitate the process of addressing and releasing them. For example, by helping patients appreciate that we cannot control which genes we pass on, it is possible to begin to address feelings of guilt or blame related to possibly having passed on "bad genes" to children. Similarly, causal explanations may underlie some behavioural responses to illness, like whether or not to take prescribed medications. For example, individuals who perceive their condition to be entirely attributable to non-biological factors (e.g., stress causing their heart disease) may find it difficult to rationalize the need for biological treatment, and not adhere to their medications. Sometimes exploring treatment non-adherence with patients can uncover beliefs such as this, exploring and addressing them could have important health implications.

Summary

In sum, the nature of the relationship between patient and nurse and the nurses' skill-set in terms of clear communication and empathy mean that in many ways, nurses are ideally positioned to take a leadership role in integrating genetics into the practice of professional health care. The main barrier to nurses integrating genetics into their daily practice relates to comfort level with the specific genetics-related knowledge. However, as we have seen, there is much that nurses can do to help their patients even without specific genetics knowledge. A nurse's awareness that for patients, understanding that genetics is important in the etiology of their conditions can potentially have a profound impact, and being willing to provide empathic support and referral to genetic counselling is already a significant contribution. For those nurses who wish to engage with these issues in a deeper and more comprehensive manner, more specialized genetics knowledge can be obtained through additional training, for which we provide some resources in Exhibit 24-2.

EXHIBIT 24-1

Biobanking

Biobanking has become a routine aspect of much biomedical science and research. Molecular advances typically require samples of tissue, body fluid, or other material that provides DNA/RNA, proteins, enzymes, etc. that can be used for diagnostic, therapeutic, and epidemiologic purposes. This allows researchers to link molecular and clinical or phenotypic information in the patient population. Biobanking is also done on a large scale with stratified random samples of the general public in order to amass a large database that can be studied by multiple groups for varying aims from basic research through clinical trials. The largest and most well known example is the UK Biobank, which has now surpassed half a million volunteers. The collection, storage, and use of biobanked materials raises many ethical, social, and legal issues that are of current importance to policymakers as well as researchers. The second edition of the Canadian Tri-Council Policy Statement (Canadian Institutes of Health Research et al. 2010) addresses many of the ethical issues related to research in the chapter on genetic research.

EXHIBIT 24-2

Resources for Nurses

Effective integration of nursing with genetic services will have curricular implications. There is a need for basic as well as more specialized education about genetics. For nurses who wish to enhance their confidence or skill set in the sorts of genetic counselling activities outlined in this chapter and engage in these issues in a deeper or more comprehensive fashion, the International Society for Nurses in Genetics (ISONG), and the Genetic Nurse Credentialing Commission offer resources. In particular, in conjunction with the American Nurses Association, ISONG produced a Statement on the Scope and Standards of Genetics Clinical Nursing Practice (1998) that reviews theories and ethical frameworks used in genetics nursing practice, the scope of basic and advanced genetics clinical nursing, and appropriate standards for professional performance. For nurses who have patients that they believe might benefit from a more in depth exploration of some of these issues, the Canadian Association of Genetic Counsellors (CAGC) and National Society of Genetic Counsellors (NSGC) both have websites that include listings of genetic counsellors, to whom referrals can be directed.

Website Resources

www.nchpeg.org

www.isong.org

www.geneticnurse.org

www.nsgc.org

www.cagc-accg.ca

www.humgen.org/int/geneinfo.cfm?&lang=1

www.ukbiobank.ac.uk/

www.pre.ethics.gc.ca/eng/

Book Resource

Uhlman, W., Schuette, J., and Yashar, B. 2009. *A guide to genetic counseling.* Hoboken, New Jersey: John Wiley and Sons, Inc.

For Reflection

1. What aspects of your nursing education and practice best equip you to assist patients and families coping with hereditary and/or genetic conditions? In what areas are you least equipped?

2. Would you want to take a genetic test revealing which conditions you are likely to develop later in life? If so, why? If not, why not? Are there some conditions that you would want to know about and others you would not? Are there some conditions that you have a responsibility to know about? Why or why not?

3. Imagine you are a prospective parent whose unborn child has just been diagnosed with trisomy 21 after amniocentesis. How would you want to be told this news? Would you wish the bearer of the news to say "I'm sorry but . . . " or take a less negative approach? Would a more neutral approach be insensitive to your feelings? What sorts of things would you most want to know about Down syndrome? Do you think it is possible for a health care provider to paint a picture of the condition that would universally be perceived to be "balanced"?

4. With many kinds of genetic testing, there is the potential for discovery of incidental findings (Kohane 2006) or information that was not expressly sought. Imagine the following scenario: You are a nurse or social worker caring for a family who has come to receive genetic test results related to cystic fibrosis. They have one child with cystic fibrosis and are considering having another child. They want to know the chances of the next child being similarly affected. The test results that you have been given clearly show that the woman's husband is not the father of their affected child. How would you approach this situation?

Endnotes

1. Mapping involves compilation of genetic linkage and physical maps indicating where an estimated 30 000 genes reside on each of the 23 pairs of human chromosomes. Sequencing, a separate but related activity, involves working out the precise order of nucleotide bases.

2. Eugenics is based on notions of racial purity and superiority and presumes that human attributes such as personality and intelligence are determined by heredity. Although eugenic thinking is most often associated with Adolf Hitler, the goals of eugenics derive from Francis Galton's (Galton, 1883) view that the governing classes should strive to control and improve the human gene pool.

3. Currently, there are tests for at least 960 genetic diseases. See the GeneTests website (www.genetests.org) for a listing of laboratories, clinics, genetics information, and educational materials.

4. Not all types of testing for hereditary or genetic conditions involve DNA analysis. For example, ultrasound is routinely used to diagnose autosomal dominant polycystic kidney disease.

5. Huntington disease (HD) is an autosomal dominant neuropsychiatric disorder. There is currently no effective prevention or cure. Onset typically occurs in mid-life, causing loss of control over voluntary movements and gradual but inexorable physical and cognitive decline (Hayden 1981).

6. Incomplete penetrance occurs where there is inconsistent phenotypic expression of a genetic variation or difference, even though the gene is present.

7. Autosomal dominant polycystic kidney disease (ADPKD) is one of the most common single-gene hereditary diseases. It typically presents in mid-life, causing progressive enlargement of the kidneys as normal tissue is replaced by fluid-filled cysts. In the absence of restorative treatment (i.e., dialysis or kidney transplant) the disease may cause renal failure and death (Qian et al. 2001).

8. The Social Construction and Clinical Management of the Hereditary Aspects of ADPKD (Principal Investigator: Rosalie C. Starzomski). Funded by the Kidney Foundation of Canada.

9. With autosomal dominant inheritance, all affected individuals have a 50 percent chance of passing the trait to each of their offspring. This is because only one copy of the variant allele is required for expression of the trait. Autosomal dominant conditions affect both women and men.

10. Autosomal recessive conditions, such as sickle cell disease, are experienced differently since gene carriers are usually unaffected by the condition.

11. Example is drawn from the study cited in endnote 9.

12. The National Coalition for Health Professional Education in Genetics is a non-profit organization that offers health professionals a range of educational resources on genetics. See the NCHPEG website: www.nchpeg.org.

13. Example is drawn from the study cited in endnote 9.

14. See also the position papers and fact sheets available through the Canadian Nurses Association website: www.cna-nurses.ca/pages/ethics/ethicsframe.htm.

References

Armstrong, D., Michie, S., and Marteau, T. 1998. Revealed identity: A study of the process of genetic counselling. *Social Science and Medicine, 47* (11), 1653–1658.

Baird, P.A. 2002. Identification of genetic susceptibility to common diseases: The case for regulation. *Perspectives in Biology and Medicine, 45* (4), 516–528.

Bloch, M., Fahy, M., Fox, S., and Hayden, M. 1989. Predictive testing for Huntington disease: Demographic characteristics, life-style patterns, attitudes, and psychological assessments of the first fifty-one test candidates. *American Journal of Medical Genetics, 32*, 217–224.

Bombard, Y., Veenstra, G., Friedman, J.M., Creighton, S., Currie, L., Paulsen, J.S., Bottorff, J.L., Hayden, M.R., Canadian Respond-HD Collaborative Research Group. 2009. Perceptions of genetic discrimination among people at risk for Huntington's disease: A cross-sectional survey. *British Medical Journal,* (Clinical research ed.), 338b, 2175.

Bottorff, J.L., Blaine, S., Carroll, J.C., Esplen, M.J., Evans, J., Nicolson Klimek, M.L., Meschino, W., and Ritvo, P. 2003. *The educational needs and professional roles of Canadian physicians and nurses regarding genetic testing and adult onset hereditary disease.* Unpublished report.

Bottorff, J.L., McCullum, M., Balneaves, L., Esplen, M.J., and Carroll, J. 2002. *Genetic services and adult onset hereditary diseases: Current and future nursing roles.* Ottawa: Canadian Institutes of Health Research.

Brock, D. 1994. The genome project and human identity. In R. Weir, S. Lawrence, and E. Fales (Eds.), *Genes and human self-knowledge: Historical and philosophical reflections on modern genetics* (pp. 18–33). Iowa City: University of Iowa Press.

Burgess, M.M. and d'Agincourt Canning, L. 2001. Genetic testing for hereditary disease: Attending to relational responsibility. *The Journal of Clinical Ethics, 12* (4), 361–372.

Canadian Nurses Association. 2002. *Code of ethics for registered nurses.* Ottawa: Canadian Nurses Association.

Caulfield, T.A., Burgess, M.M., Williams-Jones, B., Baily, M.A., Chadwick, R., Cho, M., Deber, R., Fleising, U., Flood, C., Friedman, J., Lank, R., Owen, T., and Sproule, J. 2001. Providing genetic testing through the private sector: A view from Canada. *Isuma, 2* (3), 72–81.

Canadian Institutes of Health Research, Natural Sciences and Engineering Research Council of Canada, and Social Sciences and Humanities Research Council of Canada. 2010. *Tri-Council policy statement: Ethical conduct for research involving humans.* (December).

Clayton, E.W. 2002. Bioethics of genetic testing. In *Encyclopedia of Life Sciences* (pp. 1–7). London: Macmillan Publishers Ltd.

Condit, C.M., Gronnvoll, M., Landau, J., Shen, L., Wright, L., Harris, T.M. 2009. Believing in both genetic determinism and behavioural action: A materialist framework and implications. *Public Understanding of Science, 18* (6), 730–746.

Cox, S.M. 2003. Stories in decisions: How at-risk individuals decide to request predictive testing for Huntington disease. *Qualitative Sociology, 26* (2), 257–280.

Cox, S.M. and McKellin, W.H. 1999. "There's this thing in our family": Predictive testing and the social construction of risk for Huntington disease. *Sociology of Health and Illness, 21* (5), 622–646.

Cox, S.M and Starzomski, R.C. 2004. Genes and geneticization? The social construction of auto-somal dominant polycystic kidney disease. *New Genetics and Society, 23* (2), 133–166.

Duster, T. 1990. *Backdoor to eugenics.* New York: Routledge.

Evans, J.P. Meslin, E.M, Marteau, T.M., and Caulfield, T. 2011. Deflating the genomic bubble. *Science, 1*, 8 February 2011, 861–862. [DOI:10.1126/science.1198039].

Feero, W.G., Guttmacher, A.E., and Collins, F.S. 2010. Genomic medicine: An updated primer. *New England Journal of Medicine, 362*, 2001–2011.

Galton, F. 1883. *Inquries into human faculty and its development.* London: Macmillan.

Garver, K.L. and Garver, B. 1994. The human genome project and eugenic concerns. *American Journal of Human Genetics, 54*, 148–158.

Godoy-Izquierdo, D., Lopez-Chicheri, I., Lopez-Torrecillas, F., Velez, M., and Godoy, J.F. 2007. Contents of lay illness models: Dimensions for physical and mental diseases and implications for health professionals. *Patient Education and Counseling, 67*, 196–213.

Gottlieb, L.N. 1998. The human genome project: Nursing must get on board. *Canadian Journal of Nursing Research, 30* (3), 3–4.

Guttmacher, A.E., Jenkins, J. and Uhlmann, W.R. 2001. Genomic medicine: Who will practice it? *American Journal of Medical Genetics, 106*, 216–222.

Hallowell, N., Statham, H., Murton, F., Green, J., and Richards, M. 1997. "Talking about chance": The presentation of risk information during genetic counseling for breast and ovarian cancer. *Journal of Genetic Counseling, 6* (3), 269–286.

Hayden, M. 1981. *Huntington's chorea.* Berlin: Springer-Verlag.

Hubbard, R. and Wald, E. 1993. *Exploding the gene myth: How genetic information is produced and manipulated by scientists, physicians, employers, insurance companies, educators, and law enforcers.* Boston: Beacon Press.

International Society of Nurses in Genetics. 1998. *Statement on the scope and standards of genetics clinical nursing practice.* Washington, DC: American Nurses Publishing.

Jansen, L.A. 2001. Role of the nurse in clinical genetics. In M.B. Mahowald, V.A. McKusick, A.S. Scheuerle, and T.J. Aspinwall (Eds.), *Genetics in the clinic: Clinical, ethical, and social implications for primary care* (pp. 133–141). St. Louis: Mosby.

Kenen, R. 1996. The at-risk health status and technology: A diagnostic invitation and the "gift" of knowing. *Social Science and Medicine, 42* (11), 1545–1553.

Kevles, D.J. and Hood, L. (Eds.). 1992. *The code of codes: Scientific and social issues in the human genome project.* Cambridge: Harvard University Press.

Khoury, M.J., Coates, R.J., and Evans, J.P. 2010. Evidence based classification of recommendations on use of genomic tests in clinical practice: dealing with insufficient evidence. *Genetics in Medicine,* (in press).

Kohane, I.S., Masys, D.R., and Altman, R.B. 2006. The incidentalome: A threat to genomic medicine. *Journal of the American Medical Association, 296* (2), 212–215.

Lashley, F.R. 2000. Genetics in nursing education. *Nursing Clinics of North America, 35* (3), 795–805.

Lewontin, R.C. 2000. *It ain't necessarily so: The dream of the human genome and other illusions.* New York: New York Review of Books.

Lippman, A. 1992. Led (astray) by genetic maps: The cartography of the human genome and health care. *Social Science and Medicine, 35* (12), 1469–1476.

Lippman, A. 1998. The politics of health: Geneticization versus health promotion. In S. Sherwin (Ed.), *The politics of women's health: Exploring agency and autonomy* (pp. 64–82). Philadelphia: Temple University Press.

Mccarthy Veach, P., Bartels, D.M., and LeRoy, B.S. 2007. Coming full circle: A reciprocal-engagement model of genetic counselling practice. *Journal of Genetic Counseling, 16* (6) 713–728.

McGuire, A.L. and Burke, W. 2010. Health system implications of direct-to-consumer personal genome testing. *Public Health Genomics,* (in press).

McLaren, A. 1990. *Our own master race: Eugenics in Canada, 1885–1945.* Toronto: McClelland & Stewart.

Peay, H.L. and Austin, J.C. 2011. *How to talk to families about genetics and psychiatric disorders.* New York. Wiley.

Quaid, K.A. and Morris, M. 1993. Reluctance to undergo predictive testing: The case of Huntington Disease. *American Journal of Medical Genetics, 45*, 41–45.

Reed, S. 1955. *Counseling in medical genetics.* Philadelphia: Saunders.

Resta, R., Bowles Biesecker, B., Bennett, R.L., Blum, S., Estabrooks-Hahn, S., Strecker, M.N., and Williams, J. L. 2006. A new definition of genetic counseling: National Society of Genetic Counselors' task force report. *Journal of Genetic Counseling, 15*, 77–83.

Silvers, A. 2001. Normality and functionality: A disability perspective. In M.B. Mahowald, V.A. McKusick, A.S. Scheuerle, and T.J. Aspinwall (Eds.), *Genetics in the clinic: Clinical, ethical, and social implications for primary care* (pp. 89–100). St. Louis: Mosby.

Smith, D.H., Quaid, K.A., Dworkin, R.B., Gramelspacher, G.P., Granbois, J.A., and Vance, G.H. 1998. *Early warning: Cases and ethical guidance for presymptomatic testing in genetic diseases*. Bloomington: Indiana University Press.

Thapar, A., Harold, G., Rice, F., Langley, K., and O'Donovan, M. 2007. The contribution of gene-environment interaction to psychopathology. *Development and Psychopathology, 19* (4). 989–1004.

Wade, C.H. and Wilfond, B.S. 2006. Ethical and clinical practice considerations for genetic counsellors related to direct-to-consumer marketing of genetic tests. *American Journal of Medical Genetics,* 142C, 284–292.

Walter, F.M., Emery, J., Braithwaite, D., and Marteau, T.M. 2004. Lay understanding of familial risk of common chronic diseases: A systematic review and synthesis of qualitative research. *Annals of Family Medicine, 2*, 583–594.

Weeks, S.L. 1994. From high-touch to high-tech: Hospital nursing and technological change. *Technology Studies, 1/2* (2), 153–174.

Wexler, N. 1990. *Presymptomatic testing for Huntington's disease: Harbinger of the new genetics.* Paper presented at Genetics, Ethics and Human Values: Human Genome Mapping, Genetic Screening and Gene Therapy, XXIVth Conference of CIOMS, Japan.

Wright, L. 2001. Documenting nursing expertise in genetics: Where are we going? *American Journal of Medical Genetics, 98*, 13–14.

CHAPTER 25

Neuroethics: An Emerging Field of Scholarship and Practice[1]

Eric Racine and Cynthia Forlini

[T]he ability to measure, intervene in, and alter the neural correlates of the mind raises important ethical questions. These questions are arguably weightier and more momentous than any set of questions in any other area of bioethics. This is because techniques that target the brain can reveal and directly affect the source of the mind and the deepest aspects of our selves: free will; personhood; personal identity through time; the relation between the mind and the body; the soul. (Glannon 2007, 4)

INTRODUCTION

Neuroethics is commonly considered a new field of contemporary bioethics that focuses on the ethics of neuroscience research and related clinical specialties such as neurology, neurosurgery, and psychiatry (Glannon 2007; Racine and Illes 2008; Wolpe 2004). Neuroethics addresses ethical concerns related to patients with mental health and neurological problems as well as emerging social and philosophical challenges created by advances in neuroscience and neurotechnology such as functional neuroimaging and deep brain stimulation (DBS) (Racine 2008). Nurses in advanced practice and other leadership positions need to understand this rapidly evolving field in order to join their colleagues in other disciplines as they grapple with how society *ought* to move forward in relation to neuroethics issues. The ramifications of neuroscience for research, patient care, and public health are diverse and far-reaching—and, as yet, are only beginning to be understood.

In this chapter, we first review definitions that are relevant for understanding the field of neuroethics. Second, we show how advances in neuroscience are creating ethical dilemmas at the bedside and beyond, all of which call for broader policy perspectives. Finally, we briefly discuss how neuroscientific perspectives on ethics, that is, the neuroscience of ethics, constitute a unique context of knowledge and inquiry.

PART ONE: DEFINITIONS OF AND PERSPECTIVES ON NEUROETHICS

Bioethics is a pluralistic field—pluralistic in terms of its definitions, background of its scholars and practitioners, as well as its future directions. The same holds true of neuroethics, which is in many respects a smaller and younger field. Yet, as we will sketch out in the following pages, the field of neuroethics has an interesting and pluralistic history, with many competing views of the field co-existing and suggesting different boundaries as well as, to some degree, different approaches to ethical challenges.

Harvard physician Anneliese A. Pontius was, to our knowledge, the first scholar to use the term neuroethics (actually "neuro-ethics") in print in the early 1970s (Pontius 1973). Interestingly, she used the term to condemn how certain interventions targeting young babies were both scientifically and ethically wrong. For example, at that time, interventions to accelerate walking in the first months of life were widely discussed and attracted public interest. She argued that these interventions were being attempted too early. They did not take into account that the physiology of babies was not supportive of walking. Therefore, interventions to speed up development could actually have detrimental long-term consequences and therefore constituted, in her eyes, unethical forms of experimentation (Pontius 1973). In her 1973 paper, she concluded with a call for more attention to "a new and neglected area of ethical concerns—neuro-ethics"; a general comment that some still think applicable to contemporary bioethics (Pontius 1973, 244). A few contemporary scholars have stressed that neuroethics could be valuable in bringing further attention to the challenges met by individuals, families, health care providers, and other stakeholders in the context of neurological and psychiatric care (Fins 2005; Racine 2010).

Another important scholar used the term neuroethics independently (and later the term "neuroethicist") in the 1980s. Ronald Cranford was an American neurologist who was extensively involved in discussions about ethics in neurological care at the American Academy of Neurology in particular (Bernat and Anderson 2006). In a paper published in 1989, Cranford discussed the ethical and legal cases in which the neurologist is often involved (e.g., anencephalic infants, brain death, acute brain injury, and dementia). He employed the terms "neuroethicist" or "neuroethics consultant" to designate "a neurologist who has taken a specific interest in bioethical issues and becomes an active member of [his] IEC [Institutional Ethics Committee] or becomes an individual consultant" (Cranford 1989, 700). Cranford concluded his paper by stating that, "[t]he neuroethicist, because he or she understands the neurologic facts and has extensive clinical experience in dealing with these neuroethical dilemmas at the bedside, serves in a significant educational and consultative capacity by clarifying the neurologic facts and integrating them with the ethical and legal issues" (Cranford 1989, 711).

It is unclear whether Pontius and Cranford intended for the eventual development of a distinct field of scholarship and practice dedicated to ethics in neuroscience and clinical care. However, they shared the conviction that knowledge of the inner workings of the brain, and health care related to the brain, evoke important ethical challenges that merited much more attention. The perception of a blind spot in mainstream bioethics fuelled a renewed interest in the ethical challenges of neuroscience in the early 2000s. Indeed, at a landmark conference held in 2002 in San Francisco supported by the Dana Foundation, the late *New York Times* columnist William Safire stated that the "specific ethics of brain science hits home as research on no other organ does" (Safire 2002, 6) The Dana Foundation, a private philanthropic organization that supports brain research and promotes public understanding of it, has since published several volumes dealing with neuroethics.

Shortly after the 2002 Dana Foundation meeting, philosopher Adina Roskies was one of the first to define the field of contemporary neuroethics (Roskies 2002). In "Neuroethics for the new millennium," a paper published in *Neuron,* Roskies argued that neuroethics was different from other areas of biomedical ethics because of "the intimate connection between our brains and our behaviours, as well as the peculiar relationship between our brains and our selves" (Roskies 2002, 21). Roskies also distinguished two parts of neuroethics: the *ethics of neuroscience* and the *neuroscience of ethics*. Although she acknowledged that "each of these can be pursued independently to a large extent," Roskies also stated, "most intriguing is to contemplate how progress in each will affect the other" (Roskies 2002, 21). Roskies parsed the *ethics of neuroscience* into two "divisions," that is, "the ethics of practice" and the "ethical implications of neuroscience." The neuroscience of ethics addresses fundamental concepts (e.g., free will, self-control, personal identity) and how neuroscience could change these concepts based on, for example, neuroimaging research (as discussed briefly in the third and last section of this chapter). Essentially, Roskies explains that, "[a]s we learn more about the neuroscientific basis of ethical reasoning and self-awareness, we may revise our ethical concepts" (Roskies 2002, 22). Because of its focus on the implications of neuroscience research on ethics itself, one of us has described Roskies' perspective as a *knowledge-driven perspective* (Racine 2010, 33).

Another early definition of neuroethics was provided by sociologist and bioethicist Paul Wolpe (2004) in the third edition of the *Encyclopedia of Bioethics*. In his entry, Wolpe described neuroethics as a "content field," in his words, a field "defined by the technologies it examines rather than any particular philosophical approach" (Wolpe 2004, 1894). Wolpe alluded to previous uses of the term in European neurology to discuss ethical challenges in brain disorders such as stroke or epilepsy, and to discuss ethical concerns in psychiatry, child development, and neuro-rehabilitation (Wolpe 2004). Wolpe's definition stressed that "[n]euroethics encompasses both research and clinical applications of neuro-technology, as well as social and policy issues attendant to their use" (Wolpe 2004, 1894). For Wolpe, the distinctive nature of the field derives from novel questions stemming from the application of neurotechnology because the brain is "the seat of personal identity and executive function in the human organism" (Wolpe 2004, 21) and this perspective can be labelled a *technologically driven perspective* (Racine 2010, 33).

Finally, one of us has proposed a distinct perspective on the field of neuroethics that is influenced both by a desire to integrate the pluralism inherent in neuroethics as well as influences from pragmatism (Racine 2010). As a theoretical approach, pragmatism stresses the interdisciplinary nature of ethics, the need for empirical research in ethics as well as the importance of social contexts in understanding and examining ethical behaviour (Racine 2010). According to this view, which can be labelled as a *pragmatic* or *health care–driven perspective,* the defining goal of neuroethics is to improve patient care and understanding for specific populations of neurological and psychiatric patients (Racine and Illes 2008; Racine 2010). One of the features of this definition is to consolidate some of the earlier historical meanings (e.g., Pontius and Cranford) focusing on clinical aspects with some of the contemporary views (e.g., Roskies, Wolpe) that emphasize the philosophical challenges posed by neuroscience as well as the ethical challenges of neurotechnology. Another distinct feature of this view is its description of neuroethics as both a scholarly and practical endeavour, akin to medicine, nursing, and other health care professions, which attempt to both understand and intervene. In summary, neuroethics is a new field defined by both scholarly and practical goals in order to meaningfully tackle challenges emerging in areas such as functional neuroimaging and deep brain stimulation (DBS).

PART TWO: FROM BENCH NEUROTECHNOLOGY TO BEDSIDE NEUROSCIENCE-BASED CARE

The reinvigoration of contemporary neuroethics has largely been due to the attention raised by advances in neuroscience research and neurotechnology. In the next pages, we review some of the key areas that raise important questions and have attracted the attention of scholars, clinicians, and policy makers. We focus on two areas: (1) research infunctional magnetic resonance imaging (fMRI) and (2) DBS.

Neuroimaging

Certainly, important strides have been made in the last decades with the combined insights of basic neurobiology and neurophysiology as well as other fields that approach brain function at a higher level of organization such as neuropsychology and cognitive neuroscience. However, we still lack a general understanding of brain function and what underlies the exquisite human capacity for language acquisition, fine motor behaviour, thought, and memory. In the last 20 years or so, many scholars, universities, and funding agencies have progressively come to consider the rise of advanced neuroimaging research to be a key avenue for the further development of neuroscience and our understanding of brain function. As we review this topic, it is important to understand the basic distinction between structural and functional neuroimaging modalities.

Structural neuroimaging techniques such as magnetic resonance imaging (MRI) and computed tomography (CT) scan have been around for longer than functional techniques and are well known in nursing and medicine for their diagnostic use in clinical care to detect structural anomalies. However, several more recent techniques have been grouped under the banner of functional neuroimaging since they examine—albeit indirectly—the activity of the brain (Racine and Illes 2007). These techniques currently underlie intense international research efforts in various major neurological and psychiatric conditions such as depression, schizophrenia, and attention deficit–hyperactivity disorder (Agarwal et al. 2010). For example, one of most ambitious studies is the Alzheimer's Disease Neuroimaging Initiative, led by American neuroscientists but also involving Canadian sites in Quebec, Alberta, and British Columbia (Mueller et al. 2005). The Alzheimer's Disease Neuroimaging Initiative is attempting to develop biomarkers of early onset Alzheimer's disease in elderly patients that can be detected by neuroimaging. Such developments in neuroscience have acted as a strong catalyst of hope for patients, families, and the general public (Bell et al. 2010; Kulynych 2002; Racine 2011). To date, health care billing codes for the clinical use of fMRI have been approved for the presurgical mapping of language and motor function but clinical translation in other areas awaits (Racine, Bell, and Illes 2010).

There is great enthusiasm for the clinical translation of functional neuroimaging to the bedside. Yet it is imperative to keep in mind that available functional neuroimaging techniques examine physiological processes that are *presumably* associated with brain activity. They fall short of enabling the imaging of neurons per se. To give a few examples, fMRI (at least its most common usage) relies on the measure of blood oxygenation level contrast; it enables detection of when oxygenated blood replaces deoxygenated blood in blood vessels. This measure presumes that the varying ratio of oxygenated and deoxygenated haemoglobin reflects neuronal activity. Blood oxygenation level contrast signal is thus a surrogate measure of brain activity. The same holds true of the commonly used electroencephalography (EEG), which captures electrical activity of the brain, and newer techniques like magnetoencephalography (MEG), which detects electromagnetic field changes related to neuronal activity. There are several other caveats that need to be kept in mind when contemplating the possible ethical use of these functional techniques in real world settings. Brain function measured in an artificial setting like the MRI scanner may be different than brain activity occurring in a natural setting due to potentially distinct underlying cognitive processes. For example, functional neuroimaging techniques typically rely on the comparison of (1) brain activity in a "resting state", where subjects do not engage in any active task, to (2) brain activity measured during the performance of a task (Bell and Racine 2009). Again, this qualification is important to consider since the selection of a task will depend on a study design where the objective is to capture only one part of a cognitive function or a pathological process. Although these nuances do not take away (nor should they) all the clinical interest in functional neuroimaging, they do bring to light other important points to consider in the common depiction of these devices as techniques that yield direct pictures of the brain at work or reveal the true essence of who we are because of a presumed incontestable accuracy and reliability (see Exhibit 25-1). These emerging interpretations take the distinctive shapes of *neuro-essentialism* (the belief that we are basically our brains, our self-identity lies in our brains) and *neuro-realism* (the belief that functional neuroimaging techniques provide direct pictures of the brain at work).

Popular over-interpretations of functional neuroimaging techniques create expectations in the public, patients, and families in terms of diagnostic capability. Further, the sale (mostly in the United States of America) of neuroimaging services (mostly structural but also functional) directly to consumers without medical consultation or referral builds on such expectations that promote interest in such techniques (Racine and Illes 2008; Racine, Van der Loos, and Illes 2007). Over-confidence in functional neuroimaging and other areas of neuroscience could bring unnecessary or unwelcome support to biological approaches in psychiatry. These approaches are not inherently wrong but there is a heavy reliance on biological models that may leave little room for cognitive and psychosocial interventions in nursing and other fields.

EXHIBIT 25-1

Emerging Over-interpretations of Functional Neuroimaging

Developments in functional neuroimaging, especially fMRI, have had an effect on patients, families, and the general public as progress in these conditions often comes as a strong catalyst of hope. Together with colleagues, we have discovered that these

emerging interpretations take distinctive shapes in the media and elsewhere in society (Racine, Bar-Ilan, and Illes 2005; Racine et al. 2010).

Neuro-essentialism: designates interpretations that the brain is the self-defining essence of a person, a secular equivalent to the soul (Racine, Bar-Ilan, and Illes 2005). Neuro-essentialism describes that the concept of the brain becomes shorthand for other concepts (e.g., the person, the self) that may serve to express features of the individual not ordinarily found in the concept of the brain. For example, the claim is made that "[w]ith more powerful imaging devices and new genetic information, scientists are exploring the secrets of the organ that makes humans unique" (Colburn 1999, Z12).

Neuro-realism: designates interpretations that neuroimaging research yields direct data on brain function despite the complexities of data acquisition and image processing involved (Racine, Bar-Ilan, and Illes 2005). Observed brain activation patterns are, as a result, portrayed as the ultimate proof that a phenomenon is real, objective, and effective (e.g., in the case of health interventions such as hypnosis and acupuncture). For example, "Reading the brain: New imaging technique lets doctors see inside, but some question how it is used" (Blakeslee 2000, C1).

Neuro-policy: indicates that the rapid transfer of neuroscience research is particularly appealing when neuroscience is described in neuro-essentialist and neuro-realist ways (Racine, Bar-Ilan, and Illes 2005). For example, a media report of neuroscience research on adolescent brains stated "These research findings have profound implications for policy-makers, teachers, parents and, most of all, for teenagers" (Johnstone 2004, 2).

Overall, these interpretations could shape expectations of patients and family members and distort their understanding of the true clinical capabilities of functional neuroimaging. Further research in psychology suggests that the simple presence of neuroimaging data leads non-experts to give greater value to scientific explanations (Weisberg et al. 2008).

Functional neuroimaging research has targeted an increasing number of neurological and psychiatric conditions, creating ethical challenges in current research and potential clinical uses. These ethical challenges will likely be further shaped by the contexts—be they research or clinical—in which the technologies are introduced. In addition to the challenges of clinical uses, functional neuroimaging has expanded beyond the borders of clinical neuroscience. A whole range of fascinating studies have now examined brain activity in relationship to personality traits (Kramer et al. 2007; Raine and Yang 2006), gender differences (Harenski et al. 2008), as well as processes such as decision making (Sommer et al. 2010), deception (Hayashi et al. 2010), perceptions of race (Lieberman et al. 2005), and sexual stimuli. This line of research, sometimes associated with the field of "social neuroscience," brings forth a range of possible uses both intriguing and controversial (Illes, Kirschen, and Gabrieli 2003). For example, research on cognition and emotion related to sexuality could lead to better rehabilitative treatments for emotional or affective disorders and at the same time raises questions about how far we should go with this research.

Neuroscience research could be used in non-clinical ways to gain insights into the mind for nefarious purposes (Moreno 2006). To date, we access each others' thoughts and feelings through the mediation of senses like vision and hearing and the ability to understand speech and gestures. Functional neuroimaging studies constantly bring up the prospect of accessing someone's intimate thoughts and emotions directly through the examination of brain function rather than via traditional human communication. This is well exemplified in the case of fMRI in disorders of consciousness where ground-breaking results suggest that a small minority of patients diagnosed as being in a vegetative state and a minimally conscious state could communicate their thoughts through fMRI (see Exhibit 25-2). More controversial scenarios surface in the use of functional neuroimaging in marketing research (Plassman 2007), lie detection (Giridharadas 2008), and moral decision making (see Exhibit 25-3 below). Stakeholder groups have reacted vehemently against the use of these techniques to develop more effective marketing strategies, while American courts have recently determined that fMRI is not reliable enough to be used as a lie-detection device (Madriga 2010a; 2010b). Both in clinical and non-clinical domains, the prospect of "mind reading" seems far away but the sheer possibility of establishing communication with vegetative patients is bringing novel perspectives on this patient population.

EXHIBIT 25-2

Reading Brains and Minds? Functional Magnetic Resonance Imaging (fMRI) Research in the Vegetative State and the Minimally Conscious State

In 2006, Adrian Owen and his research group in the United Kingdom published a paper in *Science* suggesting that a patient diagnosed with a vegetative state showed signs of awareness. Owen and colleagues examined brain function of a 23-year-old female vegetative patient who suffered a car accident. They then presented this patient with some mental imagery tasks such as imagining playing tennis and navigating in her house. They found that her brain activation patterns were comparable to a normal healthy individual imagining the same situations (Owen et al. 2006). Owen and colleagues concluded that "[t]hese results confirm that, despite fulfilling the clinical criteria for a diagnosis of VS, this patient retained the ability to understand spoken commands and to respond to them

through her brain activity, rather than through speech or movement" (Owen et al. 2006, 1402). In their view, this "confirmed beyond any doubt that she was consciously aware of herself and her surroundings" (Owen et al. 2006, 1402), a very controversial conclusion given standard views on the vegetative state (Royal College of Physicians 2003; The Multi-Society Task Force on PVS 1994a; 1994b). The researchers envisioned that such patients could perhaps eventually use their "residual cognitive capabilities to communicate their thoughts to those around them by modulating their own neural activity" (Owen et al. 2006, 1402). Needless to say, Owen and colleagues' paper sparked considerable discussion and debate in the scientific and public domains.

Another important issue that fMRI research has brought attention to is called "incidental findings," (Illes 2008). Incidental findings have been defined as "observations of potential clinical significance unexpectedly discovered in healthy subjects or in patients recruited to brain imaging research studies and unrelated to the purpose or variables of the study" (Illes et al. 2006, 783).

Since then, the topic of incidental findings has been introduced in the second edition of the *Tri-council policy statement: Ethical conduct for research involving humans*

(TCPS) (2010) in Canada (www.pre.ethics.gc.ca). Some of the major underlying questions raised by this issue involve: (1) clarifying who bears responsibility for establishing the clinical significance of an incidental finding; (2) how the finding will be reported to the research subject who is not necessarily a patient of the team members; (3) if ethical responsibilities of clinicians and non-clinicians as well as trainees such as graduate students would differ; and (4) what kind of support should be offered following disclosure of a clinically significant incidental finding. Some of the most recent and comprehensive guidelines agree on the obligation to inform research subjects about the potential discovery and to have a plan in place to deal with incidental findings (Illes et al. 2008; Wolf et al. 2008). This line of thinking is also captured in Article 3.4 of the second edition of the TCPS (2010) stating that "researchers have an obligation to disclose to the participant any material incidental findings discovered in the course of research" (34). The new article sets the requirement for a plan to be in place to handle incidental findings and also suggests different forms of consultation with peers and research ethics boards (REBs) to deal with these findings.

Deep Brain Stimulation (DBS)

Perhaps even more surprising than the evolution of functional neuroimaging techniques is the development of DBS and other forms of neurostimulation. DBS typically involves the implantation of at least one electrode, typically in thalamic, sub-thalamic, or the globus pallidus regions. The electrodes are connected through very small wires (leads) to an implanted pulse generator in the upper portion of the chest. DBS was approved by the United States Food and Drug Administration in 1997 for the treatment of essential tremors and in 2002 was more widely approved for the management of refractory Parkinson's disease. DBS is used for the same indications in Canada (OHTAC 2005).

DBS is now a common therapy for Parkinson's disease and essential tremors patients whose disease is severe and drug refractory (Greenberg 2002). Seemingly, over 35 000 patients worldwide have received DBS for those indications (Kuehn 2007). The current scientific and medical knowledge surrounding the mechanism of action of DBS is still incomplete but a widespread hypothesis is that DBS replicates the effects of neurosurgical lesioning (Benabid 2007). The technique changes brain function, it is believed, by disrupting the abnormal functioning of neural circuitry. However, in contrast to ablative neurosurgery, DBS is generally considered reversible and non-destructive (Larson 2008) although DBS may have some irreversible short-term (e.g., haemorrhage) and long-term effects (e.g., reshaping synaptic connectivity).

DBS is currently being investigated as an experimental treatment for some neuropsychiatric disorders in Canada and internationally. These disorders include severe refractory cases of major depressive disorder; Tourette's syndrome; obsessive-compulsive disorder; chronic pain; multiple sclerosis; and Alzheimer's disease (Kopell, Greenberg, and Rezai 2004; Hamani et al. 2008; Huff et al. 2010). There is an emerging literature documenting the promises of DBS in treating these disorders (Benabid 2007). Interestingly, case reports of DBS to treat a generalized anxiety disorder (Kuehn 2007) and obesity (Hamani et al. 2008) have led to unexpected results of relief of co-morbid alcohol dependence and memory enhancement respectively (without any effects on the anxiety disorder or the obesity). A recent working group proposed a series of recommendations to tackle ethics in the field of neuropsychiatry focusing on the design of clinical trials as well as the protection of human participants in DBS studies (Rabins et al. 2009).[2]

With the possible extension of DBS to neuropsychiatry, costs and resource allocation could become major issues. The costs of DBS devices and procedures for Parkinsonism run to several tens of thousands of dollars (approximately $50 000 for the implant; not including the expensive batteries that need to be replaced after a few years) (Fraix et al. 2006). Clearly, the costs may create significant challenges for patients, providers, and publicly funded health care services.

Obtaining consent for last-resort innovative interventions is another area of ethical significance given the enthusiastic media response to DBS in Parkinson's disease. A study of United States and United Kingdom media coverage of neuro-stimulation found increasing coverage and marked enthusiasm for the clinical translation of DBS, with many articles featuring "miracle stories" where patients were "literally cured" (Racine et al. 2007). Ethical issues of DBS have been acknowledged and are starting to be discussed by leaders in the field of DBS neurosurgery (Benabid 2007) and neurosurgical ethics (Fins 2000; Fins, Rezai, and Greenberg 2006; Kubu and Ford 2007).

PART THREE: NEUROSCIENCE OF ETHICS

One of the most intriguing and distinctive features of neuroethics is that it potentially incorporates a feedback loop between ethics and neuroscience, that is, a "neuroscience of ethics" (Roskies 2002). By this term, different authors have claimed that neuroscience will change our way of approaching ethical concepts and social behaviour because of the scientific perspectives yielded by neuroscience. Accordingly, neuroscience would provide powerful insights into the mechanisms underlying moral reasoning, co-operative behaviour, and emotional processes such as empathy. Illustrative of this, neuroscientist Michael Gazzaniga (2005, xv) writes in his book *The Ethical Brain,* that, "neuroethics is more than just bioethics for the brain. (. . .) It is—or should be—an effort to come up with a brain-based philosophy of life." Nonetheless, the neuroscience of ethics is not necessarily viewed unanimously or without controversy as an area of neuroethics and bioethics scholarship.

Where does the excitement of some ethicists, philosophers, and neuroscientists for the neuroscience of ethics come from? Why is neuroscience invested with such powerful promises to reveal the nature of ethics and of who we are? This enthusiasm is likely due, in part, to the symbolic importance of the brain as an organ that sustains crucial vital physiological functions (e.g., breathing) as well as the most complex cognitive processes (e.g., decision making, memory, language). In addition, a rising number of studies have tapped into these questions. Illustrative papers include recent articles on neural mechanisms of moral sensitivity (Harenski et al. 2008; Robertson et al. 2007) and functional neuroimaging of the evaluation of guilt and embarrassment (Takahashi et al. 2004). One landmark study (see Exhibit 25-3) examined how moral dilemmas differ in their level of emotional and personal engagement. Although the study has been criticized for different reasons, it remains an epigone of the type of research and related insights yielded by this area of research.

EXHIBIT 25-3

Case Example of a Landmark Neuroscience of Ethics Study

In a landmark fMRI study conducted at Princeton University, Joshua Greene and his collaborators examined neuronal activation in a series of ethical scenarios. They used the example of the trolley problem well known by philosopher-ethicists to illustrate how traditional moral theories poorly capture the complexity of actual moral reasoning.

Briefly, the trolley problem features a runaway trolley that will, if let free to pursue its course, kill five individuals. However, if a switch is activated to change the tracks on which the trolley is running, it will kill one individual instead of the five on the first set of tracks. Generally, most respondents would think it is ethically acceptable to activate the switch if this is the only means by which the five individuals can be saved. However, in the footbridge dilemma, a variant of the trolley scenario, one has a choice between allowing the trolley to kill the five individuals on the track or push an innocent bystander from a bridge onto the track to stop the trolley and save the five individuals. In this case, most would hesitate and say that this is not ethically acceptable.

From a theoretical perspective, it is difficult to understand why responses would differ based on traditional ethical theories (e.g., utilitarian or deontological). Greene et al. found that these dilemmas varied systematically in the extent to which they engaged emotional processing and that these variations in emotional engagement influenced moral judgment in ways that are ill-captured by conventional moral theories (Greene et al. 2001). Because the study suggested that differences in moral reasoning can be caused by the different level of emotional and personal engagement in ethical dilemmas, it brought another explanatory perspective on divergences between moral constructs. The study brings self-reflection on why we can disagree about moral dilemmas and emphasized the embodied nature of some of our ethical judgments (Greene et al. 2001).

Other researchers in the area of neuroscience of ethics hope to shed light on long-standing disputes with respect to the nature of moral reasoning and moral decision making. For example, Farah and Heberlein asked if current neuroscience informs how we define personhood and if neuroscience could help establish criteria distinguishing between persons and non-persons. The distinction between persons and non-persons is often at the root of controversial bioethics discussions (e.g., moral status of the fetus and embryo, diagnosis of disorders of consciousness, determination of death). Farah and Heberlein (2007) reviewed the neuroscience literature and found that recent studies in cognitive neuroscience point to separate systems in the brain for processing persons as being distinct from other objects, pointing to a specialized neurocognitive system for person recognition. This innate system, argue the authors, could be tricked by ambiguous categories and therefore explain cognitive hurdles in defining personhood. Our hard wiring would create trouble when we try to explicitly define borderline cases of persons and non-persons. They suggest that personhood "is a kind of illusion" (Farah and Heberlein 2007, 45) and according to them, "[r]ather than ask whether someone or something is a person, we should ask how much capacity exists for enjoying the kinds of psychological traits previously discussed (e.g., intelligence, self-awareness) and what are the consequent interests of the being" (Farah and Heberlein 2007, 46).

Other neuroscience findings have provoked discussions on the nature of moral reasoning. Neurologists Paul Eslinger and Antonio Damasio encountered in their practice a patient who after having suffered a lesion to the orbito-frontal cortex could not conduct himself in socially and ethically acceptable ways (Eslinger and Damasio, 1985). Damasio has hypothesized that "somatic markers"—markers that evaluate the emotional bodily feeling of making decisions—are absent in this patient, which leads to a form of callousness and inappropriate behaviour. Damasio has argued that emotions are key in rational decision making, contrary to rationalist claims (Damasio 1994). If Damasio is right, does this fundamentally change current views about moral decision making? Many other questions come up in trying to sort the findings of Greene cited above and the findings made earlier by Damasio within a more comprehensive neuroscience of moral decision making.

In spite of the enthusiasm for and the fascinating aspects of the neuroscience of ethics, several questions remain. First, questions about how ethics can be examined from a neuroscience standpoint bring forth a wide set of epistemological issues. For example, how do the descriptions of moral concepts like personhood really fit the understanding that neuroscientists have of persons when conducting their neuroscience studies? Does the content of the concept overlap significantly enough to ensure that different disciplines are talking about the same things? Also, given that ethics is normative, that is, concerned with value judgments, how does a descriptive discipline contribute to make our value judgments evolve? And what are the risks involved in the potential sway that neuroscience explanations can have on the public's understanding of social behaviour and cognitive phenomena?

Second, the possible implications of this field are rife with speculation. For example, literature on moral psychology in health care has suggested that nurses differ in the forms of moral reasoning they employ in comparison to physicians (Robertson 1996). One hypothesis, inspired by the neuroscience of ethics, would be that the sustained relationships that nurses engage in with their patients, in contrast to physicians, directs their moral reasoning differently than physicians who are more distanced from the daily lives and struggles of patients. The effect of being at the bedside could shape a different moral psychology because the experience of this kind of relationship activates different brain systems. What would be the implications of such observations? Would the insights help us make more sense of our personal and professional differences? Would they change how we approach multidisciplinary team work and collective discussions on difficult clinical cases? Would they command changes to how difficult ethical dilemmas are dealt with?

The emergence of the neuroscience of ethics raises questions regarding the nature of ethics (e.g., is ethics only a matter of understanding neuronal networks involved in decision making?) and the potential meaningful input of neuroscience on ethics (e.g., will this change how ethics is applied in clinical practice or how ethics is taught?). It also brings about questions concerning the potential dangers and risks of such research given the potential for misuse and misunderstanding. It is far too soon for those involved in the neuroscience of ethics to answer all these questions. Nonetheless, the neuroscience of ethics could help us to reflect on the implicit and automatic ways we have of framing ethical problems and of trying to resolve them. Further, this area is prompting discussions about the impact of neuroscience on humanity, society, and human behaviours as well as about the areas of scholarship traditionally dedicated to understanding these aspects of human life (the humanities, social science, and ethics). At the same time, we need to proceed with caution, given significant conceptual fallacies plaguing the integration of neuroscience research into ethics (Racine 2007; 2010). The risks of overly objective medicine are great and should not be minimized. Indeed part of the role of bioethics is to help voice the concerns of persons and ensure that they are respected as persons and not simply as biological systems (Andre 2002).

Summary

In this chapter, we provided an overview of the field of neuroethics by highlighting first how this burgeoning new field has interesting historical precedent. Even in the early development of neuroethics, different definitions have been proposed and different perspectives are leading to diverging research and policy programs on an international scale. Second, we presented and discussed three areas where neuroscience advances—and in particular technological developments—have led to new avenues for understanding brain function with functional neuroimaging, treating neurological and neuropsychiatric disorders (with DBS). Third and last, we discussed how neuroethics also includes a potential contribution of neuroscience research to shed light on the nature of ethics itself, that is, the neuroscience of ethics. Altogether this intriguing area of research promises to change how we view ethics or, at the minimum, bring new ways of framing older questions to the forefront of biomedical and nursing ethics.

At the outset, several questions are raised by recent advances in neuroscience and call for greater reflection from different stakeholders, including clinicians, scholars, and public stakeholders. The following case (Ethics in Practice 25-1) provides an opportunity for further reflection on different aspects of neuroethics and neuroscience raised in this chapter. Neuroethics is an exciting and challenging new field. None of us—whether we come from ethics, nursing, law, medicine, neuroscience, or other related disciplines—are ready to answer all the questions we have raised above. Nurses as individuals, and the nursing profession as a whole, should join others calling for thoughtful progress to benefit the health and well-being of individuals, families, communities, and society as a whole within the field of neuroethics.

ETHICS IN PRACTICE 25-1[3]

Tackling Neuroethics in Daily Practice

Jana Czernowski is a clinical nurse specialist in a neurological centre in a major teaching hospital. As part of her role she provides teaching and counseling support for patients and families dealing with complex chronic and acute neurological disorders, and she develops regular continuing education programs for nurses, rehabilitation professionals, and social workers. She also works closely with a team of neurologists, neurosurgeons, and neuroscientists who are engaged in an active program of research and clinical innovation.

Jana has been in her role for four and a half years. Over the past two years she has seen a rapid and dramatic acceleration of new therapies, including deep brain stimulation for patients with intractable seizures, and neuro-imaging to evaluate the effectiveness of pharmacotherapeutics. Jana finds the pace of change she is witnessing difficult to keep up with, particularly in trying to develop guidelines for safe clinical practice and for teaching staff, patients, and their families about the health implications of the new therapies. She is excited about the potential benefits of most of what she sees, but she wonders about the ethics of proceeding with treatments that patients, families, and many staff may not fully understand. She also wonders how she can keep herself current in her field of specialization, and how she can mentor other potential nurse leaders in the field.

For Reflection

1. What measures can Jana take to keep herself current in the fields of neuroscience and neuroethics?

2. How might Jana work to foster interprofessional collaboration between the diverse caregivers, professionals, and researchers in her centre?

3. What are the challenges in informed consent for patients and families undergoing new neuroscience procedures given the hope and expectations they may generate?

4. What approaches to patient and family teaching could Jana cultivate?

5. In what ways could Jana mentor nurses and other caregivers/professionals to increase their expertise in neuroscience and neuroethics?

6. How can specialty groups in nursing (such as the Canadian Association of Neuroscience Nurses) and ethics (such as the Canadian Bioethics Society) contribute to knowledge development in neuroscience and neuroethics?

7. What are some policy implications for provincial nursing associations? For the Canadian Nurses Association?

Endnotes

1. **Acknowledgments:** Our sincere thanks to the editors of this volume for exemplary constructive feedback on a previous version of this chapter. Support for the writing of this chapter comes from a New Investigator Award (E.R) from the Canadian Institutes of Health Research (E.R., States of Mind Network and New Investigator Award) from the Social Sciences and Humanities Research Council of Canada (E.R.) and a doctoral scholarship from the Fonds de la recherche en santé du Québec (C.F.) This chapter is based partly on material published in Eric Racine. 2010. *Pragmatic neuroethics: Improving understanding and treatment of the mind–brain*. Cambridge, MA: MIT Press.

2. See Rabins et al. 2009 for a summary of key recommendations from a working group on scientific and ethical issues in the application of deep brain stimulation in the treatment of mood and behavioural disorders.

3. This case was kindly contributed by Dr. Patricia Rodney.

References

Agarwal, N., Port, J.D., Bazzocchi, M., and Renshaw, P.F. 2010. Update on the use of MR for assessment and diagnosis of psychiatric diseases. *Radiology, 255* (1), 23–41.

Andre, J. 2002. Bioethics as a practice. In A.M. Brandt and L. R. Churchill (Eds.), *Studies in Social Medicine*. Chapel Hill and London: The University of North Carolina Press.

Bell, E., Maxwell, B., MacAndrews, M.P., Sadikot, A., and Racine, E. 2010. Hope and patient expectation in deep brain stimulation: Healthcare provider perspectives and approaches. *Journal of Clinical Ethics, 21* (2), 112–124.

Bell, E. and Racine, E. 2009. Enthusiasm for fMRI often overlooks its dependence on task selection and performance. *American Journal of Bioethics, 9* (1), 3–13.

Benabid, A.L. 2007. What the future holds for deep brain stimulation. *Expert Review of Medical Devices, 4* (6), 895–903.

Bernat, J.L. and Anderson, D.C. 2006. Ronald E. Cranford, MD (1940–2006). *Neurology, 67,* 1338–1339.

Blakeslee, S. 2000, March 20. Reading the brain: New imaging technique lets doctors see inside, but some question how it is used. *Plain Dealer,* p. 1F.

Brendel, D.H. 2006. *Healing psychiatry: Bridging the science/humanism divide.* Cambridge, MA: MIT Press.

Colburn, D. 1999, September 28. The infinite brain: People used to think the brain was static and inevitably declined with age. Actually, the brain never stops changing—and we never stop learning. *The Washington Post,* p. Z12.

Cranford, R.E. 1989. The neurologist as ethics consultant and as a member of the institutional ethics committee. *Neurologic Clinics, 7* (4), 697–713.

Damasio, A.R. 1994. *Descartes' error.* New Jersey, NJ: Penguin Putnam Publishers.

Downie, J. and Marshall, J. 2007. Pediatric neuroimaging ethics. *Cambridge Quarterly of Healthcare Ethics, 16* (2), 147–160.

Editorial. 2004. Brain scam? *Nature Neuroscience, 7* (7), 683.

Eslinger, P.J. and Damasio, A.R. 1985. Severe disturbance of higher cognition after bilateral frontal lobe ablation: Patient EVR. *Neurology, 35,* 1731–1741.

Farah, M.J. and Heberlein, A.S. 2007. Personhood and neuroscience: Naturalizing or nihilating? *American Journal of Bioethics, 7* (1), 37–48.

Farah, M.J. and Wolpe, P.R. 2004. Monitoring and manipulating brain function: New neuroscience technologies and their ethical implications. *Hastings Center Report, 34* (3), 35–45.

Fins, J.J. 2000. A proposed ethical framework for international cognitive neuroscience: A consideration of deep brain stimulation in impaired consciousness. *Neurological Research, 22,* 273–278.

Fins, J.J. 2005. Clinical pragmatism and the care of brain damaged patients: Toward a palliative neuroethics for disorders of consciousness. *Progress in Brain Research, 150,* 565–582.

Fins, J.J., Rezai, A.R., and Greenberg, B.D. 2006. Psychosurgery: Avoiding an ethical redux while advancing a therapeutic future. *Neurosurgery, 59* (4), 713–716.

Fraix, V., Houeto, J.L., Lagrange, C., Le Pen, C., Krystkowiak, P., Guehl, D., Ardouin, C., Welter, M.L., Maurel, F., Defebvre, L., Rougier, A., Benabid, A.L., Mesnage, V., Ligier, M., Blond, S., Burbaud, P., Bioulac, B., Destee, A., Cornu, P., and Pollak. P. 2006. Clinical and economic results of bilateral subthalamic nucleus stimulation in Parkinson's disease. *Journal of Neurology, Neurosurgery, and Psychiatry, 77* (4), 443–449.

Gazzaniga, M.S. 2005. *The ethical brain.* New York/Washington, DC: Dana Press.

Giridharadas, A. 2008, September 14. India's novel use of brain scans in courts is debated. *The New York Times,* p. A10.

Glannon, W. 2007. *Bioethics and the brain.* New York, NY: Oxford University Press.

Greenberg, B.D. 2002. Update on deep brain stimulation. *The Journal of ECT, 18* (4), 193–196.

Greene, J.D., Sommerville, R.B., Nystrom, L.E., Darley, J.M., and Cohen, J.D. 2001. An fMRI investigation of emotional engagement in moral judgment. *Science, 293* (5537), 2105–2108.

Hamani, C., McAndrews, M.P., Cohn, M., Oh, M., Zumsteg, D., Shapiro, C.M., Wennberg, R.A., and Lozano, A.M. 2008. Memory enhancement induced by hypothalamic/fornix deep brain stimulation. *Annals of Neurology, 63* (1), 119–123.

Harenski, C.L., Antonenko, O., Shane, M.S., and Kiehl, K.A. 2008. Gender differences in neural mechanisms underlying moral sensitivity. *Social Cognitive and Affective Neuroscience, 3* (4), 313–321.

Hayashi, A., Abe, N., Ueno, A., Shigemune, Y., Mori, E., Tashiro, M., and Fujii, T. 2010. Neural correlates of forgiveness for moral transgressions involving deception. *Brain Research, 1332,* 90–99.

Huff, W., Lenartz, D., Schormann, M., Lee, S.H., Kuhn, J., Koulousakis, A., Mai, J., Daumann, J., Maarouf, M., Klosterkotter, J., and Sturm, V. 2010. Unilateral deep brain stimulation of the nucleus accumbens in patients with treatment-resistant obsessive-compulsive disorder: Outcomes after one year. *Clinical Neurology & Neurosurgery, 112* (2), 137–143.

Illes, J., Kirschen, M.P., Edwards, E., Bandettini, P., Cho, M.K., Ford, P.J., Glover, G.H., Kulynych, J., Macklin, R., Michael, D.B., Wolf, S.M., Grabowski, T., and Seto, B. 2008. Practical approaches to incidental findings in brain imaging research. *Neurology, 70* (5), 384–390.

Illes, J., Kirschen, M.P., Edwards, E., Stanford, L.R., Bandettini, P., Cho, M.K., Ford, P.J., Glover, G.H., Kulynych, J., Macklin, R., Michael, D.B., and Wolf, S.M. 2006. Incidental findings in brain imaging research. *Science, 311* (5762), 783–784.

Illes, J., Kirschen, M.P., and Gabrieli, J.D. 2003. From neuroimaging to neuroethics. *Nature Neuroscience, 6* (3), 205.

Johnstone, A. 2004, November 23. A glimpse inside: It's what many parents and teachers have long suspected: Teenagers may actually go temporarily insane on the path to maturity. *The Herald,* p. 2.

Kopell, B.H., Greenberg, B., and Rezai, A.R. 2004. Deep brain stimulation for psychiatric disorders. *Journal of Clinical Neurophysiology, 21* (1), 51–67.

Kramer, U.M., Jansma, H., Tempelmann, C., and Munte, T.F. 2007. Tit-for-tat: The neural basis of reactive aggression. *Neuroimage, 38* (1), 203–211.

Kubu, C.S. and Ford, P.J. 2007. Ethics in the clinical application of neural implants. *Cambridge Quarterly of Healthcare Ethics, 16* (3), 317–321.

Kuehn, B.M. 2007. Scientists probe deep brain stimulation: Some promise for brain injury, psychiatric illness. *Journal of the American Medical Association, 298* (19), 2249–2251.

Kulynych, J. 2002. Legal and ethical issues in neuroimaging research: Human subjects protection, medical privacy, and the public communication of research results. *Brain and Cognition, 50* (3), 345–357.

Larson, P.S. 2008. Deep brain stimulation for psychiatric disorders. *Neurotherapeutics, 5* (1), 50–58.

Levy, N. 2007. *Neuroethics: Challenges for the 21st century*. Cambridge: Cambridge University Press.

Lieberman, M.D., A Hariri, J.M.J., Naomi, I.E., and Bookheimer, S.Y. 2005. An fMRI investigation of race-related amygdala activity in African-American and Caucasian-American individuals. *Nature Neuroscience, 8* (6), 720–722.

Madriga, A. 2010a, June 1. Brain scan lie-detection deemed far from ready for courtroom. *Wired*. Available at http://www.wired.com/wiredscience/2010/06/fmri-lie-detection-in-court/.

Madriga, A. 2010b, May 17. Judge issues legal opinion in Brooklyn fMRI case. *Wired*. Available at http://www.wired.com/wiredscience/2010/05/brooklyn-fmri-case/#ixzz10l5rmzkN.

Marcus, S.J. (Ed.). 2002. *Neuroethics: Mapping the field, conference proceedings*. New York, NY: Dana Press.

Moreno, J.D. 2006. *Mind wars: Brain research and national defense*. New York, NY: Dana Press.

Mueller, S.G., Weiner, M.W., Thal, L.J., Petersen, R.C., Jack, C., Jagust, W., Trojanowski, J.Q., Toga, A.W., and Beckett, L. 2005. The Alzheimer's disease neuroimaging initiative. *Neuroimaging Clinics of North America, 159* (4), 869–877.

Ontario Health and Technology Advisory Committee. 2005. *OHTAC recommendation: Deep brain stimulation in Parkinson's disease and other movement disorders*. Toronto: Ontario Health Technology Advisory Committee. Available at http://www.health.gov.on.ca/english/providers/program/ohtac/tech/recommend/rec_dbs_030205.pdf.

Owen, A.M., Coleman, M.R., Boly, M., Davis, M.H., Laureys, S., and Pickard, J.D. 2006. Detecting awareness in the vegetative state. *Science, 313* (5792), 1402.

Plassmann, H., O'Doherty, J., and Rangel, A. 2007. Orbitofrontal cortex encodes willingness to pay in everyday economic transactions. *The Journal of Neuroscience, 27* (37), 9984–9998.

Pontius, A.A. 1973. Neuro-ethics of "walking" in the newborn. *Perceptual and Motor Skills, 37* (1), 235–245.

Porta, M., Brambilla, A., Cavanna, A.E., Servello, D., Sassi, M., Rickards, H., and Robertson MM. 2009. Thalamic deep brain stimulation for treatment-refractory Tourette syndrome: Two-year outcome. *Neurology, 73* (17), 1375–1380.

Rabins, P., Appleby, B.S., Brandt, J., DeLong, M.R., Dunn, L.B., Gabriels, L., Greenberg, B.D., Haber, S.N., Holtzheimer, P.E., 3rd, Mari, Z., Mayberg, H.S., McCann, E., Mink, S.P., Rasmussen, S., Schlaepfer, T.E., Vawter, D.E., Vitek, J.L., Walkup, J., and Mathews, D.J. 2009. Scientific and ethical issues related to deep brain stimulation for disorders of mood, behavior, and thought. *Archives of General Psychiatry, 66* (9), 931–937.

Racine, E. 2007. Identifying challenges and conditions for the use of neuroscience in bioethics. *The American Journal of Bioethics Neuroscience, 7* (1), 74–76.

Racine, E. 2008. Comment on "Does it make sense to speak of neuroethics?" *European Molecular Biology Oragnization Reports, 9* (1), 2–3.

Racine, E. 2010. *Pragmatic neuroethics: Improving treatment and understanding of the mind–brain.* Cambridge, MA: MIT Press.

Racine, E. 2011. Neuroscience and the media: Ethical challenges and opportunities. In J. Illes and B.J. Sahakian (Eds.), *Oxford handbook of neuroethics* (pp. 783–802). Oxford: Oxford University Press.

Racine, E., Bar-Ilan, O., and Illes, J. 2005. fMRI in the public eye. *Nature Reviews Neuroscience, 6* (2), 159–164.

Racine, E., Bell, E., and Illes, J. 2010. Can we read minds? Ethical challenges and responsibilities in the use of neuroimaging research. In Giordano, J. and Gordijn, B. (Eds.), *Neuroethics: Scientific, philosophical, and ethical perspectives* (pp. 240–266), Cambridge: Cambridge University Press.

Racine, E. and Illes, J. 2007. Emerging ethical challenges in advanced neuroimaging research: Review, recommendations and research agenda. *Journal of Empirical Research on Human Research Ethics, 2* (2), 1–10.

Racine, E., Van der Loos, H.Z.A., and Illes, J. 2007. Internet marketing of neuroproducts: New practices and healthcare policy challenges. *Cambridge Quarterly of Healthcare Ethics, 16*, 181–194.

Racine, E., Waldman, S., Palmour, N., Risse, D., and Illes, J. 2007. Currents of hope: Neurostimulation techniques in US and UK print media. *Cambridge Quarterly of Healthcare Ethics, 16* (3), 314–318.

Racine, E., Waldman, S., Rosenberg, J., and Illes, J. Contemporary neuroscience in the media. *Social Science & Medicine, 71* (4), 725–733.

Raine, A. and Yang, Y. 2006. Neural foundations to moral reasoning and antisocial behavior. *Social Cognitive & Affective Neuroscience, 1* (3), 203–213.

Robertson, D., Snarey, J., Ousley, O., Harenski, K., DuBois Bowman, F., Gilkey, R., and Kilts, C. 2007. The neural processing of moral sensitivity to issues of justice and care. *Neuropsychologia, 45* (4), 755–766.

Robertson, D.W. 1996. Ethical theory, ethnography, and differences between doctors and nurses in approaches to patient care. *Journal of Medical Ethics, 22*, 292–299.

Rodriguez, P. 2006. Talking brains: A cognitive semantic analysis of an emerging folk neuropsychology. *Public Understanding of Neuroscience, 15*, 301–330.

Royal College of Physicians. 2003. *The vegetative state: Guidance on diagnosis and management.* London: Royal College of Physicians. Available at http://www.rcplondon.ac.uk/pubs/contents/47a262a7-350a-490a-b88d-6f58bbf076a3.pdf.

Safire, W. 2002. *Visions for a new field of neuroethics.* Paper presented at Neuroethics: Mapping the Field, San Francisco.

Sommer, M., Rothmayr, C., Dohnel, K., Meinhardt, J., Schwerdtner, J., Sodian, B., and Hajak, G. 2010. How should I decide? The neural correlates of everyday moral reasoning. *Neuropsychologia, 48* (7), 2018–2026.

Takahashi, H., Yahata, N., Koeda, M., Matsuda, T., Asai, K., and Okubo, Y. 2004. Brain activation associated with evaluative processes of guilt and embarrassment: An fMRI study. *Neuroimage, 23* (3), 967–974.

The Multi-Society Task Force on PVS. 1994a. Medical aspects of the persistent vegetative state (1). *New England Journal of Medicine, 330* (21), 1499–1508.

The Multi-Society Task Force on PVS. 1994b. Medical aspects of the persistent vegetative state (2). *New England Journal of Medicine, 330* (22), 1572–1579.

Weisberg, D.S., Keil, F.C., Goodstein, J., Rawson, E., and Gray, J.R. 2008. The seductive allure of neuroscience explanations. *Journal of Cognitive Neuroscience, 20* (3), 470–477.

Wolf, S.M., Lawrenz, F.P., Nelson, C.A., Kahn, J.P., Cho, M.K., Clayton, E.W., Fletcher, J.G., Georgieff, M.K., Hammerschmidt, D., Hudson, K., Illes, J., Kapur, V., Keane, M.A., Koenig, B.A., Leroy, B.S., McFarland, E.G., Paradise, J., Parker, L.S., Terry, S.F., Van Ness, B., and Wilfond, B.S. 2008. Managing incidental findings in human subjects research: Analysis and recommendations. *Journal of Law, Medicine & Ethics, 36* (2), 219–248.

Wolpe, P.R. 2004. Neuroethics. In S.G. Post (Ed.), *The encyclopedia of bioethics* (3rd ed., Vol. 3; pp. 1894–1898). New York, NY: MacMillan Reference.

CHAPTER 26

To Boldly Go Forward: Epilogue and Future Horizons

Janet L. Storch, Rosalie Starzomski, and Patricia Rodney

Well, we have to have some hope. And so that's how I look at it. . . . I am in no way thinking that there's not more work to be done. There definitely is. But I have seen successes and so I think it is possible. . . . [W]e need to engage everybody . . . it has to be a level playing field. So . . . all people, physicians, nurses . . . and our health care team [have] to . . . have basically the same value and mission really, about what we're trying to do. (Nurse research participant, Rodney et al. 2002, 91)

As we claimed in closing the first edition of this text, the challenges nurses face in attempting to enact the ethics of their practice are rooted in history and are unlikely to go away in the near future. While we concluded the first edition of this book (writing in 2003), the events surrounding SARS (Severe Acute Respiratory Syndrome) were unfolding. The events included a variety of occasions in which nurses spoke out about the unmistakable public safety concerns that were evident as SARS continued to spread. Specifically, nurses warned that the incidence of SARS was being underestimated and that some illnesses and deaths might have been prevented. They requested more resources to deal safely with the new cases, and, in Ontario, called for a comprehensive public inquiry into the handling of the SARS crisis. In the wake of the 2003 outbreak, we were left with some too-familiar questions. Why did it take so long for nurses to be heard as SARS continued to wreak havoc in the health care system? And why was the response only partial? Would the lessons of history ever be learned? How was it that nurses continued to be marginalized and devalued in health care when their role had always been all about the *care* in health care?

Now as we close this second edition of our text (writing in 2011), we have the benefit of the leadership and analysis provided by the Registered Nurses Association of Ontario (RNAO) and many other groups. The RNAO's Final Report (2004) on the SARS outbreak included the following warnings:

> Our report . . . argues that we—government, health organizations, and health-care professionals—were ill-prepared to tackle SARS. Not only did we need to manage an infectious disease, whose origin and transmission were initially unknown, but we had to do this from within a depleted health-care system. This is a system weakened from years of funding cuts and a workforce exhausted by a decade of relentless restructuring. SARS further challenged:
>
> * A system that is poorly connected;
> * A public health sector that is under-resourced and disintegrated;
> * A home health care sector that is destabilized;

- A hospital sector that is unprepared for major emergencies; and
- A nursing workforce that battles with dangerously low staffing levels, high workloads, and an overreliance on part-time, casual and agency staff (5).

Governments have attempted to address some of these issues, for example, establishing the Public Health Agency of Canada, and urging hospitals to ensure that plans are in place for major emergencies. However, good communication amongst hospitals and other health agencies is an ongoing challenge. Other issues, specifically nursing care concerns, prevail. Across Canada (and throughout much of the world) many of the nursing workforce problems articulated by the RNAO in 2004 are not getting better. Indeed, with the economic downturn in 2008 and to the present, some of these issues appear to be getting worse (Austin 2011; Canadian Nurses Association [CNA] and RNAO 2010; Pringle 2009; Rodney and Varcoe in press; see also Chapters 10, 11 and 18).

Yet the RNAO's Final Report (2004) also pointed to strengths—strengths to pull together from all the diverse arenas of our profession to focus on the well-being of the public and the well-being of our profession. Ensuring that nurses' voices are heard within nursing and across the health professions, by policy makers, and by governments was also emphasized as an important goal in this report. Over the eight years that have passed since our first edition, we have seen significant advances in nursing education and nursing inquiry—advances that position us to have our voices better heard during challenging events such as SARS. Indeed, in our own province (British Columbia) the Ministry of Health has convened an ongoing ethics advisory group (including nurses, physicians, ethicists, and other health care experts) to analyze and provide recommendations for pandemic planning, ethics and aging, and a host of other ethical challenges.

We do not claim that our text contains definitive answers to the multitude of ethical questions facing nurses and other health care practitioners today. But we believe that within the preceding chapters readers should find deeper and newer ways to consider what it means to engage in safe, compassionate, competent, and ethical nursing practice. Throughout the text, the authors emphasize the ways that nurses can enact their role as advocates and influence change within the health care system. Such engagement involves understanding the ethical background (the *moral terrain*), the environment (the *moral climate*), and the current and future challenges (the *moral horizon*) of nursing ethics. Together with an array of expert co-authors we have taken up the challenge laid out in Chapter 1—to promote *ethical fitness* for ourselves and our colleagues in nursing and other health care professions. Ethical fitness requires being mentally engaged by thinking, reasoning, grappling with difficult situations or their potential, on a regular basis, as well as by a commitment to finding better ways to reach good outcomes (Kidder 2009). It is our hope that every chapter in this text will promote such fitness.

WHAT WE HAVE OFFERED

Our Approach

As we indicated in Chapter 1, our approach in Part I of this book was designed to provide substantive background in ethics, including an historical sketch of nursing in order to locate our current philosophical and ethical thinking (Chapters 2 and 3); to critically examine ethical principles and theories—including foundational theories as well as narrative ethics, relational ethics, and ecological ethics (Chapters 3 through 8); and to focus on key concepts of ethical practice—specifically relational practice, moral agency, and moral climate (Chapters 7 through 11).

Following this background, in Part 2 we turned to applications of health and health care ethics and nursing ethics related to practice (Chapters 12 and 13), research (Chapter 14), education (Chapter 15), policy (Chapter 18), and particular areas of practice that are challenging to the enactment of nursing values such as hearing the voice of children (Chapter 16) and working in partnership with people at the end of their lives (Chapter 17). Overall, in this second section we focused on the current situation in which nurses and other health professionals seek to engage in ethical practice. Beginning with an analysis of health care funding and delivery in respect to health reforms (Chapter 12), we showed that health reforms involve ethical choices that cannot be considered irrelevant to nursing ethics. In the remaining chapters in this section, we focused on *how* nurses can influence practice and policy.

In Part 3: Broadening the View of Health Care Ethics/Nursing Ethics, the authors of the first four chapters challenge our thinking about the breadth of our ethical scope. In their writing about home health care (Chapter 19), public health ethics (Chapter 20), and enacting social justice in the care of marginalized people (Chapter 21), they demand that we consider the limitations of taken-for-granted current health care and enlarge our thinking about ethical practice in these areas. In the last four chapters, a wide array of ethical concerns and challenges that have major implications for scholarship and practice—and that we consider to be highly relevant to emerging frontiers in nursing ethics—are highlighted. The writers describe issues surrounding biotechnological development (Chapter 22), pregnancy and reproduction (Chapter 23), genetics (Chapter 24), and neuroethics (Chapter 25) as some of the significant developments about which nurses will need to develop greater knowledge and ethical awareness to care for people in the twenty-first century.

There are undoubtedly many chapters that could have been included in this book covering many other topics—some of which are in our current realm of thinking and some that we may not yet have recognized. Future topics we have thought about include, for example, greater attention to ethics and chronic disease management (Lohne et al. 2010), ethics and elder care (Rees, King, and Schmitz 2009; Suhonen et al. 2010), mental health (International Council of Nurses 2008), and global ethics (Austin 2001/2003; 2004; Benatar and Brock 2011; Davis 2003).

ON THE HORIZON
Challenges and Opportunities

As we close this second edition of our book, we offer a cautionary note that deals with the status of nursing as a profession in the twenty-first century and the critical need for us, as nurses, to sharpen our political acumen. The importance of achieving greater equity in whose voices are heard in health care planning and delivery cannot be over-emphasized. The health of the community depends upon equity of access to be championed in health policy. Dr. Peggy Chinn, a nursing scholar who has long been concerned with issues of equity, puts it this way:

> The most basic challenge, I believe, is to continue to make the voice of nursing stronger, louder, better understood, and heard (even among our own colleagues). . . . Our primary motive should be, and must be, a conviction that what we offer is exactly what the majority of people need the most from healthcare, regardless of where on the globe they reside. (Chinn 2009, 281)

We need to celebrate milestones over the past decade, particularly two developments in nursing. The first is the legislative mandate in most provinces to raise the educational level required for entry into registered nursing practice across Canada. This move to require a baccalaureate degree for entry to practice commenced in 2005 and has continued its momentum. Individual graduate nurses are personally richer with this broadened knowledge, patients and clients benefit from RNs preparedness, and the nursing profession is enriched. The second development is the gradual implementation of advanced practice nurses through legislation to allow nurse practitioners a fuller scope of practice in primary health care. These types of legislative developments have been long sought goals of the majority of Canadian nurses.

Notwithstanding such milestones, we recognize that many nurses continue to be limited in their ability to use their knowledge and skills by bureaucratic decisions that favour cost efficiency over cost effectiveness. In this case we mean administrators who choose to engage less prepared individuals to do "nursing tasks," seemingly oblivious to the critical thinking involved in patient assessment and care planning. At an international level this phenomenon has been called "task shifting," and at international nursing conferences it is very clear that registered nurses around the world are highly concerned about these trends that waste nursing expertise and pose a significant threat to safe, compassionate, competent, and ethical practice across Canada and globally. In a position statement published in 2000 and revised in 2008, the ICN (2008) emphasized their concern that ". . . unless planned with [registered] nurses, task shifting and adding new cadres of assistive personnel may result in fragmented, unsafe and inefficient service" (2).

In the first chapter of our book, the problem of task shifting and displacement of nurses was noted as a significant challenge to ethical practice. As new models of care are introduced by administrators, it is important for nurses to be involved in assessing impacts on patient care (Van De Velde-Coke 2009) with meaningful indicators. For example, do the indicators include holistic nursing care or do they only measure completion of a series of tasks done for the person in care? Are short term and long term outcomes for patients and their families, as well as nurses and other health care providers, being tracked? Who is being held accountable for monitoring and responding to the impacts of task shifting--locally, nationally and globally?

Also noted in the introductory chapter was the matter of patient safety, which continues to be a major concern. Principles of patient safety have included transparency and the importance of reporting unsafe practices so that learning might occur. However, in one recent study in an emergency department, researchers (Brubacher et al. 2011) found several barriers impacting the reporting of unsafe practices or 'near misses' by nursing staff and nurse managers. These included constraints on their time, a sense of futility, a fear of reprisal, being unfamiliar with the need to report, and believing their reporting was viewed as incompetence, It seems clear that the culture of the workplace environment may not have changed sufficiently to move beyond a "blame and shame" mentality (Lowe 2008) to a safety culture that rewards early reporting of safety risks and violations. The leadership of nurse managers and other nurse leaders to help change the culture of the work environment will be critical to avoiding and minimizing patient harm in health care. One positive aspect of the attention to patient safety is that increasingly the safety of staff is being recognized as a critical factor as well, particularly in home care but also in hospital care. Unsurprisingly, there is a ". . . strong link between a safety culture from a patient or client perspective and a safe work environment for employees" (Lowe 2008, 49). Our own multiple research projects on ethical climate and culture noted throughout this book, support this finding.

Safety of health care providers became a significant issue during and following the SARS epidemic referred to at the beginning of this chapter. On-going expressions of concern about health care workers vulnerability during epidemics/pandemics have been raised and, as Silas, Johnson and Rexe (2007) noted, safety is not negotiable: planning for safety of staff during pandemic planning is critical. Racette (2009) described the 3 year project initiated by the Canadian College of Health Service Executives to plan for pandemic readiness with attention to communications with health care providers, including having in place resources to help them deal with their distress. The April 2009 outbreak of a severe respiratory illness in Mexico labeled as H1N1 was quickly elevated to pandemic status by the World Health Organization June 11, 2009 with predictions of widespread morbidity and mortality. Mahon, et al. 2011.have written about the years of planning for managing a pandemic at the Izaak Walton Killam Center in Halifax, presenting the way in which the organization was able to handle the H1N1 crisis. In meeting to determine what worked well and what did not work well when it was over, they highlighted many strengths and many areas that could be enhanced. They noted that

> The evaluation process in itself became an H1N1 debrief session, often cathartic for those who had participated because it provided people with the opportunity to tell their stories and to offer their feedback and suggestions on how to do it better next time (17).

The importance of taking time to reflect and time to debrief (i.e. time for interactive debriefing) is a continuing theme throughout our book.

Charting Our Course

Nurses are positioned more effectively than ever before to take leaderships roles to maintain what is beneficial in health care and shape the changes that need to occur in the future. We know that the Canadian public holds nurses in high regard, and in the many public opinion polls that have been conducted over the last 10 years, nurses rate high in public trust. Indeed, nurses rate highest among those professions with inside knowledge of the health care system (Haines 2002, 2; *Reader's Digest* 2011). There is data available that describes the state of nursing in Canada (Canadian Nurses Association [CNA] and RNAO 2010). Recognition is being given for the complexity of the professional nursing role, and it appears that governments are interested in making changes in how health care is delivered. This suggests that nurses are in a position to be heard, both by the public and by decision makers. However, we must not be complacent. To ensure that our voices are heard, we must show vision and leadership, and at the same time, develop and use appropriate approaches to continue to influence change. To do so with integrity, nurses need sound knowledge of the current health care provisions in Canada, and Canada's somewhat unique approach to providing access to health care for all Canadians. This unique approach involves a health insurance program that allows for public funding with some room for autonomy of health professionals and organizations, as noted in Chapter 12.

Continuous critical reflection and political action are required to ensure that our messages are given prominence in the health care arena. And in this arena, we need to be very clear about *who we serve*—that is, individuals, families and communities requiring care, rather than governments and politicians. Nurses have demonstrated how keeping this focus in mind can make a major difference in the lives of Canadians. For example, Cathy Crowe in Toronto, Ontario, has worked tirelessly as a champion of the homeless, improving living standards for marginalized people dramatically, thus demonstrating the difference that nurses can make in the health of populations. Similarly, Dr. Bernadette Pauly, (our colleague and co-author from the University of Victoria School of Nursing), in her work of advocacy and policy development in Victoria B.C., has helped to enhance the lives of many street-involved people and people with addictions. Further, provincial, national, and international nursing organizations have time and again risen to the challenge of influencing change within health care.

Our political action can be well served through our national nursing associations in Canada and other countries. As we write this chapter in the fall of 2011, the Canadian Nurses Association (CNA) is consulting with nurses and others as part of a national expert commission called "The Health of Our Nation—The Future of Our Health System". The commission, led by CNA, is made up of leaders in the fields of business, law, government, academia, and health care. Co-chaired by Marlene Smadu (a former CNA president) and Maureen McTeer (a lawyer and health law expert), "the commission's mandate is to make policy recommendations to support the transformation of Canada's health system by realigning health services to meet the needs of our evolving population and investing in networks and connections that make better use of existing health resources" (CNA Press Release, May 30, 2011). Smadu and McTeer (2011) state that this is a timely and important CNA initiative since

. . . . there is the expectation that a new health accord in 2014 will replace the one from 2004. . . . Collectively . . . we are saying that this is an opportunity not just to put money into the system but to buy the kind of system change and investments that will actually create better health care in the future (14–15).

It will be essential that *ethical practice* be foregrounded in the work of the commission. To that end we three have met with commission members to urge that ethics in health care be construed as not just another interesting topic, but that ethics must become embedded in health care through use of an ethics lens in all decisions and actions.

Overall, our future horizon ought to include a more purposeful linking of ethics with politics (see Chapters 5, 13, and 18 through 21). Effecting *the good* of individuals and of society through nursing practice should never be taken for granted. As the authors in this book have illustrated, some of the most pressing ethical challenges facing us today are rooted in systemic inequities in access to resources for health and health care in Canada and around the globe (Anderson et al. 2009; Benetar and Brock 2011; Canadian Nurses Association 2009; Rodney 2011; World Health Organization 2008a; 2008b). And as the authors in this book have also illustrated, as cost constraints proliferate in health care delivery, there are serious concomitant challenges to the moral agency of nurses and other health professionals (Austin 2011; Canadian Nurses Association and Registered Nurses Association of Ontario 2010; Pringle 2009; Rodney and Varcoe in press). We therefore must continue to examine our values and our ethics and how to further them in a democracy that is founded on an egalitarian ideal and where diversity is respected. We need to be thoughtful and careful as we chart the course ahead in our current sociopolitical climate. This will require local through to global policy work and political action with communities, workplaces, governments, and professional organizations (Mason, Leavitt, and Chaffee 2007; Oulton 2007). Working with our provincial and national nursing associations will be foundational to charting our way forward.

The CNA made a bold move in 2008 to include greater attention to social inequities. In the Code of Ethics for Registered Nurses, Part II is focused on ethical endeavours. In this section, attention is drawn to the need for primary health care, health promotion, attention to the social determinants of health, greater attention to vulnerable groups and to global health, and to numerous other issues that press for a broader, more inclusive approach to health care. In creating this section, nurses were encouraged to recognize the broader context of health and health care and the social injustices so apparent in our approaches to health care (see Chapters 18, 20 and 21).

Awareness is important but it is not enough. The time has come to go beyond mere "awareness" of these social injustices. It is time for nurses to accept responsibility to work collectively to right the wrongs. Throughout this book, emphasis has been directed to *relational ethics*. As our colleague and co-author from the University of Toronto Faculty of Nursing Dr. Elizabeth Peter (2011) makes clear, moral agency from a relational standpoint can be conceptualized as a social or collective matter. Peter (2011) states,

> A social connection model of responsibility views individuals as having some responsibility for social injustices, because they contribute, through their actions, to the social processes and rules that bring about these injustices. (13)

Peter urges that we think collectively about moral agency, since this would not only foster nursing's identity and power as a profession but it could also bring about significant changes to health care and the people with whom nurses work (16).

In closing, we hope our text can contribute to the potential for nurses to make ethical and political choices knowingly and wisely. We agree with the nurse whom we cited at the outset of this chapter. As a profession, we have achieved a great deal, yet a great deal more remains to be done. We must ensure that we are able to demonstrate moral imagination and moral courage in the face of the challenges that confront us at all levels of the health system. Most importantly, we must take up the challenge to shape the future system with hope that the ethical scholarship, practice, and political action of nurses will ensure a future where health is an achievable goal for all citizens on our planet. Our colleague and co-author from the University of British Columbia School of Nursing, Dr. Joan Anderson (2009), expresses the future challenge very well:

> Generations of nurses before us harnessed opportunities and demonstrated the political skill to move the profession forward to a place of which we can all be proud. The current generation of nurses must use the knowledge we have acquired, and construct new knowledge to advance nursing practice and strengthen health-care delivery systems. We can combine our knowledge with wisdom to work within health-care systems and political systems to bring about policy change that will address the complex contexts of health and illness. (54–55)

References

Anderson, J.M. 2009. [Discourse]. Looking back, looking forward: Conceptual and methodological trends in nursing research in Canada over the past decade. *Canadian Journal of Nursing Research, 41* (1), 47–55.

Anderson, J.M., Rodney, P., Reimer-Kirkham, S., Browne, A.J., Khan, K.B., and Lynam, M.J. 2009. Inequities in health and healthcare viewed through the ethical lens of critical social justice: Contextual knowledge for the global priorities ahead. *Advances in Nursing Science, 32* (4), 282–294.

Austin, W. 2003. Using the human rights paradigm in health ethics: The problems and the possibilities. In V. Tschudin (Ed.), *Approaches to ethics: Nursing beyond boundaries* (pp.105–114) Edinburgh: Butterworth Heinmann. (Reprinted from *Nursing Ethics* 2001; *8* (13), 183–195).

Austin, W. 2004. Global health challenges, human rights, and nursing ethics. In J. Storch, P. Rodney, and R. Starzomski (Eds.) *Toward a moral horizon: Nursing ethics for leadership and practice* (pp. 339–356). Toronto: Pearson Prentice Hall.

Austin, W.J. 2011. The incommensurability of nursing as a practice and the customer service model: An evolutionary threat to the discipline. *Nursing Philosophy, 12*, 158–166.

Benatar, S. and Brock, G. 2011. *Global health and global health ethics.* Cambridge: Cambridge University Press.

Bruebacher, J.R., Hunte, G.S., Hamilton, L. and Taylor, A. 2011. Barriers and incentives for safety event reporting in emergency departments. *Healthcare Quarterly, 13* (3), 57–65.

Canadian Nurses Association. 2008. *Code of ethics for registered nurses.* Ottawa: Author.

Canadian Nurses Association. 2009. *Position statement: Determinants of health.* Ottawa, ON: Authors.

Canadian Nurses Association. 2011, Communique. *Registered nurses launch expert commission on health system renewal.* Ottawa: Author. May 26.

Canadian Nurses Association and Registered Nurses Association of Ontario. 2010. *Nurse fatigue and patient safety: Research report.* Ottawa, ON: Canadian Nurses Association.

Chinn, P.L. 2009. [From the editor] Healthy people beyond 2010. *Advances in Nursing Science, 32* (4), 281.

Davis, A. 2003. International nursing ethics: Context and concerns. In V. Tschudin (Ed.), *Approaches to nursing ethics* (pp. 95–104). London: Butterworth Heinemann.

Haines, J. 2002. The convergence of trust and concern. *Canadian Nurse, 98* (4), 2.

International Council of Nurses. 2008. *Assistive nursing personnel. Position Statement.* Geneva: Author. Available at www.icn.ch.

International Council of Nurses. 2008. *Mental health. Position Statement.* Geneva: Author. www.icn.ch.

Kidder, R.M. 2009. *How good people make tough choices: Resolving the dilemmas of ethical living.* New York: Harper.

Lohne, V., Aasgaard, T., Caspari, S., Slettebo, A. and Naden, D. 2010. The lonely battle for dignity: individuals struggling with multiple sclerosis. *Nursing Ethics, 17* (3), 301–311.

Lowe, G.S. (2008). The role of healthcare work environments in shaping a safety culture. *Healthcare Quarterly,* 11 (2), 42–51.

Mahon, K., Blackmore, N., Thibeault, M., Belliveau, B. and Burgess, S. 2011. When ordinary days become extraordinary: The response to H1N1 at the Izaak Walton Health Centre. *Healthcare Management Forum,* 24 (1), 14–19.

Mason, D.J., Leavitt, J.K., and Chaffee, M.W. 2007. Policy and politics: A framework for action. In D.J. Mason, J.K. Leavitt, and M.W. Chaffee (Eds.), *Policy & politics in nursing and health care* (5th ed.; pp. 1–20). St. Louis, MO: Saunders Elsevier.

Oulton, J. 2007, Nursing in the international community: A broader view of nursing issues. In D.J. Mason, J.K. Leavitt, and M.W. Chaffee (Eds.), *Policy & politics in nursing and health care* (5th ed.; pp. 966–981). St. Louis, MO: Saunders Elsevier.

Peter, E. 2011. Fostering social justice: The possibilities of a socially connected model of moral agency. *Canadian Journal of Nursing Research, 43* (2), 11–17.

Pringle, D. 2009. Alert—Return of 1990s healthcare reform. *Nursing Leadership, 22* (3), 14–15.

Racette, R.J. 2007. Will we be judged ready for the influenza pandemic? *Healthcare Management Forum,* 22 (2), 6–11.

Reader's Digest. 2011. Most trusted Canadians—3rd annual trust poll. Available at *http://www.readersdigest.ca/magazine/most-trusted-canadians-3rd-annual-trust-poll-results.*

Rees, J., King, L., and Schmitz, K. 2009. Nurses' perspectives of ethical issues in the care of older people. *Nursing Ethics, 16* (4), 436–452.

Registered Nurses Association of Ontario. 2004. *SARS unmasked: Celebrating resilience, exposing vulnerability.* (Final Report on the nursing experience with SARS in Ontario.) Toronto, ON: Authors.

Rodney, P. 2011. [Guest editorial]. Nursing inquiry to address pressing empirical and ethical questions. *Canadian Journal of Nursing Research, 43* (2), 7–10.

Rodney, P. and Varcoe, C. in press. Constrained agency: The social structure of nurses' work. In F. Baylis, J. Downie, B. Hoffmaster, and S. Sherwin (Eds.), *Health care ethics in Canada* (3rd ed.). Toronto, ON: Nelson. (Revision of Varcoe, C. and Rodney, P. 2009 Constrained agency: The social structure of nurses' work. In B.S. Bolaria and H.D. Dickinson (Eds.), *Health, illness, and health care in Canada* (4th ed.; pp. 122–151). Toronto, ON: Nelson Education.)

Rodney, P., Varcoe, C., Storch, J.L., McPherson, G., Mahoney, K., Brown, H., Pauly, B., Hartrick Doane, G., and Starzomski, R. 2002. Navigating toward a moral horizon: A multi-site qualitative study of nurses' enactment of ethical practice. *Canadian Journal of Nursing Research, 34* (3), 75–102.

Silas, L., Johnson, N. and Rexe, K. 2007. Safety is not negotiable: The importance of occupational health and safety to pandemic planning. *HealthcarePapers,* 8 (1), 8–16.

Smadu, M. and McTeer, M. 2011. On a mission to listen. *Canadian Nurse, 107* (7), 14–15.

Suhonen, R., Stolt, M., Launis, V., and Leino-Kilpi, H. 2010. Research on ethics in nursing of older people: A literature review. *Nursing Ethics, 17* (3), 337–352.

Van De Velde-Cook, S. 2009. A cross-country check-up in healthcare. *Canadian Journal of Nursing Leadership,* 22 (2), 20–25.

World Health Organization. 2008a. *Closing the gap in a generation: Health equity through action on the social determinants of health.* (Final Report of the Commission on Social Determinants of Health.) Geneva: Authors.

World Health Organization. 2008b. *World Health Report 2008: Primary health care: Now more than ever.* Geneva: Authors.

APPENDIX A

Storch Model for Ethical Decision-Making Guiding Questions for Clinical Decision Making

1. INFORMATION AND IDENTIFICATION

- Talk with all parties involved. From that conversation, there should emerge a central story.
- Learn about the patient's medical status and the expectations he or she or the family have for outcomes, as well as the expectations of the health care team.
- Gather non-medical information about social conditions, family roles and relationships, quality of life, and power dynamics in the situation.
- Determine level of competency/capacity.

2. CLARIFICATION AND EVALUATION

Consider the VALUES involved:

- What is the significance of the values involved—moral, religious, cultural, personal, professional?
- What is the significance of these values to the people involved?
- What is the story behind the value conflicts?

Consider the ETHICAL PRINCIPLES involved:

- Which principles might be most important in this situation?
- Are some principles in conflict with others?

Consider the SOCIAL EXPECTATIONS and the LEGAL REQUIREMENTS involved:

- Is there any institutional history on a similar situation?
- What institutional policy requirements are important?
- What legal provisions need to be considered?

Determine a RANGE OF POTENTIAL ACTIONS and their CONSEQUENCES:

- Focus on ethically acceptable courses of action.
- Build consensus around which action is most fitting for the situation.
- Ensure patient, family, and team have common understandings about the plan of action.
- Plan to meet again to consider consequences/learning.

3. ACTION AND REVIEW

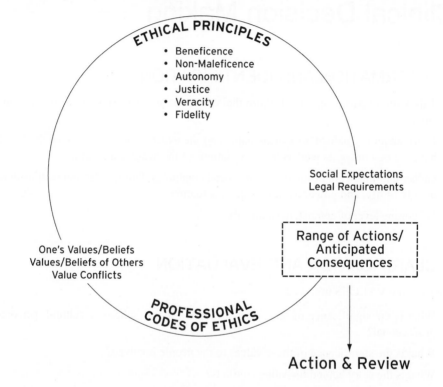

APPENDIX B

An Ethical Decision-Making Framework for Individuals (2009)[1]

Michael McDonald

Adapted by Patricia Rodney and Rosalie Starzomski

1. COLLECT INFORMATION AND IDENTIFY THE PROBLEM(S)

a) Identify what you know and *what you don't know but need to know.* Be prepared to add/update your information *throughout* the decision-making process.

b) Gather as much information as possible on the patient's physical, psychological, social, cultural, and spiritual status, including changes over time. Seek input from the patient, family, friends, and other health care team members.

c) Investigate the patient's assessment of their own quality of life and their wishes about the treatment/care decision(s) at hand. This includes determining the patient's competency as well as determining what family members the patient wants involved in discussions about and/or decision making in their treatment/care. If the patient is not competent, look for an advance directive. Identify a proxy decision maker for patients who are not competent and seek evidence of the patient's prior expressed wishes. Regardless of the patient's competence (capacity), involve the patient as much as possible in all decisions affecting him or her.

d) Include a family assessment: What are the various roles, relationships, and relevant "stories"?

e) Identify the health care team members involved, and circumstances affecting them.

f) Summarize the situation briefly but with all the relevant facts and circumstances. Try to get a sense of the patient's overall health and illness trajectory.

g) What decisions have to be made? By whom?

2. SPECIFY FEASIBLE ALTERNATIVES FOR TREATMENT AND CARE

a) Use your clinical expertise to identify a wide range and scope of alternatives. *Avoid binary thinking* (such as "treat/don't treat") and lay out carefully tailored alternatives for the problems you have identified.

b) Identify *how* various alternatives might be implemented (e.g., time trials).

3. USE YOUR ETHICS RESOURCES TO EVALUATE ALTERNATIVES

a) **Principles/Concepts**
   - **Autonomy:** What does the patient want? How well has the patient been informed and/or supported? What explicit or implicit promises have been made to the patient?
   - **Nonmaleficence:** Will this harm the patient? Others?
   - **Beneficence:** Will this benefit the patient? Others?
   - **Justice:** Consider the interests of all those (including the patient) who have to be taken into account. Are biases about the patient or family affecting your decision making? Treat like situations alike.
   - **Fidelity:** Are you fostering trust in patient/family/team relationships?
   - **Care:** Will the patient and family be supported as they deal with loss, grief, and/or uncertainty? What about any moral distress of team members? What principles of palliative care can be incorporated into the alternatives?
   - **Relational Autonomy:** What relationships and social structures are affecting the various individuals involved in the situation? How can these relationships and social structures be used to enable support of the patient, family members, and health care providers?

b) **Standards**
   Examine professional norms, standards and codes, legal precedents, health care agency policy.

c) **Personal judgments and experiences**
   Consider yours, your colleagues' and other members of the health care team's.

d) **Organized procedures for ethical consultation**
   Draw on the expertise of the resources in the health care agency. Consider a formal case conference(s), an ethics committee meeting, and/or an ethics consultant, especially if the situation is complex and/or conflicted. This could include a quick survey to see if there is relevant bioethics literature—for example, a bioethics case book or set of narratives.

4. PROPOSE AND TEST POSSIBLE RESOLUTIONS

a) Select the best alternative(s), all things considered.
b) Perform a sensitivity analysis. Consider your choice(s) critically: Which factors would have to change to get you to alter your decision(s)? Then carefully consider whether you want to maintain or change your previous choice(s).
c) Think about the effects of your choice(s) upon others' choices: Are you making it easier for others (health care providers, patients and their families, etc.) to act ethically?
d) Is this what a compassionate health care professional would do in a caring environment?

e) Formulate your choice(s) as a general maxim for all similar situations. Think of situations where it does *not* apply. Consider situations where it does apply.

f) Are you and the other decision makers still comfortable with your choice(s)? *If you do not have consensus, revisit the process.* Remember that you are not aiming at the perfect choice, but the best possible choice. If no consensus is forthcoming, is it possible to reach a compromise?

g) Ensure that there is a clear implementation plan. Ensure that the rationale for and details of the plan are clearly communicated to all those who will be affected (patient, family, and health care providers). Be sure that the implementation plan includes feedback from relevant individuals (the patient, family and friends, health care providers).

5. MAKE YOUR CHOICE

Live with it and learn from it! Seek feedback on the process from all those involved. Take the opportunity to reflect on how you will deal with other challenging situations in the future. Consider organizing follow-up debriefings and continuing education sessions and/or planning changes to related policies and procedures.

Endnote

1. The editors would like to thank Dr. Michael McDonald for his kind permission to use this version of his Ethical Decision-Making Framework for Individuals. A similar version of his Framework also appeared as an appendix in Yeo, M., Moorhouse, A., Khan, P., and Rodney, P. (Eds.). 2010. *Concepts and cases in nursing ethics* (3rd ed.; pp. 391–394). Peterborough, ON: Broadview Press.

APPENDIX C

An Ethical Framework for Making Allocation Decisions

Michael McDonald

Step 1: Consultation Process
- Will it yield useful information?
- Do all the relevant parties have a fair say?
- Is there competent representation for those who need help in presenting their interests?
- Does it avoid expert imperialism and conflicts of interest?

Step 2: Identify Distributional Issues
- What is being distributed?
- By which decision makers?
- To what persons?
- From which persons?
- For what reasons?
- Are any of the above ethically suspect?
- Make the necessary corrections.

Step 3: Look Up, Down, Around
For impacts on:
- Population health
- Particular populations and patients
- Existing and future claims
- Systemic capacity and sustainability

Step 4: Four Ethical Tests
- Fiduciary test: best interests of present and future populations
- Fair dealing test: respecting the rights of all parties
- Good stewardship: using public resources efficiently for intended purposes
- Public processes: open and accountable

Step 5: Make Your Choice
- From the remaining options
- Live with the choice
- Learn from it
- Good CQI (continuous quality improvement)
- Good consultation and feedback

Index

A

AAP. *See* American Academy of Pediatrics
aboriginal belief systems, 90
abortion, 474–477
    access to, 474–476
    barriers to, 474–476
    conscientious objection, 476–477
    debate about, 474
accessibility, 238
Accord on Health Care Renewal, 239
accountability for reasonableness, 70–71
action research, 202–204
ADPKD. *See* autosomal dominant polycystic
        kidney disease (ADPKD)
adult respiratory distress syndrome (ARDS), 480
advance care planning tracking record, 340
advance directives
    integral feature of, 341
    problems with, 340–341
    use of, 340
advantageous comparison, 172
advocacy ethics, 401
ageism, 367
AHR. *See* assisted human reproduction (AHR)
Aiken, Linda, Dr., 195
Alberta Health Services Draft Code of Ethical
        Conduct, 12
allocation decision-making model, 542
altruism, and nursing ethics, 23–24
American Academy of Pediatrics, 325
American Journal of Nursing, 31
American Nurses Association (ANA), 31
American Society of Superintendents of Training
        Schools, 31
amniocentesis, 481–482
ANA. *See* American Nurses Association (ANA)
ANA Code of Ethics for Nurses, 15
anticipating suffering, 316
"anti-establishment" movement, 64
applied ethics, 65, 401
archetypal narratives, 110
ARDS. *See* adult respiratory distress syndrome
        (ARDS)
argumentation, 41
argument-based ethics literature, 348

artificial insemination, 477
assisted human reproduction (AHR), 473, 477–481
    artificial insemination, 477
    ethical issues associated with, 478
    IVF, 477–478
        availability of, 478–479
    PGD, 478
Attig, Thomas, 322
authentic listening, promotion of, 327
authentic presence, 175, 180
    education about, 180
authoritarian communitarianism, 406
automythologies, 110
autonomy
    child, needs, 259
    ethical principles, 66–67, 72, 261
    and moral agency, 162
    relational, 93–94, 256, 264, 268, 437
autosomal dominant conditions, 496
autosomal dominant polycystic kidney disease
        (ADPKD), 496

B

BCNU. *See* British Columbia Nurses Union (BCNU)
"bed blockers," 173
beneficence, 67–69
biobanking, 502–503
bioethics, 29–30, 402, 509
    autonomy, 66–67, 72
    beneficence, 67–69
    early history/traditions of, 63–66
    early influences on, 61–62
    informed consent, 67, 68–69
    justice in, 69–71
    nonmaleficence, 67–69
    principles of, 66–71
biomedicine, and health inequities, 435
biotechnology, 29–30
    implications for nurses, 463–465
    macro-level strategies, 465
    meso-level strategies, 465
    micro-level strategies, 464
    overview, 448
    promises and pitfalls, 449–450
    xenotransplantation (*See* xenotransplantation)

Black and Blue, 108
Boal, Augusto, 118
Bovine Spongiform Encephalopathy (BSE), 449
British Columbia Cancer Agency, 203
British Columbia Nurses Union (BCNU), 195
British North America Act of 1867, 237–238
British Nurses' Association, 31
Browne, A. J., 224
BSE. *See* Bovine Spongiform Encephalopathy (BSE)
Buddhist perspective
  of compassion, 90–91
  nursing philosophy, 47
Building a Moral Community for Collaborative
    Practice in Ambulatory Oncology
    Care, 203

C
CACCN. *See* Canadian Association of Critical Care
    Nurses (CACCN)
CAGC. *See* Canadian Association of Genetic
    Counsellors (CAGC)
Canada
  health care systems, 216, 271, 370
  research ethics, evolution of, 283–286
Canada Health Act (CHA), 238
  home care services, 384
  neo-liberalism, impact of, 387
  requirements, 386
Canada Health and Social Transfer (CHST)
    Act, 238
Canadian Abortion Rights Action League
    (CARAL), 475
Canadian Association of Critical Care Nurses
    (CACCN), 116
Canadian Association of Genetic Counsellors
    (CAGC), 503
Canadian Bioethics Society, 29
Canadian Community Health Nursing Standards
    of Practice, 387
Canadian Genome and Technology (CGAT)
    Program, 492
Canadian health care system. *See also* Medicare
  background, 237–239
  enduring values, 242–243
  ethical choices, 244–245
  fairness in, 243–244
  limitations of, 239–240
  public needs/problems, 240–242
Canadian Institutes for Health Research
    (CIHR), 119
Canadian Journal of Nursing Leadership, 196
Canadian National Association of Trained Nurses
    (CNATN), 31

Canadian Nurses Association (CNA), 7, 14,
    68, 288, 362, 464
  adoption of ICN Code, 31, 32
  code of ethics (*See* CNA Code of Ethics for
    Registered Nurses)
  committee formation, 24
  The Health of Our Nation-The Future of Our
    Health System, 532
  professional associations/colleges, 246
Canadian Nurses Foundation, 203
Canadian Pandemic Influenza Plan for the
    Health Sector
  goals, 417–418
Canadian Pediatric Society, 317
  medical treatment decisions, publishes, 317
  pre-adolescent children, 318
Canadian Public Health Association (CPHA),
    461–462
Canadians for Choice, 475
Canadian Society for Medical Bioethics, 29
Canadian Society of Bioethics, 29
CARAL. *See* Canadian Abortion Rights Action
    League (CARAL)
cardio-pulmonary resuscitation, 338
  decision of, 338
  importance of, 338
caring
  concept of, 30
  in nursing, 167–168
  and spirituality, 48
"Caring Science as Sacred Science," 48
case knowledge, 164, 165
Catholic Health Association of Canada, 13
CBR. *See* community-based research (CBR)
CCAC. *See* Community Care Access Centre
    (CCAC)
CGAT Program. *See* Canadian Genome and
    Technology (CGAT) Program
CHA. *See* Canada Health Act (CHA)
Chadwick, Edwin, 405
chaos narratives, 110
chief medical officer, 296
children
  American Academy of Pediatrics, 325
  authentic listening, 325
  best-interests model, 320
  chronic illness, participation, 318
  conventional morality, 321
  co-operation, 324
  cultural and religious freedom, 319
  ethics in practice narratives, 327–328
  harm, protection, 328
  minors capacity, 318
  moral awareness of, 325

moral lives, 321, 323
moral objectification, 319
moral order, 326
moral subject to moral object, 319–320
moral worlds, 324
  assent, broad conception of, 325
  clinical care, implications for, 326–327
moral worthiness, 319
parents, 318
voice of, 320, 324
  best-interests model, adult-centredness
    of, 320–322
  "maturity" of moral reasoning recognition, 320
moral awareness, 322–323
moral responsibility, 323–324
CHN. *See* community health nurse
chorionic villus sampling (CVS), 482
Christianity, and nursing, 21
chronic obstructive pulmonary disease, 334
chronological time, 137
CHST Act. *See* Canada Health and Social Transfer
  (CHST) Act
CIHR. *See* Canadian Institutes for Health
  Research (CIHR)
Circle of care, 3
civic republicanism, 406, 407, 408
clinical learning unit, 221
  centrality of indigenous knowledge, 222–223
  cultural integrity, 223
  eco-efficiency
    value of striving, 222–223
  ecological integrity, 223
  hospital-based nursing program, 223
  inter-professional, 221
  need to cross boundaries, 222
  turbulent health system, 221
clinical nurse educator, 303
clinical services, contracting out, 242
CLU. *See* clinical learning unit
CMO. *See* chief medical officer
CNA. *See* Canadian Nurses Association; Canadian
  Nurses Association (CNA)
CNA Code of Ethics for Registered Nurses, 7–8,
  68, 147, 236–237, 246, 389, 394, 476, 479,
  498, 533
CNATN. *See* Canadian National Association of
  Trained Nurses (CNATN)
codes of ethics, 12–14, 147
  development of, 31
  nursing organizations and, 31–32
  public health nursing and, 415
Coles, Robert, 322
collaboration, 176–180
  education about, 180

collateral damage, 416
Commission for the Study of Ethical Problems in
  Medicine and Biomedical and Behavioral
  Science, 66
Commission on the Future of Health Care,
  236, 387
commitment
  ethical, 133
  nurses, to patients, 166
communal public, and public health, 400
communitarian ethics, 227
communitarianism
  different perspectives, 407–408
  feminist critiques of, 406–407
  public health ethics and, 405–406
  types of, 406–407
communities, cross-fertilization principle, 222
community-based research (CBR), 438–439
Community Care Access Centre (CCAC), 388
community health councils, 370
community health nurse, 307
compassion
  Buddhist perspective of, 90–91
  ethics, 112–114
complementary approaches, health care ethics,
  84–95
  contextualism, 84–86
  cultural ethics (*See* cultural ethics)
  feminist ethics, 91–95
comprehensiveness, 238
conscientious objection, abortion and, 476–477
constitutive narratives, 109
contemporary health care, 359
contested agency, 166–168
  caring theory, 167–168
  gender and context, 166–167
contextualism, 84–86
  defined, 84–85
  situation-specific relevance of, 85
contractarianism, 61
  public health ethics and, 405
contracting out
  non-clinical services/clinical services, 242
contractual pregnancy, 478
conventional framework, examining,
  317–319
conventional morality, 321
corporate ethos, 189, 192
corporatism, 189
  goals of, 393
counter stories, 110
CPHA. *See* Canadian Public Health
  Association (CPHA)
CPR. *See* cardio-pulmonary resuscitation

CPS. *See* Canadian Pediatric Society
Cranford, Ronald, 510
critical care settings, families, 263
critical public health ethics, 401–402
critical realism, 45
cultural competency, 439–440
cultural ethics
    Buddhist notion of compassion, 90–91
    critiques, 86–90
    cultural imperialism, 90
    possibilities, 90–91
cultural imperialism, 90
cultural integrity, 218, 219
cultural relativism, 85
culture
    broad meaning of, 87
    global corporate, 89
    and principle-based approach, 73
CVS. *See* chorionic villus sampling (CVS)

D
DALYs. *See* disability adjusted life
        years (DALYs)
Dana Foundation, 510–511
DBS. *See* deep brain stimulation (DBS)
Deaconess Institute at Kaiserswerth,
        Germany, 22
death
    death-denying society, 341
    "death talk," 339, 341
    impending, lack of truthful disclosure of, 344
deep brain stimulation (DBS), 509, 516–517
    ethical issues of, 517
    and Parkinson's disease, 516
dehumanization, 173
deinstitutionalization, 434
deliberative democracy, 408
democratic communitarianism, 406–407
democratic policy processes, 369–371
    procedural standards for, 370–371
deontology, 60–61
descriptive ethics, 65
dialogue, and relational ethics, 138–139
difficulty, nursing obligations and, 153–154
diffusion of responsibility, 172
direct to consumer (DTC) testing
        agency, 493
disability adjusted life years (DALYs), 405
displacement of responsibility, 172
distressing, symptoms, 343
distributive justice, 69, 436
DNR orders. *See* do-not-resuscitate orders
doctor-patient relationships
    metaphors/models of, 7

doctrine of informed consent, 64, 67
    collaborative decision-making, 68–69
doing more with less, 221–222
domination, 94
do-not-resuscitate orders, 338–339
    importance of, 338
Down syndrome, 482
DTC testing agency. *See* direct to consumer
        (DTC) testing agency

E
Eastern nursing philosophy, 47
ecological citizenship, 225
ecological health, rehabilitating, 216
ecological integrity, 218, 219
ecological restoration, 217
ecological sensibilities, development of, 217
ecology, 225
ecomedical disconnection syndrome, 216
ecosystem, 218
    health of, 215, 216
EEG. *See* electroencephalography (EEG)
electroencephalography (EEG), 513
Elliott, Carl, 226
ELSI program. *See* Ethical, Legal, and Social
        Implications (ELSI) program
embodiment, 131–133
empathetic imagining, 114
Encyclopedia of Bioethics, 511
end-of-life decisions, 269, 333, 346
    Canada, assisted suicide and euthanasia,
        348–349
    end-of-life care
        nurses leading and influencing change
            in, 349–351
    ethics and, 333–351
    fostering family and friend support,
        345–346
    good care at the end of life, 339–342
        living wills and advance directives,
            340–342
    information and truthfulness, 343–345
    listening, reflecting, and developing trust,
        346–347
    nurses, moral imperative for, 334–339
        do-not-resuscitate orders, 338–339
        "good death," meaning of, 335–336
        medical futility (inappropriate care),
            336–339
    nurses and palliative care, 347
    patients participate in, 346
    public policy developement, 333
    relief of pain and discomfort, 342–343
        challenges in pain/symptom control, 343

enduring values, in Canadian health care
       system, 242–243
engagement, 134–138
Engelhardt, Tristam, Jr., 67
environment, 129–131
EOL decisions. *See* end-of-life decisions
epistemological, 305
   questions, in nursing, 43
equity, meaning of, 236
Ethical, Legal, and Social Implications (ELSI)
       program, 492
ethical action, dialogic space for
       diversity, 259, 263
ethical commitments, 133, 228
ethical conflict, themes of, 193
ethical counterpoise, 219
ethical decision, 263, 264
   agreement, 255
   cultural meanings, 255
   diversity, 259
   McDonald's, 263, 270
   moral deliberation, 264
ethical decision-making frameworks, 365
   for individuals, 539–541
ethical decision-making models, 265, 270
   allocation decisions, 542
   Storch model for ethical decision-making
       guiding questions for clinical decision
       making, 537–538
ethical decision-making process, 261
ethical dilemma, 3, 6, 47
Ethical Endeavours, 415
ethical fitness, 2
ethical/moral climate, 11–14
ethical nursing practice
   complexity of, 302
   educative spaces for, 302
       nursing values and ethical obligations,
           307–308
       principles and practices, 308–312
       teaching and learning, 302, 303
   ethical endeavours of, 311
   knowledge, 304
ethical obligations, 262, 308
ethical policy analyses, 369
ethical practice
   constraints, responses to, 24–25
   moral concerns in, 24–25
   requirements of, 59
ethical principles
   autonomy, 66–67, 72
   beneficence, 67–71
   bioethics, 66–69
   and culture, 73

and feminist theorists, 73
justice, 69–71
limitations, 72
nonmaleficence, 67–69
principle-oriented approach, 72–73
role in nursing, 49
ethical principles governing research, 119
ethical relations, 223–225
ethical relativism, 85
ethical schools, 226
ethical space, 96–97
ethical theory, 227. *See also* health care ethics
   contextualism, 84–86
   cultural ethics, 86–91
ethics
   about death, 333
   applied, 65
   bioethics, original focus in, 359
   Canada, assisted suicide and euthanasia,
       348–349
   and Canadian health care system (*See* Canadian
       health care system)
   communitarian, 227
   compassion, 112–114
   culture and relationships, 227
   defined, 65
   descriptive, 65
   and development of nursing, 21–22
   end-of-life care
       nurses leading and influencing change in,
           349–351
   end-of-life decisions and, 333–351
   ethical practice, 358
   fostering family and friend support,
       345–346
   good care at the end of life, 339–342
       living wills and advance directives,
           340–342
   in Health Care Organizations and Health/Health
       Care Policy, 358–372
   impact on, nursing roles/responsibilities, 4–5
   importance of, 358
   information and truthfulness, 343–345
   law and, 72
   listening, reflecting, and developing trust,
       346–347
   narrative (*See* narratives)
   normative, 65
   nurses, moral imperative for, 334–339
       do-not-resuscitate orders, 338–339
       "good death," meaning of, 335–336
       medical futility (inappropriate care), 336–339
   nurses and palliative care, 347
   nursing (*See* Nursing ethics; nursing ethics)

ethics (*continued*)
in nursing education, 25–27
nursing ethics education, 303
organizational resources, 271–273
perspectives about, 4–5
place, 227
and politics, 246
of public health (*See* public health ethics)
in public health nursing, 414–416
relational, 96–97, 227
relief of pain and discomfort, 342–343
challenges in pain/symptom control, 343
vocabulary, 3, 6–7
vs. morality, 6
in workplace, 11–14
ethics committee
health care institutions, 271
ethics education
educative spaces, 302–312
narrative in, 114–117
readers' theatre, 115
thick narratives, 114–115
Victorian parlour game, 115–116
ethics for public health. *See* advocacy ethics
Ethics in Action, 5
Ethics in Practice
artful nurse, 50–51
being there, 500
bridging autonomy and community, 140
dialogue, 138
emergency department nursing, 167–168
engagement, 135
environment, 129–131
implications of hereditary risk, 496
limit to our knowledge, 499
managers, 194
medical unit, 191–192
moral agent, 9–10
moral community, 11
moral distress, 5, 10–11
mutual respect, 133–134
nurse-patient-family relationships, 391
nurse-patient relationship, 145–146
nurses practicing in emergency department, 88
nursing in difficult conditions, 53
objections to providing abortion care, 477
policies for accessing IVF, 480
prenatal testing, 483–484
public-private partnerships, 241–242
schizophrenia and genetics, 497
self-care/family care, 388–389
working conditions, 390
working together, 163–164
xenotransplantation, 450–451

Ethics in Practice, 32
ethics in public health. *See* applied ethics
ethics of neuroscience, 511
ethics of public health. *See* professional ethics
ethics pedagogy, feature of, 306
ethnocentrism, in Western health care ethics, 88
etiquette, nursing, 27
EUnetHTA document, 369
euphemistic language, 172
euthanasia, 335
definitions, 348
existentialism, 45
experience, 164

F
Fae, Baby, 452
fairness, in Canadian health care system, 243–244
families
caregivers, 389, 391
engagement of, 179
impact of care services on, 193
FDA. *See* Food and Drug Administration (FDA)
feminist ethics, 91–95
applications of, 92
justice, 94–95
oppression, 92
philosophical inquiry, 30–31
power inequities, 92
power relations, 92–93
process, 95
relational autonomy, 93–94
and social justice, 436–437
feminist theorists, 73, 93–94
film (video), 110–111
fiscal policy, 262
fMRI. *See* functional neuroimaging research (fMRI)
Food and Drug Administration (FDA)
and xenotransplant, 459
frog breathing, 139
From Detached Concern to Empathy, 113
full acute care, 340
functional neuroimaging research (fMRI), 512–516
developments in, 513–514
and incidental findings, 515
landmark study, 518
futility concept, 336

G
gender. *See also* women
and moral agency, 166–167
and nursing profession, 167
genetic counselling
defined, 501
and nurses, 500–502

Genetic Information Non-discrimination Act
    (GINA), 493
genetics
    Human Genome Project, 492–493
    information, 495
    knowledge about, 499
    and nursing, 491, 498–500
    and psychiatric disorders, 496–498
    testing (*See* genetic testing)
genetic testing, 494–496
    hereditary risk, 495–496
    predictive/presymptomatic, 494–496
genome mapping, 493
geriatric medicine, 261
GINA. *See* Genetic Information Non-
    discrimination Act (GINA)
global corporate culture, 89
globalization, 360
*Golubchuk v. Salvation Army Grace General
    Hospital et al.*, 352
good death
    case study, 335–336
    meaning of, 335–336
government monitoring programs, 216

H
harm-reduction approach, adoption of, 439
HCP. *See* health care providers
HD. *See* Huntington disease (HD)
healing capacities, 220
Health Canada, 119
    and xenotransplants, 459, 462
Health Canada Working Group on Public and
    Professional Educational Requirements
    Related to Genetic Testing of Late Onset
    Disease, 498
health care. *See also* nursing
    adverse events in, 8
    context, in 2012, 7–11
    funding issues in, 25
    relational ethics for (*See* relational ethics)
health care ethics, 65–66. *See also* ethical theory
    children needs, 259
    children's interests, 258
    children's participation, 258
    complementary approaches to (*See*
        complementary approaches, health
        care ethics)
    decision-making process, 261, 263–270
    developmental theories, 259
    development of, 59
    diversity in, 254–256
    ethical action, 259–263
        advanced practice nurse's account, 260

families interests, 262–263
    rights, needs, and relationships,
        260–262
ethics consultation, 272–273
ethnocentrism in, 88
history of, 60–71
landscape of, 254–273
organizational ethics resources,
    271–273
    effectiveness, evaluating, 272–273
    ethics committee, 271–272
    ethics consultants, 272
peace proposal, 73–75
PH problems and, 404–405
principle-oriented approach to, 72–73
professional knowledge, 255
reflections on interests
    considering needs, 258–259
    of families, 262–263
    honouring rights, 258
    of persons, 256–257
    respecting relationships, 259
vs. PH ethics, 402–403
health care ethics committee, 271
    culture shift, 271–272
    ethics consultant, 272–273
    institutions, 271
    interdisciplinary professional, 271
    respect for patient, 271
health care institutions
    social processes of, 362
health care organizations
    ethics in, 358–372
        democratic policy processes,
            369–371
        further reflections, ecological and
            political, 371–372
        organizational practices, 363–364
        organizational virtues, 362–363
        resource allocation, 364–366
    modernity, malaise of, 359–362
health care policy, 254, 366
    development, narratives and, 119–120
    ethics in, 358–372
        aging issues, 366–367
        democratic policy processes, 369–371
        further reflections, ecological and
            political, 371–372
        policy gaps, 367–368
        policy progress, 368–369
    framing of, issues associated with, 242
    modernity, malaise of, 359–362
    public policy in, 366
    research, narratives and, 118–119

health care professionals
  and abortion, 474–475
  challenges for, health care/nursing
      context and, 8
  codes of ethics for, 13
  education, thick narratives for, 114–115
  environment, 269
  as moral agents, 10
  traditional virtues of, 62
health care providers, 318, 340
  child-patient's interests, 319
  children's moral order, 326
  safety of, 531
health care systems
  Canada (*See* Canadian health care system)
  colonization, 229
  eco-efficient, 225
  environmental issues, 215
  ethical comportment, 216
  maladaptive management of, 216
  moral imaginations, 225–226
  place ethics, 217
    locating, 226–228
    reinhabitation, advancing, 228–229
    in twenty-first century, 217–221
  post-colonial, 224
  resource allocation/service delivery, 215
Health Council of Canada, 243, 361
Health Ethics Guide, 13
health ethics research
  narratives in, 117–120
health inequities, 431–432
  biomedicine and, 435
  housing insecurity and, 434
  identification of, 430
  inequalities *vs.,* 431
  intersectionality, 432–433
  marginalization and, 433–435
  neo-liberalism and, 433–435
  public health ethics and, 437
  racism and, 434–435
  reducing, 430, 436
  social justice perspectives, 435–437
  social positioning and, 432
The Health of Our Nation-The Future of
      Our Health System, 532
health professionals, 345
health professionals' reluctance, 341–342
health promotion, and PH development, 403–404
health restructuring, impact of, 385
health technology assessment, 368
  European document on, 368
Healthy Cities/Communities movement, 400
HEC. *See* health care ethics committee

hereditary risk, genetic testing and, 495–496
HGP. *See* Human Genome Project (HGP)
Higgs, E.S., 218–220
HIV/AIDS, PH ethics and, 403, 404
H1N1 pandemic, 416, 417
home care nurses, 385
home care organizations, 359
home health care, 384–394
  demand for, 384
  everyday ethical issues, 388–392
  expenditures for, 388
  family caregivers, 389, 391
  fiscal constraints, 385
  health restructuring, impact of, 385
  nurse-patient-family relationships, 391–392
  political context, 385–387
  recommendations, 392–394
  social/market justice, 387
homelessness, 432
home support worker, 390
Hospital Insurance and Diagnostic Services
      Act, 1957, 238, 385
hospital "visiting policies," 326
housing
  and health, 430
  insecurity, and health inequities, 434
HTA. *See* health technology assessment
Human Genome Organization, 492
Human Genome Project (HGP), 492–493
human rights, 62–63
  critiques, 71–72
  international, 63
  and nursing ethics, 28–29
Huntington disease (HD)
  and predictive genetic testing, 494
hurt in crossfire, 316
hypoplastic left heart syndrome, 452

I

ICN. *See* International Council of Nurses (ICN)
ideology of scarcity, 89
inappropriate care, 336–339
  creating tension, 338
incidental findings, fMRI and, 515–516
income, and health inequities, 430, 434
induced abortion. *See* abortion
industrialized farming practices, 225
inequalities
  defined, 243
  health inequities *vs.,* 431
inequity. *See also* health inequities
  defined, 243
infertility
  artificial insemination and, 478

informed choices
  about prenatal testing/screening, 484–485
informed consent, 64, 67, 283, 288
  collaborative decision-making, 68–69
  excellence in, 286
  issues associated with, 294–295
  need for, 284
  protection of, 89
  ramifications for, 289
  seeking, from participants, 285
  and xenotransplantation, 456–457
injurious consequences, minimizing/
      disregarding, 172
Institutional Research Boards, 284
interests, reflections
  children, 258
  conflicting, 271
  considering needs, 258–259
  ethics, caring for, 257
  of families, 262–263
  health care team, 268
  honouring rights, 258
  patients, 262
  of persons, 256–257
  respecting relationships, 259
interim summary, 61–62
International Council of Nurses (ICN), 26, 28
  adoption of, 31, 32
  formation of, 31
international research
  on nurses' workplaces, 194–196
International Society for Nurses in Genetics
      (ISONG), 503
International Xenotransplant Association, 460
interpersonal conflict, 201
intersectionality, 432–433
in vitro fertilization (IVF), 473, 477–478
  availability of, 478–479
  commodification of reproductive material, 481
  cycle, 479–480
IRBs. *See* Institutional Research Boards
ISONG. *See* International Society for Nurses
      in Genetics (ISONG)
IVF. *See in vitro* fertilization (IVF)

J
justice, 69–71
  accountability for reasonableness, 70–71
  distributive, 69, 436
  and feminist ethics, 94–95
  macro-allocation, 69–70
  market, 387
  meso-allocation, 70–71
  micro-allocation, 71

procedural rules of, 69
  social (*See* social justice)
  substantive rules of, 69

K
kairos, 137, 138
Kant, Immanuel, 60, 161
Kantian perspective, 67
Karen-Anne Quinlan case, 29
knowledge, nursing, 43–44, 164–165
  about genetics, 499
  and patient care, 164–165
  types of, 45
knowledge-driven perspective, 511
Kohlbergian morality, 322
kronos, 137, 138

L
law, and ethics, 72
Law Reform Commission, 29
leadership. *See also* nursing leadership
  in clinical practice, 179–180
  in nursing ethics, 3
Leadership for Ethical Policy and Practice
      (LEPP), 5
learning nursing, 309
legislative developments, nursing practices, 530
*Legislative Theatre: Using Performance to Make
      Politics,* 118
LEPP. *See* Leadership for Ethical Policy and
      Practice (LEPP)
liberal individualism, 360
libertarianism, in health care, 244
liberty, 408
licensed practical nurse (LPN), 195
life-preserving technologies, 339
Literature and Aging, 110
living wills, 340–342
living with the decision, 269
location, of work, 164
LPN. *See* licensed practical nurse (LPN)

M
MacIntyre, Alisdair, 62
macro-allocation, 69–70
magnetoencephalography (MEG), 513
manifestos, 110
marginalization
  and health inequities, 433–435
market justice, 387
master narratives, 110
maternal serum screening, 481
McDonald's ethical decision-making
      models, 537–540

Medical Care Act, 1967, 238, 385
medical futility, 336–339
  classifications of, 337
  defined, 337
  use of, 337
Medical Research Council, 284
Medicare, 239. *See also* Canadian health
    care system
MEG. *See* magnetoencephalography (MEG)
memoirs, 110
meso-allocation, 70–71
metaethics, 65
metaphors
  doctor-patient relationships, 7
  of moral winter, 190–194
micro-allocation, 71
Mill, John Stuart, 60
Minnesota Pandemic Ethics Project, 418
modernity
  features of, 360
  forces of, 359
  malaise of, 359–362
Montefiore-Einstein Center's bioethics
    mediation paradigm, 272
Montello, Martha, 111
moral agency, 5, 160–180
  and autonomy, 162
  conceptualizing, 161–163
  contested agency, 166–168
  defined, 162
  moral disengagement, 171–173
  moral sequelae, 168–171
  nurses' enactment, 165–173
  nurses' voices, 163–164
  relationships in particular contexts, 161
  self-condemnation and, 171
  traditional perspectives, critiques of, 161
  women and, 161–162
moral agency, responsibility, 323
moral agents, 9–10
  nurses as, supporting, 173–180
  traditional view of, 161
moral climate, of nursing practice,
    11–14
  change, 188–198
    premises and, 189–190
  defined, 188
  implications, 196–198
  improvement of, actions for, 198–204
    fostering moral communities, 198
    interdisciplinary strategies, 204
    organizational action, 198–200
    political action, 200–201
    research action, 201–204

  inquiry into, 190–196
  problems with, 196–197
Moral Code, adoption of, 26
moral community, 128–129
  defined, 11–12
  development of, 11
  establishment of, 25
  fostering, 198
  and inter-professional practice, 14
  and values-based change, 199
moral conduct, in nursing, 27
moral courage, 173
moral disengagement, 171–173
  defined, 173
  mechanisms of, 172–173
moral distress, 168–171
  defined, 169
  Ethics in Practice, 5, 10–11
  nurses and, 197
moral experience, narratives of, 315
moral good, 51–52
moral imagination, 267
morality
  ethics *vs.,* 6
moral justification, 172
moral language, coercive, 315
moral norm, for mature adults, 321
moral questions, in nursing, 43
moral residue, 168–171
moral responsibility
  degree of, 324
  nurse educators, 308
moral status
  children's, 258
moral theory, 65
moral winter, metaphors of, 190–194
moral work, of nurses, 164–165
Mount's concept, 347
MRC. *See* Medical Research Council
multiprofessional teams, 178
mutuality, 137
  in nursing relationships, 144
mutual respect, 133–134

N
NAFTA. *See* North American Free Trade
    Agreement (NAFTA)
Nancy B. (N) v. Hotel Dieu de Quebec,
    348, 352
narrative ethics, 227
narratives, 107–120. *See also* specific types
  compassion ethics, 112–114
  in ethics education, 114–117
  and health care policy, 118–120

in health ethics research, 117–120
of learning, 109
for moral exploration, 112–114
presentation forms, 110–111
purposes of, 111–117
readers' theatre, 115
for research, 117–118
for research presentation, 117
thick/thin, 109
types of, 109–111
value of, 107–109
Victorian parlour game, 115–116
"yick factor," 116–117
National Commission for the Protection of Human
    Subjects of Biomedical and Behavioral
    Research, 66
National Council on Bioethics in Human Research
    (NCBHR), 284
Nationally funded treatment program, 368
National Society of Genetic Counsellors
    (NSGC), 503
natural law, 62, 453–454
Natural Sciences and Engineering Research
    Council of Canada (NSERC), 284
neo-liberalism, 385–387
    Canada Health Act and, 387
    defined, 433
    and health inequities, 433–435
neuro-essentialism, 513–514
neuroethics, 509–521
    deep brain stimulation, 516–517
    definitions of, 509–511
    neuroimaging, 512–516
    neuroscience of ethics, 517–520
    overview, 509
    perspectives on, 509–511
neuroimaging, 509, 512–516
neuro-policy, 514
neuro-realism, 513, 514
neuroscience of ethics, 511, 517–520
New Public Management, 386
Nightingale, Florence, 22, 25–26, 53
*No Longer Patient: Feminist Ethics and
    Health Care,* 92
non-clinical services, contracting out, 242
nonfiction stories/memoirs, 108
non-linear time, 137
nonmaleficence, 67–69
    principle of, 344–345
normative ethics, 65
North American Free Trade Agreement
    (NAFTA), 242
NSGC. *See* National Society of Genetic
    Counsellors (NSGC)

numerical public, and public health, 400
nurse educators
    goal of, 310
    moral responsibility, 308, 310
    teaching for ethical practice, 309
nurse-patient relationships. *See* relationships
nurse researchers
    emic perspective, 295
    ethical challenges for, 292
    process consent, 294
    voicing concerns about protocol, 296
nurses
    anxiety, 303
    artful, 50–51
    challenge for, 349
    challenges for, health care/nursing
        context and, 8
    commitment to patients, 166
    conviction developement in patients, 334
    current shortage of, 9
    educators, 350
    ethical decision, 302
    facilitating communication, 335
    front-line nurse managers, 291
    genetic counselling and, 500–502
    good, virtue of, 52–54
    home care, 385
    information, 290
    knowledge, 164–165
    lead and influence change in, 349–351
    as leaders, 296–297
    longstanding disempowerment of, 196
    moral agency, 165–173
    and moral distress, 197
    moral imperative for, 334–339
        do-not-resuscitate orders, 338–339
        "good death," meaning of, 335–336
        medical futility (inappropriate care),
            336–339
    moral responsibility of, 53
    moral work of, 164–165, 173–174,
        245–246
    obedience and loyalty, 291
    palliative care and, 347
    personal characteristics of, 20–21, 27–28
    practicing in emergency department, 88
    private duty, 23
    professional obligation of, 28
    protest by, 25
    registered, 195, 237, 247, 438–439
    relational connections, 173–175
    relationships with clients, 7
    relationship with physicians, 28
    research in ethics, 297

nurses (*continued*)
resources for, 503
responsibility of, 296–297
and responsive relationships, 144
roles for, 282, 288–296, 350
end-of-life care, 334
senior nurse managers, 291
and social justice issues, 394
studies, 297
teaching and learning of ethics, 303
and vocabulary of ethics, 6–7
voices of, 163–164
whistle-blower, 292
workplaces, international research on,
194–196
nurse's professional judgment, 290
nurses' skills, 294
nursing. *See also* health care
ancient history, 20–21
being ethical, 304
caring in, 167–168
challenge, 304
Christianity and, 21
conceptual models of, 28–29
context, in 2012, 7–11
defined, 1, 156
development of, religion/spirituality/ethics
and, 21–22
emotional work of, 174
ethics and, 4–5
etiquette, 23
gender-based analysis of, 167
genetics and, 491, 498–500
meta-domains of, 42
moral conduct in, 27
moral conflict in, 26
ontological/epistemological/moral
questions in, 43
organizations, and code of ethics, 31–32
philosophy (*See* nursing philosophy)
relationships in (*See* relationships)
role of, 246–247
role of ethical principles in, 49
status, social changes and, 22
unique ethical perspective, 50
in United States, 24
nursing education
ethics in, 25–27
nursing ethics, 333. *See also* ethics
altruism and, 23–24
debate about, 7
human rights and, 28–29
leadership in, 3
nursing ontology and, 46–49

nursing science and, 45–46
overview of, 1–2
personal characteristics of nurse
and, 27–28
philosophical contributions to (*See* nursing
philosophy)
philosophical influences on, 44–45
vs. nursing etiquette, 27
nursing ethics education
approaches, 303
behaviourist orientation, 305–306
classroom interaction, 306
as epistemological activity, 303–305
institutional attachment, 306
principles and practices
learning how to learn, 310–311
releasing epistemologies' grasp,
308–309
teaching for ethical being, 309–310
teaching toward social justice,
311–312
teaching toward values and
obligations, 311
problem of knowledge, 303
re-personalization of ethics, 302
nursing ethics pedagogy. *See* nursing ethics
education
nursing etiquette, 23
nursing ethics *vs.*, 27
nursing leadership. *See also* leadership
ethics in, 5–6
need for, 3–4
nursing obligations
abyss of difficulty, 153–154
and different levels of care, 154–156
as external entities, 148
reflexive/intentional, 152–153
reframing, 149
relational inquiry and, 151–156
relationships and, 147–149
nursing ontology
and nursing ethics, 46–49
nursing philosophy, 30–31
Buddhist perspective, 47
defined, 42–44
Eastern, 47
knowledge and, 43–44
and nursing ethics (*See* nursing ethics)
nursing science *vs.* nursing ethics, 45–46
politics and, 52
spirituality and, 48–49
unresolved issues, 49–50
virtue of good nurse, 52–54
Western, 47

Nursing Philosophy, 43
nursing practices
    collaborative practice, 176–180
    complexity of, 308
    early, values in, 22–23
    ethics in, 5–6
    good, nature of, 50–54
    legislative developments, 530
    license, 53
    moral climate of (*See* moral climate, of nursing
        practice)
    social justice in, 430–440
*The Nursing Profession: Five Sociological
        Essays,* 4
nursing resources, 261
nursing science
    nursing ethics and, 45–46
nursing theorists, 42
nursing values, 312
    and CNA Code of Ethics for Registered
        Nurses, 7–8

O
objective sense of moral good, 52
obligations, nursing. *See* nursing obligations
Odysseus, 108
OHSS. *See* ovarian hyperstimulation
        syndrome (OHSS)
One True Thing, 108
ontological questions, in nursing, 43
opioid analgesics
    acceptability of, 342
oppression, 92, 94
    social positioning and, 432–433
Orchids: Not Necessarily a Gospel, 113
organizational action, and moral climate, 198–200
organizational ethics, 364
organizational ethics resources, 271–273
    effectiveness, evaluating, 272–273
    ethics committee, 271–272
    ethics consultants, 272
Ottawa Charter on Health Promotion, 404
ovarian hyperstimulation syndrome
        (OHSS), 480

P
PAG. *See* Public Advisory Group (PAG)
pain
    control techniques, 342
        family resistance to, 343
    challenges in pain/symptom control, 343
    relief of, 342–343
pain-management strategies, 327
palliative care, 347

Pandemic Influenza Working Group (PIWG),
        417, 418
pandemic planning, and public health, 416–419
    ethical issues in, 417
PAR. *See* participatory action research (PAR)
Parkinson's disease
    DBS and, 516
participative assessment, 326
participatory action research (PAR), 203
pathogen transmission, and xenotransplantation,
        455–457
patient-centred care (PCC), 114, 115
patients
    care, knowledge essential to, 164–165
    engagement of, 179
    impact of care services on, 193
    nurses commitment to, 166
    rights, 29
    safety, health care/nursing context, 8–10
patient safety movement, 8–10
Patient's Bills of Rights, 28
PBL. *See* problem-based learning (PBL)
PCC. *See* patient-centred care (PCC)
peace proposal, 73–75
PEPPI. *See* Public Engagement Project on
        Pandemic Influenza (PEPPI)
personal narratives, 110
person-directed attention, 137
PERVs. *See* pig endogenous retroviruses (PERVs)
PGD. *See* pre-implantation genetic
        diagnosis (PGD)
PH. *See* public health (PH)
PHAC. *See* Public Health Agency of Canada
        (PHAC)
phenylketonuria, screening for, 494
Philippine Nurses' Association, 28
philosophical inquiry, 201
philosophies of nursing. *See* nursing philosophy
philosophy
    defined, 41
    nursing (*See* nursing philosophy)
philosophy in nursing. *See* nursing philosophy
PHN. *See* public health nursing (PHN)
phronesis, 153
physicians, relationship with nurses, 28
pig endogenous retroviruses (PERVs), 455
PIWG. *See* Pandemic Influenza Working Group
        (PIWG)
place ethics, in twenty-first century, 227
    ecological integrity, 217–218
    health care systems, 217–221
    matters of integrity, 219–220
    transient technical repairs, execution of,
        218–219

poem, 111
policies, review of, 269
political action, and moral climate,
        200–201
    and levels of health care, 201
political public, and public health, 400
politics, 52
    ethics and, 246
Pontius, Anneliese A., 510
portability, 238
postmodernism, 45
poverty, 430, 431, 432, 434, 435–436
power differentials, 119
power inequities, 92, 189–190
pragmatism, 45
pregnancy
    and abortion (*See* abortion)
    AHR (*See* assisted human reproduction (AHR))
    contractual, 478
    ethical issues in, 473–485
    prenatal tests/screens, 481–485
pre-implantation genetic diagnosis (PGD),
        473, 478
prenatal testing/screening, and pregnancy,
        481–485
    access to, 482–484
    amniocentesis, 481–482
    CVS, 482
    informed choices about, 484–485
    maternal serum screening, 481
    ultrasound, 481
presentation form, narratives, 110–111
"prevention paradox," 402
primary care, 239, 247
primum non nocere, 67
principle-oriented ethics
    critiques, 72–73
Principles of Bioethics, 66
Principles of Biomedical Ethics, 30
principlism, 66
privatization, of health care
    approaches to, 241–242
problem-based learning (PBL), 114, 115
procedural rules of justice, 69
professional ethics, 400–401
professional nursing organizations, 349
professional obligation, of nurse, 28
protective secrets, 316
proxy directive, 340
psychiatric disorders, genetics and, 496–498
    treatment of, 498
public
    challenges for, health care/nursing context
        and, 8

participation, and xenotransplantation,
        460–463
    in public health, 400
public administration, 238
Public Advisory Group (PAG), 461
Public Engagement Project on Pandemic Influenza
        (PEPPI), 418
public health (PH)
    defined, 399
    ethics of (*See* public health ethics)
    features of, 402–403
    goal of, 399–400
    historical streams in, 398–399
    and pandemic planning, 416–419
    problems, and health care ethics, 404–405
    public in, 400
    success of, 416–417
Public Health Agency of Canada
        (PHAC), 418
public health ethics
    advocacy ethics, 401
    applied ethics, 401
    and contractarianism, 405
    critical, 401–402
    development stages, 403–405
    frameworks, 408–414
    health care ethics *vs.,* 402–403
    and health inequities, 437
    history of, 403–405
    perspectives on, 400–402
    philosophical/theoretical underpinnings of,
        405–408
    professional ethics, 400–401
    social change and, 406
Public Health Leadership Society, 400
public health nursing (PHN), 398
    defined, 415
    ethics in, 414–416
    role of, 415
publicly funded health care
    preservation of, 240
public policy, 367
public-private partnerships,
        241–242
    endorsement of, 245
public resistance, 341

Q
QALYs. *See* quality adjusted life years (QALYs)
quality adjusted life years (QALYs), 405
Quebec Select Committee, 348
quest narratives, 110
Quindlen, Anna, 108
Quinlan, Karen Ann, 29, 34

R

R. v. Morgentaler, 474

racism, and health inequities, 434–435

Rawls, John, 61, 69

    theory of justice, 405

readers' theatre, 115

REB. *See* research ethics board (REB)

reciprocity, 137

registered nurse (RN), 195, 237, 247, 438–439

    and social justice, 435

Registered Nurses Association of Ontario (RNAO), 362

    Final Report on SARS, 527–528

relational approaches, 162

relational autonomy, 93–94, 256, 437

relational ethics, 96–97, 227

    defined, 127

    for health care, 127–140

    intersubjectivity, 128

    self-knowledge, 139–140

    themes (*See* relational themes)

    through dialogue, 138–139

relational inquiry

    and nursing obligations, 151–156

    and relationships, 150–151

relational matrix, 174–175

    trust and, 175–176

relational solidarity, 437

relational space, 128

    for difficulty, and nursing obligations, 153–154

relational themes

    embodiment, 131–133

    engagement, 134–138

    environment, 129–131

    mutual respect, 133–134

relationships, 261

    in CLU project, 224

    connectedness in, 163

    defined, 144

    educator–learner, 312

    elements of good, 144

    ethical, 223–225, 227, 228

    ethical obligation, 312

    health care delivery system, 261

    iceberg pattern of, 150–151

    importance of, 263

    intra-organizational, 222

    and moral agency, 161

    with nature, 229

    and nursing obligations, 147–149

    relational inquiry and, 150–151

    significance of, 144–145

social, 228

trust in, 163, 224

religion. *See also* spirituality

    and development of nursing, 21–22

reproduction, ethical issues in, 473–485

research ethics

    boards responsibility, 286–287

    Canada, evolution of, 283

        guiding principles, 285–286

        Institutional Research Boards, 284

        Medical Research Council, 284

        public funding, 284

        research ethics board, 284

        Tri-Council Policy Statement, 284

        war crimes trials, 283

    inclusion and exclusion criteria, 292

    nurses, responsibility of, 296–297

    nurses, roles for, 282, 288–296

        as care provider, 289–291

        as manager, 291

        as member of review boards, 295–296

        as research assistant/coordinator, 291–292

        as researcher, 292–295

        withdrawing from clinical trial, 288–289

    respect for persons, 290

    trust in local community, 282

research ethics board (REB), 285, 295, 516

    compliance, evidence of, 286

    members, 286

    research protocols, review of, 295

    responsibility of, 286–287

    scientific merit of study, 295

research nurse, 291, 292

resource allocation, 364–366

    resource challenges, illustration of, 365

respect, characteristics of, 144

responsibility

    diffusion/displacement of, 172

restitution narratives, 109–110

RN. *See* registered nurse (RN)

RNAO. *See* Registered Nurses Association of Ontario (RNAO)

Robb, Isabel Hampton, 27

Rodriguez, Sue, 348

Rodriguez v. British Columbia (Attorney General), 352

Romanow Report, 393–394

Roskies, Adina, 510–511

S

SARS. *See* severe acute respiratory syndrome;
Sudden Acute Respiratory Syndrome
(SARS)
secular law, 62
self-condemnation, and moral
agency, 171
self-determination, 261
self-determining agents, 320
self-knowledge, relational ethics and,
139–140
severe acute respiratory syndrome, 216
Sherwin, Susan, 92, 256
Short stories, 110
Sisters of Charity, 21–22
social change
and public health ethics, 406
social cognitive theory, 171
social contract, 61
social justice, 387, 394
feminist ethics and, 436–437
and health inequities, 435–437
in nursing practices, 430–440
social knowledge, 165
social positioning
and health inequities, 432
and systems of oppression,
432–433
Social Sciences and Humanities Research
Council, 219, 284
socio-political challenges, health care/
nursing context and, 8
solidarity, 236
relational, 437
solid organ transplantation, 452
Somera Case, 28
Sourkes, Barbara, 322
spending, defined, 137–138
spirituality. *See also* religion
caring and, 48
and development of nursing, 21–22
and nursing philosophy, 48–49
SSHRC. *See* Social Sciences and Humanities
Research Council
staff learning, 222
"Stand on Guard for Thee," 417, 419
Stories of Sickness, 108
story, 108. *See also* narratives
short, 110
struggling to escape, 316
subjective sense of moral good, 52
substantive rules of justice, 69
Sudden Acute Respiratory Syndrome (SARS),
242, 405, 416, 449, 527–528

suffering, nursing obligations and, 153–154
"sustainability crisis mantra," 241
sustaining narratives, 109

T

task shifting, 530
TCPS. *See* Tri-council Policy Statement
(TCPS)
Tentative Code, 31
theatre, as way of presenting research, 117
therapeutic misconception, 289
thick narratives, 109
for health care professionals education,
114–115
"think like a system" ability, 217
thin narratives, 109
threat, 261
nurses' employment, 292
time
for quality nursing care, 192
requirements, for nurses, 179
time-full self, 137
trauma-informed care, 439
Tri-council Policy Statement (TCPS),
285, 515–516
trust
defined, 175
education about, 180
in nursing relationships, 144, 163
and relational matrix, 175–176
typal narratives, 110

U

ultrasound, 481
United States
development of nursing in, 24
universality, 238
universalizability, 60
unspoken diagnosis, 316
user fees, 241
utilitarianism, 61, 405, 409

V

values, 12–13
values-based change, 199
veil of ignorance, 69
Victorian parlour game, 115–116
virtues, 52–53
virtue theory, 62
visiting policies, hospital, 326

W

Wald, Lillian, 435
Walker, Margaret Urban, 155

wealth, inequities in
  and health, 431
Western health care ethics, 90
  ethnocentrism in, 88
Western nursing philosophy, 47
WHO. *See* World Health Organization (WHO)
Who Cares? The Crisis in Canadian Nursing, 25
Wilde, Oscar, 51
women. *See also* gender
  IVF (*See in vitro* fertilization (IVF))
  and moral agency, 161–162
  and nursing profession, 167
workplace
  ethics in, 11–14
  nurses, international research on, 194–196
World Health Organization (WHO),
    416–417, 418

X
xenograft, 452, 455
xenotransplantation, 449, 450–463
  benefits/challenges of, 454–455

  clinical application of, 452
  corporate/research influences on,
      457–459
  debates around, 451–452
  ethical implications in, 451–460
  Health Canada and, 459
  and informed consent, 456–457
  natural law, 453–454
  pathogen transmission, risk of,
      455–457
  public participation in policy
      development, 460–463
  regulatory concerns, 459–460
  science of, 452
  societal implications in, 451–460
  solid organ transplantation, 452
  source animals for, 453

Y
Yeo, Michael, 59
"yick factor," 116–117
Young, Iris Marion, 436